PALKO'S MEDICAL LABORATORY PROCEDURES

Third Edition

Phyllis Cox, MA, MT(ASCP)
Associate Professor of Allied Health Science
Director of the Medical Assistant and Medical Technology Programs
Arkansas Tech University
Russellville, Arkansas

Danielle Wilken, MS, MT(ASCP)
Associate Professor and Chair of the Health and Natural Sciences Department
Goodwin College
East Hartford, Connecticut

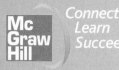

McGraw Hill

Connect
Learn
Succeed™

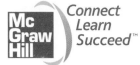
PALKO'S MEDICAL LABORATORY PROCEDURES

Published by McGraw-Hill, a business unit of The McGraw-Hill Companies, Inc., 1221 Avenue of the Americas, New York, NY, 10020. Copyright © 2011 by The McGraw-Hill Companies, Inc. All rights reserved. Previous editions © 1996 and 1999. No part of this publication may be reproduced or distributed in any form or by any means, or stored in a database or retrieval system, without the prior written consent of The McGraw-Hill Companies, Inc., including, but not limited to, in any network or other electronic storage or transmission, or broadcast for distance learning.

Some ancillaries, including electronic and print components, may not be available to customers outside the United States.

This book is printed on acid-free paper.

2 3 4 5 6 7 8 9 0 DOW/DOW 1 0 9 8 7 6 5 4 3 2 1 0

ISBN 978-0-07-340195-9
MHID 0-07-340195-1

Vice president/Editor in chief: *Elizabeth Haefele*
Vice president/Director of marketing: *John E. Biernat*
Publisher: *Kenneth S. Kasee Jr.*
Senior sponsoring editor: *Debbie Fitzgerald*
Director of development, Allied Health: *Patricia Hesse*
Executive marketing manager: *Roxan Kinsey*
Marketing manager: *Mary B. Haran*
Lead media producer: *Damian Moshak*
Media development editor: *Marc Mattson*
Director, Editing/Design/Production: *Jess Ann Kosic*
Project manager: *Marlena Pechan*
Senior production supervisor: *Janean A. Utley*
Senior designer: *Srdjan Savanovic*
Senior photo research coordinator: *Lori Hancock*
Media project manager: *Cathy L. Tepper*
Cover design: *Jessica M. Lazar*
Interior design: *Kay D. Lieberherr*
Typeface: *10/12 Melior*
Compositor: *Laserwords Private Limited*
Printer: *R. R. Donnelley*
Cover credit: specimen dipstick: © daveRN/istockphoto, samples: © www.imagesource.com, lab glasses: © Steve Allen/Brand X Pictures, microscope: © Stockbyte/PunchStock
Credits: The credits section for this book begins on page 451 and is considered an extension of the copyright page.

Library of Congress Cataloging-in-Publication Data

Cox, Phyllis.
    Palko's medical laboratory procedures.—3rd ed. / Phyllis Cox, Danielle Wilken.
      p. ; cm.
    Rev. ed. of: Glencoe medical laboratory procedures / Tom Palko, Hilda Palko. c1999.
    Includes bibliographical references and index.
    ISBN-13: 978-0-07-340195-9 (alk. paper)
    ISBN-10: 0-07-340195-1 (alk. paper)
    1. Diagnosis, Laboratory—Handbooks, manuals, etc. 2. Medical assistants—Handbooks, manuals, etc. I. Wilken, Danielle. II. Palko, Tom. III. Palko, Tom. Glencoe medical laboratory procedures. IV. Title. V. Title: Medical laboratory procedures.
    [DNLM: 1. Laboratory Techniques and Procedures. QY 25 C8776p 2011]
    RB38.2.C69 2011
    616.07'56—dc22

                                      2009019121

The Internet addresses listed in the text were accurate at the time of publication. The inclusion of a Web site does not indicate an endorsement by the authors or McGraw-Hill, and McGraw-Hill does not guarantee the accuracy of the information presented at these sites.

www.mhhe.com

About the Authors

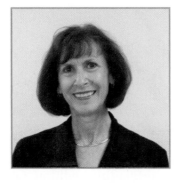

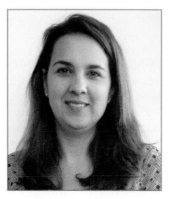

Phyllis Cox, MA, MT(ASCP) Phyllis is an associate professor of Allied Health Science and director of the Medical Assistant and Medical Technology Programs at Arkansas Tech University in Russellville, Arkansas, located in the beautiful foothills of the Ozarks.

She teaches medical laboratory science, basic pharmacology, and clinical medical assisting. Phyllis has experience in clinical laboratory medicine, beginning her career as a medical technologist working in Arkansas and Louisiana. She has been teaching for over 35 years, entering med tech education as the first director of South Louisiana Medical Center, School of Medical Technology, and achieving accreditation by NAACLS in the first year.

She enjoys any and all activities involving her beautiful grandchildren, Hayden, Addison, Peyton, and Camryn.

Danielle Wilken, MS, MT(ASCP) Danielle is an associate professor and chair of the Health and Natural Sciences Department at Goodwin College in Connecticut. She holds Bachelor degrees in Clinical Laboratory Sciences and Biology. Danielle holds a Master's degree in Health Care Policy and Management and is currently pursuing an EdD in Educational Leadership.

Danielle has worked as a medical technologist in community hospitals and a quality control laboratory for the American Red Cross. In addition to her clinical experience, she has served as faculty in medical assisting and clinical laboratory sciences departments. Danielle taught Clinical Laboratory Medicine for Physician Assistants at the State University of New York at Stony Brook and also has served as medical assisting faculty and program director for Goodwin College. In her capacity as a medical assisting faculty member, Danielle taught Clinical and Laboratory Procedures and Anatomy and Physiology. During her time as Medical Assisting Program Director, the program successfully completed the CAAHEP and ABHES self-study and site visit process.

Danielle enjoys spending time with her family.

DEDICATION

To my husband, children, grandchildren and Allied Health Science colleagues of Arkansas Tech University, I thank you and love you for your support and encouragement.

Phyllis

To Eric and Rachel—I am so proud of you. You are my inspiration. I love you both so much. To Joel—Thanks for everything. The reasons are too numerous to count. I love you. To Mom, Dad and Craig—Thanks for always being there. Love you.

Danielle

Preface

Welcome to the third edition of McGraw-Hill's *Palko's Medical Laboratory Procedures.* The origin of this text began at a time when the number of clinical laboratories in ambulatory care facilities was increasing and quality control was mandated by CLIA 1988 and laboratory safety by OSHA. Since then, challenges in the labs have been met with additional requirements and many advances have been made in testing. This text includes theory and principles of clinical laboratory science; laboratory testing procedures, manual and automated, that have been around for decades; as well as current automated and point-of-care laboratory procedures.

This edition is revised, rearranged, and updated in honor of the late Tom Palko and his widow, Hilda, who both worked for many years in the medical laboratory field; Tom then spent over 25 years teaching in the allied health sciences, including medical technology and medical assisting.

This text can serve in the following ways:

- as a textbook for an orientation course in laboratory medicine for students beginning the study in medical technology or clinical laboratory science.

- as a textbook in the clinical laboratory portion of the curriculum for students of allied health sciences, especially medical assisting programs and medical technician programs.

- as a source of reference for personnel working in a clinical laboratory, particularly an ambulatory care facility.

Because this text can be utilized by so many different health professionals, for the purpose of this book, anyone performing laboratory tests will be referred to as lab personnel.

Effective clinical laboratory personnel must understand the theory, principle, and pathology behind the testing procedures. Knowing about the conditions and diseases that alter the lab test results, medical personnel will contribute even more to the care of the patient and thus make the job more meaningful and enjoyable. Due to advances in laboratory instrumentation, microtesting, and simplified testing procedures, today many laboratory tests are run in the physician's

office laboratory. Quality assurance programs are so explicit that the physicians can rely on the accuracy of test results for both diagnosis and treatment of the patient. The more knowledge and practice the lab personnel has about all areas of the clinical laboratory, the more enhanced the contribution is to total patient care.

Instructors will find great improvements and new features in this third edition. Obviously, the first noticeable feature will be addition of color, making, for example, cellular differentiation, testing procedures, and general visuals much easier to learn, teach, and read. Safety regulations from OSHA and total quality assurance have been updated and used throughout the text. Current HIPAA regulations appropriate to the laboratory, along with proper record keeping, have been updated and expanded. Review of math and statistical calculations is again included but with additional problems for those students who need more practice. The section on blood collection has been extended and examples of current testing procedures in hematology, urinalysis, chemistry, immunology, and microbiology are included. Laboratory procedures have been modified to include performance standards and evaluation scores. Common laboratory equipment can now be found in the appendix along with laboratory vocabulary, reference values for common laboratory tests, and CLIA levels of certification.

ORGANIZATION

This is a competency-based textbook and reference that functions also as a workbook and laboratory manual. The book is organized into six units.

Unit I, Introduction to the Physician's Office Laboratory, is the introduction to the laboratory and includes safety, math, statistics, quality control, and record keeping.

Unit II, Urinalysis, includes the urinary system and collection and analysis of urine specimens.

Unit III, Blood Collection, is new and covers blood collection including capillary, venipuncture, and advanced venipuncture procedures.

Unit IV, Hematology, is on hematology and hematology testing of whole blood components and also includes coagulation principles and testing.

Unit V, Blood Chemistry, is the section on complications of diabetes and glucose testing, along with other chemistry analytes.

Unit VI, Immunology and Microbiology, includes the immunology and microbiology chapters.

WHAT'S NEW

Chapter-specific changes are

- **Laboratory Safety**—Updates and requirements from CDC and OSHA can be found in Chapter 1, along with the addition of information on new safety devices, standard precautions, hepatitis C, and how to locate current information on issues that lab personnel may encounter. OSHA Bloodborne Pathogen Standards have been added to the appendix, as well as an example of an exposure report form.

- **Microscopy**—Details of the compound microscope are again included in Chapter 2 with color photos of microscope parts and the proper use.

- **Math Review**—The addition of a section in Chapter 3 teaching the dimensional analysis process of converting from one unit to another will be helpful for English to metric or metric to metric conversions. Also, adding 60 extra problems with fractions, equations, percents, and making solutions will help those students needing further practice.

- **Statistics**—Chapter 4 remains important in the course because of quality control calculations. It simplifies statistical calculations that are used each day by lab techs. In accredited med tech programs, students are required to take a separate course in statistics.

- **Quality Assurance and Quality Control**—Chapter 5 has been revised to include current terminology that is being utilized today.

- **Record Keeping in the POL**—Chapter 6 has included information on HIPAA as it relates to the laboratory. In addition, it includes information about oral communication in the laboratory.

- **Urinary System—Anatomy and Physiology**—Chapter 7 has been reorganized to focus on the anatomy and physiology most critical to understand urinalysis testing and patient test results.

- **Urine Collection and Preservation and Physical, Chemical, and Microscopic Analysis of Urine Specimens**—The entire Urinalysis unit (Chapters 8–10) has been reorganized for better correlation and understanding.

- **Blood Collection: Routine Venipuncture and Advanced Venipuncture Techniques**—This new unit (Chapters 11 and 12) provides detailed instruction on how to perform routine venipuncture, venipuncture utilizing a syringe, venipuncture utilizing a butterfly needle, as well as capillary specimen collection. The chapters include updated safety procedures.

- **Hematology**—Chapters 13–17 include manual and updated automated methods of counting, measuring, and analyzing whole blood, either capillary or venous blood, for all components of CBCs, platelet counts, sedimentation rates, reticulocyte counts, and other hematology techniques. Principles of blood formation, the body's responses to disease processes, and comparing test results have been enhanced and expanded.

- **Coagulation**—Current information about coagulation studies and disorders has been included in Chapter 18. Also, point-of-care (POC) instruments using capillary blood to test prothrombin times to monitor patients on coumadin therapy have been included and the use of INR results has been added.

- **Blood Glucose and Other Chemistry Tests**—These chapters (Chapters 19 and 20) remain essential to the student as a core of laboratory testing and include updated diabetes terminology and guidelines and information about POC testing.

- **Immunology Tests**—This is an area of the laboratory where advances in sensitivity and specificity have made available on-the-spot testing for a variety of disorders or conditions from HCG to HIV. Many CLIA-waived kits are now available and allow the physician to evaluate and treat patients earlier. Numerous examples are given in Chapter 21 along with sample procedures.

- **Microbiology**—Chapter 22 has been expanded to include examples of automated bacterial identification systems used in larger clinic laboratories. More photos and diagrams of microbes, both normal and pathogenic, have been added, along with diagrams to show collection of specimens for culturing.

TEACHING AND LEARNING SUPPLEMENTS

For the Instructor

- The Instructor's Manual to accompany this text, which is posted to the Online Learning Center, www.mhhe.com/CoxPalkoMedLab3e, includes many items that will assist the instructor, enhance the presentation, and help with evaluation of learning. Chapter-by-chapter teaching strategies, cognitive and performance objectives, and procedure checklists are included.

- Other instructor resources posted to the Online Learning Center include chapter PowerPoint presentations that can be modified to fit the instructor's lesson plans and an electronic testing program (EZTest), allowing instructors to create tests from book-specific items.

For the Student

- Each chapter includes a review section that allows students to assess what information presented in the chapter they have mastered and determine their weaknesses. All chapters have been revised to include review questions in multiple formats including multiple choice, short answer, and critical thinking questions.

- In addition, for all chapters with performance objectives, students are provided with a competency checklist for the performance objective. Each checklist has been updated to determine the number of points each step is worth, as well as determining which steps are critical steps and must be performed correctly in order to pass the competency. Students can now determine in advance what skills and steps they need to master in order to succeed.

- The Online Learning Center, www.mhhe.com/CoxPalkoMedLab3e, provides additional quizzes, flashcards, and learning activities.

WHAT EVERY STUDENT NEEDS TO KNOW

Many tools to help you learn have been integrated into your text.

CHAPTER FEATURES

Cognitive Objectives

present a list of the key points you should focus on in the chapter.

Performance Objectives

outline the tasks that you should be able to complete after studying the chapter.

Terminology

highlights important chapter terms and definitions that will assist you in understanding the content.

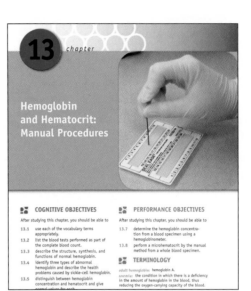

13 *chapter*

Hemoglobin and Hematocrit: Manual Procedures

COGNITIVE OBJECTIVES

After studying this chapter, you should be able to

13.1 use each of the vocabulary terms appropriately.
13.2 list the blood tests performed as part of the complete blood count.
13.3 describe the structure, synthesis, and functions of normal hemoglobin.
13.4 identify three types of abnormal hemoglobin and describe the health problems caused by sickle-cell hemoglobin.
13.5 distinguish between hemoglobin concentration and hematocrit and give normal values for each.

PERFORMANCE OBJECTIVES

After studying this chapter, you should be able to

13.7 determine the hemoglobin concentration from a blood specimen using a hemoglobinometer.
13.8 perform a microhematocrit by the manual method from a whole blood specimen.

TERMINOLOGY

adult hemoglobin: hemoglobin A.
anemia: the condition in which there is a deficiency in the amount of hemoglobin in the blood, thus reducing the oxygen-carrying capacity of the blood.

Reminder Boxes, Information Boxes, Note Boxes

provide focus and helpful hints on key chapter information.

Phlebotomy Supply Checklist

It is important that you remember to check the supplies in your phlebotomy tray every day to ensure that you have the items you need for each procedure. The following checklist should be used as a template. Modify as needed to meet the needs of your own POL, including maintaining minimums.

Tables

summarize data and help organize concepts.

Performance Standards	Points Awarded	Maximum Points
1. Wash your hands with disinfectant, dry them, and put on gloves, face shield, and apron or lab coat.		5
2. Follow standard precautions.		5
3. Assemble and prepare the appropriate equipment and supplies.		5
4. *Prepare the hemoglobinometer according to the manual supplied, checking calibration and/or optical self-test and hemoglobin controls.		15
5. *Inspect the EDTA-anticoagulated blood for proper labeling.		15
6. Mix the tube of EDTA-anticoagulated blood thoroughly.		5
7. Remove the cap from the tube of blood, using a tissue or cap remover; take care to avoid splattering blood.		5
8. *Load the microcuvettes, or other measuring device supplied or recommended by the manufacturer of the hemoglobinometer, with blood and wipe off any excess blood from the outside of the cuvette.		10
9. Load the cuvette into the holder of the photometric reader and push the measuring position.		5
10. Read the hemoglobin value from the display and record.		10

Figures

Colorful illustrations and photos add to the understanding of topics.

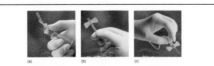

Figure 11-4 Various needles with safety mechanisms: (a) hinged cap; (b) protective shield; (c) retractable needle.

hurt more but are less likely to cause a hemolyzed specimen, thus requiring the specimen to be recollected; (2) smaller needles are less painful but tend to take longer to collect a specimen and are more likely to cause hemolysis in the specimen. Needles should be sterile—never use a needle in which someone other than you has broken the seal at the time of collection. Needles can only be used once and must be discarded in a biohazardous sharps container after they have been used. Never bend, break, or recap needles. In addition, the Needlestick Safety and Prevention Act signed by former President Clinton in 2000 requires that all needles have a safety mechanism to help avoid accidental **needlesticks.** Each manufacturer uses its own safety mechanism, so be sure to familiarize yourself with the mechanism PRIOR to the use of the needle.

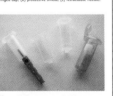

Figure 11-5 Examples of needle holders.

Procedure Competency Checklists

provide detailed lists and expectations for competency performance.

End-of-Chapter Review (Matching, Multiple Choice, Applying Knowledge)

checks your understanding and mastery of chapter content.

Appendices

offer additional information that is pertinent to the medical laboratory.

Online Learning Center

www.mhhe.com/CoxPalkoMedLab3e
offers additional learning and teaching tools.

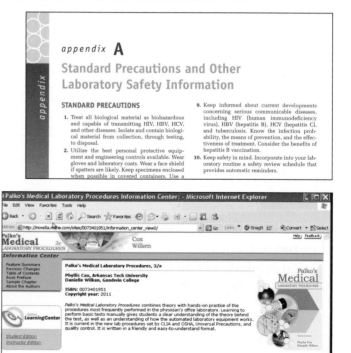

Brief Contents

Contents

ACKNOWLEDGMENTS

For insightful reviews, criticisms, helpful suggestions, and information, we would like to acknowledge the following:

Cindy A. Abel, BS, CMA(AAMA), COLT, PBT(ASCP)
Ivy Tech Community College of Indiana

Marcia A. Armstrong, MS, CLS(NCA)
University of Hawaii, Kapiolani Community College

Rhonda M. Asher, MT(ASCP), CMA
Pitt Community College

Kaye F. Bathe
Tri County Technical College

Michelle L. Blesi
Century College

Becky M. Clark, M.Ed., MT(ASCP)
J. Sargeant Reynolds Community College

Joyce Combs, CMA (AAMA), MS
Bluegrass Community & Technical College

Michele Crissman, JD, MS, BS
Colorado Technical University

Amber Cox Joachim, JD
Houston Christian

Holly Crouch Gerard, BS
Arkansas Tech University

Jane P. Dunlap
Zane State College

Cathy Flores
Central Piedmont Community College

Steve Forshier, M.Ed.
Pima Medical Institute

Brenda K. Frerichs
Colorado Technical University

Tammy T. Gant, RHIT, CMA, CAHI
Surry Community College

Stefanie Goodman, MSN, RN, CMA (AAMA)
Ivy Tech Community College

Darlene S. Grayson Harmon MA, BS
Remington College

Debra J. Hessell, SEN, RGN, DipN, BSc(Hons), APSN
Sawyer School

Dolly Horton, CMA, BS, M.Ed.
Mayland Community College

Eugenia Ilisei, MD
IIA College

Cassandra D. James
College of Marin

Rhonda S. Jost, MSH, MT(ASCP)
Florida Community College at Jacksonville

Art Keehnle
Beufort County Community College

Deanna Klosinski, Ph.D., MS, MT(ASCP), DLM
The College of Allied Health Sciences, Michigan State University

Gideon Labiner, MS, MT(ASCP), CLS(NCA)
University of Cincinnati

Michelle Mantooth, M.Sc., MT(ASCP), CLS(NCA), CLSp(CYG)
Trident Technical College

Richard H. Miller, Ph.D., MRA, MT(ASCP), CM, CLS(NGA)
Southwest Georgia Technical College

Bridgit R. Moore, EdD, MT(ASCP), CLS (NCA)
McLennan Community College

Melissa Munoz, BS
Dorsey Schools

Patrice M. Nadeau, MS, MT(ASCP)
Dakota County Technical College

Lisa Riojas-Smithart, A.S., RMA, NRCPT
Richland College

George H. Roberts, Ed.D., CLS(NCA)
South Arkansas Community College

Patricia Rock, LPN
Brevard Community College

Melanie E. Schmidt
College America

Tara S. Shepherd, AAB, BS, CMA(AAMA)
Apollo Career Centre

Rosalyn H. Singleton, BS, MT(ASCP)
Northeast Mississippi Community College

Lauren I. Strader, MT(ASCP), M.Ed.
North Georgia Technical College

Cindy Thompson, RN, RMA, MA
Davenport Univeristy

Tamra L. West, B.S., M.Ed.
Forest Institute

Accrediting Bureau of Health Education Schools
ABHES

Evaluation Standards for Medical Laboratory Technology

Correlation Chart

Medical Laboratory Procedures	Chapters
To provide for student attainment of entry-level competencies, the curriculum must include, but not necessarily be limited to, the following:	
a. Orientation	
OSHA compliance rules and regulations	1
Laboratory equipment and maintenance	2, 16, 17, 18, 19
Biohazard safety	1, 8, 9, 10, 11, 12, 13, 14, 15, 17, 18, 19, 21,22
Fire safety	1
Use and care of microscope	2
Requisition processing	6, 11
b. Urinalysis	
Specimen collection and study	8
Physical, chemical, and microscopic properties	8, 9, 10
c. Hematology Specimen Collection and Study	
Venipuncture and finger puncture	11, 12
Hemoglobin and hematocrit	13
RBC and WBC counts	14
Blood smears and differentials	15
d. Blood Chemistries	
Chemistry analyzers—principles and procedures	19, 20
Electrolytes	
Blood and body fluid analytes—normal values and indications	19, 20
e. Immunology and Serology	
Selected test procedures	21
Titering and dilutions	21
f. Microbiology	
Staining techniques—gram, acid fast, negative, and variations	22
Use of culture media	22
Culture methods—aerobic, anaerobic, microaerophilic	22
Normal flora v. significant growth	22
Multitest methods of ID	22
Serological ID methods	21, 22
Antibiograms	22
Phage typing	

unit

I

INTRODUCTION TO THE PHYSICIAN'S OFFICE LABORATORY

chapter

1

Safety in the Laboratory

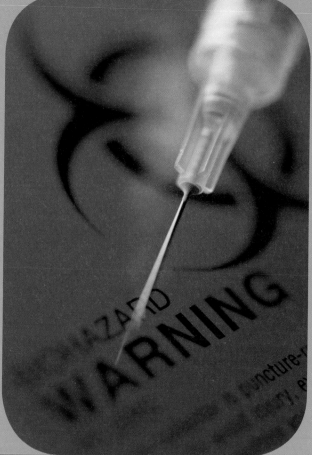

COGNITIVE OBJECTIVES

After studying this chapter, you should be able to

1.1 use each of the vocabulary terms appropriately.

1.2 identify the agencies primarily responsible for regulating lab safety.

1.3 list three major types of laboratory hazards and give examples of each.

1.4 identify four types of control methods used to promote lab personnel safety and describe one example of each.

1.5 discuss the role of HBV vaccination in promoting lab personnel safety.

1.6 describe how lab personnel are evaluated and the follow-up after exposure to a biohazard in the lab.

1.7 explain how biohazardous materials can be safely disposed of in laboratories.

1.8 discuss the role of good housekeeping practices in maintaining a safe work environment in the lab.

1.9 describe the areas in which lab personnel should be educated in order to be safe on the job.

1.10 identify four safety tips for using lab chemicals.

1.11 describe how reagents should be labeled and stored.

1.12 explain why acids and bases pose special risks for lab personnel.

1.13 describe how to prevent injury from electrical, fire, weather, and personal hazards.

1.14 explain why a professional attitude is important for safety in the lab.

1.15 list seven reasons for lab accidents that are related to personnel characteristics.

1.16 discuss steps that can be taken to alleviate stress on the job.

PERFORMANCE OBJECTIVES

After studying this chapter, you should be able to

1.17 plan a lab safety orientation program for new employees.

1.18 devise a waste-disposal plan for a physician's office laboratory.

1.19 develop an accident-proofing program for the lab.

1.20 plan fire and severe weather drills for lab personnel.

1.21 design posters that remind lab personnel to follow important safety guidelines and procedures.

1.22 evaluate a lab on campus for safety and prepare a report listing ways in which safety can be enhanced.

1.23 locate Internet sources for OSHA and CDC updates and recommendations.

TERMINOLOGY

acid: a chemical that donates hydrogen ions (H^+), lowers the pH of solutions, and reacts with bases to form water and chemical salts.

aerosolization: the conversion of a liquid, such as blood or blood products, or a solid, such as a powdered chemical, into a fine mist that travels through the air.

autoclave: a device utilizing steam under pressure to sterilize medical instruments and laboratory specimens.

base: a chemical that yields hydroxide ions (OH^-) when dissolved in water (e.g., sodium hydroxide). Bases raise the pH of a solution and react with acids to form chemical salts and water.

biohazard: a biological specimen containing blood or other body fluid that has the potential for transmitting disease.

biological specimen: a specimen that originates from a living organism. Examples are blood, blood products, other body fluids such as cerebrospinal fluid or urine, biopsy samples, bacterial smears, and bacterial cultures.

bloodborne pathogens: microorganisms that cause disease and can be transmitted through blood or other body fluids. HIV is an example.

caustic: burning or corrosive; usually destructive to living tissue.

CDC: Centers for Disease Control and Prevention.

chain of transmission: the unbroken line of transmission of a disease from one host with the disease to a new host.

chemical hazard: a source of danger from exposure to chemicals.

contamination: the pollution of an area or substance with unwanted extraneous material such as pathogens or hazardous chemicals.

disinfection: any practical procedure for reducing the pathogen contamination in the inanimate environment, as in the air, on work counters, or on equipment.

engineering control: a device that keeps biohazards away from laboratory personnel.

exposure incident: a situation in which laboratory personnel are exposed to a potentially hazardous substance, such as blood or a toxic chemical.

hazardous chemical list: a list maintained by OSHA that identifies toxic chemicals used in laboratories. It may be consulted to determine the toxicity of a chemical.

HBV (hepatitis B virus): the virus that causes hepatitis B, a type of severe hepatitis transmitted by sexual contact, by needle sharing, or through contaminated blood, blood products, or other body fluids.

HCV (hepatitis C virus): previously known as Non-A Non-B hepatitis virus; the virus that causes hepatitis C, a serious type of hepatitis transmitted by contaminated blood and blood products, needles, and sexual contact. There is presently no vaccine for HCV.

HIV (human immunodeficiency virus): the virus that causes AIDS (acquired immunodeficiency syndrome).

ICP (infection control program): a program that provides the maximum protection for health care workers against occupational sources of disease.

MSDS (Material Safety Data Sheet): included with all chemical shipments describing precautions and disposal information.

NFPA Diamond: a symbol, issued by the National Fire Protection Association, in the shape of a diamond with four colored quadrants that can be used in laboratories to label hazardous materials to show the type and level of hazard.

OSHA (Occupational Safety and Health Administration): a federal agency within the U.S. Department of Labor. OSHA works to assure the safety and health of workers.

pathogen: disease-causing microorganism.

physical hazard: a source of danger in the environment, such as shock, housekeeping accidents, and falls.

POL: physician's office laboratory.

post-exposure evaluation: a set of procedures required by OSHA as a follow-up to exposure incidents.

post-exposure prophylaxis: preventive treatment for exposure to possible pathogenic microorganisms, HIV, HBV, and HCV, for example.

PPE (personal protective equipment): clothing and other equipment that shield health care workers from outside contaminants. PPE includes gloves, uniforms, fluid-proof aprons, masks, and eye-shields.

specimen: a small amount of body tissue (e.g., urine, blood, or tumor biopsy) taken for purposes of examination. The sample is assumed to represent the whole and to provide meaningful results for the total individual.

Standard Precautions: guidelines that use the CDC Universal Precautions and OSHA Bloodborne Pathogen Standards to direct health care workers in protection against pathogens transmitted by infectious patients.

STD: sexually transmitted disease.

toxic: poisonous.

Universal Precautions: a set of recommendations formulated by the CDC to protect workers against HIV and other pathogens. The precautions impose isolation of all specimens of blood, blood products, and other body fluids capable of transmitting pathogens.

vector: a carrier, such as an insect, of a pathogen.

work-practice control: a method that incorporates safety into laboratory procedures.

INTRODUCTION

Safety in the **POL,** physician's office laboratory, is an essential part of all laboratory work. No laboratory procedure is complete unless it includes controls against infection, chemical toxicity, and physical hazards.

WORKING TOWARD A SAFE LABORATORY

Laboratory safety requires knowledge of laboratory procedures, equipment, and reagents, as well as constant watchfulness for danger. One careless worker can undo all the safety practices followed by coworkers in the lab.

Regulating Lab Safety

A major concern for personnel in the medical laboratory is infectious disease and exposure to infectious microorganisms from patient **specimens.** This concern stems largely from the epidemic of AIDS, a fatal bloodborne disease caused by human immunodeficiency virus (HIV), and from the spread of hepatitis B virus and hepatitis C virus. Legislation to enforce laboratory standards of safety has been passed, and as a result clinical laboratories are safer now than they were in the past when disease prevention received less emphasis.

Two government agencies have had primary responsibility in monitoring medical lab safety: **Centers for Disease Control and Prevention (CDC),** which is within the U.S. Department of Health and Human Services (www.hhs.gov), and the **Occupational Safety and Health Administration (OSHA),** which is within the U.S. Department of Labor (www.dol.gov). These two agencies formulated important regulations and guidelines for laboratory safety. The CDC developed a set of principles called **Universal Precautions** that heighten awareness of the potential risk that medical laboratory specimens pose to the personnel who handle them. This led OSHA to develop a set of guidelines known as Bloodborne Pathogens Standards for the protection of health care workers at risk for exposure to bloodborne pathogens. CDC extended these standards and issued the Guide to **Standard Precautions** for Infection Control to control hospital infections, to protect health care personnel, and also to protect the patients.

Hazards

Potential hazards in POLs fall into three categories:

- **Biohazards** are sources of danger from living ("bio") specimens, including blood and other body fluids, microbiology specimens, and cultures.
- **Chemical hazards** are sources of danger from exposure to laboratory chemicals, including immediate and long-term effects on the health of workers.
- **Physical hazards** are sources of danger in the environment, including electrical shock, housekeeping accidents, and falls.

The federal government mandates addressing all three types of potential hazards in the procedure manuals of POLs. You should familiarize yourself with the procedure manual in any lab where you work. The rest of this chapter describes potential dangers and how to deal with them for each of these three types of hazards.

BIOHAZARDS

Lab specimens sometimes contain disease-causing microorganisms, called **pathogens.** Exposure of lab personnel to pathogens is likely to vary from one medical practice to another. A small rural family practice clinic will have a much different patient population with different health problems than will a specialty practice in a large metropolitan area. Nonetheless, general principles of hygiene and safety should be followed in all POLs to decrease the risk of disease transmission.

Safety and Procedure Manuals

Specific safety procedures addressed in POL procedure manuals include the following:

- safe workplace practices
- disinfection
- hepatitis B vaccine
- avoiding and reporting needlestick injuries
- spills and cleanups
- labeling of hazardous materials
- waste disposal
- hygienic practices
- OSHA accident log (for reporting accidents)
- safety education
- storage, inventory, and handling of chemicals
- first aid
- fire prevention and use of fire blankets

Biohazards

Potentially infective biospecimens encountered in clinical laboratories include the following:

- blood
- body fluids
- body tissue biopsies
- urine
- exudates (pus, mucus, sputum)
- bacterial smears
- bacterial cultures

How Diseases Are Transmitted

To know how to avoid disease transmission in the lab, you first must understand how diseases are transmitted. Most infectious disease pathogens gain entry to the body through one of the body's systems, most commonly the skin, respiratory system, or gastrointestinal tract (see Table 1-1). In order to cause disease in a susceptible person, the pathogen must leave the first host and enter an uninfected individual in an

Table 1-1 Major Routes of Disease Transmission

Type of Contact*	Infections
Direct skin contact	Staph, strep, measles, colds, influenza, tuberculosis
Mucus-to-mucus contact	Strep, syphilis, gonorrhea, herpes, HIV, HCV, other **STDs**
Aerosols and dust	Colds, influenza, measles, tuberculosis, chicken pox
Food and water	Food poisoning, typhoid, hepatitis A, cholera, intestinal parasites
Blood and other body fluids	HIV, HBV, HCV
Animal **vectors**	Tularemia, malaria, Rocky Mountain spotted fever, Lyme disease

*This list is not inclusive. For example, rabies can be transferred by a rabid animal's bite or by infected tissue in surgical transplants.

unbroken **chain of transmission.** Pathogens in test specimens and on contaminated equipment may infect laboratory personnel who handle them. To prevent infection in the lab, barriers must be maintained between workers and biohazardous material, thereby breaking the chain of transmission.

Disease Risks in the Lab

Because blood is so frequently encountered, bloodborne diseases are a special risk for lab personnel, but almost any type of infection can pose a risk for those who work in a medical lab. (See Figure 1-1.)

Bloodborne Infections. Even though they usually cannot survive for long outside body fluids or tissues, **bloodborne pathogens** pose the greatest

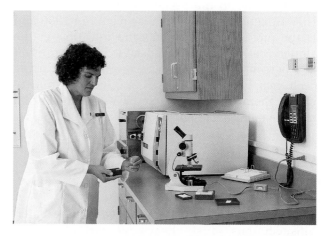

Figure 1-1 To avoid the risk of infection in the POL, keep it clean and orderly at all times.

potential risk to lab personnel. Most important of these are **HIV, human immunodeficiency virus; HBV, hepatitis B virus; and HCV, hepatitis C virus.** They are usually transmitted by the direct contact of body fluids, such as blood or semen, from one person to another in some manner, most often through sexual activity or use of contaminated needles. These viruses may cause infection in which the virus is present in body tissues and fluids even though the patient has no symptoms of disease. Because clues may not be apparent from patients or specimens to warn the laboratory personnel of infection, all **biological specimens** should be considered potentially infectious and handled as such. Needlesticks are the leading cause of bloodborne infections of lab personnel. Improper handling of sharps, such as broken glass tubes, slides, or lancets, may result in cuts to lab personnel.

The actual number of people contracting HIV through work in clinical laboratories is very small. There are only a few documented cases of HIV being transmitted through occupational exposure of health workers.

The number of people infected with HIV remains high, so exposure of health workers is still a concern. In 2008, the U.S. Public Health Service reported that at the end of 2003, approximately one million persons in the United States were living with HIV infection, including approximately 250,000 who do not know they are infected (www.cdc.gov). AIDS, the disease caused by HIV, results when the virus damages the immune system, allowing other diseases to ravage the body. There is no cure for AIDS, thus preventive measures must be 100 percent effective to ensure the safety of lab personnel.

There is a higher risk of infection of health care workers from HBV and HCV. The good news is there has been a significant decrease in the number of HBV infections, 260,000 in the 1980s to 46,000 in 2006, due to the vaccine available to prevent HBV infections. HCV was discovered in 1990 and is the most chronic bloodborne infection in the United States. Workers exposed to blood represent 2–4 percent of total new cases of HCV occurring each year (www.cdc.gov/NIOSH/topics). Unfortunately, there is no vaccine for HCV and prevention must be completely effective.

WORKING SAFELY WITH BIOHAZARDS

Although hazards such as disease-contaminated biospecimens must always be part of laboratory work, they need not pose a serious threat to the safety of lab personnel. Personal protective equipment, if properly worn, is an important safeguard. In addition, automation has greatly reduced the need to handle contaminated specimens and toxic chemicals. Microtesting procedures using very small amounts of specimens and chemicals also make clinical laboratories safer.

OSHA has established laboratory guidelines and procedures to reduce the risk of infection from biohazards. OSHA's Infection Control Program details procedures to be used in the following areas, each of which is addressed in the remainder of this section:

- control methods
- HBV vaccination
- post-exposure treatment, evaluation, and follow-up
- disposal of infectious waste and biohazardous material
- housekeeping practices
- employee education

Control Methods

Control methods refer to procedures and devices meant to eliminate or prevent **exposure incidents** in POLs. They include Universal/Standard Precautions, engineering controls, work-practice controls, and personal protective equipment.

Universal/Standard Precautions. CDC's guidelines use Universal Precautions, which are based on the premise that all body fluids and tissues are potentially infected with HIV, HBV, HCV, or other pathogens and lab personnel are safe only when they are completely isolated from direct contact with biological specimens. These precautions, in combination with the Bloodborne Pathogens Standards by OSHA, help ensure that all human blood and other potentially infectious materials are isolated to protect workers from infection. The Bloodborne Pathogens Standard issued by OSHA can be found in Appendix B.

Engineering Controls. Devices that provide a safer laboratory environment are called **engineering controls.** These are meant to eliminate or minimize worker exposure to biohazards. They may enclose the biohazard completely, shield the biohazard from aerosolization and spattering, clean and disinfect contaminated equipment, or identify and enclose hazardous waste. It is imperative for worker safety that all engineering control devices be inspected on a regularly scheduled basis and repaired or replaced as needed.

Body Fluids and Disease

Body fluids capable of transmitting HIV and HBV include the following:

- blood and blood products
- semen
- vaginal secretions
- spinal fluid
- pleural fluid
- synovial fluid
- peritoneal fluid
- pericardial fluid
- amniotic fluid

   Some body secretions, such as urine, saliva, sputum, and tears may be capable of transmitting HIV if they contain blood. It is important to remember that minute amounts of blood in body fluids may not be obvious or easily detected. These body fluids may carry other pathogens as well. The fact that the body fluid is being tested in a clinical laboratory suggests that it is likely to have a higher than average probability of disease.

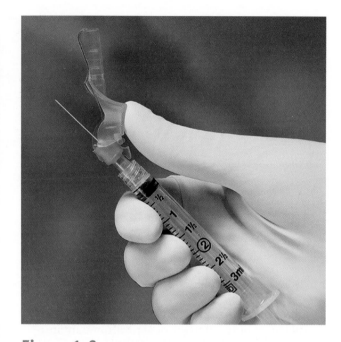

Figure 1-2 Safety needles now reduce the risk of needle injuries.

Following are descriptions of engineering controls that you should employ to ensure safety in the medical lab:

- *Needlestick safety.* In response to The Needlestick Safety and Prevention Act passed in 2000, OSHA now requires employers to use new safety needles that decrease the risk of needle injuries. Safety needles provide shields permitting lab personnel to dispose of contaminated needles without recapping or touching the needles, thus reducing the risk of needlestick injuries. (See Figure 1-2.)

- *Specimen containment.* Confine and transfer body fluids within closed containers whenever possible. Place specimens in well-constructed containers with secure lids to prevent leakage during mailing or transport. Do not contaminate either the laboratory request form or the outside of the container during collection.

- *Prevention of **aerosolization.*** When minute amounts of body fluids or bacterial cultures are sprayed or swept into the air by spillage, laboratory procedures, or wind currents within the room, aerosols are formed. Aerosol droplets cannot be seen by the naked eye, but they can carry disease and penetrate to the depths of the respiratory tract, causing infection of lab personnel. Avoid aerosolization of biohazards by covering all specimens. Cap or cover urine containers and tubes of blood when they are not undergoing actual testing.

- *Vented hoods or biohazard cabinets with filters.* Use this equipment when working with bacteria or hazardous material that may generate aerosols. Always inoculate microbiological specimens onto culture media and streak and isolate cultures inside a hood or biohazard cabinet because minute amounts of microscopic organisms may be infectious.

- *Safe use of centrifuges.* Stopper or cap specimens and centrifuge them with the lid closed. An open lid is unsafe because of occasional accidental breakage. Flying glass fragments and spattering or aerosolization of biological specimens can result in both cuts and contamination at once. Never stop centrifuges by hand or open them before spinning stops because these actions encourage spattering and aerosolization of contents.

- *Barriers between body fluids and laboratory personnel.* In addition to needle safety shields, other devices serve as barriers between laboratory personnel and the biohazard. Devices that remove test tube stoppers prevent aerosols from escaping and eliminate direct handling of contaminated stoppers. Plexiglass shields also can be placed as needed between the specimens and technicians. Figure 1-3 shows examples of barrier devices.

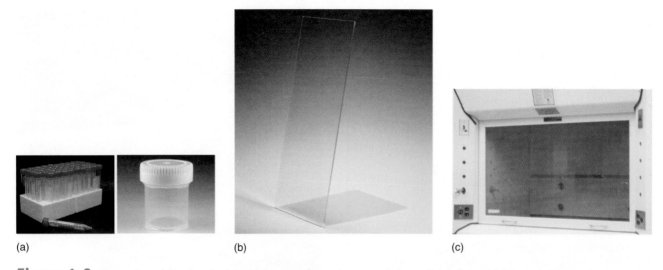

Figure 1-3 Examples of barrier devices: (a) capped specimen container; (b) safety shield; and (c) hood.

- *Safe pipetting.* Pipetting by mouth is unsafe because of the danger of aspirating contaminated body fluids and hazardous chemicals. Instead, use mechanical suction devices to uptake and release fluids from pipettes.

- *Disposable equipment.* The less often contaminated equipment is handled, the less likely there is exposure to disease organisms. Disposable equipment, which does not have to be washed and disinfected for reuse, provides a safer laboratory environment. Using disposables is also usually cheaper than cleaning and sterilizing used equipment. A wide variety of disposable products are available, including glassware, needles, lancets, and transfer pipettes.

Work-Practice Controls. Any technique or procedure that makes lab work safer falls into this category. Most **work-practice controls** are simple but proven methods of protecting oneself from disease. All require self-discipline if they are to be effective. To keep yourself as safe as possible in the lab, you should follow these important rules:

- *Wash your hands frequently with antimicrobial soap or an alcohol-based gel or foam.* The importance of hand hygiene cannot be overemphasized. Direct contact is the most common method for transmission of microorganisms that cause disease. Wash your hands using antimicrobial soap or an alcohol-based disinfectant gel or foam (see Figure 1-4). After drying your hands, apply lotion to prevent skin from cracking and leaving open wounds.

- *Avoid wearing false fingernails.* Many labs have rules regarding false fingernails, tips and overlays because they may harbor bacteria and they increase the puncture risk to gloves which could leave the skin exposed to biohazardous substances.

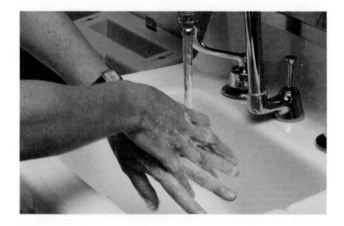

Figure 1-4 Wash your hands thoroughly between patients, after handling hazardous chemicals, between laboratory and nonlaboratory activities, and before and after using the restroom.

- *Keep objects away from your face.* The mouth is the entrance to the body's digestive and respiratory systems. The mucous membranes of the nose and eyes also are pathways for infection. Absentmindedly chewing on pencils or fingernails, rubbing your face, or putting on makeup in the lab can breach the barrier between pathogen and worker. In order to avoid possible contamination with biospecimens and chemicals, do not store or consume food and drink in the laboratory. Take coffee breaks and meals outside the laboratory after washing your hands.

- *Keep personal items in storage.* A closet or locker near the laboratory should house personal effects such as jewelry and purses or extra clothing worn to and from work. Carrying such personal items into and out of the lab increases the risk of spreading pathogens and other hazards outside the lab environment.

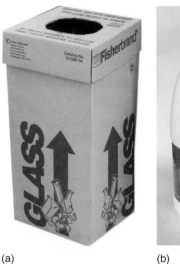
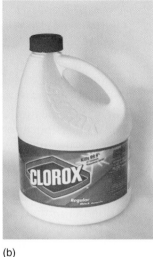

(a)   (b)

Figure 1-5 (a) Clean up broken glass with care and place in proper container; (b) Freshly prepared solutions of 10% household bleach may be used to sanitize the area or commercially available spill kits may be used.

- *Clean up spills immediately.* In the event of potentially infectious spills, pour a 1:10 bleach solution liberally, cover the spill with paper towels to prevent spreading, and allow the spill to soak for 5 minutes before wiping it up. If glass is broken, never pick up the pieces by hand because of the danger of cuts. Instead, scoop broken glass into a dustpan or box and dispose of it in a puncture-proof container (see Figure 1-5). Dispose of items used in the wipe-up, including gloves, aprons, and other barrier items, in another plastic bag. Label these bags with a biohazard indicator. Always wash your hands after cleaning up a spill.

- *Decontaminate equipment.* Decontaminate equipment that comes into contact with blood or other body fluids on a daily basis with disinfectant, such as a bleach solution. Equipment that may corrode from daily wiping with a bleach solution may be wiped with alcohol.

- *Prevent splashing or spraying of materials.* Analyze all procedures for better ways to control mishaps that may contaminate equipment or the lab environment.

Personal Protective Equipment (PPE). PPE refers to specialized clothing and other gear that help shield laboratory personnel from contaminants. Examples include fluid repellant, high-collar laboratory jackets and coats, vinyl or latex dispos-

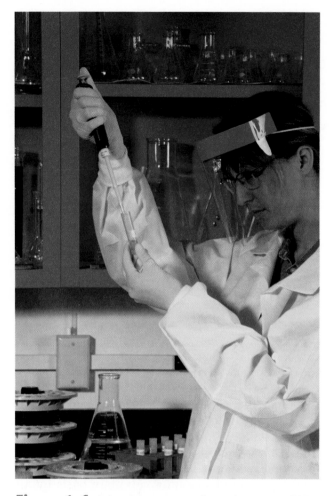

Figure 1-6 Laboratory personnel wearing proper PPE.

able gloves (see Figure 1-6), fluid-proof aprons, enclosed shoes, face shields, masks, and goggles. PPE should be exchanged for street clothing before lab personnel leave the medical office and placed in a designated area for storage, laundry, decontamination, or disposal. OSHA stipulates that medical labs must provide these items and that the equipment must be replaced or repaired when necessary to maintain its effectiveness.

Always wearing disposable, protective gloves is especially important when working with biohazardous material. Wearing gloves helps prevent the entrance of pathogens into abrasions that may not be obvious if they are very small. Gloves used in venipuncture and laboratory procedures should be discarded after specimen processing. Gloves also should be changed after each patient contact, and hands should be washed with antimicrobial soap or sanitized with alcohol-based hand gel or foam between each glove change. Gloves should not be disinfected and reused because disinfected gloves may disintegrate and allow fluid to pass through undetected holes. At the end of the day, gloves should be discarded and hands washed again before leaving the office. Note that frequent hand washing dries and cracks the skin. Always use a hand lotion after washing your hands to help maintain skin integrity.

To properly remove contaminated gloves, remove the first glove and hold it in your hand with the second glove while you pull down the second glove over the hand holding the first glove. The gloves are inside out, with contaminants inside. Discard the gloves in the biohazardous waste container.

Latex Allergy

The occurrence of allergic reactions to latex is increasing and health care facilities provide both latex and nonlatex gloves for personnel. Allergic reactions could be in the form of a simple rash or more serious reaction of anaphylaxis.

HBV Vaccination

Although there is no proven vaccine to prevent HIV or HCV infection, a safe and effective vaccine is available for the prevention of HBV infection. This vaccine is recommended for laboratory personnel who are at risk of HBV infection. It is offered free of charge on a voluntary basis by all employers and employees refusing the vaccine must sign a waiver.

Post-Exposure Evaluation and Follow-Up

Even when control measures are followed, exposure accidents sometimes occur. If you receive a needlestick or other exposure to potentially hazardous biomaterial, you should immediately wash or flush the area with water and then submit a written report of the incident to your employer. As a **post-exposure evaluation** and follow-up, your employer must then do the following:

- Track the exposure incident to blood or other potentially infectious material.
- Report the injury on the OSHA Occupational Injury and Illness Log if **post-exposure prophylaxis** (PEP) is prescribed and administered by licensed medical personnel. An injury report form can be found in Appendix C.
- Record HBV, HIV, or HCV exposure if the infection can be traced to an injury or other biohazard exposure incident.
- Make available to the exposed worker a confidential medical evaluation and follow-up.

- Document the route of exposure; the HBV, HCV, and HIV status of the source patient, if known; and the circumstances of the exposure.
- Notify the source patient of the incident and ask for consent to collect and test his or her blood for the presence of HIV, HBV, and HCV.
- Collect blood samples from the worker as soon as possible after exposure for HIV, HBV, and HCV testing.
- Repeat HIV testing for the exposed worker at 6 weeks, 12 weeks, and 6 months after the exposure. Extended HIV testing is recommended (12 months) for health care personnel who become infected with HCV following exposure to a source infected with both HIV and HCV.
- Provide counseling to the exposed worker and medical evaluation of any acute febrile illness occurring within 12 weeks after exposure.

This system of record keeping and data collection ensures that exposed workers receive the best possible treatment for potential health problems relating to the accident. OSHA requires employers to train employees in preventing possible exposure to diseases such as HIV, HBV, and HCV. OSHA compiles similar information on the incidence of chemical exposures and other laboratory accidents.

Disposal of Biohazardous Material

One of the most important aspects of safe handling of biohazardous material is appropriate decontamination and/or disposal of contaminated equipment, especially sharp instruments, and of used biospecimens and other contaminated waste. The laboratory waste-disposal system should provide safe, quick disposal of all items used in collecting and testing body specimens, following federal, state, and local regulations. The aim is to prevent contamination of the lab environment and possible infection of lab personnel.

Bagging, Tagging, and Labeling Biohazardous Materials. To protect from the possibility of infection, all lab personnel must be aware of the location of biohazardous materials—whether they are blood samples, dirty glassware, or used needles. To this end, it is crucial that biohazards be marked with the word *biohazard* or the red or orange biohazard symbol (see Figure 1-7), or simply color-coded red or orange. The identifying mark must be recognizable from a distance of 5 feet. If using identifying tags or labels, fasten them as closely as possible to

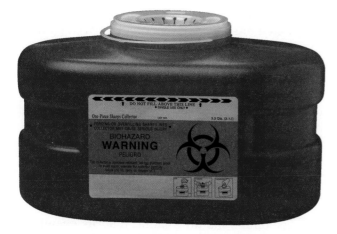

Figure 1-7 This symbol in orange or red permits quick identification of biohazardous material.

the hazard with string, wire, or adhesive to prevent their loss or unintentional removal. Before working in any lab, it is important to familiarize yourself with the location of all biohazardous materials. You must be constantly aware of biohazards as you work. In addition, maintenance crews and other nonmedical personnel should be instructed on proper safety and handling of lab wastes.

Cleaning or Disposal of Contaminated Equipment. Reusable pieces of equipment such as hemacytometers and pipettes should be placed immediately after use in a suitable disinfectant such as diluted solution of household bleach. This reduces risk of further **contamination** and makes the equipment easier to clean. Larger pieces of equipment should be washed by hand or in an automatic washer and then disinfected with diluted solution of bleach or sterilized in a drying oven. Contaminated disposable supplies like plastic tubing should be disinfected with germicide or bleach prior to disposal.

Disposal of Sharp Instruments. All disposable sharp instruments, including needles, lancets, and syringes with attached needles, should be placed in a sharps container immediately after use. The sharps container should be located where these items are most often used. The container should be disposed of when the fill line has been reached. (See Figure 1-8.)

You should be especially careful when discarding contaminated needles. A significant number of infections of lab personnel have been documented from needlesticks received while discarding needles.

Disposal of Biohazardous Waste. Discarded lab specimens, blood, and other contaminated waste must be placed in containers or bags that are sturdy and leak proof. They also must be labeled, tagged,

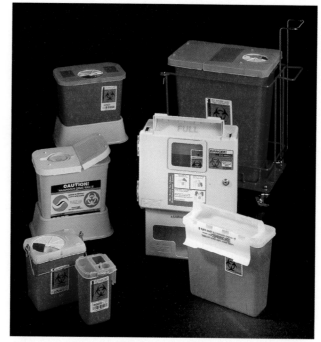

Figure 1-8 These laboratory safety devices are designed to help laboratory personnel avoid skin puncture from contaminated needles, lancets, and other sharp objects. Sharps containers accommodate different needs in the laboratory.

or color-coded so that the danger of their contents is apparent to anyone who may handle them. If the outside of the bag is contaminated with blood or other potentially infectious material, the waste must be double bagged—one bag inside another. Contaminated waste that will be placed in a landfill must be **autoclaved** or incinerated first.

> **Note**
> Under no circumstances should you recap, bend, break, or handle a needle in any unnecessary manner.

Housekeeping Practices

Safe medical laboratories have smooth, seamless surfaces on floors and countertops so that they are easily washed and disinfected. Floors should be covered with vinyl, not carpeting, to facilitate thorough cleaning and **disinfection.** The entire laboratory should be well lighted and well ventilated with adequate room for work areas and storage of supplies and equipment. Cleaning should be scheduled as often as necessary to maintain a sanitary workplace. When cleaning, workers should use appropriate PPE including gloves.

Disinfection. For general cleanup, an approved hospital disinfectant, a chemical germicide that is tuberculocidal, or a fresh bleach solution should be used each day on counters, work surfaces, and accessible machine parts that are subject to contamination. Because bleach solutions lose their potency over time, they should be prepared daily. A 1:10 dilution of household bleach, such as 5 percent sodium hypochlorite in water, is effective against HIV and other pathogens.

Laundry. Laundry that is contaminated with blood or other potentially infectious material should be treated as if it were HBV, HCV, or HIV infectious and handled as little as possible, with minimum agitation. It should be bagged at the location where it is used and transported in biohazard-identified bags. A solution of 1:10 to 1:100 bleach can be used to disinfect the garments before laundering. Many laboratories use disposable lab coats, but these are expensive.

Laboratory Personnel Education

Training and education of employees are required by law for everyone whose work exposes them to blood or other potentially infectious materials (OPIM). An education program should include maintenance crews who do general after-hours cleaning and/or repairs. The program must explain the following:

* epidemiology, transmission, and symptoms of HBV, HCV, and HIV
* effectiveness, safety, and benefits of HBV vaccination
* employer's **infection-control program (ICP),** including procedures to follow if an exposure incident occurs and labeling of biohazards
* methods of control that may prevent or reduce exposure to biohazards, including Standard Precautions, engineering controls, work-practice controls, and personal protective equipment

WORKING SAFELY WITH CHEMICAL HAZARDS

Safety in POLs requires knowledge of and respect for chemicals. The current trend is using very small amounts of premixed chemicals embedded in plastic or dissolved in some other medium in order to eliminate most mixing and handling of reagents. Test kits with these small amounts of chemicals are not hazardous if used correctly.

Unfortunately, hazardous chemicals cannot be eliminated entirely from medical labs. Chemicals such as methyl alcohol and acetone are required as preservatives, stains, drying agents, and cleaners. These and other lab chemicals may be flammable, caustic, carcinogenic, or **toxic** in other ways. This is true of their fumes as well as their liquid or solid forms. Therefore, it is important to be familiar with the rules of safety concerning lab chemicals.

Safety Tips for Using Lab Chemicals

Lab personnel should assume that all chemicals are harmful until they learn otherwise and should never taste or sniff an unknown chemical in order to identify it. OSHA maintains a **hazardous chemical list** used in medical labs that may be checked if there is any question about toxicity. OSHA also requires chemical manufacturers and distributors to furnish a **Material Safety Data Sheet (MSDS)** with all shipments of hazardous chemicals (see Figure 1-9). The MSDS provides usage precautions, among other information. For safety's sake, familiarize yourself with all precautions for chemicals that you use in the lab.

> **Right-to-Know**
>
> OSHA developed the Right-to-Know Law, which requires employers to make certain that all employees are informed of any possible chemical hazards in the workplace. This is accomplished by proper chemical container labeling, MSDS, and employee training.

When using hazardous chemicals, it is especially important to keep your workstation free of excess reagents and equipment. This will help prevent spills and mistakes. Manipulate chemicals that generate fumes or a cloud of powder under a vented hood. Avoid direct contact of lab chemicals with skin or clothes, and wash your hands after each use.

Always place covers from reagent containers top down on a clean counter to prevent contaminating both the counter and reagent container cover. Replace the cover and return the reagent to its storage place as soon as possible.

Most reagents may be safely flushed down the laboratory sink unless otherwise specified. Place these directly into the drain to prevent spattering and flush with plenty of water. Refer to MSDS for proper disposal.

MATERIAL SAFETY DATA SHEET **WAVICIDE-01**   Date Issued:

SECTION 1	IDENTIFICATION

Manufacturers Name and Address: Wave Energy Systems, Inc.   Phone: 1-800-252-1125
25 Mansard Court   Fax: (201) 633-1023
Wayne, NJ 07470

Hazardous Chemicals: *Glutaraldehyde*
Routes of entry: Inhalation ✓ Skin/Eye ✓ Ingestion ✓

Product Name: WAVICIDE-01 (2.5% aqueous glutaraldehyde solution)

PRECAUTIONARY LABELING
(HMIS Rating System)

Product Code: 0104 (case of 4 gallons) or 0112 (case of 12 quarts)

Health	3
Flammability:	0
Reactivity:	0
Physical Hazard:	None

Product Type/General Information: Chemical Sterilant/Disinfectant

EPA Registration Number: 15136-1

Chemical Name: (active ingredient) 2.5% glutaraldehyde

The New Jersey Poison Control Center has been provided information for use in medical emergencies involving this product. Call 1-800-962-1253.

SECTION 2	HAZARDOUS INGREDIENTS/IDENTITY INFORMATION

WAVICIDE-01 contains the following hazardous ingredients at concentrations greater than 1.0%:

CHEMICAL COMPONENTS	CAS%	% w/v	OSHA PEL	ACGIH TLV
Glutaraldehyde (active ingredient)	111-30-8	2.5	0.2 ppm[1]	0.2 ppm

WAVICIDE-01 contains no hazardous ingredients listed as carcinogens or potential carcinogens by the National Toxicology Program (NTP), International Agency on Cancer (IARC) or OSHA, and present at a concentration greater than 0.1%:

[1] The OSHA Permissible Exposure Level (PEL) for glutaraldehyde was invalidated in 1992 by court order. However, the PEL may remain valid in some OSHA approved state plans, and also can be enforced by federal OSHA under its General Duty Clause.

SECTION 3	PHYSICAL/CHEMICAL CHARACTERISTICS

Boiling Point:	100°C/212°F	Evaporation Rate:	0.81 (Butyl Acetate = 1)
Specific Gravity:	1.005 - 1.013	Solubility (H_2O):	Complete
Vapor Pressure:	16.9 mm Hg	Appearance & Color:	A clear, slightly yellow liquid with typical aldehyde odor and added lemon scent.
Melting point:	N/A	pH:	Approximately 6.30
Vapor Density:	1.1 (air = 1)	Molecular Weight:	100.11 (glutaraldehyde)
Freezing Point:	0°C/32°F (same as water)	Odor Threshold:	0.04 ppm, detectable (ACGIH)

SECTION 4	FIRE AND EXPLOSION HAZARD DATA

Flash Point (Test Method):	None (Tag Closed Cup ASTM D 56)		
Special Fire Fighting Procedures:	Self-Contained Breathing Apparatus (SCBA) and protective clothing should be worn when fighting chemical fires.		
Unusual Fire and Explosion Hazards:	None known	Extinguishing Media:	Carbon dioxide, foam, dry chemical.

SECTION 5	REACTIVITY DATA

Stability: Unstable_____ Stable___✓___   Hazardous Polymerization: May Occur_____ Will Not Occur___✓___

Hazardous Decomposition Products: Thermal decomposition may produce carbon dioxide and or carbon monoxide.

Conditions and Materials to Avoid: Alkaline (pH > 10) and acidic (pH < 3) materials catalyze an aldol-type condensation (exothermic but not expected to be violent). Avoid High temperatures above 40°C/104°F and or evaporation of H_2O.

Date Issued:

SECTION 6	HEALTH HAZARD DATA

Routes of Entry: *Inhalation:* ✓ *Skin:* ✓ *Ingestion:* ✓ *Eyes:* ✓

Signs and Symptoms Associated With Overexposure (one-time or repeated):

Ingestion:	May cause irritation and possibly chemical burns of the mouth, throat, stomach and esophagus. May produce discomfort in the mouth, throat, chest and abdomen, nausea, vomiting, diarrhea, dizziness, faintness, drowsiness, thirst and weakness.
Eyes:	Solution contact may cause damage, including severe corneal injury, which could permanently impair vision if prompt first-aid and medical treatment are not obtained. Vapors may cause stinging sensation in the eye with excess tear production, blinking, and redness of the conjuntiva.
Skin:	Direct solution contact may cause skin irritation or aggravation of an existing dermatitis. May also cause skin to turn a harmless yellow or brown color.
Inhalation:	Vapor is irritating to the respiratory tract. May cause stinging sensations in the nose and throat, chest discomfort and tightening, difficulty with breathing and headache. May also aggravate pre-existing asthma and pulmonary disease.

Emergency and First Aid Procedure:

Ingestion:	DO NOT INDUCE VOMITING. Drink large quantities of water and call a physician immediately NOTE TO PHYSICIAN: Probable mucosal damage from oral exposure may contraindicate the use of gastric lavage.
Eyes:	Immediately flush eyes with water and continue washing for at least 15 minutes. Obtain medical attention immediately, and follow up with an ophthalmologist.
Skin:	Immediately remove contaminated clothing and flush skin with soap and water for a minimum of 15 minutes. If irritation persists, seek medical attention. Wash or discard contaminated clothing.
Inhalation:	Remove to fresh air. Give artificial respiration if not breathing. If breathing is difficult, oxygen may be given by qualified personnel. If irritation persists, seek medical help.

Medical Conditions Generally Aggravated by Overexposure: See above.

SECTION 7	PRECAUTIONS FOR SAFE HANDLING AND USE

Steps to be Taken if Material is Released or Spilled: Wear suitable protective equipment, including nitrile gloves, chemically resistant gown or apron, and protective eyewear (safety glasses or shield). A full face respirator , or half-face respirator with gas proof goggles, both worn with organic vapor cartridges, is recommended for small spills. A respirator is essential for large spills, or if you experience discomfort watery eyes, nasal or respiratory irritation) due to inadequate ventilation. For small spills of 1 gallon or less, gather up a bucket, household ammonia, and a sponge or mop. Don protective equipment and mix approximately 1 cup of ammonia with 1 cup of water in the bucket. Mop or sponge the ammonia mixture into the spill until thoroughly combined (about 2 minutes). Wipe or mop up resulting mixture and discard down the drain with a copious amount of water. Rinse bucket, mop or sponge with water, and give spill area a final wipe or mop with fresh water. Re-rinse all equipment, and allow spill area to dry. For large spills of more than 1 gallon, remove people from immediate spill area, and isolate until cleaned up. Don protective equipment including a respirator with organic vapor cartridges. Contain spill with absorbent material, ie. towels. Add approximately 228 grams of sodium bisulfite powder per gallon of WAVICIDE-01 spilled (aqueous sodium hydroxide and ammonium will also neutralize glutaraldehyde). With a sponge, mix neutralizing chemical into spill, and allow 5 minutes for deactivation to occur. Discard resulting mixture according to your facility's waste disposal guidelines. Mop spill area with fresh water. Rinse out all equipment (bucket, mop, towels) with large amounts of water. If paper towels were used, dispose of in a tightly closed trash bag. Let spill area dry, and if possible increase ventilation. Once glutaraldehyde odor is below allowable levels (TLV), the area may be released from isolation.

Waste Disposal Method: Dispose of WAVICIDE-01 after 30 days of re-use, or the MEC Indicator shows the solution is below it's minimum effective concentration (1.7% w/v), which ever is sooner. This may be accomplished by pouring solution down drain in accordance with state and local regulations. Flush with a large quantity of water. Do not reuse empty containers. Rinse thoroughly with water and dispose of in trash.

Precautions to be Taken in Handling and Storing: WAVICIDE-01 should be stored in it's original sealed container at controlled room temperature (15°C/50°F to 30°C/85°F).

Precautionary Labeling: Avoid contact with eyes, prolonged and repeated contact with skin, and contamination with food.

SECTION 8	TRANSPORTATION DATA & ADDITIONAL INFORMATION

Proper Shipping Name:	2.5% Glutaraldehyde Solution	DOT (ground): Not regulated	IATA (air): Not Regulated	IMO (ocean): Not Regulated
Hazard Class: None	Labels: None needed	Packaging: None	ID#: None	Special Instructions: None	Reportable Quantity: None

SECTION 9	CONTROL MEASURES

Eye Protection: Safety glasses, goggles or face shield recommended when working with WAVICIDE-01. An eye wash, and full face respirator with organic vapor cartridges or half face respirator with gas proof goggles and organic vapor cartridges should be available for emergency situations.

Ventilation: WAVICIDE-01 should be used in closed containers with tight fitting lids. The working area should be large enough with ventilation necessary to keep the level of atmospheric glutaraldehyde below the Threshold Limit Value (TLV). If the solution vapors are irritating to eyes and nose, the TLV is probably being exceeded, and additional ventilation may be necessary. A fume hood or self contained fume absorber may be appropriate for this purpose. Any ventilation should pull fumes away from worker and towards the floor.

Skin Protection: Nitrile gloves and a chemical resistant gown or apron should be worn when working with WAVICIDE-01. Rubber boots may be needed to contain large spills.

Respiratory Protection: None required if glutaraldehyde vapor levels are below the TLV. A full face respirator with organic vapor cartridges or SCBA should be available for emergencies.

SECTION 10	SPECIAL REQUIREMENTS

None

Figure 1-9 An example of a Material Safety Data Sheet (MSDS) that includes proper handling, storage, and disposal of hazardous chemicals.

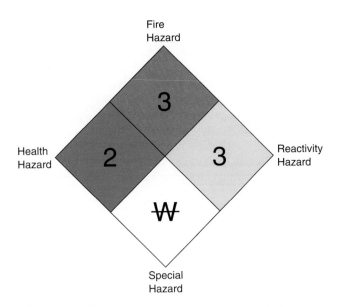

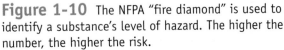

Figure 1-10 The NFPA "fire diamond" is used to identify a substance's level of hazard. The higher the number, the higher the risk.

Labeling and Storing Reagents

OSHA requires that all reagent containers be clearly and prominently labeled with the chemical's name and pertinent information about hazards, such as toxicity and flammability. The date of receipt or preparation of chemicals, their expiration date, and any special storage requirements also should be noted. Discard reagents with missing or unreadable labels to prevent potential misuse. As an extra safety measure, it is a good idea to label all caustic reagents with a brightly colored sticker or easily recognized symbol.

The National Fire Protection Association has standardized a method of labeling hazardous materials using colors and symbols to identify a substance's level of hazard. It is sometimes referred to as the "**NFPA diamond.**" The symbol is divided into four colored quadrants, each quadrant representing a hazard and level of that hazard. (See Figure 1-10.)

All reagents should be stored away from heat and sunlight in a dry location because heat, light, and moisture often cause chemicals to react. Reagents may be stored at room temperature unless storage directions indicate the need for refrigeration. Reagents that react together should be stored in isolation from one another in safety containers, and flammable reagents should be stored in a fireproof metal cabinet. The smallest amount of all necessary chemicals should be kept in stock to keep the potential for contamination and injury at a minimum.

Acids and Bases—Special Concerns

Two groups of chemicals requiring special caution are **acids** and **bases.** Both are **caustic,** generate heat when they come into contact with water, and react quickly with other chemicals and each other. Even the fumes of acids and bases react together. Acids and bases are prone to spattering and can cause serious burns to the eyes and skin. Protective eyewear is recommended when working with acids, bases, and other chemicals that may spatter.

Acids always should be added to water—not water to acids—because there is less chance of spattering and burns. When water is added to acid, it remains on top because it is less dense. There, it reacts and generates heat, potentially spattering the workstation and lab personnel.

Acids and bases neutralize each other; therefore, a base is used to neutralize acid spills and an acid to neutralize base spills. A large amount of a weak base will neutralize a strong acid as effectively as a smaller amount of a stronger base but in a safer manner. Similarly, a large amount of a weak acid is safer to neutralize a strong base than is a stronger acid.

First Aid for Chemical Spills

No matter how careful laboratory personnel are, the possibility of an accident with hazardous chemicals still exists. Therefore, every laboratory should have a designated sink where chemical spills can be washed off quickly. An eyewash station should be installed at a sink that is quickly accessible (see Figure 1-11). Check your lab's manual for more explicit procedures to follow when chemical spills occur.

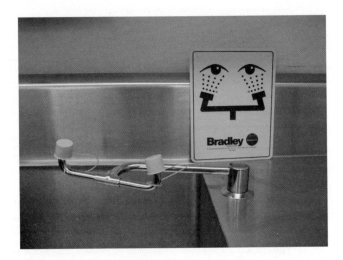

Figure 1-11 An eyewash station is an instant source of water for a quick rinse when an accident occurs. A quick response can be crucial.

SAFETY FROM PHYSICAL HAZARDS

Physical hazards such as slippery floors and falling objects may present risks to workers in most workplaces, but are especially dangerous in laboratories where biohazardous materials are at hand. Good housekeeping and time management are important to help prevent accidents of this nature. The best way for lab personnel to avoid injury from physical hazards is to follow basic rules for physical safety. These are described next for electrical, fire, weather, and personal hazards.

Electrical Hazards

Always use common sense when using electricity. For example, always unplug electrical appliances before changing bulbs or servicing. Be careful to keep water and chemicals away from outlets and electrical equipment to avoid dangerous shorts that can start fires and cause electrocution.

The electrical wiring system of the laboratory should be adequate for the amount of electricity used—extension cords and multiple tap plugs are not safe and usually indicate an inadequate electrical wiring system. There should be safety devices such as three-prong grounded plugs, current breakers or fuses, and a master switch that is accessible in case of emergency.

Any malfunctioning electrical equipment should be checked by a professional. If the malfunction is major, unplug the machine until it can be repaired or replaced. Check cords periodically for breaks and frays.

Fire Hazards

Any situation that is a potential fire hazard should be remedied before an accident occurs. For example, long hair or loose clothing presents a fire hazard around open flames such as laboratory burners. Situations like this are easily avoided.

Even when precautions are taken to prevent fires, they may still occur. All lab personnel should know how to report a fire. Each lab should have a multiple-use fire extinguisher conveniently mounted on a wall ready for use. Know how to use it. The fire extinguisher should be in good condition and checked periodically. A fire blanket at a convenient location is essential to smother flames.

The POL manual should include a fire escape plan. Dual exits should be included in the plan in case one exit is blocked by fire. Exits to be used as fire escapes should be clearly marked and accessible at all times during work hours.

Weather Hazards

In some parts of the country, weather emergencies are relatively common. For example, hurricanes are a potential risk in the Southeast and tornadoes in the Midwest. The places to take cover in case of severe weather in your area should be described in the POL manual. Learn where they are.

Personal Hazards

Wherever you work, you should analyze your work environment for personal safety hazards such as theft and assault. To maximize your personal safety in the lab, in the parking lot, and on route to and from work, follow these safety tips recommended by police:

- When you arrive at work, park in a well-lighted area and lock your car.
- At work, keep your purse or other valuables out of sight, preferably in a locked place such as a desk or filing cabinet.
- Avoid working alone, especially at night.
- When you leave work, particularly after dark, stay alert, leave the building with coworkers, have your keys handy, and drive on well-lighted streets.

LABORATORY PERSONNEL CHARACTERISTICS AFFECTING LAB SAFETY

Safety rules and regulations and specialized equipment and gear cannot ensure lab safety unless personnel use care and common sense on the job everyday.

Personnel Attitudes

In POLs, as elsewhere, worker attitudes can contribute to an unsafe work environment. Workers who take shortcuts and are inconsiderate of others may undermine everyone's safety. Attitudes that may contribute to a safer laboratory, on the other hand, include awareness of potential danger, willingness to learn and use safe methods, and concern for the welfare of coworkers. Professionalism in medical laboratories is a combination of positive attitudes that put a high priority on personnel safety.

To ensure safety on the job, lab personnel should avoid taking unnecessary risks. Sometimes, even experienced workers take risks that can cause lab accidents. Indeed, experienced workers sometimes take unnecessary risks because they have performed these tasks without incident so many times in the past. Other common reasons for lab accidents include

- hurrying to meet deadlines or goals
- carelessness and fatigue
- preoccupation with nonwork matters
- excessive stress

Keep in mind that working under these conditions may lead to accidents.

Chronic Injury to Muscles and Bones

Muscles and bones, if overused over a period of time, can develop chronic injuries classified as occupational diseases. Two examples are carpal tunnel syndrome of the wrist, which affects keyboard operators, and neck torsion disorder, which may occur from long periods of microscope use.

The following suggestions can help you prevent these injuries. Examine your work activities, furniture, and lighting for stressful elements. Use good posture; comfortable chairs; good lighting; large, padded grip and handle surfaces; and cushioned hand/wrist rests. Alternate between high- and low-risk activities and take brief breaks to stretch muscles during tedious tasks. Try to eliminate awkward or stressful motions such as extending beyond your usual reach. Use minimal, not excessive, force to operate keyboards and instruments. If the microscope is not at a comfortable height, try placing books under it to raise it to a level that does not require you to bend your neck tightly.

More About Stress

While some stress may be helpful in maintaining alertness, too much stress may cause work quality to deteriorate and lead to accidents on the job. Stress may originate off the job—a too busy lifestyle, for example—or work conditions may be the cause. It is not uncommon for lab personnel to feel pressure to work faster. Whatever the cause, excessive stress should be brought under control before injury or ill health results. Following are some ways to help control job-related stress:

- Prioritize your job tasks each day and schedule your work assignments by the day, week, and month. Work piling up on your desk may create job stress. If you develop a plan to deal with all of the work, you will feel less stressed.
- Try to resolve job-related stress by first discussing problems with your supervisor. For example, be realistic with your time. Tell your supervisor if you have more work than you can handle.
- Develop a personal wellness program—eat a well-balanced diet, get plenty of rest, and exercise regularly.

PROCEDURE 1-1

Hand Washing

Goal

After successfully completing this procedure, you will be able to wash your hands with soap and running water to sanitize your skin prior to gloving before hazardous laboratory procedures and also after completing such procedures.

Completion Time

2 minutes

Equipment and Supplies

- A sink with running water
- Liquid soap in a dispenser (preferably an antiseptic soap)
- Paper towels in a dispenser
- Hand lotion

Instructions

Read through the list of equipment and supplies you will need and the steps of the procedure. Be sure you understand each step correctly and in the proper order.

*Steps marked with (*) are critical and must have the maximum points to pass.

Performance Standards	Points Awarded	Maximum Points
1. Remove all jewelry such as rings (except for a plain gold band), bracelets, and your wristwatch because these may harbor microorganisms in the crevices. Wristwatches worn at work in the POL should be sanitized separately.		10
2. Turn on the faucet and regulate the water temperature to a desired warm temperature. Soap will suds better in warm water.		5
3. Wet your hands with water. Hold your hands lower than your elbows to prevent water running past your elbows. Microorganisms and debris will be washed away into the sink instead of traveling up your arms.		5
4. Apply approximately 2–4 mL of liquid soap to your hands and arms up to your mid forearm. Suds the soap with about 10 circular motions of your hands.		10
5. Use friction along with the circular motions to suds your palms, the backs of your hands, and your forearms.		10
6. Wash your fingers with 10 circular motions, interfacing your fingers and rubbing them back and forth with friction.		10
7. Rinse your hands well, making sure to hold your hands lower than your elbows. Then rinse your wrists and forearms until no soap remains.		10
8. Repeat the soaping and rinse process to be sure that your hands are clean.		5
9. Dry your hands gently and thoroughly with paper towels. Drying your hands well will help prevent chapping, which causes crevices and breaks in skin.		5
10. Turn off the water using a paper towel. The faucet handles are considered contaminated.		5
11. Inspect your hands for cuts and abrasions. Cover any hangnails or open wounds with bandages.		5
12. Put lotion on your hands.		5
13. If this is your last hand wash of the day before leaving work, clean your nails thoroughly with an orange stick. Nails harbor microorganisms in the debris lodged underneath them.		5
14. If work is to continue with hazardous material, put on nonsterile gloves.		5
15. Wipe the sink area with a paper towel to remove water and debris. Keep the paper towel between your hands and the sink. The sink is considered contaminated.		5
Total Points		**100**

Overall Procedural Evaluation

Student's Name _____

Signature of Instructor _____ Date _____

Comments _____

_____

PROCEDURE 1-2

Practicing Lab Safety

Goal

After successfully completing this procedure, you will be able to properly use equipment to safely handle and dispose of biohazardous materials in the laboratory.

Completion Time

45 minutes

Equipment and Supplies

- Disposable gloves
- Hand disinfectant
- Face shield or goggles
- Surface disinfectant
- Paper towels
- Biohazard container
- Sharps container
- Pipette and suction device
- Personal protective gear
- Bags and tags for biohazardous waste
- Needle and needle remover or forceps
- Tap water

Instructions

Read through the list of equipment and supplies you will need and the steps of the procedure. Be sure you understand each step before you begin. Then complete each step correctly and in the proper order. If your completion time is too long, repeat the procedure until you increase your speed.

Steps marked with (*) are critical and must have the maximum points to pass.

Performance Standards	Points Awarded	Maximum Points
1. Collect or locate the appropriate equipment.		10
2. Wash your hands thoroughly with hand disinfectant.		20
3. Dry your hands completely.		10
4. Put on disposable gloves.		5
5. Assemble and correctly put on a complete outfit of protective gear.		10
6. Remove all gear, except the gloves, and return to storage.		10
7. Use the pipette suction device to pipette a small amount of tap water into a disposable pipette.		10
8. Empty the pipette and repeat step 7.		5
9. Pour a small amount of tap water on the floor to simulate a biohazardous spill.		5
10. Pour surface disinfectant liberally on the spill. Cover the spill with paper towels to prevent spreading, and let the spill soak for 5 minutes.		10
11. Wipe up the spill thoroughly with paper towels.		5
12. Dispose of the paper towels in a plastic bag. Label the bag with a biohazard indicator.		10
13. *Remove your gloves, wash your hands with disinfectant, dry your hands, and put on clean gloves.		20
14. Thoroughly wipe a piece of equipment such as a centrifuge with disinfectant or alcohol and paper towels.		10
15. Dispose of the paper towels in a plastic bag and label the bag with a biohazard indicator.		10

16.	*Remove your gloves, wash your hands with disinfectant, dry your hands, and put on clean gloves.	20
17.	*Dispose of the needle and syringe safely in the sharps container.	20
18.	Disinfect work counters and tables with surface disinfectant.	10
19.	*Clean the work area following Standard Precautions.	20
20.	*Remove your gloves, wash your hands with disinfectant, and dry them.	20
	Total Points	**240**

Overall Procedural Evaluation

Student's Name _____

Signature of Instructor _____ Date _____

Comments _____

_____

chapter 1 REVIEW

Using Terminology

Define the following terms as they apply to laboratory safety.

1. Aerosolization _____

2. Biohazard _____

3. Exposure incident _____

4. Chain of transmission _____

5. Material Safety Data Sheet _____

6. Infection Control Program _____

7. Post-exposure prophylaxis _____

8. Universal Precautions _____

Match the following terms to the most appropriate meaning.

____ **9.** Biological specimen

____ **10.** Engineering control

____ **11.** HBV

____ **12.** HCV

____ **13.** HIV

____ **14.** PPE

____ **15.** OSHA

____ **16.** Vector

a. hepatitis B virus

b. federal agency that ensures safety and health of workers

c. virus that causes AIDS

d. an animal, such as an insect, that carries a pathogen

e. includes gloves, face shields, aprons, uniforms

f. lab samples originating from living organisms

g. safety devices used in the laboratory

h. hepatitis C virus

Acquiring Knowledge

Answer the following questions in the spaces provided.

17. How do the Universal Precautions protect laboratory personnel against infection?

_____

_____

_____

18. List five medical problems or diseases that may be encountered in a laboratory.

_____

_____

_____

19. Discuss appropriate ways to manage a high level of stress at work.

_____

_____

_____

20. How should you apply the rule of placing a barrier between you and the possible source of contamination or disease in the laboratory? Give examples for

Pipetting

_____

_____

_____

Disposing of used needles and lancets

_____

_____

_____

Working with biohazards that may splatter

_____

_____

_____

21. Why are biohazards labeled with an easily read label, whether they are test specimens or waste material?

_____

_____

_____

22. Why do the Universal Precautions dictate that all biospecimens be regarded as hazardous?

_____

_____

_____

23. Which of the following may transmit HIV?

_____ a. blood

_____ b. amniotic fluid

_____ c. semen

_____ d. synovial fluid

24. What protection against HBV is available to laboratory personnel?

_____

_____

_____

25. What records are kept of reported laboratory accidents involving biohazards and toxic chemicals?

_____

_____

_____

26. List seven ways to prevent exposure to toxic chemicals in the laboratory.

_____

_____

_____

27. In a safety education program provided by the employer, what information should be provided to new lab personnel?

_____

_____

_____

28. What are some physical hazards in the laboratory and how are they best controlled?

_____

_____

_____

29. What is an acceptable dilution of household bleach prepared daily for the purpose of decontaminating counters, equipment, and floors?

_____

_____

_____

30. What part does attitude play in laboratory safety?

_____

_____

_____

31. When should laboratory personnel wash their hands?

_____

_____

_____

32. What rule should laboratory personnel follow regarding facial contamination?

_____

_____

_____

33. How should laboratory personnel dispose of waste contaminated with biohazards or chemicals?

_____

_____

_____

34. Why should fire escape routes be posted and exits not blocked with supplies or furniture?

_____

_____

_____

35. How can lab personnel avoid being exposed to needlesticks from contaminated needles?

_____

_____

_____

36. When should lab personnel wear gloves in the laboratory?

_____

_____

_____

Applying Knowledge—On the Job

Answer the following questions in the spaces provided.

37. Mary and Jane were working as a team in the POL. The schedule for that day was very busy. Mary had just drawn blood. As she attempted to dispose of the contaminated needle into the sharps container, Jane reached for a reagent and was accidentally stuck. Write the report that Jane must submit to her employer and list the post-exposure procedure steps that her employer must follow.

_____

_____

_____

38. A patient infected with HIV is having a blood test in the POL. What precautions should you take when you draw his blood? When you perform the blood test?

_____

_____

_____

39. Joseph, a student, is instructed to visit a lab to see how safety rules are being observed. Make a list of at least eight safety rules that Joseph could easily observe when he visits the lab.

_____

_____

_____

40. Anna, a lab technician, performs the following tasks in the following order. After which tasks should she wash her hands?

_____ a. entering the lab for her work shift

_____ b. putting on disposable gloves

_____ c. performing a test using a test tube of blood

_____ d. removing gloves

_____ e. taking the lab report to the receptionist

_____ f. putting on gloves

_____ g. drawing blood from a patient for a blood test

_____ h. performing the blood test

_____ i. removing the gloves

_____ j. putting the cover on the microscope

_____ k. making a phone call

_____ l. going to the waiting room to call a patient to come to the lab for a timed blood test

_____ m. verifying that the test request is for the right patient

41. A laboratory fails a fire safety inspection only because an exit in the lab is partially blocked. List three other safety requirements that it must have met.

_____

_____

_____

42. Web Research: Go to **www.cdc.gov/mmwr** and search for the updated U.S. Public Health Service Guidelines for the Management of Occupational Exposure to HBV, HCV, and HIV. Report to the class the recommendations for post-exposure prophylaxis for health care personnel to these three infections.

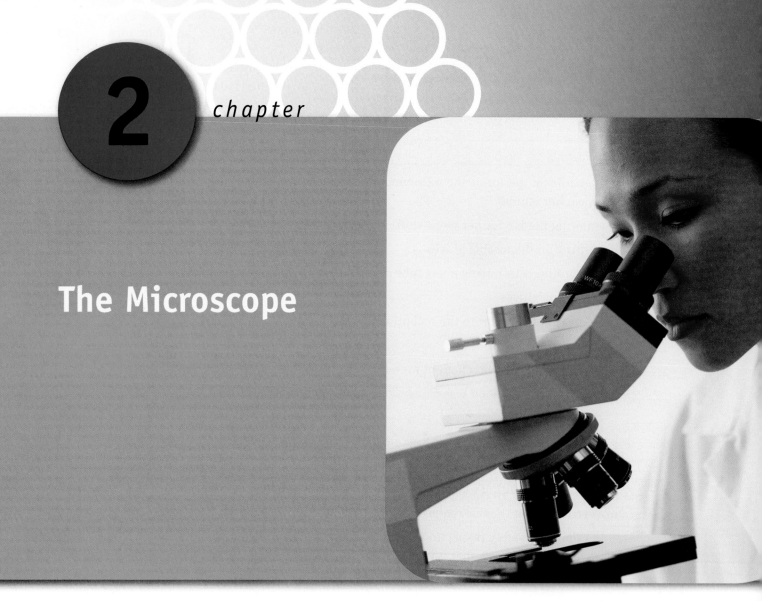

2 *chapter*

The Microscope

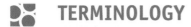

TERMINOLOGY

adjustable ocular: usually, the eyepiece on the left. It can be adjusted to correct the focus for the individual's visual acuity.

aperture: in a microscope, the opening through which the light passes such as in the stage or iris diaphragm.

artifact: an extraneous, nontissue feature that contaminates specimen slides.

binocular: literally, pertaining to two eyes; a microscope with two eyepieces, one for each eye.

coarse adjustment: the first step in focusing, in which the distance between the specimen and the lens (working distance) is covered very quickly, either by lowering the objective or raising the stage.

condenser: also called the substage. Located just below the opening in the mechanical stage and above the light source, the condenser controls the amount of light.

eyepiece: *see* ocular.

fine adjustment: the step in focusing in which only small changes are made in the working distance between the lens and the specimen.

iris diaphragm: located in the condenser, the iris diaphragm is the aperture that controls the amount of light entering through the opening in the stage by contracting or enlarging like the iris of the eye.

mechanical stage: a platform that holds the slide. The mechanical stage can be moved in four directions so that any part of the slide may be viewed.

microscope: an instrument that uses a lens or combination of lenses to enlarge very small objects for viewing.

microscopy: the use of a microscope.

monocular: literally, pertaining to one eye; a microscope in which there is only one eyepiece.

nosepiece: a rotating, circular apparatus on the microscope that holds the objectives and moves them into position as needed.

objective: the lens of the microscope that collects the image from the slide, magnifies it, and transmits it to the eyepiece lens, or ocular.

ocular: also called eyepiece. The ocular lens collects the image from the objective lens and magnifies it 10X in most oculars.

oil-immersion objective: the lens with the highest power of magnification (about 100X). The oil-immersion objective clarifies the image by using a layer of oil between the specimen and the objective to refract the light into the lens.

reagent: a substance used to produce a chemical reaction.

resolution: the ability of a set of lenses to distinguish fine detail; the most important gauge of a microscope's quality.

rheostat: a device that controls the amount of current entering an electrical circuit. A rheostat controls the light on a microscope.

stage: the platform on a microscope that supports the glass slide and specimen for viewing. The stage may move up and down for focusing.

stationary ocular: usually, the eyepiece for the right eye. It is adjusted for focus first using the coarse and fine adjustment knobs.

visual acuity: clarity of vision.

working distance: the distance between the specimen and the objective. It is important to check this distance frequently to avoid bringing the lens into contact with the slide.

INTRODUCTION

This chapter describes why the **microscope** is an important tool in medical laboratories and how the microscope works. It also explains how to use, care for, and select a microscope.

MICROSCOPY

Microscopes are used in all POLs to obtain valuable information about patients by viewing structures invisible to the naked eye. Many abnormalities in blood and other body tissues and many types of disease-causing microorganisms can be identified when they are viewed under the magnification of a microscope.

The Role of the Microscope

Lab personnel often use the microscope (see Figure 2-1) for a diversity of tasks. They may test blood for anemia or leukemia, which requires them to magnify a blood specimen so that they can recognize blood cell maturation stages. To identify a particular type of microorganism such as bacteria, lab personnel must magnify specimens to see their shape, size, and stain and growth characteristics.

Quality Control

As valuable as it is, **microscopy** is the most variable aspect of laboratory testing. For example, slide specimens require special preparation, which may produce variable results unless timing and quality

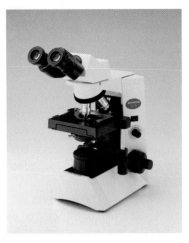

Figure 2-1 Binocular microscope with a built-in graduated mechanical stage and four objectives: 4X, 10X, 40X, and 100X.

of **reagents** are monitored closely. Slides may be contaminated with **artifacts** that mimic biological structures. Interpreting slides may be difficult, requiring lab personnel to recognize complicated patterns of blood cell structure, urine sediment composition, and microorganisms. These and other factors may introduce error in test results.

Mastering the Microscope

Mastering the essentials of microscope use takes practice. It is not as easy as it looks. The microscope requires extended training to utilize its different functions. In addition, identifying differences among microorganisms and cell structures takes much study and practice viewing them under magnification.

HOW THE MICROSCOPE WORKS

Before learning how to use the microscope, it is important to understand how the microscope works. This section describes the different features of the microscope and the role that they play in magnifying specimens. While reading this section, refer to Figure 2-2, which shows the microscope and its parts.

All of the following parts of the microscope are mounted in a stand, which consists of an arm and a base. The stand must be sturdy enough to resist vibrations and jars. It supports the lens system, the accessories needed to operate it, and the **stage**

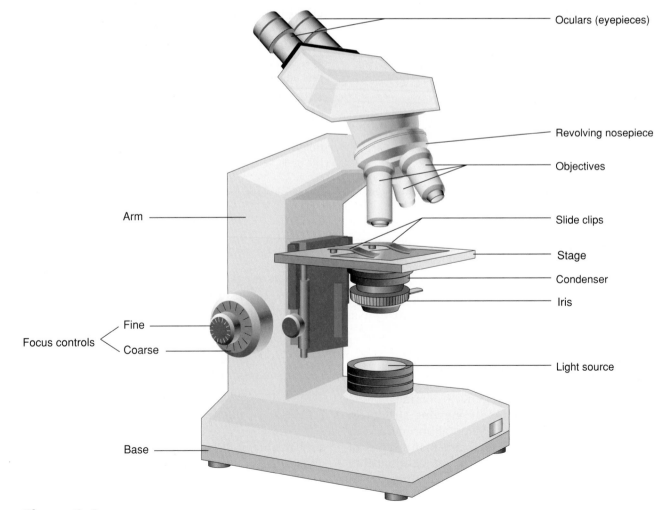

Figure 2-2 The parts of a microscope.

upon which the specimen is mounted on its slide. The base usually contains the light source necessary to operate the microscope.

The Lens System

The compound microscope, which is the type most commonly used in POLs, has two lenses mounted on opposite ends of a closed tube, called the barrel. These two lenses, the **ocular** and the **objective,** work together to magnify the specimen.

Ocular. The lens nearest the eye is called the ocular, or **eyepiece. Monocular** microscopes have one eyepiece; **binocular** microscopes have two. Most oculars magnify the specimen by a power of ten (10X), meaning that the ocular increases the diameter of the specimen to 10 times its actual size.

Objectives. The lens farthest from the eye and closest to the specimen is called the objective. A microscope may have three or four objectives offering different powers of magnification (usually 4X, 10X, 40X, and 100X). (See Figure 2-3.) Only one objective is used at a time. The objectives are screwed into a circular **nosepiece** that is revolved by hand until the objective with the desired magnification is reached and clicked into place. Each objective is stamped with its power of magnification. It also has a different-colored band around it for quick identification.

The 4X objective is used for scanning a slide for areas to examine under higher magnification. The 10X objective is referred to as low power, and it is used extensively in the initial steps of focusing, to count cells, and to scan urine sediment. The 40X

(43X or 45X on some microscopes) objective is referred to as high power. It is used extensively for red and white blood cell counts, scanning differential smears, and viewing urine sediment. The 4X, 10X, and 40X objectives are called dry lenses because they do not require oil to assist in magnification. In fact, if oil touches these objectives, it should be removed immediately because it softens the cement that holds the lenses in place.

> **Note**
>
> High dry objectives may range from 40X to 43X or 45X, with 40X the most common in clinical laboratories.

The 100X (95X or 97X on some microscopes) is an **oil-immersion objective,** which uses a layer of oil between the specimen and the objective to refract light into the lens. Because this oil is a relatively dense medium with about the same refractive index as glass, the light rays do not diffuse through it as they do through air, which is less dense. The 100X oil-immersion objective has the greatest power of magnification. Only under this objective are the identifying characteristics of the different types of bacteria and white blood cells revealed. Blood differential smears are routinely counted under the oil-immersion objective. The oil should be wiped from the 100X objective after each slide is viewed to prevent the oil from damaging the cement around the lens.

Magnification and Resolution. Total magnification of a microscope is the product of the magnification of the ocular and the magnification of the objective. If the ocular magnifies 10X and the objective 10X, for example, the total magnification is 100 times actual size (10X × 10X = 100X). A 10X ocular with a 43X objective would give a total magnification of 430 times actual size (10X × 43X). With the 100X objective, the magnification would be 1000 times actual size (10X × 100X).

The **resolution** of the microscope is its ability to distinguish fine details. This ability depends on not only the power of magnification but also the quality of the microscope. For the same level of magnification, a better quality of microscope will have higher resolution. Resolution can best be assessed by viewing a familiar slide and noting the details discernable with different microscopes.

The Stage

The stage is the platform that holds the slide to be viewed. The stage provides a secure grip on the slide, which is placed over a circular or oval hole in its center. The hole allows light to enter from below,

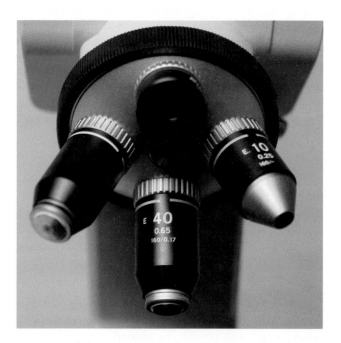

Figure 2-3 Four objectives can be seen: 4X, 10X, 40X, and 100X.

passing through the specimen to the lens system. On some microscopes, the platform stage may be raised or lowered to focus the specimen with the objective. On other models, the stage is stationary, and the objective moves up and down instead.

Fastened onto the platform stage, a smaller optional stage allows movement of the slide in four directions along the *x* and *y* axes. This smaller stage is usually referred to as the **mechanical stage.** Etched markings on a scale on the mechanical stage denote the position of a field on the slide.

Light

In order for the microscope to work, light must pass upward through the material being viewed and into the objective lens. Then, the light must travel to the ocular lens and to the eyes of the lab personnel viewing the specimen. The light is changed by the lens of the microscope so that the rays reaching the eyes show a magnified image of the specimen.

The light source usually is located in the base of the microscope stand. It has a filter to change wavelengths. Generally, blue daylight is used because it provides the most comfortable viewing, but other filters may be used for special purposes. Light intensity may be controlled with a **rheostat.** The **condenser,** also called the substage, is located just below the opening in the mechanical stage and above the light source. It controls the stream of light. The condenser

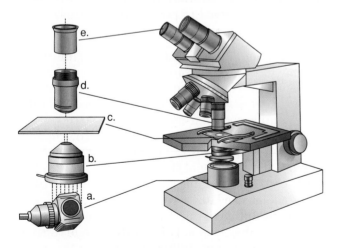

Figure 2-4 The path of light through the microscope: (a) The light originates at the base of the microscope, where it is adjusted with a rheostat. A lens directs it upward to the condenser. (b) The condenser concentrates the light in an intense cone of light. It may be raised or lowered. The iris diaphragm, part of the condenser, will open and close to control the light. (c) The light passes through the glass slide and specimen and into the objective. (d) The objective magnifies the image on the glass and passes the image into the eyepiece. (e) The eyepiece again magnifies the image, which enters the user's eye.

may be lowered or raised and its aperture narrowed or widened to control the amount of light passing through to the specimen on the slide. The **aperture** in the condenser is called the **iris diaphragm** because it resembles the iris of the eye.

Because the light shines up through the specimen to the viewer (see Figure 2-4), the specimen must be thin enough to allow light to pass through it without being diffused. This also is why specimens are always viewed on glass slides. In addition, there must be enough contrast in light and dark shades and different colors among structures for the structures to be visible. Most specimens do not have the natural level of contrast or color needed for effective viewing; therefore, stains and dyes are used to prepare specimens. Also, the specimen must be only one-cell-layer thick in order to show cellular structures clearly.

HOW TO USE A MICROSCOPE

Using a microscope primarily involves focusing the image by moving the objective closer to the specimen (or the specimen closer to the objective) and attaining the correct level of illumination from the light source. Although this chapter describes focusing and adjusting the light source separately, they actually are done together as part of the same process.

Focusing

Focusing the microscope is done by moving the objective up or down relative to the stage (or the stage relative to the objective). Movement of the objective (or stage) is controlled by round knobs, usually located on both sides of the microscope and near enough to the base of the microscope to permit resting your arms on the table while focusing.

Working Distance. The distance between the specimen on the stage and the objective lens is referred to as the **working distance.** The working distance is longest at lower magnification (4X and 10X) and gets shorter as the magnification increases. With the 100X objective, the working distance is very small, about the same thickness as a piece of heavy paper. At this distance, the oil on the oil-immersion lens touches both the glass slide and the objective. Because the objective is so close to the slide under high-power magnification, you should check the working distance by looking at the microscope from the side when changing from 40X to 100X. If you move the objective too close to the stage, you can grind it into the slide and ruin the lens.

Coarse and Fine Adjustments. The **coarse adjustment** focus knob moves the objective quickly; that is, it moves the objective a great distance with one revolution. This knob is used first to bring the specimen into approximate focus. The **fine adjustment** focus knob then brings the specimen into sharper focus. It moves the objective much more slowly because the knob moves the objective only a short distance with one revolution.

In order to prevent damage to the lens, it is especially important to use the fine adjustment knob at high power when the objective is close to the slide. For the same reason, the specimen should be focused first under the 4X or 10X objective because, on most microscopes, these low-power objectives usually cannot touch the slide even when they are moved as close as possible to the stage. Only then should the objective be changed to 40X or 100X, when further focusing should require only a partial turn of the fine adjustment focus knob.

Eyepiece Adjustment

When using a binocular microscope, it is necessary to adjust the eyepieces to your own eye span and **visual acuity.** A gentle push inward or pull outward will adjust the distance between the eyepieces to accommodate your eye span.

To adjust the eyepieces to the visual acuity of each of your eyes, first bring the specimen into focus with the **stationary ocular.** The stationary ocular is usually on the right, and you should look through it with your right eye, your left eye closed. Use the coarse and fine adjustment knobs on low power to obtain a clear image with the right eye. Then, close your right eye and use your left eye on the **adjustable ocular.** The latter will have a collar of ridges or beads around it. Adjust this eyepiece to correct the focus for the visual acuity of your left eye. Then, check the focus using both eyes. Repeat these steps if necessary until you obtain a clear focus when viewing the specimen through both oculars simultaneously.

Light Adjustment

The right level of light is essential for a clear image. Too little light will obscure details in darkness, while too much light will produce a blinding glare without the contrast necessary to distinguish features. As a general rule, less light is required at lower levels of magnification. As higher power objectives are used, the light must be increased accordingly. Some specimens also require more light than others. A darkly stained slide requires more light than does an unstained one.

The level of light is adjusted by raising or lowering the condenser, narrowing or widening the iris diaphragm, or adjusting the rheostat. The higher the condenser and the wider the iris, the greater the level of light.

> **Note**
> Never force the leaves of the diaphragm.

Putting It All Together

To focus the microscope for lab work using the 10X objective:

- With the maximum distance between the stage and objective, clamp the slide on the stage, specimen side up, to prevent it from moving.
- Turn on the light.
- Raise the condenser to its highest position with the control knob and open the iris diaphragm to its maximum extent.
- Looking at the microscope from the side, not through the oculars, rotate the low-power (10X) objective into viewing position in the center of the stage.
- Still looking at the microscope from the side and using the coarse adjustment knob, lower the objective until it nears the stage or stops.

> **Note**
> When handling slides of biospecimens such as blood smears, remember to follow the Standard Precautions and other biohazard safety procedures to prevent possible contamination. Remember to coverslip liquid specimens of urine to prevent damage to the objectives and biohazardous contamination of the POL.

- Look through the eyepiece and reverse the direction of the coarse focus adjustment knob until the slide comes into focus.
- Still looking through the eyepiece, turn the fine focus adjustment knob back and forth until you attain the clearest possible image.
- Adjust the condenser and light source until the image is clear and the light level is comfortable.
- Adjust the oculars for your eye span and visual acuity.
- Scan the slide to observe the entire specimen, using the knobs on the mechanical stage to move the slide in four directions.

To focus the microscope for lab work using the 40X objective:

- Again viewing the microscope from the side, rotate the 40X objective into place.
- Looking through the eyepiece, turn the fine adjustment focus knob to focus clearly.

- Adjust the condenser and light source until the image is clear and the light level is comfortable.
- Scan the slide to observe the entire specimen, using the mechanical stage to move the slide.

To focus the microscope for lab work using the 100X objective:

- Return to the side view and rotate the 100X power objective into position.
- Look through the ocular and turn the fine focus adjustment knob to focus clearly.
- Adjust the condenser and light source until the image is clear and the light level is comfortable.
- Rotate the oil immersion objective slightly out of the way. Taking care that the 40X objective does not touch the oil, add one drop of oil to the center of the slide over the condenser.
- Carefully rotate the 100X lens back into place over the slide.
- Turn the fine focus adjustment knob back and forth a fraction of a turn, until the image is clear. If you lose the focus, you must return to the 10X objective and start focusing all over again.
- Scan the slide to observe the entire specimen, using the mechanical stage to move the slide.

MICROSCOPE CARE

The microscope is a delicate, expensive instrument that is easily damaged by dust, excess oil and light, vibrations, and falls. It must be stored in a safe place, cleaned carefully after each use, and otherwise treated as the sensitive device it is. If properly cared for, most microscopes require very little service and work well for years.

Service and Parts

As with any other piece of expensive equipment, records should be kept of routine maintenance and other service procedures performed on the microscope. The microscope should be cleaned and serviced annually by a professional microscope service company. Likewise, only a professional should disassemble the microscope or try to clean the back of the objectives or adjust any interior part of the microscope.

Because parts may differ from one manufacturer to another, they should be purchased from the original manufacturer whenever possible. For example, only the bulb and illuminator recommended by the microscope's manufacturer should be used—others may produce too much heat. Use only recommended brands of immersion oil, never cedar wood oil.

Location and Storage

The microscope should be assigned a permanent space on a counter where it is not likely to vibrate or be knocked off. It should be kept away from extremes of heat and cold and sudden temperature changes because these extremes may injure the lens cement and damage the alignment of the lens system. The microscope should not get wet or sit in liquid on the counter—electric shock could result.

When not in use, the microscope should be kept in a cabinet or under a plastic cover. This will help protect it from dust and excess light, both of which may damage the lenses. This also will lessen the likelihood of its being struck by other objects or knocked over. Security precautions should be taken to prevent theft of the microscope, such as keeping the cabinet or room locked when not in use.

Cleaning

Use a magnifying glass if necessary to examine the lenses when cleaning them. Blow dust from the glass surfaces with an infant's ear syringe or a similar device that does not touch the lens.

Clean only the outside surfaces of the lenses, using a circular motion from the center outward. Use a piece of lens paper slightly moistened with 70 percent isopropyl alcohol or lens cleaning solution. Never substitute Kimwipes or other tissues to clean the lenses—they may leave behind a residue or scratch the lenses. Many microscope warranties may be voided by the manufacturer if lens paper is not used. Do not use xylene to clean the lenses because it is toxic and may loosen the lens cement. If you used the 100X objective, take special care to clean the oil from the objective and all other parts of the microscope immediately after use.

After Using the Microscope

After using the microscope, you should follow these steps in cleaning and storing it:

- Looking at the microscope from the side, rotate the 10X power objective back into place in the center. Take care that the 40X objective does not touch the oil if the 100X objective was used.
- Remove the slide from the microscope. If it is to be saved, wipe it with a piece of lens paper to remove the oil.
- Clean the outside of all the lenses with lens paper, taking particular care to remove all traces of oil from the 100X lens.
- Clean the stage, condenser, and other accessible parts of the microscope.
- Using the coarse adjustment focus knob, move the 10X objective to the lowest position in

Other criteria to consider when selecting a microscope for the POL include

- objectives in the powers of 10X, 40X, and 100X.
- parfocal objectives for easy focusing.
- a mechanical stage (on the platform stage) that moves easily and enables methodical, efficient viewing of specimens.
- a built-in light source.

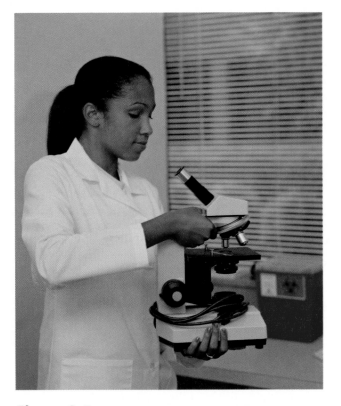

Figure 2-5 When carrying a microscope, always support it underneath with one hand and grasp the arm fully with the other hand.

preparation for the next use of the microscope. Cover the microscope with a plastic cover or return it to its storage cabinet. See Figure 2-5 for instructions for carrying a microscope.

- Follow the procedures outlined in Chapter 1 to clean and disinfect the work area, other equipment that was used, and your hands.

SELECTING A MICROSCOPE

There are several important considerations in selecting a microscope for the POL. A demonstration before purchase is essential. A familiar slide should be used to test the quality of the microscope by focusing and viewing its features. Differentiation of detail, that is, the microscope's resolution, is the most important criterion for microscopic work in medical labs.

While monocular microscopes are sometimes used in schools because they cost less, binocular microscopes are preferred in labs because viewing a magnified specimen with both eyes (through two eyepieces) is less stressful. This is an important consideration in POLs, where much time is spent studying specimens through a microscope. For the same reason, eyepieces should be in a comfortable position and focusing adjustments should allow the arms to rest comfortably on the table.

Troubleshooting

Following are nine common microscope problems. For each problem, the probable cause or causes and remedies are given.

- *Problem:* the light will not come on. *Probable cause:* the light bulb may be burned out or the light may not be plugged in. *Remedy:* check the light bulb and plug.
- *Problem:* the bulb burns out often. *Probable cause:* the bulb may not be a standard bulb or the voltage switch of the light does not match the local mainline voltage. *Remedy:* use a bulb recommended by the manufacturer or replace the voltage switch.
- *Problem:* the lamp flickers or goes off and on. *Probable cause:* the lamp may be about to burn out or there may be a loose electrical connection. *Remedy:* change the light bulb or check the electrical connections.
- *Problem:* the light is too bright or too dark and cannot be adjusted. *Probable cause:* the line voltage switch may not be suitable for the local mainline voltage. *Remedy:* change the selector switch.
- *Problem:* the field of vision remains too dark after increasing the voltage. *Probable cause:* the condenser may not be high enough or it may not be positioned correctly. *Remedy:* raise or reposition the condenser.
- *Problem:* the field of vision is dark even with the light switched on. *Probable cause:* the iris diaphragm may be closed. *Remedy:* open the diaphragm.
- *Problem:* too much contrast of the image. *Probable cause:* the condenser may be too low. *Remedy:* raise the condenser.
- *Problem:* the image cannot be focused without blurs. *Probable cause:* the lenses may not be clean. *Remedy:* clean the lenses with lens paper and alcohol.
- *Problem:* dust is visible on the lens. *Probable cause:* the lenses may not be clean. *Remedy:* blow dust away with an infant ear syringe. If dust specks remain, wipe the lens with lens paper dampened in lens cleaner.

PROCEDURE 2-1

Focusing the Microscope

Goal

After successfully completing this procedure, you will be able to focus the microscope at 10X, 40X, and 100X magnification.

Completion Time

30 minutes

Equipment and Supplies

- Disposable gloves, impermeable apron, lab jacket, or gown
- Hand disinfectant
- Surface disinfectant
- Paper towels and tissues
- Biohazard container
- Microscope, accessories, and immersion oil
- Blood-stained smear
- Lens paper
- 70% isopropyl alcohol or lens cleaner

Instructions

Read through the list of equipment and supplies that you will need and the steps of the procedure. Be sure that you understand each step before you begin. Then complete each step correctly and in the proper order. If your completion time is too long, repeat the procedure until you improve your speed.

*Steps marked with (*) are critical and must have the maximum points to pass.

Performance Standards	Points Awarded	Maximum Points
1. Wash your hands with disinfectant, dry them, and put on gloves, apron, jacket, or gown.		10
2. Follow the Universal Precautions.		10
3. Collect and prepare the appropriate equipment.		5
4. Clean the ocular and objective lenses with lens paper slightly moistened with 70% isopropyl alcohol or lens cleaner.		5
5. Observing the microscope from the side:		
a. Raise the condenser to its highest position by turning its control knob.		5
b. Open the diaphragm to the maximum extent and turn on the light.		5
c. Increase the distance between the stage and objective.		5
d. Secure the slide on the stage with the specimen side up and fasten it with clips to prevent movement.		5
e. Rotate the 10X objective into viewing position in the center of the stage.		5
f. Turn the coarse adjustment focus knob to decrease the distance of the slide to the objective until it stops or is just above the slide.		5
6. Looking through the eyepiece:		
a. Reverse the direction of the coarse adjustment focus knob, increasing the distance between the objective and the stage until the slide comes into focus.		5
b. Use the fine adjustment focus knob by turning it back and forth for short distances until you obtain the best image.		5
c. Adjust the condenser and light controls until the image is clear and the level of illumination is comfortable for viewing.		5

d.	Adjust the ocular lenses to each eye.	5
e.	Scan the slide using the stage controls to move it in four directions.	5
7.	Observe the microscope from the side and rotate the 40X objective into place.	5
8.	Look through the eyepiece and repeat steps 6b, 6c, and 6e.	5
9.	Observe the microscope from the side and rotate the 100X objective into place.	5
10.	Look through the ocular lenses and repeat steps 6b, 6c, and 6e.	5
11.	Observe the microscope from the side and rotate the 100X objective slightly out of the way. Add one drop of oil to the center of the slide over the condenser and then carefully rotate the 100X lens back into place over the slide.	10
12.	Look through the ocular lenses and repeat steps 6b, 6c, and 6e.	5
13.	Rotate the 10X objective back into place in the center, taking care that the 40X lens does not touch the immersion oil.	5
14.	Remove the slide from the microscope, wiping it with a piece of lens paper to remove the oil if the slide is to be saved.	5
15.	Clean the lenses with lens paper, including the oculars and all objectives, going from lowest to highest power.	5
16.	Clean the 100X oil-immersion lens with lens paper to remove all traces of oil.	5
17.	Clean the stage, condenser, and other parts of the microscope.	10
18.	Move the 10X objective to the lowest position in preparation for the next use of the microscope.	10
19.	Cover the microscope with a plastic cover or place it in its cabinet and return it to storage.	10
20.	Discard disposable supplies.	5
21.	Disinfect and return other equipment to storage.	5
22.	Clean your work area following the Universal Precautions.	10
23.	Remove your gloves and apron, jacket, or gown; wash your hands with disinfectant and dry them.	10
	Total Points	**200**

Overall Procedural Evaluation

Student's Name _____

Signature of Instructor _____ Date _____

Comments _____

_____

chapter 2 REVIEW

Using Terminology

Match the terms in the right column with the appropriate definition in the left column.

_____ **1.** eyepiece of microscope

_____ **2.** rotates the objectives

_____ **3.** controls the amount of light

_____ **4.** moves a shorter distance

_____ **5.** microscope with two eyepieces

_____ **6.** determines the quality of a microscope

_____ **7.** has the highest magnification

a. binocular

b. condenser

c. fine adjustment focus knob

d. nosepiece

e. ocular

f. oil-immersion lens

g. resolution

Acquiring Knowledge

8. Label the parts of the microscope in the figure as indicated.

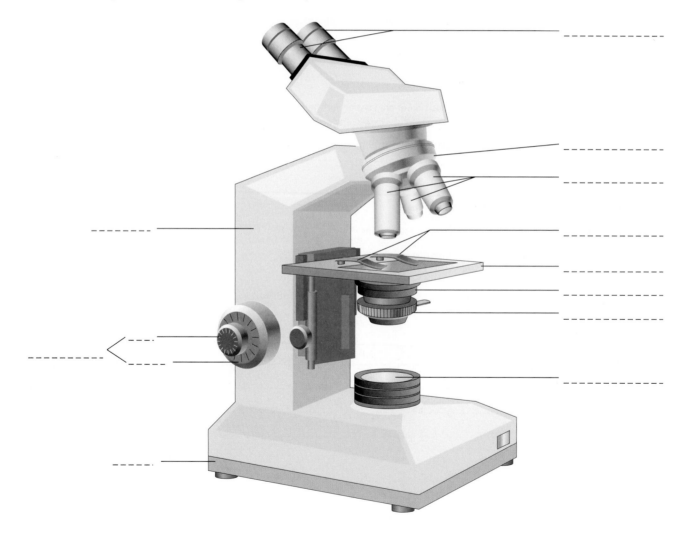

Choose the best answer for the following questions.

9. Which of the following objectives would have the highest magnification?
    a. scanning power
    b. high dry power
    c. oil immersion
    d. low power

10. What would be the total magnification if using the 40X objective to view blood cells?
    a. 10
    b. 100
    c. 400
    d. 4000

11. How many lenses in the compound microscope act together as one to make a clear image of a magnified specimen?
    a. 1
    b. 2
    c. 3
    d. 4

12. The ability of a microscope to distinguish fine details in a stained slide is referred to as
    a. visual acuity
    b. resolution
    c. light refraction
    d. magnification

13. When viewing a slide through the microscope, which of the following objectives would create the greatest working distance?
    a. 4X
    b. 10X
    c. 40X
    d. 100X

Answer the following questions in the spaces provided.

14. Explain why you must be careful when focusing the oil-immersion objective.

    _____

    _____

    _____

15. Name the type of compound microscope that has two oculars (eyepieces) and is therefore less tiring and preferred for lengthy viewing of specimens.

    _____

    _____

    _____

16. Where is the lens magnification system of the compound microscope mounted?

    _____

    _____

    _____

17. What result is obtained when the power of the objective you are using is multiplied by the power of the eyepiece of the microscope?

_____

_____

_____

18. In order to receive the best-quality and best-fitting replacements, what specification should you include when ordering light bulbs and other replacements for the microscope?

_____

_____

_____

19. What is the total magnification of a red cell in a urine specimen viewed under a 10X ocular and a 40X high dry objective?

_____

_____

_____

20. Staining a specimen allows you to distinguish the details more clearly. Name the two qualities that staining enhances.

_____

_____

_____

21. When you view a prepared slide under the microscope, how many layers can you see clearly with distinct details?

_____

_____

_____

22. When you focus a slide under the microscope, why should you alternate between looking through the oculars and looking at the objectives from the side of the microscope?

_____

_____

_____

23. What is the technical term for the hole in the microscope stage that permits light to pass from the condenser to the objective?

_____

_____

_____

24. When using the microscope, you must always be aware of the space between the objective and the specimen in order to prevent damage to the objective. What term describes this space?

_____

_____

_____

25. Which focus adjustment knob should you use to begin the focusing process?

_____

_____

_____

26. Which focus adjustment knob should you always use finally to adjust the details of a fuzzy focus?

_____

_____

_____

27. Which focus adjustment knob should you always use to focus the oil-immersion lens?

_____

_____

_____

28. What objective has a very short working distance and therefore requires the fine focus adjustment knob for focusing?

_____

_____

_____

29. Why must you always use special lens paper for cleaning the microscope lenses instead of ordinary facial tissue?

_____

_____

_____

30. How and when do you clean a microscope lens in order to keep the microscope in good order?

_____

_____

_____

31. How and where should you store a microscope when it is not in use?

_____

_____

_____

Directions: Place a + in the space at the left of each true statement. Place a 0 in the space at the left of each false statement. Rewrite each false statement so that it is true.

32. _____ A rheostat is a device that controls the size of the magnification of an objective.

_____

_____

_____

33. ____ A microscope specimen consists of a part or product of the human body or a microbe. A specimen is examined microscopically in order to learn about the health of the whole body.

_____

_____

_____

34. ____ The oil-immersion objective has a very high power of magnification and therefore requires oil to produce a clear image of the specimen.

_____

_____

_____

35. ____ The working distance is the distance between the oculars and the specimen.

_____

_____

_____

36. ____ Lab personnel using the microscope must learn to recognize complicated patterns of blood cell structures, urine sediment composition, and microorganisms.

_____

_____

_____

37. ____ Most microscopes require very little maintenance except for routine care and a yearly inspection by a professional microscope technician.

_____

_____

_____

38. ____ In the term 40X, the X means times or magnification.

_____

_____

_____

39. ____ A mechanical stage is attached to the platform stage.

_____

_____

_____

40. ____ Resolution refers to the fact that when objectives are changed, the object in the center of the magnified field should remain centered in the field of view.

_____

_____

_____

41. ____ Located in the condenser, the rheostat controls the amount of light entering through the aperture in the stage.

_____

_____

_____

42. ____ The higher the magnification, the more light is required for viewing a specimen.

_____

_____

_____

43. ____ The higher the magnification, the longer the working distance.

_____

_____

_____

44. ____ With a mechanical stage, you can control much more easily the direction of the slide movement.

_____

_____

_____

45. ____ When moving from the 40X objective to the oil-immersion objective, you should remove your eyes from the oculars and look from the side at the microscope objectives.

_____

_____

_____

46. ____ On a mechanical stage, the range of motion between the _x_ axis and the _y_ axis permits movement in four directions.

_____

_____

_____

47. ____ If you lose your focus on a higher-powered objective, you must return to the 10X objective and start the focusing process from the beginning.

_____

_____

_____

Applying Knowledge—On the Job

Answer the following questions in the spaces provided.

48. Melissa performs some blood cell differential counts under the oil-immersion objective of the laboratory's binocular microscope. She has to leave the microscope, and while she is gone, Susan (a coworker) views urines under the 10X and 40X objectives. When Melissa tries to resume her blood-cell differential work, she finds that she cannot bring one of the oculars into focus. What is the problem? How can it be solved?

_____

_____

_____

49. LaTasha looks over the service records of the microscope at the laboratory where she has begun work. The microscope does not focus well and she finds that a professional has not inspected it for several years. What should she do?

_____

_____

_____

50. Brenda observes that her coworker does not coverslip the urine sediment specimen when she views it under the microscope. Is this practice acceptable? If not, what should Brenda do about it?

_____

_____

_____

51. One of your coworkers has placed the POL's microscope next to the centrifuge and near the laboratory entrance for convenience. There is a sturdy table that would accommodate the microscope in the back of the laboratory. Should you mention this to your supervisor? Why or why not?

_____

_____

_____

52. Your coworker, Jamie, is trying to focus the microscope onto a urine sediment specimen, but all that she can see is a black hole down the oculars. What advice would you give Jamie?

_____

_____

_____

53. In the laboratory where you work, a blood smear is focused under the oil-immersion lens by a coworker. She asks you why the slide is dark with indistinct cells. What do you tell her?

_____

_____

_____

54. Tim is counting and identifying the white blood cells on a stained blood smear under a microscope with a mechanical stage. Several of the white cells are abnormal, so he lays the slide aside until later, when the doctor will be in and can view them. When he reinserts the slide, he has to search for 10 minutes to find the blood cells that he had viewed before. How could Tim have found the cells quickly on the second viewing?

_____

_____

_____

55. Maria, an employee in the laboratory, wipes the oculars of the microscope with her laboratory coat sleeve to clean them. She does not bother to clean the objectives between uses. What long-term effects will this type of care have on the microscope?

_____

_____

_____

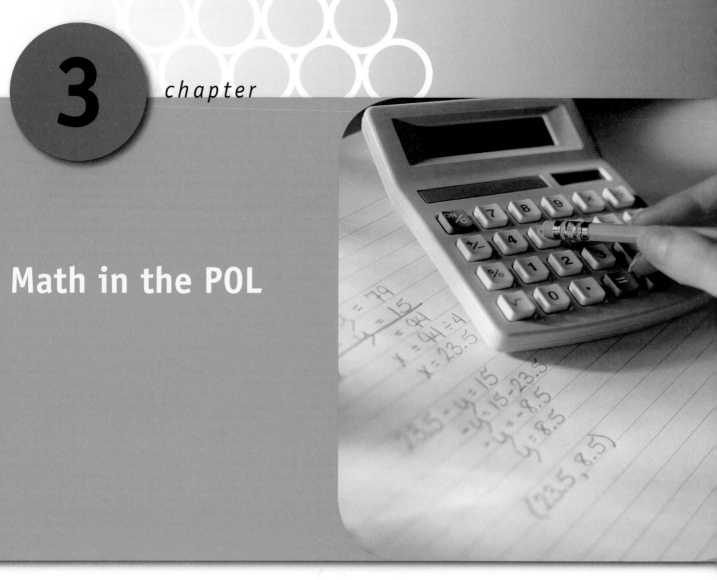

3 chapter

chapter

Math in the POL

COGNITIVE OBJECTIVES

After studying this chapter, you should be able to

3.1 use each of the vocabulary terms appropriately.

3.2 distinguish among numbers expressed as fractions, decimals, and percents, and list ways in which each type of number is used in the POL.

3.3 give examples of equivalent fractions and explain why they are equal.

3.4 explain how and why scientific notation is used.

3.5 identify the differences between the English and metric systems of measurement and explain why the metric system is preferred for use in the POL.

3.6 give examples of metric units used in the POL.

3.7 distinguish which formulas are used to solve common POL problems.

3.8 list the steps that lab personnel should take if they are having problems with math in the POL.

PERFORMANCE OBJECTIVES

After studying this chapter, you should be able to

3.9 multiply, divide, add, and subtract fractions.

3.10 find common denominators and simplify fractions.

3.11 convert fractions to decimals, round correctly, and calculate with decimals.

3.12   measure length, mass, and volume in metric units.

3.13   solve simple POL formulas.

3.14   prepare solutions and dilutions as described in procedures and manufacturer's instructions.

3.15   convert from one unit of measure to another using dimensional analysis.

TERMINOLOGY

colorimeter: an instrument for measuring intensity of color. It identifies the wavelengths of colored light in nanometers.

common denominator: a common multiple of the denominators of two or more fractions.

concentrate: a substance, either liquid or solid, that is strong because it has had fluid removed from it.

concentration: the strength of a chemical in a solution.

conversion factor: a ratio that relates the same measure in the systems of units; used to convert from one unit to another.

decimal: any number expressed in base 10, or a fraction in which the denominator is a power of 10.

denominator: the part of a fraction that is at the bottom of a fraction. It functions as a divisor.

diluent: an agent that reduces the strength of a substance to which it is added.

dilution: a solution that has been weakened by addition of a diluent.

dimensional analysis: a method of problem solving in which units of measure are carried through all calculations. This method ensures the answer has the desired units.

dividend: a number to be divided.

divisor: the number by which a dividend is divided.

English system: the foot–pound–ounce system of units of measurement that most of us use every day.

equation: a mathematical statement that expresses equality between two expressions on either side of an equals sign.

equivalent fractions: fractions that look different but have the same quantity.

exponent: a symbol written above and to the right of a number. An exponent indicates how many times the number is multiplied by itself.

formula: a rule written in mathematical symbols and numbers. A formula expresses the relationship between two or more quantities.

fraction: a numerical representation of the quotient of two numbers.

gram (g): the basic metric unit for weight or mass. A gram equals 0.03527 ounce in the English system.

International System of Units (SI): the world's most widely used modern form of the metric system of units.

inverse: opposite or reverse. The inverse of a fraction is created by turning it upside down.

kilogram (kg): the metric unit of weight or mass that is equal to 1,000 grams and to 2.2 pounds in the English system.

kilometer (km): the metric unit of length that equals 1,000 meters. A kilometer equals 0.62137 mile in the English system.

liter (L): the basic unit of volume in the metric system. A liter equals 1.0567 quarts in the English system.

meter (m): the basic unit of length in the metric system. A meter equals 1.0936 yards in the English system.

metric system: the system of measurement based on the meter, in which each unit is related to a basic unit of volume, length, or mass by a power of 10.

milligram (mg): the metric unit of weight or mass obtained by dividing the gram by 1,000.

millimeter (mm): the metric unit of length obtained by dividing the meter by 1,000.

numerator: in any fraction or ratio, the number at the top of a fraction.

percent: "out of a hundred"; a fraction with 100 as the denominator.

quotient: the number resulting from the division of one number by another.

ratio: the relationship in size or quantity between two things.

reconstitute: to add liquid to a dried powder to return it to its original liquid form.

scientific notation: a system of writing decimals. In scientific notation, 10 raised to some power is used to specify where the decimal should be placed.

simplify: to express a fraction as a ratio between smaller numbers.

solute: the substance dissolved in a liquid to form a solution.

solution: the liquid containing a dissolved substance or substances.

solvent: the liquid in which substances are dissolved to form a solution.

total volume: the amount of a solution, including both solute and solvent.

INTRODUCTION

Medical laboratories are more technologically advanced today and the need to perform lengthy complex calculations for test results, standards, or controls is no longer necessary. However, it is essential that laboratory personnel understand the mathematics involved in preparing reagents and solutions needed for laboratory testing, converting units to metric, and performing the calculations of quality control in the lab.

This chapter reviews basic math, outlines how to use formulas, introduces the metric system, and explains how to calculate solutions and dilutions. You may want to skip the first section if you already feel comfortable using fractions, decimals, and percents. However, if math is not your strong point, read on and take time to work through the examples to make sure that you understand the material.

REVIEW OF BASIC MATH

Fractions, decimals, and **percents** are different ways of expressing the same thing, a proportion or ratio. The same quantity, say half an inch, can be expressed using a fraction ($\frac{1}{2}$ inch), a decimal (0.5 inch), or a percent (50 percent of an inch). Most people have enough familiarity with math to realize that $\frac{1}{2}$, 0.5, and 50 percent are equal, but they may not know how to figure out the decimal and percentage equivalence of fractions such as $\frac{8}{9}$ or $\frac{11}{32}$. The next sections demonstrate how to convert from fractions to decimals and percents and how to use these different quantities.

Fractions

Many people find fractions difficult. The following discussion should help clarify them for you.

What a Fraction Is. A fraction is a way of expressing the **ratio,** or relationship in size or quantity of two things. The ratio of 3 to 4, for example, is the fraction $\frac{3}{4}$. The bar (− or /) represents division, so the fraction really means 3 divided by 4. It may also be written as 3 ÷ 4, or as 3/4. In any fraction or ratio, the number at the top is called the **numerator** and the number at the bottom is called the **denominator** (see Figure 3-1). In the case of $\frac{3}{4}$, the numerator is 3 and the denominator is 4.

Most people are familiar with fractions as parts of wholes. If a pie is divided into six pieces, for

$$\frac{\text{Numerator}}{\text{Denominator}}$$

Figure 3-1 Parts of a fraction.

example, the part of the pie represented by three of the pieces is three-sixths, written as the fraction $\frac{3}{6}$, or in words, three out of six. As another example, the ratio of two chapters in a book to the total of 20 chapters would be represented by the fraction $\frac{2}{20}$. In these two examples, the fractions $\frac{3}{6}$ and $\frac{2}{20}$ each represents a part of the total. In other words, each of these fractions is less than one.

Because fractions are ratios between any two numbers, they also can have values greater than one. Whenever the numerator is larger than the denominator, the value of the fraction is greater than one. The larger the numerator relative to the denominator, the greater the value of the fraction. When the numerator and denominator of a fraction are the same, as in $\frac{2}{2}$ or $\frac{3}{3}$, the value of the fraction is one. This is because any number divided by itself equals one. Use your calculator and several different numbers to verify that this is true.

Multiplying and Dividing Fractions. Multiplying and dividing fractions are easier than you might think if you follow a few simple rules. To multiply two fractions, just multiply the two numerators and then the two denominators, as in the following example:

$$\frac{1}{2} \times \frac{3}{4} = \frac{1 \times 3}{2 \times 4} = \frac{3}{8}$$

This rule also applies to multiplication of fractions by whole numbers. For example:

$$\frac{1}{2} \times 20 = \frac{1}{2} \times \frac{20}{1} = \frac{1 \times 20}{2 \times 1} = \frac{20}{2} = 10$$

Dividing fractions requires an additional step. To divide one fraction by another, you first must change the **divisor** (the denominator, or the one being "divided into" the other) into its inverse, or opposite. To change a fraction into its **inverse,** simply flip-flop the fraction. For example, the inverse of $\frac{3}{4}$ is $\frac{4}{3}$, the inverse of $\frac{4}{5}$ is $\frac{5}{4}$, and the inverse of $\frac{1}{2}$ is $\frac{2}{1}$.

To divide two fractions, multiply the dividend fraction by the inverse of the divisor fraction, as in the following example:

$$\frac{1}{2} \div \frac{3}{4} = \frac{1}{2} \times \frac{4}{3} = \frac{1 \times 4}{2 \times 3} = \frac{4}{6} = \frac{2}{3}$$

Equivalent Fractions and Common Denominators. Because $\frac{3}{3}$ and $\frac{2}{2}$ both equal one, these two fractions are **equivalent fractions;** they are two different ways of writing the same quantity. Common sense tells us that three out of six pieces of pie is half a pie—in other words, $\frac{3}{6}$ equals $\frac{1}{2}$ —but it is not so easy to tell if other fractions are equal. For example, is the fraction $\frac{2}{3}$ equal to $\frac{4}{6}$? Is $\frac{3}{4}$ equal to $\frac{9}{12}$? Is $\frac{3}{8}$ equal to $\frac{12}{32}$?

In order to compare any two fractions to determine if they are equivalent, you must rewrite them so that they have the same denominator, called a **common denominator.** A common denominator is also required for adding and subtracting fractions.

Take the example of $\frac{2}{3}$ and $\frac{4}{6}$. It is easy to see that if you multiply the denominator of $\frac{2}{3}$ by 2, it will be 6, the same as the denominator of $\frac{4}{6}$. To write $\frac{2}{3}$ as a fraction with denominator of 6, you also must multiply the numerator by 2. This is because the denominator was multiplied by 2, and, to preserve the value of the fraction, both numerator and denominator must be multiplied by the same number. In other words, the fraction $\frac{2}{3}$ must be multiplied by the fraction $\frac{2}{2}$, producing $\frac{4}{6}$.

For more difficult fractions, you can find a common denominator by multiplying the denominator of one fraction by the denominator of the other. Take the fractions $\frac{2}{3}$ and $\frac{4}{6}$ again. Their denominators are 3 and 6, respectively. Multiplying 3×6 yields a common denominator of 18. To write $\frac{2}{3}$ as a fraction with a denominator of 18, multiply the numerator by 6 to preserve the value of the fraction:

$$\frac{2}{3} \times \frac{6}{6} = \frac{2 \times 6}{3 \times 6} = \frac{12}{18}$$

To change $\frac{4}{6}$ to a fraction with a denominator of 18, multiply the denominator of 6 by 3. Also multiply the numerator by 3:

$$\frac{4}{6} \times \frac{3}{3} = \frac{4 \times 3}{6 \times 3} = \frac{12}{18}$$

Now that $\frac{2}{3}$ and $\frac{4}{6}$ have the same denominator, 18, you can see that they are equivalent—both equal the same amount, $\frac{12}{18}$.

Adding and Subtracting Fractions. To add and subtract fractions, make sure that they have the same denominator. Once they do, adding and subtracting is simple. To add two or more fractions with the same denominator, just add the numerators, as follows:

$$\frac{3}{4} + \frac{2}{4} = \frac{5}{4}$$

To subtract fractions with the same denominator, just subtract the numerators:

$$\frac{3}{4} - \frac{2}{4} = \frac{1}{4}$$

Simplifying Fractions. You can multiply the numerator and denominator of a fraction by the same number without changing the value of the fraction when you wish to compare fractions or to add or subtract them. Sometimes it is useful to divide the numerator and denominator of a fraction by the same number to **simplify** it (to express a fraction as a ratio between smaller numbers).

Consider the fraction $\frac{10}{20}$. Are there any numbers that will divide the numerator of 10 and the denominator of 20 without producing a remainder? Three numbers, 2, 5, and 10, will:

$$\frac{10 \div 2}{20 \div 2} = \frac{5}{10}$$

$$\frac{10 \div 5}{20 \div 5} = \frac{2}{4}$$

$$\frac{10 \div 10}{20 \div 10} = \frac{1}{2}$$

Because the value of the fraction $\frac{10}{20}$ is unchanged when you divide both its numerator and its denominator by the same number (2, 5, or 10), $\frac{10}{20}$ has the same value as $\frac{5}{10}, \frac{2}{4}$, and $\frac{1}{2}$. For most purposes, $\frac{1}{2}$, which is the most simplified form of the fraction $\frac{10}{20}$, is preferred.

Decimals

Everyone is familiar with decimals, whether they realize it or not, because our money system works on the decimal principle. Decimal means "based on the number 10," that is, divided into units of 10 (or 100 or some other power of 10). A dollar is divided into 100 cents, and dollar amounts are expressed using a decimal point. Half a dollar, for example, is written as $0.50, and one dollar and seventy cents is written as $1.70. From your experience with money, you know that anything to the right of the decimal point is less than one, while anything to the left of the decimal point is one or more.

Studying the fractions and decimal equivalents will help you understand decimal notation. The first position to the right of the decimal place is tenths, the second position hundredths, the third position thousandths, and so on (see Table 3-1). Each time you increase the denominator of a fraction by a power of 10, you add a zero to the right of the decimal point. The more zeros to the right of the decimal point in front of a digit, the smaller the number.

Table 3-1   Decimal Equivalents

Fraction	Decimal Equivalent
$\dfrac{1}{10}$	0.1
$\dfrac{1}{100}$	0.01
$\dfrac{1}{1000}$	0.001
$\dfrac{1}{10,000}$	0.0001
$\dfrac{1}{100,000}$	0.00001
$\dfrac{1}{1,000,000}$	0.000001

Note

To reduce errors in reading and transcribing decimal numbers of less than one, always add a zero to the left of the decimal point. For example, .5 should be written as 0.5 to avoid errors.

Converting Fractions to Decimals. Every fraction can be converted to a decimal. Two obvious examples are $\frac{1}{2} = 0.5$ and $\frac{1}{4} = 0.25$. Some are not so obvious, like $\frac{255}{425}$. Fortunately, converting fractions to decimals is easy with a calculator. Just remember that the bar in the fraction represents division. To convert $\frac{255}{425}$ to a decimal, divide 255 by 425 on your calculator. You should get 0.6 for the answer. Convert the following fractions to decimals using your calculator to be sure that you understand the method:

$$\frac{79}{85} = 0.93 \qquad \frac{22}{345} = 0.064 \qquad \frac{3}{999} = 0.003$$

Rounding. In each of the examples just given, the answer on your calculator actually was a longer number than the answer shown above. For example, when you divided 79 by 85 on your calculator, your answer should have been 0.9294117. Round this off to 0.93, meaning that you express it with fewer digits to the right of the decimal point. Calculators usually carry out division (and most other calculations) to more digits than are needed for the answer, so rounding is a procedure that is done repeatedly in

POL work. It is crucial for standardizing results that everyone rounds off the same way. When rounding off numbers, always follow these rules:

- Never express an answer with more digits than the original measurements contain. For example, if you multiply the numbers 0.788 and 2.334, your answer should have three digits to the right of the decimal point (1.839). To include more digits in the answer than in the original measurements suggests a degree of precision that is bogus. The answer cannot be more precise than the numbers entered into the calculation.
- Always round up if the next digit is 5 or greater, and always round down if it is 4 or less. For example, to express 2.82513 with just two digits to the right of the decimal point, look at the third digit to the right of the decimal point (in this case 5) and round up if it is 5 or more (as here) and down if it is 4 or less.

To be sure that you understand how to round off numbers, convert the following fractions to decimals, each with the correct number of digits. You should get the same answers as those given here:

$$\frac{2}{45} = 0.04 \qquad \frac{31}{669} = 0.046 \qquad \frac{75}{59} = 1.3$$

Calculating with Decimals. You should convert difficult fractions to decimals, rounding when necessary, before doing further calculations. This greatly simplifies subsequent work. Follow these guidelines when adding decimals:

- Write the numbers in a column, lining up the decimal points. Put a decimal point on the right of any whole number.
- Add the numbers.
- Bring the decimal point straight down into the answer.

$$\begin{array}{r} 1.3 \\ + \ 0.25 \\ \hline 1.55 \end{array}$$

Follow these guidelines when subtracting decimals:

- Write the numbers in a column, lining up the decimal points. Put the larger number on top.
- If necessary, add zeros as place holders.
- Subtract.
- Bring the decimal point straight down into the answer.

$$\begin{array}{r} 1.3 \\ - \ 0.25 \\ \hline \end{array} \quad = \quad \begin{array}{r} 1.30 \\ - \ 0.25 \\ \hline \end{array} \quad = \quad 1.05$$

Follow these guidelines when multiplying decimals:

- Multiply the numbers.
- Count the total number of places to the right of each decimal point. Add them together.
- Count off this total number of decimal places in the answer. Count from right to left.

1.3	1 place
× 0.25	2 places
65	
26	
.325	3 places
.325 = 0.325	

Follow these guidelines when dividing decimals:

- Make the divisor a whole number by moving the decimal point to the right of the last digit.
- In the **dividend,** move the decimal point to the right the same number of places.
- Place the decimal point directly above in the **quotient,** or answer.
- Divide.
- Round off if necessary.

$$\begin{array}{r} 5.2 \\ .25\overline{)1.30} \\ 125 \\ \overline{0050} \\ 0050 \end{array}$$

See Figure 3-2.

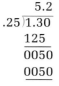

Quotient
———————
Divisor)Dividend

Figure 3-2 Parts of a division problem.

> **Note**
>
> If the answer is less than 1, add a zero to the left of the decimal point.

Scientific Notation. Expressing very small quantities with decimals can lead to error. Numbers with many zeros after the decimal point, such as 0.000000001, are difficult to read and transcribe. It is easy to misplace decimal points and change values by a power of 10 or more. To help reduce errors, a system of writing decimals called **scientific notation** is often used with very small and very large numbers.

Scientific notation uses **exponents,** which are symbols written above and to the right of a number. Exponents tell how many times the number is to be multiplied by itself. For example, the number 10^2 is 10×10, or 100. The number 10^3 is $10 \times 10 \times 10$, or 1,000. The notation 10^{-1} is the inverse of 10^1. It means $1/10^1$, which is 1/10 or 0.1. The number 10^{-2} is the inverse of 10^2, or $1/10^2$, which is 1/100 or 0.01. Using scientific notation, the number 0.1 is expressed as 1×10^{-1}, 0.01 as 1×10^{-2}, and 0.001 as 1×10^{-3}.

Here is an easy way to convert numbers to their equivalents in scientific notation, using as an example the number $0.000001234 = 1.234 \times 10^{-6}$.

- Place the decimal point to the right of the first nonzero digit: 1.234.
- Multiply this number by 10: 1.234×10.
- Use as the exponent of 10 the number of places the decimal point was moved in step one: 1.234×10^6.
- The exponent is positive if you moved the decimal point to the left and negative if you moved it to the right: 1.234×10^{-6}.

More about Exponents. Any number raised to the zero power, that is, with an exponent of zero, equals one. A number raised to the first power, that is, with an exponent of one, equals itself. A fractional exponent takes a root of a number. For example, the exponent $\frac{1}{2}$ takes the square root and the exponent $\frac{1}{3}$ takes the cube root.

To multiply or divide exponents, make sure the base is the same, such as 5^2, 5^4, or other exponents of the base number 5. To multiply these numbers, simply add the exponents: $5^2 \times 5^4 = 5^6$. To divide them, subtract the exponents: $5^2 / 5^4 = 5^{-2}$. Use your calculator to perform the calculations to verify to yourself that the method produces correct answers.

Percents

Percent literally means "out of a hundred," so a number expressed as a percent is a fraction with 100 as the denominator. Fifty percent, also written 50%, means 50 out of 100 or $\frac{50}{100}$. Likewise, 10 percent means 10 out of 100, or $\frac{10}{100}$. Because the denominator is always 100, it is easy to convert percents to decimals and decimals to percents even without a calculator. Just remember that any number followed by the word percent or the percent sign, %, is divided by 100.

Study the following examples to be sure that you understand the relationship between percents, fractions, and decimals:

- $50\% = \dfrac{50}{100} = 0.50$

- $6\% = \dfrac{6}{100} = 0.06$

- $99.5\% = \dfrac{99.5}{100} = 0.995$

- $0.1\% = \dfrac{0.1}{100} = 0.001.$

In general, to convert numbers from percents to decimals, move the decimal point two places to the left and drop the percent sign. To convert numbers from decimals to percents, move the decimal point two places to the right and add a percent sign.

USING FORMULAS

Formulas are rules that are written in mathematical symbols and numbers. They express the relationship between two or more quantities, such as temperature in Celsius and temperature in Fahrenheit. Most formulas are written in the form of **equations,** which are mathematical statements that express equality between two expressions on either side of an equal sign, such as $C = \dfrac{5}{9}(F - 32)$, which is the formula for converting temperature in Fahrenheit, represented by the letter F, into temperature in Celsius, represented by the letter C. The left side of an equation (everything to the left of the equal sign, =) is always equal to the right side of the equation (everything to the right of the equal sign).

In addition to temperature conversion, formulas are used in POLs to calculate cell counts, calibrate instruments, and establish quality control limits, among other uses. The best way to learn how to use POL formulas is by working through them. Follow the instructions step by step and remember these three rules about all mathematical equations:

- If part of an equation is enclosed in parentheses, as in the temperature conversion equation above, complete that part before solving the rest of the equation.
- In order to preserve the equality of expressions on both sides of the equal sign, treat both sides of any equation equally. For example, if you multiply the right side of an equation by 2, you also must multiply the left side of the equation by 2 to preserve the equality.
- When you solve equations, always use and carry through with the correct units of measurement (for example, degrees or mm^3). If you do, your answer should be in the correct units; if it is not, then you may have made an error in your calculations.

Work through the following two examples for a better understanding of how to use formulas:

- The formula for converting Fahrenheit to Celsius was given above as:

$$C = \frac{5}{9} \times (F - 32°)$$

where

C = temperature in Celsius
F = temperature in Fahrenheit.

Calculate the temperature in Celsius when it is 72 degrees Fahrenheit. Substitute 72 degrees for F into the formula:

$$C = \frac{5}{9} \times (72° - 32°)$$

$$C = \frac{5}{9} \times 40°$$

$$C = \frac{200°}{9} = 22° \text{ C}$$

- The formula for calculating platelet counts is

$$\text{Platelet count} = \frac{\text{Average number of platelets} \times \text{Depth factor} \times \text{Dilution factor}}{\text{Area counted}}$$

Assume that the values to be substituted into the formula for the platelet count are

Average number of platelets = 170
Depth factor = 10
Dilution factor = 100
Area counted = 1 mm^3

Substituting into the formula, you get

$$\text{Platelet count} = \frac{170 \times 10 \times 100}{1 \text{ mm}^3}$$

$$= 170{,}000 \text{ / mm}^3$$

THE METRIC SYSTEM

In your day-to-day life, most of you use the **English system** of measurement. For example, you measure length in inches and feet, weight in ounces and pounds, and volume in cups and quarts. The English system has two major drawbacks for use in POLs. One drawback is that it lacks precise units for measuring very small quantities, which are required for medications, transfusions, and accurate test procedures. The second drawback is that it is very difficult to convert from one unit of measurement to another. For example, there are 12 inches in a foot, 16 ounces in a pound, and 4 cups in a quart. Because the English system evolved over many generations of practical use, it has no systematic basis.

The **metric system** in contrast, is ordered, methodical, and easy to use. It was designed by scientists in the late eighteenth century in Europe to replace the confusing patchwork of measuring systems then in use. The basic original metric units include the **meter** (m) for length, the **gram** (g) for weight, and the **liter** (L) for volume. All other units are obtained by multiplying or dividing these basic units by 10 or some power of 10 (one hundred, one thousand, one million, and so on). These derived units are distinguished by prefixes, and each has its own abbreviations (see Table 3-2).

Converting to the Metric System

Converting from one unit to another is easy with the metric system, and some units are extremely small, making the metric system particularly useful for POLs.

Some examples will help clarify how metric prefixes are used. Multiplying the gram by 1,000 produces a unit called the **kilogram (kg).** Dividing the gram by 1,000 produces a unit called the **milligram (mg).** Similarly, multiplying a meter by 1,000 produces the **kilometer (km),** and dividing a meter by 1,000 produces the **millimeter (mm).** For very small units, scientific notation usually is used to express the power of 10. For example, the prefix *micro-* can be expressed as 10^{-6}, *nano-* as 10^{-9}, *pico-* as 10^{-12}, and *femto-* as 10^{-15}.

Comparison of the English and Metric Systems of Measurement

1 centimeter = 0.3937 inch
1 meter = 1.0936 yards
1 kilometer = 0.62137 mile
1 cubic centimeter = 0.061 cubic inch
1 gram = 0.03527 ounce
1 kilogram = 2.2046 pounds
1 liter = 1.0567 quarts

Examples of POL Metric Measurements

- Most cylinders, beakers, flasks, syringes, and test tubes measure fluid in milliliters.
- Large flasks measure fluid in liters.
- Pipettes measure fluids in milliliters or microliters.
- Solid reagents are measured in grams.
- The hemacytometer has a fluid depth of 0.10 millimeter.
- Erythrocyte sedimentation rate tubes are read in millimeters.
- The **colorimeter,** an instrument for measuring intensity of color, identifies the wavelengths of colored light in nanometers (nm).

Table 3-2 Prefixes in the Metric System

Prefix	Abbreviation	Factor	Power of 10
giga-	G	1,000,000,000	1×10^9
mega-	M	1,000,000	1×10^6
kilo-	k	1,000	1×10^3
hecto-	h	100	1×10^2
deka-	dk	10	1×10^1
deci-	d	0.1	1×10^{-1}
centi-	c	0.01	1×10^{-2}
milli-	m	0.001	1×10^{-3}
micro-	μ	0.000001	1×10^{-6}
nano-	n	0.000000001	1×10^{-9}
pico-	p	0.000000000001	1×10^{-12}
femto-	f	0.000000000000001	1×10^{-15}

In 1960, the **International System of Units (SI)** modernized the metric system to include newer scientific measurements such as the candela, which measures light intensity, and the ampere, which measures electric current. Other changes also were introduced at that time, including substitution of the kilogram for the gram as the basic unit of weight and capitalization of the abbreviation for liter (L). Since medical laboratories have not completed the changeover to SI yet, some tests are reported in both metric and SI units in some textbooks.

> **Meter Facts**
>
> The name *metric* comes from the word *meter,* the system's basic unit of length, which was set equal to 0.1 millionth of the distance from the North Pole to the Equator through Paris, France. Other units in the metric system are referenced to the meter. For example, a kilogram weighs the same as one cubic decimeter (dm^3) of water at 4 degrees Celsius and an atmospheric pressure of 760 mm of mercury. A milliliter (mL) is virtually the same as a cubic centimeter (cm^3), although the milliliter is the preferred unit of volume in POLs.

Because the metric system is used exclusively in POLs, you will need to convert between the English and metric systems when you move into the clinical setting. For example, you may need to convert a patient's body weight from pounds to kilograms to calculate drug doses, or to convert doses of medications from milliliters to teaspoons.

To convert from one unit to another, a technique called **dimensional analysis** or factor-label method is used with conversion factors. A **conversion factor** is described as a numerical ratio of one unit that is used to convert to another unit. For example, 1 kilogram = 1000 grams is a conversion factor. The units of measure are systematically set up in the problem and the unit given is canceled in the equation and the unit needed remains. Metric conversion charts can usually be found in medical dictionaries or similar references in the POL.

Consider these examples using dimensional analysis to convert from one unit to another:

- 125 pounds to kilograms

$$125 \; \text{pounds} \times \frac{1 \; \text{kg}}{2.20 \; \text{pounds}} = \frac{125}{2.20} = 56.8 \; \text{kg}$$

- 27.0 kg to pounds

$$27.0 \; \text{kg} \times \frac{2.20 \; \text{pounds}}{1 \; \text{kg}} = 59.4 \; \text{pounds}$$

- ½ inch to centimeters

First, change the fraction to a decimal: ½ inch = 0.50 inch

$$0.50 \; \text{inch} \times \frac{2.54 \; \text{cm}}{1 \; \text{inch}} = 1.27 \; \text{cm}$$

- 1.25 grams to milligrams

$$1.25 \; \text{g} \times \frac{1000 \; \text{mg}}{1 \; \text{g}} = 1250 \; \text{mg}$$

- 4.5×10^{10} nanometers to meters

$$4.5 \times 10^{10} \; \text{nm} \times \frac{1 \times 10^{-9} \; \text{m}}{1 \; \text{nm}} = 4.5 \times 10^{1} \; \text{m}$$

SOLUTIONS AND DILUTIONS

Preparing **solutions,** liquids containing dissolved substances, to exact specifications is a task that is done repeatedly in the POL. Most solutions are prepared in one of two ways:

- making a weaker solution from a stronger one, that is, making a **dilution.**
- adding liquid to **reconstitute** a dried powder, that is, to return it to its original liquid form.

Dilution refers to the strength, or **concentration,** of a chemical in a solution, not to the volume of the solution. For example, a very small amount of solution, measured in microliters, and a very large

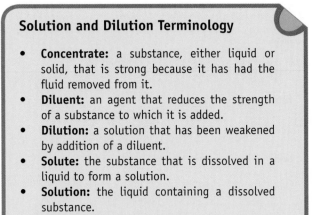

> **Solution and Dilution Terminology**
>
> - **Concentrate:** a substance, either liquid or solid, that is strong because it has had the fluid removed from it.
> - **Diluent:** an agent that reduces the strength of a substance to which it is added.
> - **Dilution:** a solution that has been weakened by addition of a diluent.
> - **Solute:** the substance that is dissolved in a liquid to form a solution.
> - **Solution:** the liquid containing a dissolved substance.
> - **Solvent:** the liquid in which substances are dissolved to form a solution.
> - **Total volume:** the amount of a solution, including both solute and solvent.

amount, measured in liters, may have the same concentration of chemicals and therefore the same dilution. The phrase "make a dilution" often is seen in manufacturers' directions, and many dilutions are used in test procedures.

Specimens for manual blood cell counts require dilution in order to be seen under the microscope. Blood, serum, or plasma is diluted with chemical solutions to produce colored reactions that are measured by a colorimeter.

The concentration of a solution may be specified in one of two equivalent ways: as a ratio or as a percent. Ratios are used for dilutions. For example, a 1 to 10 (or 1:10 or $\frac{1}{10}$) dilution and a 10 percent solution both describe the same concentration. In either case, the amount of solute is represented by the numerator and the total volume of the solution, not the amount of solvent, is represented by the denominator.

Whenever a dilution is used to specify the concentration of a solution, the numerator is set equal to one. When a percent is used, the denominator is 100 units of volume. The numerator may be measured as weight for solids or volume for liquids in a percent but only as volume in a dilution ratio. Consider these two examples:

- 0.2 L of 100 percent bleach is diluted up to a total volume of 2 L. This is expressed as a 1:10 solution: $\frac{0.2}{2} = \frac{0.1}{1} = 0.1$.

- 0.20 gram of solute is diluted to a total volume of 2 mL. This is expressed as a 10 percent solution: $\frac{0.2}{2} = \frac{0.1}{1} = 10\%$.

Making Solutions

To calculate the amount of solute needed for a particular solution, you need to know the concentration and total volume required. Assume you are to prepare a 1:7 dilution with a total

> **Note**
>
> When making solutions and dilutions, always follow the manufacturer's instructions on the package insert. Using different methods may produce solutions with different concentrations and introduce error to test results. (See also Figure 3-3.)

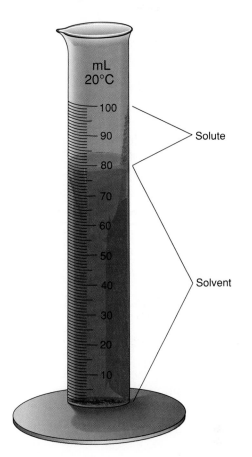

Figure 3-3 Directions for making the same solution may vary from one procedure to another and from one manufacturer to another. Twenty mL of solute added to 80 mL of solvent can be expressed as a dilution of 1:5; a ratio of 1:4, solute to solvent; or a 20 percent solution.

volume of 20 mL. Use this formula, in which the amount of solute required is represented by the letter x:

$$\frac{1}{7} = \frac{x}{20 \text{ mL}}$$

This equation means that the solution represented by $\frac{x}{20}$ mL has an unknown amount of solute, a total volume of 20 mL, and a concentration of 1:7.

To solve for x, or the amount of solute needed, you must change the equation so that x appears by itself on one side of the equal sign. Do this by multiplying both sides of the equation by 20 mL. Recall that to preserve equality, you must treat both sides of the equation equally.

$$x = \frac{20 \text{ mL}}{7}$$

Then, rewrite $\frac{20 \text{ mL}}{7}$ as a decimal by dividing 20 by 7:

$$x = 2.9 \text{ mL}$$

In words, 2.9 mL of solute are required to produce a 1:7 solution with a total volume 20 mL.

> **Note**
>
> When the solute and solvent are both liquids, they must be in the same units of measurement unless otherwise specified.

Making Dilutions

To dilute a solution from a stronger to a weaker one, use this formula:

$$C_1 \times V_1 = C_2 \times V_2$$

where,

C_1 = concentration of solution 1
V_1 = volume of solution 1
C_2 = concentration of solution 2
V_2 = volume of solution 2

Three out of the four factors in this formula must be known to solve for the fourth. Consider the following examples:

EXAMPLE 1: Determine how much 100 percent bleach is needed to make 500 mL of 10 percent bleach solution.

SOLUTION 1: Substituting in the above formula, you get

$$100\% \times V_1 = 10\% \times 500 \text{ mL}$$

Solve for V_1 by dividing both sides of the equation by 100%:

$$V_1 = \frac{10\%}{100\%} \times 500 \text{ mL}$$

Simplify the right side of the equation:

$$V_1 = 0.1 \times 500 \text{ mL, or } V_1 = 50 \text{ mL}$$

In words, 50 mL of 100 percent bleach are needed to make a 500 mL solution of 10 percent bleach.

EXAMPLE 2: Determine how much of a 1:10 solution is needed to make a 50 mL solution with a 1:50 concentration.

SOLUTION 2: For ease in calculation, first convert the ratios to percents:

$$1 : 10 = \frac{1}{10} = 0.10 = 10\%$$

$$1 : 50 = \frac{1}{50} = 0.02 = 2\%$$

Then substitute into the above formula:

$$10\% \times V_1 = 2\% \times 50 \text{ mL}$$

Solve for V_1:

$$V_1 = \frac{2\%}{10\%} \times 50 \text{ mL}$$

Simplify:

$$V_1 = 0.20 \times 50 \text{ mL, or } V_1 = 10 \text{ mL}$$

WHEN THINGS GO WRONG

Calculations in POLs must be accurate. Life or death decisions may depend upon them. You always should ask if the answers you calculate are logical and reasonable. For example, are the figures in the expected units and in the expected range? If not, check and recheck for errors. Misplaced decimal points are common errors that are easy to detect if you use common sense and good judgment.

Never proceed with calculations that you do not understand completely or that are producing illogical results. Use the following steps when you run into problems:

- Reread the instructions, several times if necessary.
- If the method still is unclear, look for an explanation in the appropriate POL manual or reference book or ask a qualified individual for assistance. Use diplomacy and follow the line of authority in your lab. Do not bypass your supervisor by getting information from an outside source.
- To be sure that you thoroughly understand the explanation, write it down, read it back, and see if it makes sense. Then enter the new information in the POL manual or your personal notebook so that you will be prepared the next time you do the procedure or calculation. Be sure to phrase the explanation in clear, understandable terms that you can decipher later.

PROCEDURE 3-1

Measuring and Mixing with Metric

Goal

After successfully completing this procedure, you will be able to use metric equipment to measure and to calculate and mix solutions.

Completion Time

30 minutes

Equipment and Supplies

- Metric ruler
- Colorimeter
- Sedimentation rate tube
- Suction device for pipettes
- Graduated flasks, cylinders, and pipettes in assorted sizes
- Scale
- Celsius thermometer
- Fahrenheit thermometer
- Paper clip
- Table salt (NaCl)
- Tap water (ice water, tepid water, and boiling water)
- Calculator
- Pen and paper

Instructions

Read through the list of equipment and supplies that you will need and the steps of the procedure. Be sure that you understand each step before you begin. Then complete each step correctly and in the proper order. If your completion time is too long, repeat the procedure until you increase your speed.

*Steps marked with (*) are critical and must have the maximum points to pass.

Performance Standards	Points Awarded	Maximum Points
1. Collect and prepare appropriate equipment.		10
2. Use the metric ruler to draw straight lines of 6, 10, 15, and 25 millimeters.		10
3. Reading the sedimentation rate tube from the top down, find these same markings, which are typical readings for erythrocyte sedimentation rates.		10
4. Inspect the colorimeter to see how wavelengths of light are designated and write the length of the shortest and longest wavelengths listed.		10
5. Convert the wavelength measurements into meters, using scientific notation. (*Possible answer:* 240 nanometers = 240×10^{-9} meters.)		20
6. Using the tap water and an appropriate flask, cylinder, or pipette, measure each of the following amounts. Always read the measurement at the bottom of the meniscus and use the suction device to pipette.		10
a. One liter in a cylinder—this amount of household bleach might be measured to prepare a dilution for general-purpose disinfecting in the lab.		5
b. One-half liter in a flask—this amount of reagent might be measured to prepare a dilution for patient tests.		5
c. One milliliter in a pipette—this amount of blood might be measured for a serological test.		5
d. One hundred microliters in a pipette—this amount of blood might be measured for a blood analyte.		5
7. Weigh samples of 1 and 10 grams of table salt.		10

—*table continued*

Performance Standards	Points Awarded	Maximum Points
8. Weigh a paper clip and record your answer in grams: _____		10
9. Place both thermometers in ice water and record their temperatures: C _____ ; F _____ *Caution:* Do not put thermometers directly into boiling water from ice water or vice versa—they may shatter.		10
10. Place both thermometers in tepid water and record their temperatures: C _____ ; F _____		10
11. Place both thermometers in boiling water and record their temperatures: C _____ ; F _____		10
12. Mix a 10 percent solution of table salt and tap water.		10
13. Mix a 1:10 dilution of table salt and tap water.		10
14. Discard the disposable equipment.		10
15. Wash the other equipment and return it to storage.		20
Total Points		**180**

Overall Procedural Evaluation

Student's Name _____

Signature of Instructor _____ Date _____

Comments _____

_____

chapter 3 REVIEW

Using Terminology

Match the terms in the right column with the appropriate definition in the left column.

_____ **1.** 1×10^{-16} a. concentration

_____ **2.** bottom of fraction   b. scientific notation

_____ **3.** one millionth   c. denominator

_____ **4.** one thousandth   d. diluent

_____ **5.** per 100   e. gram

_____ **6.** metric unit of length   f. liter

_____ **7.** metric unit of weight   g. meter

_____ **8.** metric unit of volume   h. milli-

_____ **9.** weakens solution   i. micro-

_____ **10.** strength   j. percent

Match the units of measurement in the left column with the correct abbreviation in the right column.

____ **11.** liter

____ **12.** kilogram

____ **13.** gram

____ **14.** microliter

____ **15.** milliliter

____ **16.** femtoliter

____ **17.** meter

____ **18.** millimeter

____ **19.** centimeter

a. cm

b. fL

c. g

d. kg

e. L

f. m

g. mL

h. mm

i. μ L

Using Terminology

Define the following terms in the spaces provided.

20. Concentrate _____

_____

_____

21. Diluent _____

_____

_____

22. Dilution _____

_____

_____

23. Solute _____

_____

_____

24. Solvent _____

_____

_____

25. Total volume _____

_____

_____

Acquiring Knowledge

Answer the following questions in the spaces provided.

26. What metric unit would you use to measure a person's body weight? The wavelengths of light? The POL disinfectant? A blood specimen?

_____

_____

_____

27. Arrange the following prefixes in order from large to small: deci-, kilo-, micro-, milli-, centi-, femto-. For each prefix, give the multiple or fraction that it represents.

_____

_____

_____

28. Change these dilutions to percent solutions: 1:8, 1:4, and 1:10.

_____

_____

_____

29. Convert the following measurements using dimensional analysis and the correct conversion factors.

0.002 gram to milligrams _____

0.000015 liter to milliliters _____

1.0×10^{-10} m to nanometers _____

110 pounds to kilograms _____

30. What equation is used to calculate a larger volume of a solution of the same strength? Which variable should be solved for?

_____

_____

_____

31. What equation is used to calculate a dilute solution from a concentrated solution?

_____

_____

_____

32. Why is it important to round off decimal fractions after multiplying or dividing?

_____

_____

_____

33. What general rules should be followed in rounding? Why?

_____

_____

_____

34. What fractions are the same as the following powers of 10: 10^{-2}; 10^{-3}?

_____

_____

_____

35. What is the best way to learn and become comfortable with the metric system?

_____

_____

_____

36. What is the easiest way to add the following fractions: $\frac{1}{2}, \frac{1}{4}, \frac{1}{10}, \frac{1}{20}$, and $\frac{1}{25}$? What is their sum?

_____

_____

_____

37. Which of the systems, English or metric, is the most accurate, especially for small amounts? Why?

_____

_____

_____

38. What are the three original basic units in the metric system? What does each measure? How are prefixes used with them?

_____

_____

_____

39. How can a more dilute solution be made from a concentrated solution?

_____

_____

_____

Applying Knowledge—On the Job

Answer the following questions in the spaces provided.

40. A test often performed in POLs is an erythrocyte sedimentation rate (ESR). It measures the tendency of red cells to settle together at the bottom of a column of blood. While it is not specific for any one disorder, it gives valuable information when combined with a patient's physical symptoms. Patient A had an erythrocyte sedimentation rate (ESR) of 39 mm/hr. Patient B had an ESR of 9 mm/hr. What does the unit "mm" signify? What is each patient's rate in meters? What is the difference in their rates? Use your school library or your own reference books to determine which patient's result is normal and which is abnormal.

_____

_____

_____

41. Mr. Dugal had a reticulocyte count that resulted in 4 reticulocytes for 500 red blood cells (RBC). Using the following formula, calculate the percent of reticulocytes on the stained blood smear:

$$\text{Percent retic.} = \frac{\text{Number of reticulocytes counted} \times 100}{\text{Number of RBC counted}}$$

_____

_____

_____

42. A while ago, your laboratory supervisor assigned you the task of calibrating the spectrophotometer with a new batch of reagents. She went through the procedure with you and you understood it at the time. The old batch of reagents is almost gone, and the supervisor has reminded you that it is time to recalibrate. You feel a little shaky about the task. What should you do?

_____

_____

_____

43. You have calculated a patient's data with a test formula. The answer you get for the patient's test result is abnormal. It is a very busy day. What should you do?

_____

_____

_____

44. In the POL where you work, you have been asked to give a tour to a group of students. You are to explain to them why the POL relies solely on metric measurements. What should you say?

_____

_____

_____

45. You have been instructed to take a blood sample from an infant for a microbilirubin test. The pipette measures a very small amount. You will use a heel stick to obtain the specimen. What metric unit will you use to measure the amount of blood collected?

_____

_____

_____

ADDITIONAL MATH PRACTICE

Fractions

Perform the given operations on the following fractions.

1. $\frac{1}{2} + \frac{1}{2} =$ _____

2. $\frac{3}{8} + \frac{1}{2} + \frac{1}{4} =$ _____

3. $\frac{1}{3} + \frac{1}{2} =$ _____

4. $2\frac{1}{2} + 3\frac{1}{3} =$ _____

5. $\frac{3}{16} + 3\frac{1}{8} + 1\frac{3}{4} =$ _____

6. $\frac{1}{2} - \frac{1}{8} =$ _____

7. $\frac{4}{5} - \frac{7}{15} =$ _____

8. $2\frac{1}{2} - \frac{3}{8} =$ _____

9. $\frac{6}{10} - \frac{3}{10} =$ _____

10. $1\frac{7}{8} - \frac{2}{5} =$ _____

11. $\frac{1}{2} \times \frac{1}{3} =$ _____

12. $\frac{3}{7} \times \frac{1}{2} =$ _____

13. $\frac{7}{8} \times \frac{2}{8} =$ _____

14. $\frac{5}{6} \times \frac{2}{3} =$ _____

15. $\frac{4}{5} \times \frac{2}{5} =$ _____

16. $\frac{1}{2} \div \frac{1}{2} =$ _____

17. $\frac{2}{3} \div \frac{1}{16} =$ _____

18. $\frac{1}{2} \div \frac{1}{4} =$ _____

19. $\frac{1}{3} \div \frac{7}{9} =$ _____

20. $\frac{3}{8} \div \frac{1}{2} =$ _____

Convert the fractions to decimals.

21. $\frac{85}{210} =$ _____

22. $\frac{79}{105} =$ _____

23. $\frac{3}{66} =$ _____

24. $\frac{2}{45} =$ _____

25. $\frac{1}{5} =$ _____

Decimals

Convert to scientific notation.

26. $0.00000045 =$ _____

27. $450,000,000 =$ _____

28. $0.000012 =$ _____

29. $8,000 =$ _____

30. $0.04 =$ _____

Convert to percentage.

31. $0.002 = $ _____

32. $0.99 = $ _____

33. $0.50 = $ _____

34. $0.12 = $ _____

35. $\frac{1}{5} = $ _____

Dimensional Analysis

Convert units using dimensional analysis.

36. 23 pounds to kg _____

37. 130 pounds to kg _____

38. 61 pounds to kg _____

39. 200 pounds to kg _____

40. 0.25 L to mL _____

41. 1.3 mL to L _____

42. 500 mL to L _____

43. 100 mL to L _____

44. 250 mg to g _____

45. 0.08 g to mg _____

46. 0.1 mg to g _____

47. 40 µL to mL _____

48. 1×10^{-4} L to µL _____

49. 2.5×10^{-5} L to µL _____

50. 1.0×10^{8} pm to m _____

51. 875 nm to m _____

52. 425 nm to m _____

53. $\frac{1}{5}$ g to mg _____

54. $\frac{1}{2}$ inch to cm _____

55. 6.5 cm to inches _____

Solutions and Dilutions

Prepare the following solutions and dilutions.

56. 1000 mL of 15% bleach solution _____

57. 500 mL of 1:5 _____

58. 750 mL of 1:10 _____

59. 1 L of 10% solution from a 50% solution _____

60. 0.50 L of 5% solution from a 10% solution _____

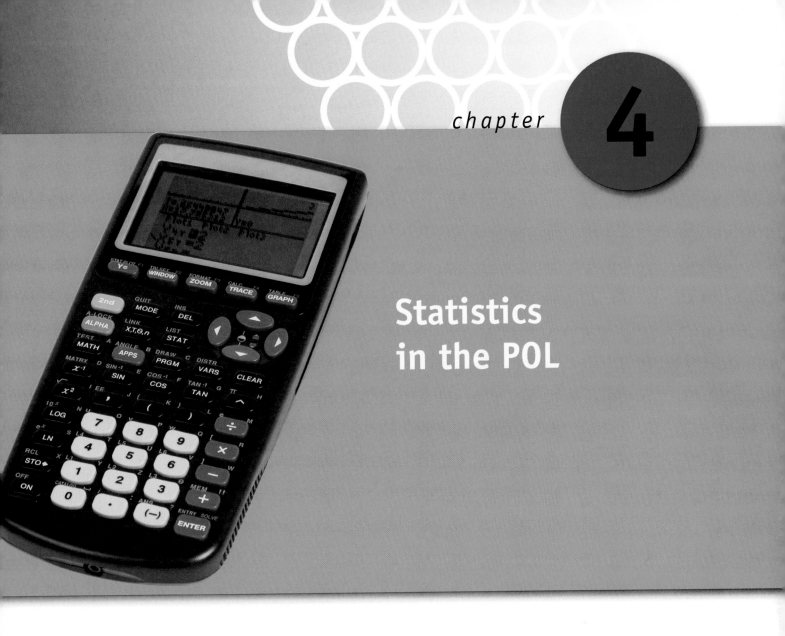

chapter **4**

Statistics
in the POL

COGNITIVE OBJECTIVES

After studying this chapter, you should be able to

4.1   use each of the vocabulary terms appropriately.

4.2   differentiate mean, mode, median, and range.

4.3   explain why the mean is the preferred measure of location.

4.4   explain how the standard deviation is used to assess variation within a sample of test results.

4.5   discuss how the coefficient of variation can be used to assess precision and accuracy of procedures and instruments.

PERFORMANCE OBJECTIVES

After studying this chapter, you should be able to

4.6   calculate the mean, standard deviation, and coefficient of variation for a sample of test results.

4.7   assess which of two procedures or instruments is more accurate based on their coefficients of variation.

TERMINOLOGY

coefficient of variation (CV): also called the relative standard deviation; the standard deviation expressed as a percent of the mean.

index: the small i under the summation sign. The index indicates the range over which the summation is to be performed.

mean: the arithmetic average of a sample of values.

median: the middle value in an ordered sample of values, with the same number of values below and above it.

mode: the value that occurs most often in a sample.

range: the difference between the largest and smallest values in a sample.

sigma (Σ, σ): the eighteenth letter in the Greek alphabet; used in statistics to represent the standard deviation (lowercase, σ) or summation (uppercase, Σ).

standard deviation (s or σ): a measurement of the variation from the mean in a sample of values.

statistics: the branch of mathematics that deals with the collection, analysis, and interpretation of numerical data.

summation: represented by uppercase sigma, Σ; indicates addition of the numbers or variables that follow.

INTRODUCTION

Statistics is one of the most important mathematical tools used in science and medicine to collect and analyze data. Medical laboratories, small and large, rely heavily on statistics to organize and compare data. This allows labs to classify test results and assess the accuracy of test controls and patient tests.

This chapter introduces you to three of the most widely used statistical measures in laboratories: the mean, the standard deviation, and the coefficient of variation. Although you will learn how to calculate these important measures, when doing statistical calculations of laboratory data you should use a scientific calculator or computer software to save time and effort and reduce the chance of errors. Many manufacturers of laboratory testing instruments have incorporated programs that perform statistical analysis to attain the mean, standard deviation, and coefficient of variation.

THE SUMMATION SIGN, Σ

In order to understand the statistical formulas in this chapter, you need to be familiar with the **summation** sign, Σ, which is the Greek letter **sigma.** The summation sign tells you to add the numbers or variables that follow it. To add the numbers 1 through 4, for example, write

$$\sum_{i=1}^{4} i = 1 + 2 + 3 + 4 = 10$$

The small i under the summation sign is called the **index.** The small numbers, 1 and 4, indicate the **range** over which summation is to be performed. Most often, the index starts with 0 or 1, but it may start at any number. Consider these additional examples:

$$\sum_{i=2}^{4} (3 + i) = (3 + 2) + (3 + 3)(3 + 4) = 18$$

$$\sum_{i=0}^{3} 2^i = 2^0 + 2^1 + 2^2 + 2^3 = 15$$

The index often is used to distinguish numbers in a set of numbers, such as in a sample of test results. Then, it is written as a subscript, x_i, read "x sub-i." When $i = 1$, $x_i = x_1$, the first number in the sample. Assume that in a sample of test results, the first test had a result of 23, the second had a result of 14, the third had a result of 5, the fourth had a result of 2, and the fifth had a result of 10. This is written

$$x = (23, 14, 5, 2, 10)$$

For this sample, x_1 refers to 23, x_2 refers to 14, and so on.

To calculate basic statistical measures like the mean for any sample, such as this one, first add up the test results. Represent addition of the numbers in this sample as

$$\sum_{i=1}^{5} x_i = 23 + 14 + 5 + 2 + 10 = 54$$

MEASURES OF LOCATION

To interpret any set of test results, first figure a statistic of location or central tendency, which is a single representative value that describes the entire sample. A measure of location gives a general sense of where the results fall. There are three such measures: the mode, the median, and the mean. The **mode** is the test result that occurs most often, such as 5 in the set 3, 4, 5, 5, 6, 7. The

median is the value that falls in the middle of all of the values obtained, which is again 5 in the set 3, 4, 5, 5, 6, 7. The **mean** is the arithmetic average, calculated by summing all of the individual test results and dividing by the number of tests. The symbol for the mean is $\bar{x}$, read "x bar," and the formula for the mean is

$$\bar{x} = \frac{\sum_{i=1}^{n} x_i}{n}$$

where,

n = the number of observations in the set

x_i = the individual observations

Returning to the set of values 3, 4, 5, 5, 6, 7, calculate the mean as

$$\bar{x} = \frac{(3 + 4 + 5 + 5 + 6 + 7)}{6} = \frac{30}{6} = 5$$

In this example, the mode, median, and mean are the same, but this is not always the case. Consider an actual example. In a series of blood glucose tests, the readings were 60, 90, 90, 91, 92, 93, and 94. The mode is 90, the median is 91, and the mean is 87. Because the mean weights all of the values equally, it is pulled down by the lowest value of 60. The mode and median, on the other hand, are unaffected by the extremely low-end value. For this reason, the mean usually is the preferred measure of location for describing test results in POLs.

MEASURES OF DISPERSION

To adequately describe a sample of test results, you need more than just the mean because the mean does not tell much about the distribution of a sample; that is, the mean does not tell how the results are spread around it. Compare the following hypothetical samples of blood glucose test results:

SAMPLE 1: 87, 88, 89, 90, 90, 91, 92, 93
SAMPLE 2: 80, 80, 81, 85, 95, 99, 100, 100

Both samples have the same mean, 90, but the test values have very different distributions. The values for the first sample are bunched around the mean, while the values for the second sample are much more spread out. A measure of dispersion describes each sample and reflects this difference in distribution. Measures of dispersion are important in POLs for evaluating procedures and instruments. The more variation in test results, the less accurate and less precise the results are likely to be.

Range

The simplest measure of the dispersion is the range, the difference between the largest and smallest values in the sample. The problem is that the range depends solely on two observations. An unusually extreme value can greatly influence the results. A better measure of dispersion uses all of the observations and therefore is less sensitive to one or two values. The standard deviation fits the bill.

Standard Deviation

The **standard deviation (s or σ)** is the most frequently used statistical measure for describing the dispersion of a sample around its mean.

> **Note**
>
> The abbreviation for standard deviation is not standardized. SD, S.D., sd, *s*, and σ are used as abbreviations for standard deviation.

The standard deviation is calculated as the average difference of each of the observations from the mean value. Generally speaking, the larger the standard deviation, the greater the spread of values around the mean, or the greater the sample's variability. The formula for the standard deviation is

$$s = \sqrt{\frac{\sum_{i=1}^{n} (x_i - \bar{x})^2}{n - 1}}$$

> **Note**
>
> In calculating the standard deviation, divide by $n - 1$ instead of n. This is due to a statistical artifact, the explanation of which is beyond the scope of this book.

In other words, the formula for the standard deviation tells you first to find the difference between each observation and the mean. Some of the differences will be negative and some will be positive. In fact, the negative and positive differences will cancel each other out. To avoid this, square the differences because any number squared, even a negative one, is positive.

Then add the squared differences and divide by the number of observations minus one to find the average squared difference. Finally, take the square root to return the answer to the original units of measurement. For ease in calculation, the formula for standard deviation is often written as

$$ s = \sqrt{\dfrac{\sum\limits_{i=1}^{n} x_i^2 - \dfrac{\left(\sum\limits_{i=1}^{n} x_i\right)^2}{n}}{n-1}} $$

Work through the following example to be sure that you understand how to calculate the standard deviation:

$$ x_i = (3, 5, 7, 12) $$

$$ \sum_{i=1}^{n} x_i = 3 + 5 + 7 + 2 = 17 $$

$$ \left(\sum_{i=1}^{n} x_i\right)^2 = (17)^2 = 289 $$

$$ \sum_{i=1}^{n} x_i^2 = 3^2 + 5^2 + 7^2 + 2^2 $$
$$ = 9 + 25 + 49 + 4 = 87 $$

$$ s = \sqrt{\dfrac{87 - \dfrac{289}{4}}{3}} = \sqrt{\dfrac{87 - 72.25}{3}} = \sqrt{\dfrac{14.75}{3}} $$

$$ = \sqrt{4.9167} = 2.2 $$

> **Note**
>
> Microsoft Excel™ spreadsheet program offers functions to calculate the sum (Σ), the mean (average), and the standard deviation.

Graphing scientific calculators include statistical functions such as the mean and standard deviation. If your calculator has these functions, the manual will explain how to use them. The standard deviation also can be estimated from the range if the sample contains between 20 and 40 observations, using the formula:

$$ s = \dfrac{\text{range}}{4} $$

The standard deviation is used to set limits on the range of values within which test results are considered to be normal. Most often, test results that fall within two standard deviations on either side of the mean ($\bar{x} \pm 2s$) are considered to be close enough to the mean to be normal. This use of standard deviation is explained more fully in Chapter 5.

Coefficient of Variation

Both the mean and the standard deviation are measured in centimeters, grams, degrees, or whatever units are used to measure the original data. For most situations, the original units are the most convenient and meaningful to work with. However, a problem arises when you wish to compare the amount of variation in two samples that are measured in different units or that have very different means. A 2 mm standard deviation is much more important when the mean is 4 mm, for example, than when the mean is 4 cm. A measure of dispersion must take into account differences in mean values and units of measurement among different samples.

One such measure is the **coefficient of variation (CV)**, also called the relative standard deviation. The coefficient of variation is the standard deviation relative to the mean for the same sample. It is calculated as follows:

$$ CV = \dfrac{s}{\bar{X}} \times 100 $$

The coefficient of variation is expressed as a percent and is unitless. It is just a number. The units in the mean and standard deviation cancel each other when they are divided. Because the coefficient of variation has been standardized for the mean, any two coefficients of variation can be compared meaningfully, even when they represent samples with very different means.

The coefficient of variation is used commonly in POLs as a measure of precision. It may be used to check the precision of two different methods for the same substances, or it may be used to check the precision of a given procedure using two different instruments. Most manufacturers of lab instruments provide the coefficient of variation of their instruments compared with instruments from other manufacturers. In general, the larger the coefficient, the poorer the precision; the smaller the coefficient, the greater the precision. Consider the following example:

METHOD 1: Mean = 100 mg/dL; s = 2.4 mg/dL
METHOD 2: Mean = 92 mg/dL; s = 2.8 mg/dL

Which method produces results with less variation; that is, which method is more precise? Compare the coefficient of variation for each sample:

METHOD 1: $CV = \dfrac{2.4}{100} \times 100 = 2.4\%$

METHOD 2: $CV = \dfrac{2.8}{92} \times 100 = 3.0\%$

Method 1 has a smaller coefficient of variation. Because it produces less variation, it is more precise.

PROCEDURE 4-1

Computing the Mean, Mode, Range, Standard Deviation, and Coefficient of Variation with a Calculator

Goal

After successfully completing this procedure, you will be able to use a calculator to compute the mean, the mode, the range, the standard deviation, and the coefficient of variation for any small sample of test results.

Completion Time

30 minutes

Equipment and Supplies

- Statistical function calculator
- Calculator manual
- Pen or pencil

Data

The following results were obtained in repeated tests on a control specimen in the POL:

78 82 89 91 88 89 95 75 88 93
93 86 78 89 90 91 92 92 94 95

Instructions

Read through the list of equipment and supplies that you will need and the steps of the procedure. Be sure that you understand each step before you begin. Then complete each step correctly and in the proper order. If your completion time is too long, repeat the procedure until you increase your speed.

Select a partner to work with on this procedure. Each of you should do the calculations independently and then check your answers against each other's. If there are discrepancies, work through the calculations together to find the error. If necessary, ask your instructor for assistance.

*Steps marked with (*) are critical and must have the maximum points to pass.

Performance Standards	Points Awarded	Maximum Points
1. Familiarize yourself with the mean and standard deviation functions on your calculator. Refer to the manual if necessary.		5
2. Enter the data on the calculator. Be sure that the calculator is in the statistical mode.		10
3. Following the steps outlined in the calculator manual, compute the sample mean.		10
4. Following the steps outlined in the calculator manual, compute the standard deviation.		10
5. Calculate the range of the sample by subtracting the lowest value from the highest value.		10
6. Estimate the standard deviation from the range using the formula $s = \dfrac{\text{Range}}{4}$ (applicable because n is between 20 and 40).		10
7. Determine the mode of the sample.		5
8. Calculate the coefficient of variation (CV) using the formula $CV = \dfrac{s}{\bar{x}} \times 100$		5
Total Points		**65**

Overall Procedural Evaluation

Student's Name _____

Signature of Instructor _____ Date _____

Comments _____

_____

chapter 4 REVIEW

Using Terminology

Define the following terms in the spaces provided.

1. Mode _____

   _____

2. Coefficient of variation (*CV*) _____

   _____

3. Median _____

   _____

4. Index _____

   _____

5. Sigma (Σ, σ) _____

   _____

6. Mean _____

   _____

7. Summation _____

   _____

8. Range _____

   _____

9. Standard deviation (*s* or σ) _____

   _____

10. Statistics _____

    _____

Acquiring Knowledge

Answer the following questions in the spaces provided.

11. When a test result falls more than two standard deviations from the mean, how should you interpret it?

    _____

    _____

12. What term tells you where the middle of a set of samples falls?

    _____

    _____

13. Calculate the range of the following samples: 88.3, 88.9, 88.9, 88.2, 98.1, 93.3, 98.2.

    _____

    _____

    _____

14. What two values must you calculate in order to set limits for the normal range of test results?

_____

_____

_____

15. What is sigma? What does it mean in statistics?

_____

_____

_____

16. How is the mean represented? How is it calculated? What is the math symbol for the term *mean?*

_____

_____

_____

17. Why is the range not used to measure variation of test results in POLs?

_____

_____

_____

18. What units are used for the mean and standard deviation?

_____

_____

_____

19. What is the formula for the coefficient of variation?

_____

_____

_____

20. What is the purpose of calculating the coefficient of variation?

_____

_____

_____

21. What is another term for the coefficient of variation?

_____

_____

_____

22. In what mathematical measurement is the coefficient of variation reported in the laboratory?

_____

_____

_____

23. What do these symbols mean? Σ; n; $\overline{x}$; $\sqrt{\ }$

_____

_____

_____

Match the terms in the right column with the appropriate definition in the left column.

_____ **24.** x bar ($\overline{x}$)   a. mean

_____ **25.** relative standard deviation   b. mode

_____ **26.** middle value   c. sigma

_____ **27.** Greek letter   d. three standard deviations

_____ **28.** large variation   e. statistics

_____ **29.** data analysis   f. median

_____ **30.** most frequent   g. CV

Applying Knowledge—On the Job

Answer the following questions in the spaces provided.

31. Your laboratory supervisor has assigned you the task of calculating the mean, standard deviation, and coefficient of variation for a new procedure being considered as a replacement for an older, more complicated procedure. You have not done these calculations in a long time, and you are not sure that you remember how to do them. What should you do?

_____

_____

_____

32. Anne, a coworker in the POL, says that she sees no point in doing the extra work of calculating coefficients of variation. "Why not just compare standard deviations?" she asks. Explain to Anne why comparing coefficients of variation is more valid than is comparing standard deviations.

_____

_____

_____

33. A novice coworker in your POL is having trouble understanding standard deviation. He cannot understand how the working formula for standard deviation can give the same result as the "regular" formula. How would you explain it to him?

_____

_____

_____

34. Your lab supervisor has given you the following two samples of test results and asked you to find the coefficient of variation for each. Without working through the calculations, show how you would set up the problem.

SAMPLE 1: 98, 99, 88, 85, 93, 96
SAMPLE 2: 79, 84, 86, 90, 91, 80

_____

_____

_____

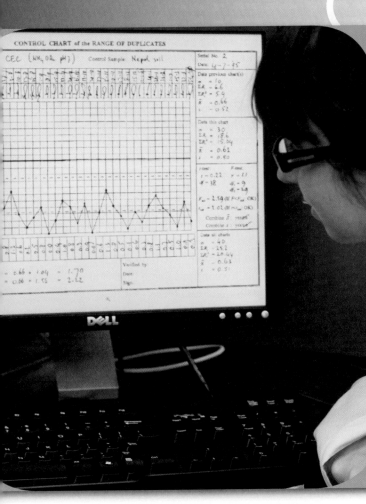

Quality Assurance and Quality Control

COGNITIVE OBJECTIVES

After studying this chapter, you should be able to

5.1   use each of the vocabulary terms appropriately.

5.2   discuss why accurate laboratory test results are necessary for quality patient treatment.

5.3   describe how accuracy in patient test results is enhanced by continuous comparisons to known standards.

5.4   describe CLIA.

5.5   explain the significance of CLIA in the clinical lab.

5.6   discuss the legal requirements of CLIA.

5.7   describe quality assessment and its role in the clinical laboratory.

5.8   describe standard deviation and its importance in the laboratory.

5.9   describe the role of statistics in evaluation quality control.

5.10   define normal ranges and describe their importance in interpreting test results.

PERFORMANCE OBJECTIVES

After studying this chapter, you should be able to

5.11   show how information is compiled in POLs to satisfy legal requirements.

5.12   calculate the mean, standard deviation, and upper and lower limits of acceptability for quality control test results.

TERMINOLOGY

accuracy: how close a test result comes to the true value of the substance being measured. Asks the question—are the results correct?

analyte: a substance that is tested for in a laboratory procedure for its presence or quantity in a patient or quality control specimen.

bias: the skewing of test results away from the true value.

calibration: the testing and adjustment of an instrument to establish that the results reported by the test reflect the actual concentration of the sample.

calibration verification: testing calibrators (known substances) in the same manner as patient specimens to ensure the accuracy of the results throughout the reportable range.

calibrator: a known solution of an analyte obtained from a manufacturer or professional organization and used as a measuring stick to set instruments to read test results correctly. Calibrators are used during calibration procedures.

Certificate for Provider-Performed Microscopy Procedures (PPMP): a certificate issued to a laboratory in which a physician, midlevel practitioner, or dentist performs only microscopy procedures. This certificate permits the laboratory to also perform waived tests.

Certificate of Accreditation: a certificate issued to a laboratory on the basis of the laboratory's accreditation by an accreditation organization approved by the Health Care Financing Administration (HCFA).

Certificate of Compliance: a certificate issued to a laboratory after an inspection finds the laboratory to be in compliance with all applicable CLIA requirements.

Certificate of Registration: a certificate issued to a laboratory that enables the entity to conduct moderate or high-complexity laboratory testing or both until the entity is determined by survey to be in compliance with the CLIA regulations.

Certificate of Waiver: certificate that allows a laboratory to only perform waived tests.

control: a sample used to maintain accuracy and quality in a procedure. Its concentration is known within very accurate limits and its variability is ascertained by the manufacturer. It is used as part of daily quality control procedures.

in-control: a phrase used to indicate that the quality system that measures the accuracy of a procedure is within acceptable limits.

Levey-Jennings chart: a chart on which control values are plotted daily. It is divided into areas of acceptable, low, and high values, enabling lab workers to easily assess the normalcy of test results.

linearity: a measure of an instrument's ability to measure test results in an accurate manner. Test results plotted in a straight line on a graph indicate accuracy.

nonwaived tests: tests with more complicated steps and procedures in which the risk of erroneous results is higher. Previously defined as "moderate" or "high-complexity" tests.

out-of-control: the description given to a quality system when test results are beyond the upper or lower limits of the accepted range or when they are on only one side of the mean, showing a shift or trend pattern.

precision: the ability to repeatedly get the same result.

primary standard: a quality control sample that is of the highest possible quality and accuracy.

proficiency testing: a component of the quality control system that tests the accuracy of laboratory procedures and staff.

quality assessment: a set of policies implemented to give patients the very best medical care possible. Quality assessment covers every aspect of medical care.

quality control (QC): any measure that ensures consistent laboratory procedures and accurate test results.

quality system: all of the laboratory's policies, processes, procedures, and resources needed to achieve quality testing.

random error: unpredictable error with no obvious pattern.

reference range: also called normal, or expected, values. The range of values that are expected in a healthy person. About 95 percent of normal, healthy individuals will test in this range.

reliability: the accuracy and precision of a testing procedure or instrument.

reproducibility: the ability to repeat test results.

secondary standard: a quality control sample that is developed in comparison with a primary standard.

standard: a rule by which test results are measured; a quality control sample manufactured and analyzed to very exact measurements.

standard deviation (s or σ): a measurement of the variation from the mean in a sample of values.

systematic error: a noticeable pattern of errors.

target value: the value given by the manufacturer of a quality control sample as the expected quality control result.

true value or gold standard: the value for a test result that is based on the results obtained from the best qualified laboratories using the purest reagents, the most refined methods, and the best technology.

validity: ability of a test to correctly determine those who have a disease or condition and those patients who do not have the disease or condition.

variability: the tendency for objects and procedures to change, or deviate, from their original state or from some standard.

waived test: defined by CLIA as "simple laboratory examination and procedures that have an insignificant risk of erroneous results."

INTRODUCTION

Every day, patients and physicians rely on laboratory test results to guide diagnosis and treatment of disease. It is the awesome responsibility of laboratory professionals to ensure that the test results reported are accurate test results. This chapter reviews quality assessment—the systems that ensure patients are receiving the highest level of health care possible, as well as the statistical methods utilized to evaluate quality control systems.

Quality Assessment

Quality assessment is the pledge of health professionals to work to achieve the highest degree of excellence in the health care given to every patient. It includes all aspects of health care, from the best possible clinical treatment to accurate financial billing.

There are three major aspects of quality assessment.

1. Constant and ongoing monitoring and review of all tests to ensure errors and potential problems are identified.
2. Taking corrective action when errors or potential problems are identified.
3. Evaluating the corrective action to ensure they will prevent future problems.

VARIABILITY

Unfortunately, variability is an innate part of laboratory testing as it is of any scientific research. **Variability** is the tendency for objects and procedures to change or deviate from their original state or from some **standard.** Variability in labs refers mainly to variability in test results. The same test done on the same patient on different days, for example, can show variable results. The reasons could range from changes in the state of the patient to differences in the skill of lab personnel.

Consider something as simple as taking a blood pressure reading. Several factors may vary in taking a blood pressure reading from one time to another. Factors that contribute to the variability include the sphygmomanometer and its accuracy, the patient's physical and emotional state, and the hearing acuity and training of the individual taking the blood pressure reading.

Clinical test procedures are affected by a variety of patient and testing factors. Test results for glucose levels, for example, may vary greatly because of patient diet. A fasting specimen of blood glucose will give a very different reading than a glucose level measured 30 minutes after eating a sugary dessert. The test result also is affected by the manner in which the blood was collected and processed prior to testing. A blood glucose determination on whole blood may be falsely low if collected by a capillary tube from a cut that was not bleeding freely. If the glucose determination is on plasma, the plasma must be separated from the red cells soon after collection. Otherwise, red cells that are still alive may deplete the plasma glucose, using it for food. A urine glucose determination may be falsely low due to outside bacterial contamination occurring at collection or afterward because bacteria digest urine glucose for food.

For many different lab tests, variation in temperature of the testing instruments and the room where the test is performed may affect test results. Worn or failing instrument parts can be a major source of variation in readings. Worker error and contaminated or decomposed reagents and standards also can affect results.

The role of a **quality control (QC)** program is to monitor such variability in test results, assessing whether the degree of variability is too great to be acceptable. An "acceptable" degree of variation can be attributed to random factors, such as the health care worker's hearing acuity in the case of blood pressure, that are not clinically significant in producing the results.

To assess the variability of patient test results, you first need to know the **true value** (or **gold standard**) for the control test you are monitoring.

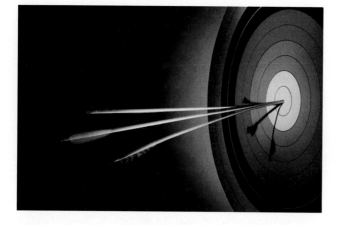

Figure 5-1 The goal of quality laboratory testing is to find the true value, similar to shooting an arrow into the center of a bull's eye.

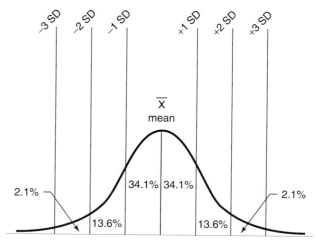

Figure 5-2 Normal distribution. The bell-shaped curve shows the ideal, or expected, distribution of test results from a single lot of control serum.

The true value is based on the results obtained from the best qualified laboratories using the purest reagents, the most refined methods, and the best technology. An accurate result of a test on a control is one that is in agreement with the true value. A quality lab test will control for variability with **precision** and **accuracy.** Precision is the ability to get the same result repeatedly and accuracy is the ability to obtain the correct, target value. (See Figure 5-1.)

The question that you must answer is how much variation away from the true value can be allowed without negatively affecting patient treatment. A variation in a red blood cell count, for example, of a few cells will not affect patient care. But how much variation will? The permissible variation from the true value must be defined.

THE STATISTICAL BASIS OF QUALITY CONTROL

The answer to the question of how much variability is acceptable lies with statistics. For any given test or procedure, you can use statistics to predict, with a given likelihood, the range of variation within which most results from multiple analyses of one control test sample will fall. Variability within this range can largely be ignored. Such test results are said to be **in-control,** that is, within a range of accuracy that permits physicians to use them in making a proper diagnosis and treatment decision. Test results outside of this range are said to be **out-of-control.**

The **standard deviation (s or σ)** is a summary measure that describes the extent to which the values are scattered around the mean. If control test

results vary only randomly, then they should show a normal distribution. If you plotted the number of times each value resulted when the control test was performed, you would get a bell-shaped curve (see Figure 5-2). This is the ideal, which is only likely in a very large number of repetitions of the test. For a normally distributed sample of test results, one standard deviation on both sides of the mean incorporates about 99 percent of test results. About 95 percent of test results fall within two standard deviations around the mean, and about 68 percent fall within three standard deviations around the mean.

The standard deviation can be used to establish an acceptable range of values around the mean. Control test results falling within this range are considered by the manufacturer or reference laboratory to be near enough to the mean to be useful for clinical purposes. A lab also may compute its own acceptable control test range using the standard deviation formula.

The acceptable **reference range** of values is usually considered to be the range between two standard deviations above and two standard deviations below the mean value ($\bar{x} \pm 2s$). Note that this use of the term *range* is different from its use as the difference between the highest and lowest values in a sample. Values within this range are referred to as *reference values*. Most healthy individuals will have test results within the range of reference values. Keep in mind, however, that age, gender, activity levels, and other factors may have a profound effect on an individual's test result and whether or not it falls within the range of reference values.

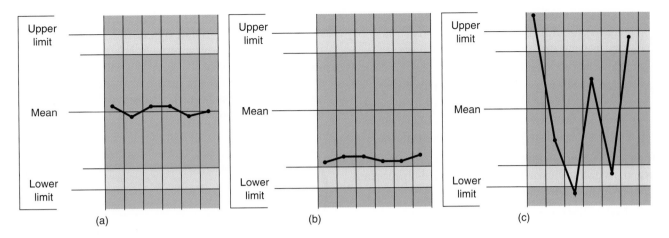

Figure 5-3 The concepts of accuracy, precision, and bias are demonstrated by the first two examples of daily quality control test results plotted on Levey-Jennings charts. (a) The quality control daily test results have close proximity to the desired mean value. They show both accuracy and precision. (b) The test results are all far below the mean and are therefore inaccurate. However, they are precise because there is little variation. (c) Extreme variability indicates that the test results are both inaccurate and imprecise. The values range out-of-control from above the upper limit to below the lower limit.

> **Reminder**
>
> The abbreviation for standard deviation is not standardized. SD, S.D., sd, *s*, and σ are used as abbreviations for standard deviation.

Other Statistical Concepts Related to Quality Control

Precision, bias, reliability, and reproducibility are other important concepts related to quality control. Precision is the closeness of test results from multiple analyses of the same sample. While accurate results are always precise, there may be precision without accuracy. This would occur, for example, if faulty equipment or improper technique led to a consistent overestimate or underestimate of the true value of a test. All of the test results would be inaccurate, but they still would be precise if they were close in value. This is an example of **bias,** which is the skewing of test results away from the true value. Bias, a measure of the amount of inaccuracy of a procedure, is apparent when values repeatedly fall on only one side of the mean of the quality control values. Potential causes of bias include contaminated controls and weak reagents. Figure 5-3 illustrates the concepts of precision and bias. When test results show extreme variability, they are both inaccurate and imprecise.

Reliability is the accuracy and precision of a testing procedure or instrument. It is closely related to **reproducibility,** the ability to repeat test results. Reproducibility is one of the most important attributes of a clinical procedure. Without reproducibility, the data are useless because they cannot be trusted.

QUALITY SYSTEM

POLs play a vital part in quality assessment because patient treatment is often based on or reinforced by results of laboratory tests. To achieve the valid or correct test results, a system of monitoring the laboratory, known as **quality systems,** has been developed. Quality control measures ensure consistent laboratory procedures and accurate test results. Quality system measures also provide laboratory personnel with an early warning of developing problems.

Without quality systems, laboratory error is difficult to detect unless physicians notice test results are inconsistent with the patient's history or clinical condition. Undetected lab errors may harm patients by delaying appropriate treatment or leading to inappropriate treatment. The result could aggravate the patient's condition, resulting in unnecessary time off from work, hospitalization, and/or a malpractice suit.

General guidelines for maintaining an effective quality system include

- **calibration,** or standardization, of instruments at least every six months and as recommended by the manufacturer.
- daily testing of control samples.

- proficiency testing of lab personnel at least every three months or more frequently as required by individual state requirements.
- accurate record keeping.
- correct patient preparation, such as fasting.
- proper specimen handling, including collection, identification, and preparation, as well as elimination of specimens unsuitable for analysis.

Even with a good quality system, errors may still occur. When an error is discovered, it is important to take immediate action by

- discontinuing patient testing for that procedure until the cause of the problem has been identified.
- investigating what, if any, erroneous results have been reported for other patients and notifying the physicians who received an erroneous report.
- documenting all of the steps taken to correct the problem and prove that the problem has been fixed (for example, showing that daily controls are within acceptable limits prior to resuming patient testing).

Legal Requirements

The Clinical Laboratory Improvement Amendment of 1988, CLIA 1988, mandates that all laboratories meet acceptable standards of quality. Test results of patients and quality controls must be recorded daily and must be kept on file for inspection. Laboratories also must enroll in an approved **proficiency testing** program and receive unknown samples for analysis every three months. These samples are tested and the results are sent back to the administering agency. The test results are then compared to those of other laboratories using the same methodology. To pass proficiency testing requirements, a laboratory must achieve results that fall within an accepted value range.

Waived versus Nonwaived Tests

CLIA defines all laboratory tests as either **waived,** "simple laboratory examinations and procedures that have an insignificant risk of erroneous result," or **nonwaived,** tests with more complicated steps and procedures in which the risk of erroneous results is higher. Nonwaived tests were previously referred to as moderate or high-complexity tests.

It is important to know whether the tests you are performing are classified as waived or nonwaived. This information can be determined by reviewing

the Federal Food and Drug Administration (FDA) Web site. Tests are listed by analyte at http://www.accessdata.fda.gov/scripts/cdrh/cfdocs/cfClia/analyteswaived.cfm.

You also can sort the tests by test name system at http://www.accessdata.fda.gov/scripts/cdrh.cfdocs/cfClia/testswaived.cfm.

CLIA History

CLIA is the federal legislation that establishes minimum standards for all laboratories to follow. It was initiated in the 1960s in response to a number of misread cytology reports that led to the death or injury of many women. In 1967, the initial Clinical Laboratory Improvement Amendment was passed. In 1988, a second amendment was passed; however, the regulations did not go into effect until 1992 when they were approved.

Summary of Key CLIA Requirements

1. At least two levels of controls must be performed daily or every day that the test is performed. If state or instrument requirements state that controls must be performed more often, the higher standard prevails.
2. Calibration verification must be performed at least every six months. If state or instrument requirements state that calibration must be performed more often, the higher standard prevails.
3. Calibration must include at least three levels of calibrators that are included in the reported patient range.
4. Proficiency testing must occur at least every three months.

If a laboratory is ONLY performing waived tests, they can apply for a **Certificate of Waiver.** This certificate allows the laboratory to perform only waived tests. The advantage of the certificate is that the laboratory is not subject to routine surveys or inspection. However, if a surveyor does come to the office, you must permit the inspection.

To apply for a Certificate of Waiver, you must complete the application (Form CMS-116) and pay the associated fee. (See Figure 5-4.)

DEPARTMENT OF HEALTH AND HUMAN SERVICES
CENTERS FOR MEDICARE & MEDICAID SERVICES

Form Approved
OMB No. 0938-0581

CLINICAL LABORATORY IMPROVEMENT AMENDMENTS (CLIA)
APPLICATION FOR CERTIFICATION

I. GENERAL INFORMATION

❏ Initial Application   ❏ Survey

❏ Change in Certification Type   ❏ Other Changes

CLIA Identification Number

_____ D _____

(If an initial application leave blank, a number will be assigned)

Facility Name

Federal Tax Identification Number

Telephone No. *(Include area code)* Fax No. *(Include area code)*

Facility Address — *Physical Location of Laboratory*
(Building, Floor, Suite if applicable.) Fee Coupon/Certificate will be
mailed to this Address unless mailing address is specified

Mailing/Billing Address *(If different from street address, include*
attention line and/or Building, Floor, Suite)

Number, Street *(No P.O. Boxes)*

Number, Street

City   State   ZIP Code

City   State   ZIP Code

Name of Director *(Last, First, Middle Initial)*

For Office Use Only
Date Received _____

II. TYPE OF CERTIFICATE REQUESTED *(Check one)*

❏ Certificate of Waiver *(Complete Sections I – VI and IX – X)*

❏ Certificate for Provider Performed Microscopy Procedures *(PPM) (Complete Sections I – X)*

❏ Certificate of Compliance *(Complete Sections I – X)*

❏ Certificate of Accreditation (Complete Sections I through X) and indicate which of the following
organization(s) your laboratory is accredited by for CLIA purposes, or for which you have
applied for accreditation for CLIA purposes

❏ The Joint Commission ❏ AOA   ❏ AABB
❏ CAP   ❏ COLA   ❏ ASHI

**If you are applying for a Certificate of Accreditation, you must provide evidence of accreditation for your
laboratory by an approved accreditation organization for CLIA purposes or evidence of application for such
accreditation within 11 months after receipt of your Certificate of Registration.**

Form CMS-116 (10/07)

Figure 5-4 Partial example of Certificate of Waiver (Form CMS-116).

Types of CLIA Certificates

- **Certificate of Waiver.** This certificate is issued to a laboratory to perform only waived tests.
- **Certificate for Provider-Performed Microscopy Procedures (PPMP).** This certificate is issued to a laboratory in which a physician, midlevel practitioner, or dentist performs no tests other than the microscopy procedures. This certificate permits the laboratory to also perform waived tests.
- **Certificate of Registration.** This certificate is issued to a laboratory that enables the entity to conduct moderate or high complexity laboratory testing or both until the entity is determined by survey to be in compliance with the CLIA regulations.
- **Certificate of Compliance.** This certificate is issued to a laboratory after an inspection that finds the laboratory to be in compliance with all applicable CLIA requirements.
- **Certificate of Accreditation.** This is a certificate that is issued to a laboratory on the basis of the laboratory's accreditation by an accreditation organization approved by the Health Care Financing Administration (HCFA).

To obtain further information, please contact your State Survey Agency or CMS Regional Office.

Taken directly from U.S. Department of Health and Human Services, Centers for Medicare and Medicaid, Clinical Laboratory Improvement Amendments (CLIA), Types of CLIA Certificate, http://www.cms.hhs.gov/CLIA/downloads/TYPES_OF_CLIA_CERTIFICATES.pdf.

TOOLS AND TECHNIQUES OF QUALITY CONTROL

Maintaining a successful quality system requires special tools and techniques. You must become familiar with these before you know how to apply quality control measures in the lab.

Controls, Calibrators, and Standards

The key to quality laboratory test results is to ensure that all of the steps of the process are "in-control" and working as expected. A quality control system is considered to be "in-control" when the accuracy of the test results are within acceptable limits. There are a variety of different tools and techniques to ensure that the testing process is "in-control."

Daily control testing before you begin patient testing is both good practice and a CLIA requirement. **Controls** are samples of known concentration that are tested in the same manner as patient samples. They are tested prior to beginning patient testing and the results are compared to the known results to see if the system is working properly. All results must be documented in the Quality Control Log. Quality control results that are "out-of-control" or not within the acceptable range also must be documented, along with any corrective action taken. (See Figures 5-5 and 5-6.)

A minimum of two levels of controls must be used daily for each day that patient testing is performed, unless a more rigorous standard is set by the state or the instrument's manufacturer. For example, if an analyzer requires that two levels of controls must be run every eight hours, you must adhere to the higher, more demanding requirement. In addition, quality control must be performed

1. when all of the reagents are changed to a new lot number.
2. when major preventive maintenance or replacement of critical parts is performed.
3. after calibration procedures.

Safety Note

Quality control samples should be treated as biological hazards because they may contain human body fluids.

MASTER LABORATORY LOG

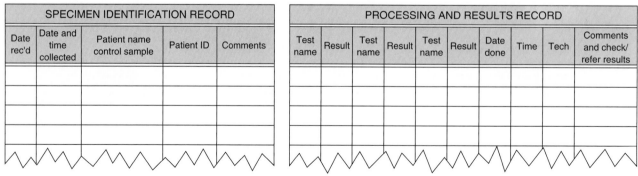

	SPECIMEN IDENTIFICATION RECORD						PROCESSING AND RESULTS RECORD								
Date rec'd	Date and time collected	Patient name control sample	Patient ID	Comments		Test name	Result	Test name	Result	Test name	Result	Date done	Time	Tech	Comments and check/ refer results

Figure 5-5 A master laboratory log has forms for recording the laboratory test information required to satisfy legal regulations.

Glucometer Daily Control Chart

Reagent Strip Name _____
Control Name _____
Low Control Result Range: 45–55 mg/dL
High Control Result Range: 135–150 mg/dL

Date	Control	Control Lot #	Control Expiration Date	Result	Comments	Initials
10/26/2012	Low	1257L	11/18/2012	54	OK	DSW
10/26/2012	High	1257H	11/18/2012	156	Out of range, open new bottle of control and rerun	DSW
10/26/2012	High	1257H	11/18/2012	148	OK – acceptable to perform patient testing	DSW

Figure 5-6 An example of a glucometer daily control chart.

Standards are quality controls manufactured and analyzed to very exact measurements for a particular method of analysis. **Primary standards** are of the highest possible quality and accuracy. **Secondary standards** are controls that are developed in comparison with primary standards. **Target values** (see Figure 5-7) are the values given by the manufacturer as the expected control test result. Actual values attained in POLs will cluster around the target value rather than duplicate it exactly. The manufacturer will usually specify the acceptable range of variation for particular test procedures using their quality control samples. Variability may be expressed as percentages or as standard deviations. This information is usually based on extensive testing of the quality control product by the manufacturer.

Quality control samples may be purchased from commercial vendors or professional associates. The purest controls available are expensive, but they are certified to have purity in excess of 99 percent. Control samples may come in either of two forms. Lyophilized (freeze-dried) controls are powdered and must be liquefied with a carefully measured amount of distilled water. Liquid controls are ready-to-use control materials. Quality control samples should not be purchased in excessive amounts. Reagents that deteriorate or expire before use are wasteful, expensive, and inefficient to store. On the other hand, purchasing a large

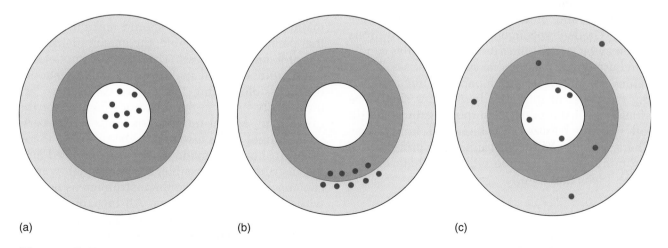

(a)   (b)   (c)

Figure 5-7 Target values. The desired target value is represented by the bull's eye in the target center. (a) The test values show good quality control. (b) The test values are biased and inaccurate. They show a consistent pattern of an error that is being repeated. (c) The test values show a pattern of random error. The quality is "out-of-control."

supply of the same lot of a QC reagent will prevent time-consuming restandardization due to frequent changing of the QC lot.

In addition to daily controls, calibration and calibration verification must be performed. **Calibrators** are known solutions of **analytes,** substances being analyzed, used as measuring sticks to set instruments to read solutions correctly. Calibrators can be obtained from a medical supply company or professional organization.

Calibration verification is the process of testing the system with calibrators and ensuring that the results determined by the test accurately reflect the actual concentration in the substance. **Calibration** is the process of making adjustments to the system when bias is determined by the calibration verification. Calibration verification must be performed at least every six months and whenever one of the following events occurs:

1. when all of the reagents are changed to a new lot number.

2. when major preventive maintenance or replacement of critical parts occurs.

3. when controls indicate an unusual trend or if controls fall outside of the acceptable limits and no other means of correcting and identifying the problem are possible.

4. when the laboratory determines the need for more frequent calibration verification.

Like control testing, calibration verification and calibration activities must be documented and available for review during inspections.

Linearity

The ability of an instrument or procedure to produce accurate test results can be assessed by measuring the **linearity** of the results. High-value, low-value, and midpoint control samples are tested. Graded specimens with more dilutions also may be made. Linearity check samples can be purchased from commercial supply houses. These values are plotted on graph paper. A line connecting the pools of high and low values should be straight, and the pool of midpoint values should fall halfway between the high and low values. There is a bias in the instrument or procedure if the midpoint is closer to either the high or low value. (See Figure 5-8.)

Instrumentation

Most lab procedures require some sort of instrument or instruments, so the correct use and upkeep

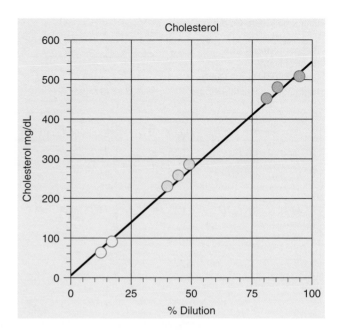

Figure 5-8 Example of linearity graph.

of lab instruments is another important aspect of quality assessment.

Instrument Maintenance. Well-functioning instruments are essential for accurate laboratory procedures. Instrument major maintenance should be the responsibility of one person, preferably the one who is most familiar with the instrument. However, everyone is responsible for performing daily maintenance and ensuring that the instrument is in good order before and during use.

The steps suggested by the manufacturer for preventive maintenance should be followed. If the instrument malfunctions, check the operator's manual to see if you can resolve the problem. If not, then the manufacturer or service company should be called. If possible, the person who usually maintains the instrument should make the call. If that person is not available, the person identifying the problem should call. The warranty, model and serial numbers, and maintenance records should be accessible during the phone call. These are most likely listed in the operator's manual for the instrument. Model numbers of replacement parts such as light bulbs also should be recorded there. The call should be made from a phone placed near the instrument, if possible, so that the lab worker can check or manipulate the instrument as needed while talking on the phone. All breakdowns and repairs should be recorded in an instrument maintenance log. Figure 5-9 is an example of an instrument maintenance record.

MAINTENANCE, REPAIR, AND PROBLEM RESOLUTION RECORD

Testing System _____ **Page No.** _____

Date	Initials	Test	Description: problem identification and resolution, actions taken, service and repairs done

Figure 5-9 Example of an instrument maintenance record.

Using New Instruments. When a new instrument is purchased, the manufacturer usually provides the assistance of a technical representative who explains the use of the instrument and its capabilities. Onsite training, a thorough explanation of the operator's manual, and a day-to-day plan for using the instrument should be provided. The operator's manual should contain detailed descriptions of procedures, including routine maintenance, troubleshooting, and the technical support that is available for problems. The manual also should explain the use of quality control. Software may be available to calculate the mean, standard deviation, and other quality control measures, for example, or quality control analysis may be built into the instrument. While the manufacturer's representative is at the lab, both patient and quality control samples should be assayed to test the instrument and familiarize the lab workers with the procedures.

Before using the new instrument routinely, another 20 to 30 patient specimens that span the analytical range from low to high should be tested. These may be obtained from a reference lab, if necessary. By the time these specimens are tested, lab workers should feel comfortable with the equipment. During this time, a manufacturer's representative should be available by phone for consultation if any questions or problems arise. If the manufacturer does not provide such assistance free of charge, another manufacturer should

be selected. Some manufacturers even provide free proficiency testing on new instruments and reagents. It is also a good idea to check references. Ask for the name of a local POL using the new piece of equipment and call that lab. Arrange for a visit, at their lab's convenience, to see the equipment. Also, get the opinions of the staff that use the equipment.

Record Keeping

Accurate record keeping is essential to quality control. A variety of forms, such as the master laboratory log, are used to record lab data. Each procedure performed in the POL requires a separate quality control record. Every record, for patients and for quality control results, must be entered into the master laboratory log with dates clearly shown. Every day that patient tests are performed there also must be quality control tests performed and the results of those tests recorded. The results of calibration tests and dates when new control vials are begun must be entered as well. Expiration dates of controls also should be entered.

Dated quality control records along with patient reports establish proof that clinical tests are performed in a reliable and valid manner. The records must be retained for a period of years, the exact number specified by state laws and CLIA 1988 mandate. Under no circumstances should out-of-control results be omitted from the records. Instead, be sure to include the out-of-control results with subsequent corrective action and in-control results. Other pertinent information that should be included in the records are

- the date of introduction of new lots of reagents.
- the initials of staff members performing each test.
- the remedies that were instigated for out-of-control results.
- the dates of instrument maintenance.

The results of each quality control test may be plotted as a daily point on specially printed graph paper called a **Levey-Jennings chart,** on which is printed the mean and the high and low ends of the acceptable range of variation around the mean, usually ± two standard deviations (see Figure 5-10). The graph also may be hand drawn. Usually, two controls a day are tested and recorded for each procedure, one a normal value and the other an abnormal value. Forms for plotting test results for both

values on the same page make the procedure more convenient. Use of a Levey-Jennings chart greatly simplifies the record keeping and mathematics of quality control. (See Figure 5-11.)

LAB PERSONNEL

The Role of Lab Personnel

The most important factor affecting quality control in POLs is the laboratory staff. The welfare of patients depends on the care and responsibility of lab personnel, who must be dedicated to achieving the highest accuracy in performing lab tests and recording and reporting results. Lab personnel also must have the honesty and courage to admit errors when they occur. Lab workers should speak out if test results are questionable. If their work schedule is too fast paced to guarantee care and accuracy, it is up to lab workers to inform their supervisors.

As stated previously, labs must apply for CLIA certificates prior to initiation of laboratory testing. The type of certificate issued, as well as state

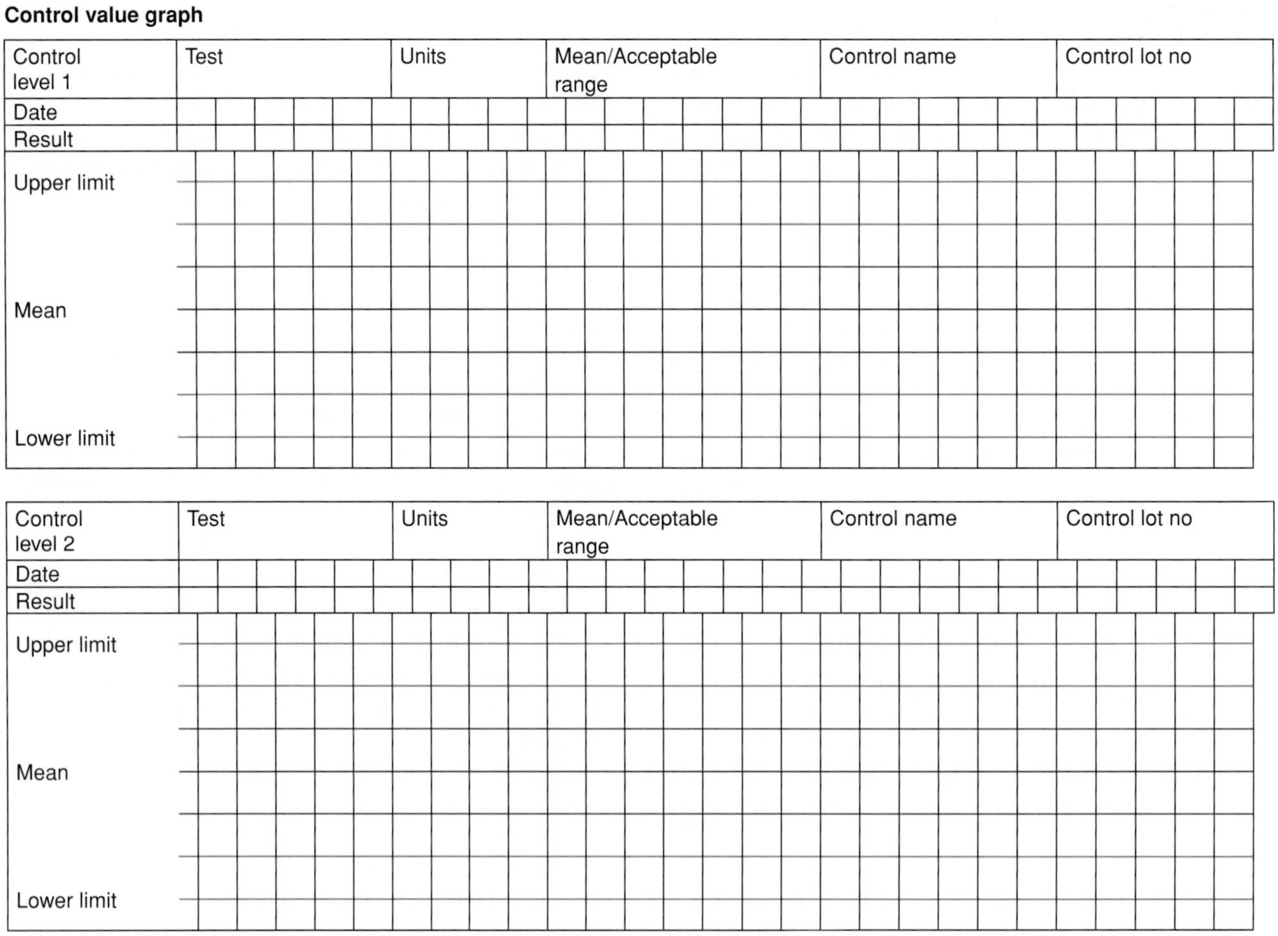

Control value graph

Figure 5-10 Levey-Jennings chart.

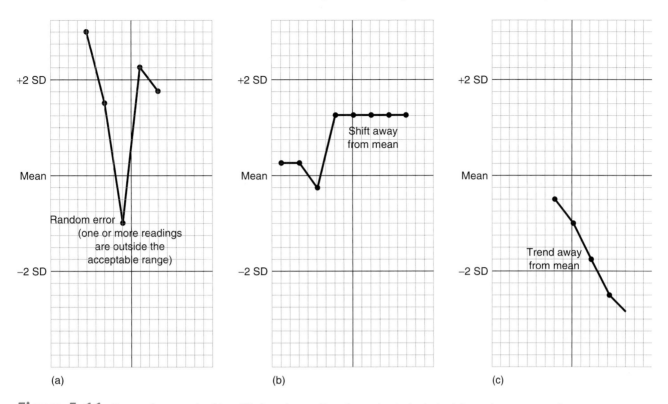

(a)   (b)   (c)

Figure 5-11 Errors that can be identified on Levey-Jennings charts include (a) random errors, where one or more readings are outside the acceptable range specified by the manufacturer or calculated in the POL; (b) a shift, where the values are consistently higher or lower than the mean or target value; and (c) a trend, where the values move farther and farther away from the target value specified by the manufacturer or the mean calculated in the POL.

regulations, will determine what tests can be performed and by whom. The varying degree of difficulty of the test determines what education and training are required in order to perform that test.

The knowledge and skill of the lab personnel has a great impact on the accuracy of test results. New workers usually receive initial orientation in all aspects of the lab work in which they will be involved. This is likely to include specimen collection and preparation, laboratory safety, record keeping, equipment operation and care, and test reporting. Competency in these areas may be tested quarterly. New employees should keep a special lab notebook for any questions that they may have about laboratory procedures.

It is a good idea to record more detailed descriptions of procedures than are outlined in lab manuals. Procedures that seem complicated and difficult to you as a new lab worker may seem boringly routine to your lab supervisor or instructor. With practice, they will seem that way to you, too. In the meantime, do not be afraid to ask questions if instructions are not clear. (See Figure 5-12.)

In addition to the qualifications mentioned above, CLIA has specific requirements for laboratory personnel depending on the type of certificate possessed by the laboratory. This is based on the

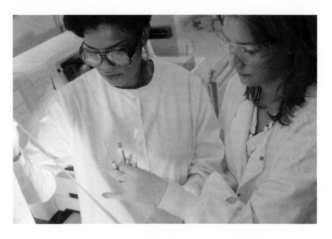

Figure 5-12 Lab technicians consulting.

type of testing performed in the laboratory. It is the responsibility of the laboratory director to determine which tests individual staff members are qualified to perform.

Proficiency Testing

CLIA also requires that laboratory personnel participate in **proficiency testing,** a procedure that tests the accuracy of the laboratory procedures and personnel.

While daily testing of known value controls is a good way to monitor day-to-day variability of test results with POLs, it does not assess how closely a particular POL's procedures match the results of other labs. Proficiency testing is required for this.

In a proficiency testing program, control samples with unknown values are received by mail and analyzed, and the results returned to the proficiency testing center. A report is received back indicating how closely the POL's results were to those of other participating labs using the same testing method. If the results of one POL are significantly different from those of other labs, this difference suggests a problem with the procedure, sample, reagent, or instrumentation. Most proficiency testing reports include suggestions for identifying and correcting problem results.

PUTTING QUALITY ASSESSMENT TO WORK

The purpose of quality assessment measures is to detect errors in test results that are significant enough to affect patient care. Any errors must be diagnosed and corrected immediately to prevent reporting of inaccurate patient results.

> ### Quality Assurance Note
> Whenever quality control test results are questionable, you should *not* report patient test results until the problem is resolved.

Errors

Use of a **Levey-Jennings chart** makes it easy to see when results are out-of-control. Values for a quality control test should fall uniformly on both sides of the mean when plotted. The more test results that appear on one side of the mean than the other, the greater the likelihood that the deviation is due to problems of bias, such as defective reagents, defective controls, defective instruments, or errors in staff performance. As explained, quality control results should fall within ± two standard deviations of the mean 95 percent of the time. The farther the result is away from the mean, the greater the error of that individual test and the more unacceptable the results.

A complete investigation of error is required if any of the following events occur because their individual probabilities are very low in an accurate test series:

- five consecutive test results fall on one side of the mean.
- two consecutive test results fall outside two standard deviations.
- one test result falls outside three standard deviations.

Three types of errors are readily identified using Levey-Jennings charts: random errors, shifts, and trends. Shifts and trends are examples of systematic errors (see Figure 5-11).

Random Errors. Random error is unpredictable error with no obvious pattern. It is characterized by large deviations from the mean. Random errors may have many different causes, including

- operator inattention due to boredom, fatigue, or distraction.
- interfering substances in reagents.
- electronic or optical variations in instruments.
- manufacturer's defects in pipettes or other equipment.
- clerical errors, such as misidentification, delays in testing, mislabeling, incorrect transcriptions, and faulty transfers of results. Clerical errors are almost entirely preventable if the staff is well trained.

Systematic Errors. Systematic error, a noticeable pattern of error, is evident when test results vary from the mean value in one direction to the other, although the results may not extend past the upper or lower acceptable limits. Systematic error may be caused by differences among staff members in performing a specific function, such as reading the meniscus or rounding off numbers. There are two types of systematic error:

- Shifts show a sudden move away from the mean and then continue in a line parallel to the mean. They may be due to a sudden change in some aspect of the procedure that remains permanent afterward, such as a change in the instrument or reagent.
- Trends show a pattern of moving continuously farther away from the mean in just one direction. Trends often indicate a failing instrument or part of a deteriorating reagent.

Finding the Source of Error

When quality control test results are out-of-control, a systematic method of analyzing the components of quality control is the most efficient approach to finding the source of the error. A checklist such as the following should be used:

STEP 1: Clerical errors.

a. Was the correct control tested?

b. Were letters or numbers omitted or transposed when they were copied into the record?

c. Were the results entered for the correct control sample level? For example, were the results for the low control entered into the high control column?

STEP 2: Reagent errors—refer to the package insert and written test procedure.

a. Were the control samples reconstituted and prepared as directed?

b. Was the temperature at the recommended level?

c. Were any reagents, calibrators, or controls past their expiration date or use date?

Quality Assurance Note

Many reagents have an expiration date from the manufacturer and a use date.

A use date is the new expiration date assigned by the user after opening the reagent. The use date supersedes the expiration date. You can determine the use date by reading the package insert that comes with the reagent. The expiration date is similar to food. If you purchase a bottle of soda, it comes with a "Best if used by date" assigned by the manufacturer. This is similar to the expiration date. Once you open the bottle of soda, you know it is only good for a much shorter period of time. This is the use date.

STEP 3: Procedural errors.

a. Were written procedures followed exactly?

b. Is the type of error listed in the troubleshooting section of the operator's manual or package insert for kits?

If steps 1, 2, and 3 do not identify the problem, then proceed to step 4.

STEP 4: Retest the control sample and record the new result in the master laboratory log and the quality control journal. If the quality control result is satisfactory, stop here and begin patient testing. If the test result is not satisfactory, go to step 5.

STEP 5: Test a fresh control sample using fresh reagent. Record the result in the master laboratory log and quality control journal, noting that fresh reagent was used. If the quality control test is satisfactory, begin patient testing. Otherwise, proceed to step 6.

STEP 6: Recalibrate the instrument and test a fresh control sample. Record the new quality control result, noting that the instrument was recalibrated. If the quality control result is unsatisfactory, go to step 7.

STEP 7: Contact a source of technical support, such as the lab director or advisor, a reference laboratory, or a hotline of the instrument or reagent manufacturer. Do not begin or report patient test results until the problem is resolved.

CONSTRUCTING A LEVEY-JENNINGS CHART—A WORKED EXAMPLE

Many instruments create Levey-Jennings charts automatically based on the control results that are run each day of testing. These same instruments will automatically flag the results that are out-of-control or identify when trends are occurring. For those instruments that don't possess this automated feature, it is up to the user to create Levey-Jennings charts and monitor the trends manually.

This example assumes that two different samples have been tested for glucose concentration. One sample is a normal control and the other is an abnormally high control. Although manufacturers usually provide the mean, standard deviation, and upper and lower limits for their quality control products, some labs calculate their own values. Calculating values will help you better understand the statistical basis of quality control. For each control sample, you will calculate the mean, standard deviation, and upper and lower limits, constructing a Levey-Jennings quality control chart for use in testing patient samples.

Samples and Test Results

The normal control was Lot # 02091, with expiration date April 23, 2010. The mean value supplied by the manufacturer was 91 mg/dL, with a standard deviation of 7, an upper limit of 105 ($\bar{x} + 2s$), and a lower limit of 77 ($\bar{x} - 2s$). The following test results were obtained in the POL for the normal control: 91, 91, 93, 88, 88, 106, 84, 85, 80, 92, 91, 96, 91, 92, 95.

The abnormal control was Lot # 020951, with expiration date April 23, 2010. The mean value supplied by the manufacturer was 302 mg/dL, with a standard deviation of 15, an upper limit of

332 ($\bar{x} + 2s$), and lower limit of 272 ($\bar{x} - 2s$). For the abnormal control, the test results obtained in the POL were 334, 249, 303, 322, 300, 297, 305, 315, 307, 282, 287, 303, 311, 292, 325.

Inspecting and Recording the Data

First, scan the test results to see if they appear reasonable. A value of 5 for the normal control and of 500 for the abnormal control, for example, would be unreasonable. Also, check the calculated values to see if they are logical. The mean cannot be greater or less than all of the test values. A check for logical values is the best protection against clerical errors in calculations.

A visual inspection of the test results shows that all of the normal control tests are within the expected range except one (106), which deviates by only 1 mg/dL. For the abnormal control, on the other hand, the first two test results (334 and 249) are outside the acceptable range. The second test result is very far from the recommended range and assumed to be subject to random error. As a consequence, you will discard that result when calculating the mean and standard deviation. Note that in an already established quality control procedure, this marked deviation would require a complete investigation using the preceding checklist. However, discarding very deviant control test results creates a tighter control for future tests because it leads to a smaller standard deviation and narrower limits of acceptability. On the other hand, using such a deviant value to calculate the mean and standard deviation leads to a larger standard deviation and wider limits of acceptability, producing greater tolerance of imprecision and inaccuracy. When the test results in a POL have much more variation than the manufacturer's recommended guidelines, the POL must "tighten up" the precision or use a different and more precise test.

Calculating the Mean and Standard Deviation

The mean and standard deviation can be calculated by hand, as here, or with a calculator or computer. The mean, $\bar{x}$, is the sum of the test results for each sample, divided by the number of tests. For the normal control, the sum of test results is 1,363. The number of tests is 15. The mean is therefore $\frac{1,363}{15}$ = 91 mg/dL. The mean for the abnormal control, calculated in the same way, is 306. Perform these calculations yourself to verify that you understand the method if you are unsure. Do not forget to discard the second test result for the abnormal sample.

To calculate the standard deviation, use the following formula:

$$S = \sqrt{\frac{\sum\limits_{i=1}^{n}(x_i - \bar{x})^2}{n - 1}}$$

where

$\bar{x}$ = the mean
x_i = each of the individual test results
n = the number of test results

In words, subtract each individual test result from the mean for that sample and square the result. Then add the differences and divide the sum by the number of tests less one ($n - 1$).

For the normal sample, the sum of squared differences is 496 and $n - 1 = 14$. The standard deviation for this sample is 5.9. For the abnormal sample, the sum of squared differences is 2,777 and $n - 1 = 13$. The standard deviation is 14.6. Using Figures 5-13 and 5-14 as worksheets, perform these calculations to be sure that you understand the method. Then plot the mean and standard deviation for each sample on the Levey-Jennings chart in Figure 5-15.

Control level _____	Test _____	Lot # _____	Units _____

Manufacturer's
Mean/Acceptable range _____   Expiration date _____

Test results	Deviation	Deviation squared
1. _____	_____	_____
2. _____	_____	_____
3. _____	_____	_____
4. _____	_____	_____
5. _____	_____	_____
6. _____	_____	_____
7. _____	_____	_____
8. _____	_____	_____
Totals _____	_____	_____

Figure 5-13 A chart for reporting data.

$\bar{x}$ (mean) = summation of test results ÷ number of tests

$\bar{x}$ = _____

$$SD = \sqrt{\frac{\Sigma(x_i - \bar{x})^2}{n - 1}} \qquad SD = \sqrt{\frac{\rule{2cm}{0.4pt}}{\rule{2cm}{0.4pt}}}$$

SD = _____   SD × 2 = _____ = ±2 SD

Figure 5-14 A formula for calculating the standard deviation.

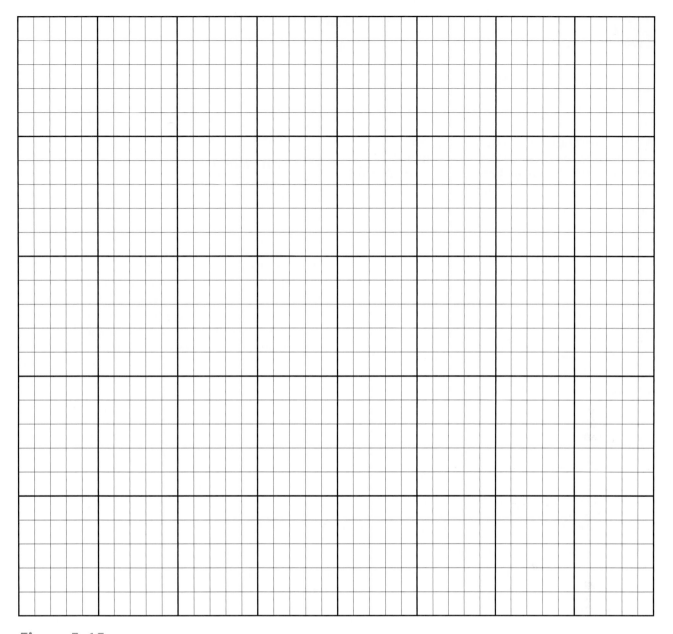

Figure 5-15 A graph for constructing a Levey-Jennings chart.

Setting Upper and Lower Limits

Next set upper and lower limits of acceptability on the range of test values for each sample by calculating $\bar{x} \pm 2s$. For the normal sample, the calculation is $91 \pm 2(5.9)$, or 79.2 mg/dL for the lower limit and 102.8 mg/dL for the upper limit. For the abnormal sample, the calculation is $306 \pm 2(14.6)$, or 276.8 mg/dL for the lower limit and 335.2 mg/dL for the upper limit. Plot the upper and lower limits for both samples on the Levey-Jennings chart in Figure 5-15.

Compare the results of your calculations with the manufacturer's recommended guidelines. The POL's range of acceptable values for the normal control is tighter than the manufacturer's. The POL's range of acceptable values for the abnormal control is about 4 mg/dL wider than the recommended values.

> **Note**
>
> The answers in the standard deviation problems may vary slightly due to rounding of the figures during calculation.
>
> References: Clinical & Laboratory Standard Institute Harmonized Terminology Database, http://www.clsi.org

PROCEDURE 5-1

Control Sample Statistics

Goal

After successfully completing this procedure, you will be able to calculate control sample statistics and construct a Levey-Jennings quality control chart for use in testing patient samples.

Completion Time

30 minutes

Equipment and Supplies

- Calculator
- Pen and paper
- Graph paper (optional)

Data

Normal Control

- Lot number: 12245
- Expiration date: January 15, 2014
- Test results: 90, 95, 89, 88, 106, 85, 86, 81, 92, 91

Abnormal Control

- Lot number: 12583
- Expiration date: February 15, 2014
- Test results: 340, 288, 303, 324, 301, 317, 306, 315, 308, 285

Instructions

Read through the list of equipment and supplies that you will need and the steps of the procedure. Be sure that you understand each step before you begin. Then complete each step correctly and in the proper order. If your completion time is too long, repeat the procedure until you increase your speed.

*Steps marked with (*) are critical and must have the maximum points to pass.

Performance Standards	Points Awarded	Maximum Points
1. Collect the needed equipment and supplies.		5
2. Scan the test results to see if they appear reasonable. Omit any that are far out of range.		5
3. Make a recording chart and a Levey-Jennings chart.		5
4. Copy the lot numbers and expiration dates onto the charts, which should show both the normal and abnormal control results on the same page for easy comparison.		5
5. Calculate the means.		5
6. Calculate the standard deviations using the following formula: $$S = \sqrt{\dfrac{\sum\limits_{i=1}^{n}(x_i - \overline{x})^2}{n - 1}}$$		15
7. Record the mean and standard deviation for both samples on the charts.		5
8. Set upper and lower limits of acceptability on the range of test values for each sample by calculating $\overline{x} \pm 2s$.		10
9. Plot the upper and lower limits for both samples on the Levey-Jennings chart.		10
Total Points		65

Overall Procedural Evaluation

Student Name _____

Signature of the Instructor _____ Date _____

Comments _____

_____

chapter 5 REVIEW

Review Questions

Match the following terms.

_____ **1.** analyte

_____ **2.** Levey-Jennings chart

_____ **3.** nonwaived test

_____ **4.** waived test

_____ **5.** reproducibility

a. chart for plotting controls

b. test were there is a low probability of erroneous results

c. the ability to repeat test results

d. substance that is tested for in a procedure

e. previously referred to as "moderate" and "high-complexity" tests

Choose the best answer for the following questions.

6. A quality assessment includes
   a. continuous monitoring of the test results
   b. taking corrective action when problems are identified
   c. reviewing the corrective action and ensuring it is working
   d. all of the above

7. The **best** method of testing laboratory personnel skills is
   a. daily quality control testing
   b. calibration testing
   c. proficiency testing
   d. none of the above

8. CLIA requires that quality control must be performed
   a. as often as the lab deems necessary
   b. once every six months
   c. every day that patient testing is performed
   d. none of the above

9. The process of testing the system with calibrators and ensuring that the results determined by the test accurately reflect the actual concentration in the substance is known as
   a. quality control testing
   b. calibration verification
   c. proficiency testing
   d. patient testing

10. The ability to get the same result repeatedly is known as
    a. variability
    b. precision
    c. true value
    d. none of the above

11. When there is a problem with an instrument, you should
    a. refer to the operator's manual for advice
    b. seek out the person in the lab who is most familiar with the instrument
    c. contact the manufacturer through the instrument hotline
    d. all of the above

12. Information included on the quality control log includes the
    a. initials of the person performing the test
    b. date the control expires
    c. date the controls were put into use
    d. all of the above

13. How often is proficiency testing required by CLIA?

    a. once every month

    b. once every three months

    c. once every six months

    d. once a year

14. Plus or minus two standard deviations includes how much of the data?

    a. 5 percent

    b. 68 percent

    c. 95 percent

    d. 99 percent

15. CLIA requires that calibration verification must be performed

    a. once every month

    b. once every three months

    c. once every six months

    d. once a year

16. List four components of a quality system

    a. _____

    b. _____

    c. _____

    d. _____

17. List five steps that should be taken when trying to find the source of error in laboratory tests

    a. _____

    b. _____

    c. _____

    d. _____

    e. _____

Define the following terms in the spaces provided.

18. Accuracy

_____

_____

_____

19. Variance

_____

_____

_____

20. Normal value

_____

_____

_____

21. Bias

_____

_____

_____

Answer the following questions in the spaces provided.

22. Give the formula calculating the standard deviation of a sample of test results.

_____

_____

_____

23. Describe the Levey-Jennings charts used to record quality control results. Why are they so useful?

_____

_____

_____

24. Identify the types of errors that are quickly noted on a Levey-Jennings chart.

_____

_____

_____

Applying Knowledge—On the Job

Answer the following questions in the spaces provided.

25. Your laboratory supervisor informs you that there is too much bias in your quality control test results although your precision is excellent. What does she mean?

_____

_____

_____

26. Your coworker wants to post the quality control test results weekly instead of daily in order to save time. Why is this not a good idea?

_____

_____

_____

27. Quality control results for a POL test that you perform regularly have always indicated accurate test results. One day, you get a control result that is more that three standard deviations from the mean. What might cause this reading and what should you do?

_____

_____

_____

28. Mrs. Smith, a patient who is prone to worry, questions the accuracy of lab tests performed "just in the doctor's office" instead of in a "big, fancy lab." What do you say?

_____

_____

_____

29. On various days, three different workers in your POL perform the same quality control test and record the results. Worker A is consistently nearest the mean, worker B is consistently a little above the mean, and worker C has results that vary widely both above and below the mean. How would you explain these results?

_____

_____

_____

30. A senior coworker has a heavy work load at the clinic as well as heavy home responsibilities. She suggests that both of you take shortcuts and fabricate an occasional quality control result. What is your response?

_____

_____

31. You have been working in a small POL for just a few months. Suddenly, you find yourself responsible for the entire POL due to your supervisor's serious illness. The glucometer is not functioning properly. What should you do?

_____

_____

_____

32. Dr. Arewa, your employer, has decided to purchase another machine to perform blood chemistries. He is considering two options: (a) an inexpensive, off-brand, used machine without a guarantee and (b) a new, more expensive machine with extended quality control and service support from the manufacturer. Which machine do you believe is the better buy? Why?

_____

_____

_____

33. A coworker in the POL is in the process of reconstituting a dehydrated control with distilled water. She accidentally adds an extra drop or two of water from the volumetric pipette into the bottle of control. What should she do?

_____

_____

_____

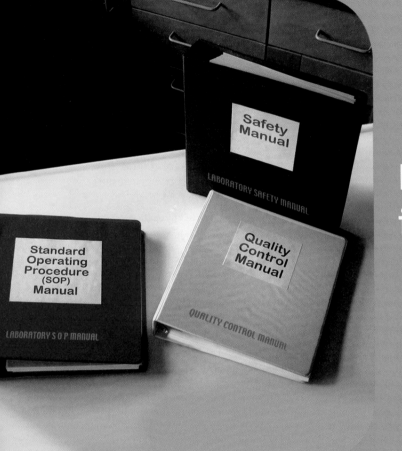

 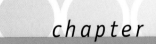

Record Keeping in the Lab

⠿ COGNITIVE OBJECTIVES

After studying this chapter, you should be able to

6.1 use each of the vocabulary terms appropriately.

6.2 list several reasons why written records are necessary in POLs.

6.3 explain how written records meet the legal requirements of accuracy, safety, and confidentiality.

6.4 discuss how the use of quality control records safeguards the accuracy of laboratory test results.

6.5 describe the role of written instructions in assuring accurate and reliable test results.

6.6 list the contents of a typical requisition form and explain how requisitions are used.

6.7 identify several manuals used in the POL and describe the information and records contained in each.

6.8 explain the impact of HIPAA in the POL.

6.9 explain how the specimen log and the patient test log serve as a backup record of all laboratory functions.

6.10 describe the clinical and legal significance of action values.

6.11 discuss legal considerations regarding patient test results and other documents.

6.12 describe the role of oral communication in the laboratory.

6.13 list which of the health care providers are authorized to order laboratory tests.

6.14 describe the safety records related to the laboratory.

6.15 describe the path of the patient test.

After studying this chapter, you should be able to

6.16   design a plan to orient new lab employees to the recordkeeping system of a POL.

6.17   trace the path of a patient's test requisition through the laboratory to the posting of the result in the patient's chart.

TERMINOLOGY

action value: also called panic value or critical value; a patient lab test result requiring immediate medical attention. Action values fall outside the normal test value range, although not all abnormal values require immediate action.

general policy manual: a laboratory manual that contains the overall policies for every aspect of laboratory operation, particularly as they relate to employees, their qualifications, job duties, and job benefits.

Health Insurance Portability and Accountability Act (HIPAA): federal regulation that established a national baseline for protecting patient's health information.

instrument calibration and maintenance manual: a laboratory manual that contains instructions and dated records of laboratory instrument calibration and maintenance.

inventory control manual: a laboratory manual that contains a file of supply house contact information and orders and a calendar for keeping a tally of supplies on hand.

manual: a laboratory handbook that contains instructions and recording forms for a particular aspect of laboratory work. Examples include safety and quality control manuals.

patient testing log: daily, chronological journal of all of the work that is performed in the lab. Logs can be either manual or computerized.

policy: a management plan based on the goals of the lab or of particular aspects of lab work. Policies guide decision making and plans of action.

procedure: the steps of a particular test or assay. They should be written so someone doing the test the first time can accurately perform the test.

proficiency testing manual: a permanent record of proficiency test results that augment the quality control record.

quality control manual: a laboratory manual that contains written descriptions of quality control procedures and records of quality control test results, the latter usually recorded on Levey-Jennings charts.

record: a written account of a procedure or past event.

requisition: a printed form used by a physician to request a laboratory test for a patient.

safety manual: a laboratory manual containing safety regulations, safety procedures, and policies, particularly as they relate to biological and chemical hazards, exposure incidents, and waste disposal.

specimen collection manual: a laboratory manual containing all of the information needed to collect specimens for the various tests performed in the POL or its referral laboratory, including the types of collection apparatus required for each test and special handling requirements for specimens. The same information is often found in a chart posted near the specimen collection site.

specimen log: a daily, chronological log of all of the specimens collected and received by the laboratory.

standard operating procedure (SOP) manual: a lab manual containing instructions for each procedure performed in the POL. Includes detailed instructions that standardize the way a test is performed.

INTRODUCTION

CLIA requires that all POLs must maintain written **policies** (management plans), **procedures** (test instructions), and **records** (written accounts) of patient test results, quality control measures, and other aspects of laboratory work. The use of written policies and instructions is necessary to ensure that testing complies exactly with the correct protocol and to ensure safety and accuracy. Written records of patient and quality control test results provide legal documentation that they were performed correctly. This chapter reviews the variety of different records that are maintained in the POL.

LEGAL AND ETHICAL CONSIDERATIONS

Laboratory test records of patients are subject to the same laws of confidentiality that apply to other medical records. Only the patient's physician has the right to receive and interpret the results of lab tests. The results can be released to other authorized persons with the written permission of the patient, but test results should not be released to the patient until the physician has reviewed them. Furthermore, the office and/or laboratory may have specific policies about who can release lab results to patients. If patients ask about the meaning of their laboratory test results, they should be referred to the physician. Discussing test results with patients risks potential accusations of illegally practicing medicine. Nor should similar cases be discussed with patients. This may infringe on other patients' privacy or be misinterpreted. For the same reasons, laboratory records, especially those that identify individual patients, never should be left in public areas where they may be read by unauthorized persons.

The federal government requires that POLs maintain and make available upon request by an inspector or other authorized person their records of quality control, proficiency testing, occupational safety, and Medicare and Medicaid reports and charges. Because federal regulations in this area are subject to change, professional medical organizations sponsor workshops, and government agencies publish documents to keep lab personnel abreast of current requirements.

In the event of a malpractice suit, lab records can be used to establish that proper procedures were used for collecting and testing specimens, reporting the results, and assuring accuracy through quality control measures. If such records do not exist, there is no way to prove that the laboratory was not negligent. State level statute-of-limitation laws define the length of time that a physician is liable to malpractice suits after treating patients. All laboratory records should be kept for at least that long.

In summary, the records kept in POLs are valuable legal documents that must be protected from fire, theft, and other potential means of destruction or loss. For this reason, it is important to store backup copies of lab records in an area different from the area where the day-to-day records are used.

HEALTH INFORMATION PORTABILITY AND ACCOUNTABILITY ACT (HIPAA)—PRIVACY STANDARDS

In 1996, the **Health Insurance Portability and Accountability Act** was written. The legislation went into effect April 14, 2003. This landmark legislation was the first federal privacy standard that dictates how patient information must be protected. HIPAA established a national baseline for protecting patient's health information. In the situations where the state sets a higher standard, the state standard must be adhered to.

This legislation applies to most health insurers, health care clearinghouses, hospitals, clinics, nursing homes, pharmacies, doctors, and other health care providers.

HIPAA established a number of patient protections. These include

1. **Medical record access.** Patients can request to see their medical records and request corrections be made if the patient identifies an error. The organization maintaining the medical record should provide the patient with a copy of the medical record within 30 days of receiving the request. The organization has the right to charge the patient for the cost of the copies and any cost associated with delivering the copies.

2. **Notice of privacy practices.** Covered organizations must provide written notification about how they may use a patient's medical information and what rights a patient has under the new HIPAA standards. For organizations providing patient care, this information is generally provided on the first visit or the first visit after April 14, 2003, for current patients. Patients are asked to sign or initial that they have received this information. Health plans must mail their Notice of Privacy to their clients upon enrollment and again if the notice changes significantly.

   Under the HIPAA standards, patients have the right to request that the covered entity further restrict the dissemination of their medical information; however, the organization is not required to comply with these requests. (See Figure 6-1.)

3. **Restrictions on the use of personal medical information.** Health professionals can still freely share patient information about patients they are caring for. HIPAA ensures that patient medical information cannot be used for any other purpose without the patient's consent.

4. **Mechanism for filing complaints.** HIPAA provides a system for patients to file a complaint when they believe their privacy rights have been violated. Complaints can be made directly to the provider or through the Health and Human Services' Office for Civil Rights. The Office for Civil Rights is responsible for enforcement of privacy regulating and determining when a violation has occurred.

Patient Name: _____

Health Record Number: _____

Date of Birth: _____

1. I authorize the use or disclosure of the above named individual's health information as described below.

2. The following individual(s) or organization(s) are authorized to make the disclosure: _____

3. The type of information to be used or disclosed is as follows (check the appropriate boxes and include other information where indicated)

☐ problem list
☐ medication list
☐ list of allergies
☐ immunization records
☐ most recent history
☐ most recent discharge summary
☐ lab results (please describe the dates or types of lab tests you would like disclosed): _____
☐ x-ray and imaging reports (please describe the dates or types of x-rays or images you would like disclosed): _____
☐ consultation reports from (please supply doctors' names): _____
☐ entire record
☐ other (please describe): _____

4. I understand that the information in my health record may include information relating to sexually transmitted disease, acquired immunodeficiency syndrome (AIDS), or human immunodeficiency virus (HIV). It may also include information about behavioral or mental health services, and treatment for alcohol and drug abuse.

5. The information identified above may be used by or disclosed to the following individuals or organization(s):

Name: _____

Address: _____

Name: _____

Address: _____

6. This information for which I'm authorizing disclosure will be used for the following purpose:

☐ my personal records
☐ sharing with other health care providers as needed/other (please describe): _____

7. I understand that I have a right to revoke this authorization at any time. I understand that if I revoke this authorization, I must do so in writing and present my written revocation to the health information management department. I understand that the revocation will not apply to information that has already been released in response to this authorization. I understand that the revocation will not apply to my insurance company when the law provides my insurer with the right to contest a claim under my policy.

8. This authorization will expire (insert date or event): _____

If I fail to specify an expiration date or event, this authorization will expire six months from the date on which it was signed.

9. I understand that once the above information is disclosed, it may be redisclosed by the recipient and the information may not be protected by federal privacy laws or regulations.

10. I understand authorizing the use or disclosure of the information identified above is voluntary. I need not sign this form to ensure health care treatment.

Signature of patient or legal representative: _____ Date: _____

If signed by legal representative, relationship to patient

Signature of witness: _____ Date: _____

Distribution of copies: Original to provider; copy to patient; copy to accompany use or disclosure

Note: This sample form was developed by the American Health Information Management Association for discussion purposes. It should not be used without review by the issuing organization's legal counsel to ensure compliance with other federal and state laws and regulations.

Figure 6-1 Example of a HIPAA Privacy Notice form.

Patients are entitled to additional rights under HIPAA that have not been covered in this text.

Oral Communication in the POL

This chapter focuses on the written records that are maintained in the POL. However, oral communication is another vital component of how information is communicated in the POL.

Oral transmission of information is often a necessary and helpful way of communicating patient information. However, that information should always be recorded in writing as a means of ensuring that information is not lost. For example, it may be necessary to notify the doctor that the patient has an **action value,** a value that requires immediate medical attention. It is important to communicate that information directly to ensure the information has been received. This should be followed up by documenting the information in the record to make sure that the information is not lost over time. Without a backup written record, the accuracy of oral reports may be compromised because of misunderstandings or memory lapses. In addition, written reports also reduce the possibility of patient confidentiality being compromised due to someone overhearing the conversation.

Physicians often orally will request laboratory tests for their patients, especially when there is an urgent need for the test to be performed quickly. When taking an oral request, be sure to put the information in writing. A notepad and pen should always be kept by the phone for this purpose. In addition, many states require that the physician submit the request in writing within a certain period of time to satisfy documentation and chart requirements.

Another example of utilizing oral communication is during "sign-out." When one laboratory person takes over for another, there is generally a "sign-out" when the person who has been overseeing the testing tells the person coming on any significant events with the patients, instruments, or other important information. Oral communication in this situation is important because it provides an opportunity for feedback and questions. It is also good practice to write the key points of sign-out in a shared journal that is kept in the laboratory so that the information is not lost or forgotten.

HOW RECORDS ARE KEPT

While many laboratory records still are written by hand, computers are becoming more important in laboratories because of the ease, speed, and convenience they bring to record keeping.

Computerized Records

Some laboratories use microcomputers to store and print out patient test results and identify data as well as quality control results and calibration records. These are easy to retrieve when stored in the computer. **Manuals** are laboratory handbooks that contain instructions and recording forms for a particular aspect of laboratory work. Manuals are much easier to revise if their contents are saved on computer files. Just how computers are utilized varies from one lab to another, so their specific functions must be learned on the job. Students should strive for computer literacy and be familiar with word processing and database programs because their future employment is likely to require these skills.

TYPES OF RECORDS

Records and other written documents in POLs can be divided into four types, each of which is described below: specimen log, patient requisitions, patient testing log, and laboratory manuals.

Types of Records in POLs

The following types of records are found in POLs:

- specimen log
- patient requisitions
- patient testing log
- laboratory manuals

  - general policy manual
  - standard operating procedure manual
  - safety manual
  - specimen collection manual
  - quality control manual
  - proficiency testing manual
  - instrument calibration and maintenance manual
  - inventory control manual

Specimen Log

The **specimen log** is a daily, chronological log of all of the specimens collected and received by the laboratory. Included in the log are the date and time the specimen was collected or received by the lab, the patient's name, the patient's medical record number or other identifying number, the type of specimen or the specimen source, and what tests are to be performed. If the specimen is sent to a reference lab, then the specimen log will include information about when it was sent and to which lab. In general, the specimen log is updated throughout the day and until specimen testing is complete. This allows the laboratory workers to monitor the work progress and identify specimens that require attention, creating a pending log. Specimen logs can be manually updated, though larger laboratories use electronic laboratory software to track this information. See Figure 6-2 for a sample specimen log.

Patient Requisitions

Requisitions are preprinted forms used by physicians to request laboratory tests for patients. Only the patient's physician or other authorized health care providers such as physician assistants or nurse practitioners have the right to requisition lab tests for the patient. A patient cannot order his or her own tests. This is regulated by state laws. (See Figure 6-3.)

Depending on the size and specific operating procedures of the POL, there may be just one requisition form, which lists all of the tests performed in the POL, or several different forms, each for a different category of tests. After the requested test is completed, the requisition form is posted in the patient's chart. Other copies of the form may be filed elsewhere for backup or financial records.

The requisition form should be filled out accurately, completely, and legibly. It should contain three types of information: (1) information about the patient, (2) specimen information such as the specimen source, and (3) information about the tests ordered. The requisition should record the patient's name, the medical record number (chart number) or other identifying number such as Social Security number, the type of test requested, the date and time the test was ordered, and the physician giving the order. Also noted should be the date and time the specimen was collected, the name of the individual who collected the specimen, and the date and time the test was completed. The timing of specimen collection and testing is especially important in some tests, such as blood glucose and fasting blood chemistries. Unusual observations about the patient or test specimen also should be entered onto the requisition form. For example, if blood appears jaundiced, this should be noted.

Date and Time Specimen Collected or Received	Patient's Name	Patient's MR#	Specimen Type	Test Orderd
10/26/2012 10:15 am	Smith, John	52786	1 blue top – blood	PT/INR
10/26/2012 11:00 am	Caso, Wanda	87596	Clean-catch urine	UA C & S
10/26/2012 2:15 pm	Rodriguez, Pedro	12358	1 lavender – blood 1 marble — blood	CBC Lipid Profile

Figure 6-2 Example of a specimen log.

LAB USE ONLY		Laboratory Name & Address					Requesting Physician Information	
Acct #								
DATE							Address	
TIME								

Patient Information Patient Name (Last)	(First)		(MI)	Date of Birth / /		Phone Number	
Address	City, State		Zip	Phone Number			
Patient I.D. Number	Responsible Party (Last)	(First)	(Phone)	Male			
				Female			
Social Security Number	Physician			Date Time Specimen Collection			

Bill: Check One
Our account   Medicare
Insurance Co./Patient

Complete the Following Information for Billing a Patient and/or a Third Party Agency

Policy Holder Name	Policy Holder Address:	Relation
	Policy Holder Phone Number:	Self Spouse Child Other _____
Insurance Co. Name	Address Insurance Co.	City , State, Zip
Employer		
Policy	Group #	
	PATIENT or GUARDIAN SIGNATURE:	DATE:

CHECK DESIRED TESTS   **PLEASE PROVIDE ICD=9-CM#**

√	ORGAN DISEASE PANELS, BLOOD	ICD-9	√	TEST, BLOOD	ICD-9	√	TEST, BLOOD	ICD-9	√	TEST, URINE	ICD-9
	ACUTE HEP. A,B,C			ESR			WBC with diff			U/A Routine	
	BASIC METABOLIC			EBV			PT				
	THYROID			FBS			PTT				
	ELECTROLYTES			Grp A β-hem strep			Bleeding time				
	HEPATIC FUNCTION			Hgb			PCO_2				
	LIPID PROFILE			Hct			PO_2				
	RENAL FUNCTION			HgbA1c			CO_2				
	TEST, BLOOD			HIV antibodies			HCO_3			**MICROBIOLOGY**	
	ACE			Insulin			Ca^{++}			AFB culture	
	ADH			Iron			Cl^-			C & S	
	ALT			Ketone bodies						Chlamydia screen	
	AFP			LD						Endocervical culture	
	Amylase			pH						GC screen	
	Acetone			Phenylalanine						Gram stain	
	AST			K^+ and Na^+			**TEST, URINE**			O & P	
	Bilirubin			Proteins, Albumin			Cys			Strep A culture	
	BUN			Proteins, Fibrinogen			CrCl			Throat culture	
	CEA			PSA			Glucose			Urine culture	
	Calcium, total			RBC			HCG			Viral culture	
	Carbon dioxide, total			Sickle cells			UBG			Wound culture	
	Cholesterol, total			TSH			UFC				
	Cholesterol, HDLs			T3			UK				
	Cholesterol, LDLs			T4			UNA				
	CK			Uric Acid			Uosm				
	CMV			WBC			UUN				

Figure 6-3 An example of a laboratory requisition.

Patient Testing Log

All patient laboratory testing must be documented in a manual patient testing log or entered into a computerized laboratory information system. **Patient testing logs** create a daily, chronological journal of all of the work that is performed in the lab. Included in this journal is patient results and the quality control testing performed prior to beginning patient testing. Proficiency samples and calibrations also may be recorded here, when appropriate. These journals serve as a backup file for information recorded in the patient's chart.

Ames Urine Pregnancy Kit

Lot Number: AYG 1245

Expiration Date: 5/27/2013

Date and Time Specimen Tested	Patient's Name	Patient Medical Record	Results
11/27/2012 8:10 am	Positive Control	AYG 1245 P	Positive
11/27/2012 8:10 am	Negative Control	AYG 1245 N	Negative
11/27/2012 8:10 am	Garcia, Kelly	158652	Negative
11/27/2012 9:18 am	Jones, Suzie	953684	Positive

Figure 6-4 An example of a patient test log.

Information that must be included in the patient testing log is the patient's name, patient's medical record number, date and time the tests were performed, the tests performed, the results, the reagent lot number, expiration date of the reagents, and the name or initials of the individual performing the testing. (See Figure 6-4.)

Laboratory Manuals

There are several different laboratory manuals, each containing the information, detailed instructions, and records necessary for the day-to-day operation of a particular aspect of laboratory work. There are manuals on safety, specimen collection, quality control, and proficiency testing, among others. The contents of the manuals for a POL are the responsibility of the physician(s) or lab director, who should review them periodically, usually every six months, to confirm that they accurately reflect current policies and procedures. Lab consultants and supply companies may offer workshops and instructions for creating and maintaining lab manuals.

Lab manuals are an excellent means of educating new employees, but even experienced workers should refer to them to ensure that they are following exactly all laboratory procedures. Some manuals also contain troubleshooting sections that help locate equipment malfunctions and clerical and procedural errors.

Manuals help POLs meet government regulations by providing up-to-date sources of lab policies and procedures and a record of test results and other relevant data. For example, by federal mandate, daily quality control records must be kept for three years. This information as well

as descriptions of quality control procedures is recorded in the lab's **quality control manual.** Part of a government inspection of the lab may include a review of the **standard operating procedure (SOP) manual.** The SOP manual contains instructions for each of the procedures performed in the laboratory. It includes detailed instructions that standardize the way in which the procedure is performed. OSHA requires that safety regulations, procedures, and policies be accessible to all lab personnel. These can be found in the lab's **safety manual.**

Laboratory manuals usually are kept in three-ring notebooks with removable, laminated pages that are waterproof to protect them from spills and washing. Several manuals may be placed together in one large binder or each may be maintained separately for convenience. The contents should be typewritten for legibility. An index is needed to make retrieval of information easier. Each new subject or procedure should begin on a new page, which should be tabbed for ease in locating it. Manual contents must be dated as to when data were entered and procedures revised. The name of the individual who wrote and/or reviewed the procedures also must be included.

General Policy Manual. The **general policy manual** states the overall policies, or management plans, for every aspect of laboratory operation, particularly as they relate to employees, their qualifications and expectations, job duties, and job benefits. The general policy manual should contain a listing of the technical expertise and personal characteristics expected of employees. Dress code and professional behavior in the office may be included. The employer's policies with regard to salary reviews, paid holidays and vacation, sick leave, insurance and medical benefits, and hiring and termination procedures also should be explained.

The general policy manual provides the background necessary to understand the job, particularly as it relates to work in the lab. Some policy manuals are broader in scope, familiarizing the employee with the overall operation of the office or clinic. The contents of the manual and the records and written instructions that the employee is responsible for vary with the size and complexity of the physician's office. The clinical assistant in a small, one-physician office, for example, may be responsible for all the clinical records and laboratory records entered into the patients' charts. The laboratory assistant in a large practice with several physicians, on the other hand, may have only a few types of specialized laboratory test records and quality control entries to coordinate with other records.

Standard Operating Procedure (SOP) Manual. The standard operating procedure (SOP) manual provides written instructions for each laboratory procedure performed in the POL. The SOP manual incorporates several other records, including quality control, safety, proficiency testing, and instrument maintenance. For example, quality control and calibration procedures are either described in the SOP or referenced to their location in other manuals, such as the instrument's operator's manual. Wherever calculations are necessary, formulas and explanations are included. Manufacturers' instructions may be substituted for typewritten instructions where applicable, as long as any irrelevant text is deleted. Each procedure should begin on a new page and be dated with its most recent revision or review.

Standard operating procedures are specific to the laboratory that is doing the testing. Therefore, it should include locations and other laboratory-specific information. In addition, SOPs should be written in such a manner that a new employee who has completed his or her orientation could perform the procedure by him- or herself if necessary.

> **Quality Assurance Note**
>
> No lab worker, no matter how experienced, should rely on memory for the wide variety of laboratory procedures used in POLs. Always refer to the SOP.

SOP manuals should include

- The name of the procedure
- The purpose of the procedure
- Specimen requirements, including
  - Any patient preparation, if necessary
  - Proper specimen collection requirements
  - Minimum specimen amount required
  - Criteria for ruling a specimen unsuitable for testing (such as a nonfasting specimen for a fasting blood glucose test)
  - Requirements for storing the specimen if immediate testing is not possible
  - Centrifugation guidelines
  - Time limitations
- Special precautions, if applicable
- Brief description of the method
- Supplies, including
  - Reagents
  - Instruments
  - Other required items, such as a stopwatch
- Step-by-step list of the tasks of the procedure

- Interpretation of the results
  - An explanation of how to interpret the results
  - Normal range
  - Action values (abnormal patient test results that require immediate medical attention and notification of the physician)

Safety Manual. New employees are required by law to be oriented to safety concerns in the lab. The safety manual provides a written review of this orientation. It contains a description of biological and chemical hazards found in the lab, infection control methods, and procedures for reporting exposure incidents. Safety tips and legal waste disposal requirements also are outlined, as are emergency procedures such as those for fire and evacuation.

As part of the safety manual, OSHA requires that the employer develop an Exposure Control Plan, in which the employer identifies methods to reduce the possibility of an occupational exposure. This plan must be reviewed annually and anytime the lab implements a new safety procedure.

In addition to the safety manual, the employer must keep several employee records related to safety and occupational exposure to hazards. These records include training records and HBV and HIV records. Training records include an employee's orientation training and subsequent annual sessions, including the dates of the training, the topics covered, and the name and qualifications of the individual performing the training. Employee HBV records include the vaccination status, including dates of vaccination, positive titer, or employee refusing the vaccination. Each of these records must be maintained for a specific amount of time, as indicated by OSHA or state requirements. Though the training records and HBV records are related to the safety manual, these records are maintained in a separate, secure area.

Specimen Collection Manual. The **specimen collection manual** provides the information needed to collect specimens for the various tests performed in the POL or its referral laboratory. It includes a list of names of the tests and their synonyms, types of collection apparatus required for each test, and a description of any special collection techniques. Also included are special handling requirements and transportation and storage needs for each type of specimen. Often, this information is presented in a large, easily read chart that is posted above the specimen collection site. The information given in the chart should be complete enough to enable lab workers to collect any specimen shown using the appropriate technique.

Quality Control Manual. This manual contains written descriptions of quality control procedures and records of quality control test results. The quality control manual describes how to perform quality control, as well how to troubleshoot controls that do not fall within the acceptable range. The accuracy of test results is monitored daily by analyzing the control specimens (artificial specimens with known values of the tested substance). Usually, two control samples are analyzed, one in the normal range and the other with an abnormally high or low value. If the test results fall within an acceptable range, as provided by the manufacturer in the package insert, then the system of instruments and reagents used in the test procedure are presumed to function properly. If the control sample falls outside the accepted range, on the other hand, then the cause must be determined.

Test values of control samples are recorded on graphs in the quality control manual. They also may be recorded in the patient testing log or entered into the computerized laboratory information system log. The graphs provide a quick and easy way of observing quality control results over time and spotting any values that fall outside the acceptable range. Federal law requires that these graphs be kept for three years. They also must be produced at onsite inspections if requested. Daily temperature controls of the freezer, refrigerator, and bacteria incubator also are maintained. The records support the assertion that specimens received proper storage in case of inspection or lawsuits.

Proficiency Testing Manual. The **proficiency testing manual** is a permanent record of proficiency test results that augment the quality control record. Unlike quality control procedures that test known controls, proficiency testing uses unknown samples that have been evaluated by outside agencies. Proficiency testing may involve an agency-run proficiency testing program or split-specimen testing. Both types of testing provide a check of the quality of testing procedures, reagents, and laboratory personnel's skills. Proficiency test results are often plotted on graphs with colored zones that indicate acceptable and unacceptable ranges of results.

Instrument Calibration and Maintenance Manual. The **instrument calibration and maintenance manual** contains instructions and dated records of laboratory instrument calibration and maintenance. Although most lab instruments are easy to use, many are complex systems that must receive regular maintenance to prevent wear and reduce instrument failure. Manufacturers provide written guidelines for periodic maintenance of their instruments. The guidelines help to ensure that the instruments are serviced as needed so that they will perform accurately in testing procedures.

Instruments must be calibrated using calibration standards at least every six months or whenever new lots of reagents are introduced.

Inventory Control Manual. In order for POLs to operate smoothly, they must have an adequate supply of necessary reagents and other supplies. The **inventory control manual** maintains records of the routine inventory of supplies on hand and orders that have been placed. It generally consists of two parts: (a) a file containing supply house contact information and orders and (b) a calendar for keeping a daily tally of supplies on hand.

PATH OF PATIENT'S TEST—FROM START TO FINISH

The most important record in POLs is the patient's test result. All other records and documents support the patient test records. Figure 6-5 shows the path of the patient's test, beginning with the physician's requisition and ending with posting of the result in the patient's chart.

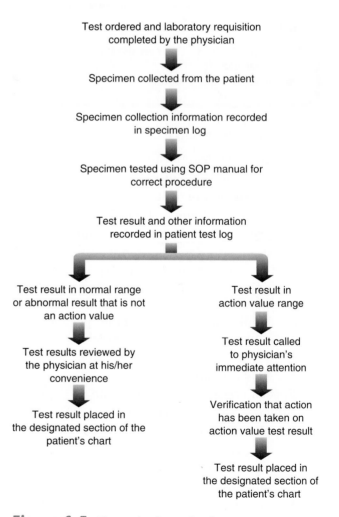

Figure 6-5 The path of a patient's test.

An Important Note on Filing Patient Test Results

When completed, test results are recorded in the patient's chart for the physician's review. Each test result should be reported with its normal range for the average, healthy individual. This way, the physician can see at a glance if a patient's test result is abnormal.

While all test results should be posted to the patient's chart as soon as possible, some test results must be called to the attention of the physician immediately. There are test results that indicate the need for prompt medical screening or treatment. Action, critical, or panic test values are those that call for immediate ("stat") medical attention. Not all abnormal test results are action values. It is up to the physician to decide for each lab test how far outside the normal range of values a test result must fall before it is considered to be an action value. A chart of action value ranges for testing procedures carried out in the POL should be posted in an obvious place so that such test results are not overlooked. In addition, many laboratory information systems are designed to "flag" the laboratory technician to take action when a patient test result falls within the action value range.

There should be an established procedure for dealing with action values in the POL, including delegation of responsibility for reporting results. A sign-off procedure such as a written report initialed by both the responsible lab personnel and the physician may be used to ensure that the physician has received the report and taken the necessary action.

PROCEDURE 6-1

Documenting in the Specimen Log

Goal

To successfully document specimens in the specimen log

Completion Time

30 minutes

Equipment and Supplies

- Pen and paper

Data—Specimen Information

- Urine for Suzie Jones. Her medical record number is 589563. Collected at 10:30 am on July 5, 2010. Doctor ordered urinalysis. Test performed at the POL. Throat swab collected at 10:35 am on July 5, 2010. Doctor ordered rapid strep test. Test performed at the POL.
- Marble top tube for Pedro Gonzales. His medical record number is 125876. Specimen was collected at 8:00 am on July 5, 2010. Doctor ordered lipid profile and a basic metabolic profile. Tests performed at the POL.
- Throat swab for Kim Lee. Her medical record number is 896352. Collected at 9:15 am on July 5, 2010. Doctor ordered rapid strep test. Test performed at the POL.
- Blue top tubes for Ekaterina Posinki. Her medical record number is 658932. Collected at 11:20 am on July 5, 2010. Doctor ordered PT/INR studies. Test performed at the reference lab.

Instructions

Read though the list of equipment and supplies that you will need. Read the steps of the procedure. Be sure that you understand each step before you begin. Then complete each step correctly and in the proper order. If your completion time is too long, repeat the procedure until you increase your speed.

Steps marked with (*) are critical and must have the maximum points possible to pass.

Performance Standards	Point Awarded	Maximum Points
1. Create a specimen log, including the following categories: Date and Time Specimen Collected or Received, Patient's Name, Patient's Medical Record Number, Specimen Type, Test Ordered, Testing Location, and Initials.		30
2. Enter the specimen information into the chart, in chronological order		20
Total Points		50

Overall Procedural Evaluation

Student Name _____

Signature of Instructor _____ Date _____

Comments _____

_____

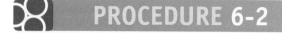

PROCEDURE 6-2

Documenting in the Patient Testing Log

Goal
To successfully document results in the patient log

Completion Time
30 minutes

Equipment and Supplies
- Pen and paper

Data
- Kit manufacturer: Advanced Testing Kits
- Kit lot number: XGB 537
- Kit expiration date: March 12, 2012
- Negative rapid strep control: Lot number XGB 537-N; Result—negative
- Positive rapid strep control: Lot number XGB 537-P; Result—positive
- Throat swab for Kim Lee. Her medical record number is 896352. Collected at 9:15 am on July 5, 2010. Doctor ordered rapid strep test. Test performed at the POL. Test result is negative
- Throat swab for Ekaterina Posinki. Her medical record number is 658932. Collected at 11:20 am on July 5, 2010. Doctor ordered coagulation studies. Test performed at the reference lab. Test result is positive.
- Throat swab for Suzie Jones. Her medical record number is 589563. Collected at 10:30 am on July 5, 2010. Doctor ordered rapid strep test. Test performed at the POL. Test result is positive.

Instructions
Read though the list of equipment and supplies that you will need. Read the steps of the procedure. Be sure that you understand each step before you begin. Then complete each step correctly and in the proper order. If your completion time is too long, repeat the procedure until you increase your speed.

Steps marked with (*) are critical and must have the maximum points possible to pass.

Performance Standards	Point Awarded	Maximum Points
1. Create a patient testing log, including the following categories: Kit Manufacturer, Kit Lot Number, Kit Expiration Date, Date and Time Specimen Tested, Patient's Name, Patient's Medical Record Number, Results, and Initials		30
2. Enter the testing information into the chart, in chronological order		20
Total Points		50

Overall Procedural Evaluation

Student Name _____

Signature of Instructor _____ Date _____

Comments _____

_____

chapter 6 REVIEW

Using Terminology

Match the term in the right column with the appropriate definition or description in the left column.

____ **1.** Action value

____ **2.** Manual

____ **3.** Procedure

____ **4.** Standard operating procedure (SOP) manual

____ **5.** Requisition

____ **6.** Specimen log

____ **7.** Patient testing log

a. series of steps taken to complete a particular task

b. form on which patient test requests are written

c. document that records information about all of the specimens received or collected by the laboratory

d. document that records all of the patient test results

e. patient test value that requires immediate medical attention

f. laboratory handbook that contains instructions for a particular aspect of the laboratory

g. lab manual containing detailed instructions for each procedure performed in the laboratory

Choose the best answer for the following questions.

8. Daily quality control results are recorded in the
   a. specimen log
   b. standard operating procedure (SOP) manual
   c. patient test log
   d. test requisition form

9. What information should NOT be recorded in the specimen log?
   a. patient name
   b. date and time the specimen was collected
   c. type of specimen
   d. patient test results

10. What information should NOT be recorded in the patient test log?
   a. patient name
   b. type of specimen
   c. date and time the specimen was tested
   d. patient test results

11. Which medical professional(s) can order laboratory tests for a patient?
   a. doctors
   b. physician assistants
   c. nurse practitioners
   d. all of the above

12. Which manual contains information about vacation, sick leave, and hiring and termination practices?
   a. general policy manual
   b. standard operating procedure (SOP) manual
   c. specimen collection manual
   d. proficiency testing manual

13. What information is found in a typical patient requisition form?
   a.   patient name
   b.   patient medical record number
   c.   tests ordered
   d.   all of the above

14. Who has the ultimate authority and responsibility for the policies in the POL?
   a.   doctor/medical director
   b.   medical assistant
   c.   lab personnel
   d.   phlebotomists

15. Under HIPAA, what rights does a patient have?
   a.   the right to request changes to his or her medical record
   b.   the right to have his or her medical information protected
   c.   the right to request copies of his or her medical record
   d.   all of the above

16. Who decides at what level of abnormality to treat patient test results as action values?
   a.   doctor/medical director
   b.   medical assistant
   c.   lab personnel
   d.   phlebotomists

17. When is oral communication an important method of communicating information?
   a.   when giving sign-out
   b.   when communicating action values
   c.   it is always a good means of communicating information
   d.   a and b

Acquiring Knowledge

Answer the following questions in the spaces provided.

18. What are some advantages of computerized record keeping in POLs?

_____

_____

_____

19. Why should even experienced laboratory personnel refer to the appropriate manual when performing lab tests?

_____

_____

_____

20. From legal, malpractice, and quality control perspectives, why is the daily recording of the temperature controls in the POL important?

_____

_____

_____

21. Describe the path of a patient's test in the POL (when results are normal)—from the doctor's requisition to recording the result in the patient's chart.

_____

_____

_____

22. What is the best way to prove that a POL is not negligent in a malpractice suit?

_____

_____

_____

23. How is a statute-of-limitations law related to POL records?

_____

_____

_____

24. When can a patient's laboratory test results be released to insurance companies or other individuals who request them?

_____

_____

_____

25. Why is it crucial that POL records be protected against loss by theft, fire, and other disasters?

_____

_____

_____

26. How do quality control records safeguard the accuracy of laboratory test results?

_____

_____

_____

27. What information does the SOP manual contain?

_____

_____

_____

Applying Knowledge—On the Job

Answer the following questions in the spaces provided.

28. Dr. Singh is very upset. Mrs. Levy, one of his patients, just informed him that a neighbor had started a rumor that Mrs. Levy's 13-year-old daughter is pregnant. The neighbor had seen the 13-year-old's name recorded with a positive pregnancy test result in the POL's patient test log. The log had been left open on a table near the test collection site where the neighbor had a blood specimen drawn.

In fact, the pregnancy test report belonged to a 30-year-old woman with the same name as the 13-year-old. Why should this mix-up never have occurred? How could it have been prevented?

_____

_____

_____

29. Dr. Paro had lunch with some friends who told her that they overheard her POL staff gossiping about her patients at a local restaurant. How should Dr. Paro deal with this problem?

_____

_____

_____

30. Jera has been asked to collect a fasting blood specimen from a patient named Mr. Boroughs. When she checks to be sure that he has fasted according to instructions, he tells her that he had only a doughnut for breakfast instead of his usual bacon and eggs. When Jera tries to explain that fasting means no food at all, Mr. Boroughs becomes angry and tells her that she had better take his blood now anyway because he is not going to miss any more work. What should Jera do?

_____

_____

_____

31. Anne, a new worker in the POL, has been told by a coworker that she lacks seniority and has to take whatever shifts the other lab personnel do not want. During her job interview, Anne had been assured of fair rotation. How can she find out which is the correct policy of the POL?

_____

_____

_____

32. Isabella has just completed a patient urinalysis. The urine contained many bacteria and had a high level of glucose and protein. She is not sure if she should call it to the physician's attention because he is having a very busy morning. What do you think Isabella should do?

_____

_____

_____

33. Mrs. Bond is upset because she has been asked to return to the doctor's office this morning for another blood test. The lab personnel failed to draw enough blood yesterday for all of the tests that were requested. How could this problem have been avoided?

_____

_____

_____

34. The POL where Tony works has been accused of reporting an erroneous positive result for a syphilis test to an insurance company. The report embarrassed the patient and caused him to lose a job. How should the POL staff determine if they were negligent?

_____

_____

_____

35. The mother of a child with a birth defect believes that her doctor's office lab failed to report a positive test for protein in her urine before the child was born. The mother is suing the clinic for malpractice in causing the birth defect of her child. What evidence is needed to determine if the POL met acceptable medical standards?

_____

_____

_____

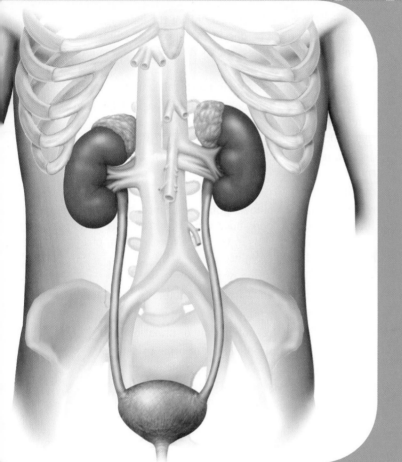

Anatomy and Physiology of the Urinary System

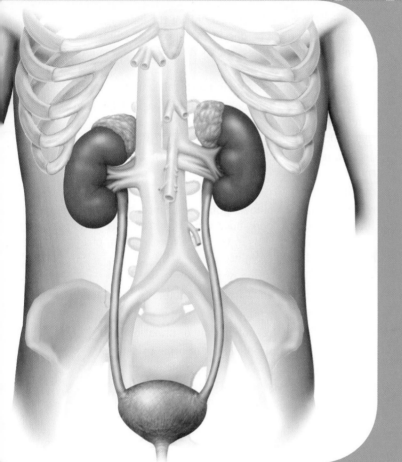

COGNITIVE OBJECTIVES

After studying this chapter, you should be able to

7.1 use each of the vocabulary terms appropriately.

7.2 explain why urine specimens are important in the POL.

7.3 describe the structure and function of the organs of the urinary system.

7.4 discuss the role of the kidneys in maintaining body homeostasis.

7.5 describe the formation and flow of urine.

7.6 describe the physiological basis for several diseases that involve the urinary system.

7.7 identify the factors that affect the volume and composition of urine.

PERFORMANCE OBJECTIVE

After studying this chapter, you should be able to:

7.8 develop a model that shows the path of urine formation, from arterial blood through the kidneys, ureters, and bladder, to micturition.

TERMINOLOGY

bladder: stores the urine produced by the kidneys.

cystitis: inflammation of the urinary bladder.

dehydration: the loss of body water in excess of intake, resulting in a net deficiency of water in the tissues. Dehydration is caused by either decreased intake or increased loss of water and may be due to excessive vomiting, diarrhea, sweating, or uncontrolled diabetes.

distal convoluted tubule: the part of the coiled renal tubule that begins after the loop of Henle.

electrolyte: ion that is positively or negatively charged.

glomerular filtrate: fluid formed in the kidneys when the entering, or afferent, arteriole is larger than the exiting, or efferent, arteriole, thus creating a higher blood pressure than is found in most capillaries. The hydrostatic pressure forces water and other substances out of the blood, forming the glomerular filtrate. The glomerular filtrate has about the same composition as tissue fluid elsewhere in the body.

glomerulonephritis: a condition in which the glomerular capillaries are inflamed and become permeable to protein.

glucosuria (glycosuria): the condition in which there is glucose in the urine.

homeostasis: an equilibrium state of the body maintained by feedback and internal regulation of body processes. Homeostasis helps keep individuals healthy by returning their physical state to normal following stress or trauma.

kidney: structure responsible for forming the urine. Most individuals are born with two.

kidney stone (calculus): a hard stone that forms in the hollow passages of the urinary system in some individuals.

micturition: also called urination; the voiding, or passing, of urine from the bladder through the urethra.

nephrology: the study of the structure and function of kidneys.

nephron: the basic functional unit of the kidneys, composed of a renal corpuscle and proximal and distal convoluted renal tubules. Each kidney has over a million nephrons.

peritoneum: a membrane lining the abdominal cavity.

pH: the degree of acidity or alkalinity (basic) expressed in hydrogen ion concentration. Acids have a pH less than 7.0. Bases have a pH greater than 7.0.

proteinuria: a condition in which protein appears in the urine.

renal: pertaining to the kidney.

renal threshold: spillover point; the concentration of a substance in the blood above which the substance is not reabsorbed and remains in the urine for excretion; often used with reference to glucose.

ureteritis: inflammation of the ureters.

ureters: carry the urine from the kidneys to the bladder.

urethra: carries the urine out of the body.

-uria: a suffix that denotes urine or urination.

urinalysis: the clinical analysis of urine to determine its physical, chemical, and microscopic properties.

urinary tract infections (UTIs): infections of the organs of the urinary tract system.

INTRODUCTION

Urine is one of the easiest specimens to collect in the POL. In addition, urine provides great diagnostic information. As a result, **urinalysis,** or the clinical analysis of urine, is the most frequently performed patient test in POLs. The urinary system is composed of the organs that produce, store, and excrete urine. Due to the importance of urinalysis in the POL, familiarity with the structure and function of the urinary system is important for greater understanding of the test and its results.

THE URINARY SYSTEM

The urinary system consists of two kidneys, two ureters, the bladder, and the urethra. These structures are shown in Figure 7-1. The **kidneys** are responsible for forming the urine, the **ureters** carry the urine from the kidneys to the bladder, and the **bladder** stores the urine. The **urethra** carries the urine out of the body. Therefore, the flow of urine is as follows: it forms in the two kidneys, flows into the two ureters, collects in the bladder, and leaves the body by way of the urethra.

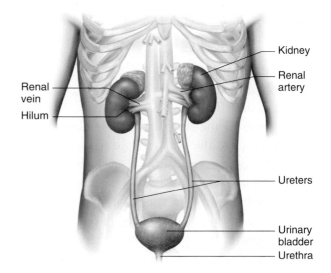

Figure 7-1 Organs of the urinary system.

110

The Kidneys

> ### Nephrology
>
> **Nephrology** is the study of the structure and function of the kidneys.

The kidneys are the organs responsible for urine production. They remove unwanted waste products from the blood. They help maintain body **homeostasis,** or equilibrium, by selectively excreting or retaining various substances according to the body's needs. The kidneys also play a role in water, **electrolyte,** and **pH** balance.

> ### Renal
>
> **Renal** is the medical term that means "pertaining to the kidney(s)."

> ### Electrolytes
>
> Electrolytes are ions that are positively or negatively charged. Examples of ions found in the blood and urine are sodium, potassium, hydrogen, chloride, and many others.

> ### pH
>
> pH is the degree of acidity or alkalinity (basic) expressed in hydrogen concentration. Acids have a pH less than 7.0. Bases have a pH greater than 7.0.

When the blood concentration of a particular substance rises, it may reach a point at which the kidney can no longer reabsorb the substance. At this point, the substance begins to appear in the urine for excretion. This point is known as the **renal threshold.**

> ### Glucosuria
>
> An example of an analyte exceeding renal threshold is a condition called glucosuria. **Glucosuria,** or glycosuria, is the condition in which there is glucose in the urine. It may occur in healthy patients following ingestion of large amounts of sugar or after intravenous administration of glucose. In patients with diabetes mellitus, who have inadequate production or utilization of insulin, glucose may spill over into the urine when blood sugar escalates. Checking for the presence of glucose in the urine is one of the ways diabetes is screened for.

The kidneys are dark red, bean-shaped organs about the size of an adult's fist. They are located within the back wall of the abdominal cavity, just below and behind the liver. The kidneys are positioned outside the **peritoneum,** which lines the abdominal cavity, and against the deep muscles of the back on either side of the spinal column. They are held in place by connective tissue. Masses of adipose tissue, or fat, surround them and help protect them from injury.

The inner region of each kidney is called the medulla, and the outer region is the cortex. The lateral side of each kidney is convex and the medial side concave. In the middle of the side of the kidney that curves inward begins the chamber called the renal sinus. The entrance to the renal sinus is called the hilum. Through the hilum pass various blood and lymphatic vessels, nerves, and the ureter. The renal pelvis is the expanded proximal end of the ureter that lies within the renal sinus. It is divided into cuplike cavities called calyces (singular, *calyx*).

> ### Diseases of the Kidney
>
> Patients who are tested in POLs may have several different kidney diseases and conditions with which you should be familiar:
>
> - nephropathy: any disease of the kidney.
> - nephrotic syndrome: any kidney disease characterized by chronic protein loss in urine.
> - nephrosis: protein loss due to noninflammatory degeneration of the kidney.
> - nephritis: any inflammation of the kidney.
> - nephrocystitis: inflammation of the kidney and bladder.
> - pyelonephritis: inflammation of the kidney and pelvis.
> - renal failure: when the kidney no longer functions.
> - renal insufficiency: when the kidney is no longer capable of functioning adequately to maintain health.

Blood is supplied to the kidneys by the renal arteries, which branch from the main abdominal artery, the aorta. About 1,200 mL of blood per minute enter the renal arteries. This is about 25 percent of total cardiac output. The renal arteries enter the kidneys through the hilum and further subdivide as they pass through to the cortex, where the **nephrons** are located.

Venous blood is returned through a series of blood vessels that correspond generally to the arterial pathway. These vessels join to form the renal vein, which leaves each kidney through the hilum. The renal veins join the inferior vena cava, the principal vein of the lower part of the body.

Nephrons are the structural and functional units of the kidneys. They remove waste products from the blood and regulate water and electrolyte concentrations in blood and other body fluids. There are an astonishing one million nephrons per kidney. Not all of these nephrons are actively functioning in healthy individuals, but they can be called into action to maintain normal kidney function if an individual loses a kidney. The loss of a kidney can occur due to disease, injury, or sometimes organ donation.

Each nephron consists of a renal corpuscle and renal tubule. The renal corpuscle is composed of a tangled cluster of capillaries called a glomerulus, which is surrounded by a thin-walled, saclike structure called the Bowman's capsule. The tubule leading away from the Bowman's capsule becomes highly coiled and is called the proximal convoluted tubule. The tubule then follows a straight path, forming the loop of Henle (descending and ascending), and finally becomes highly coiled again, at which point it is called the **distal convoluted tubule.** Distal convoluted tubules merge from several nephrons and drain into a collecting tubule.

A number of collecting tubules, in turn, coalesce in the renal cortex to form a collecting duct. The collecting ducts increase in size as they join together into papillae (singular, *papilla)* and ultimately empty into calyces that drain first into the funnel-shaped renal pelvis and then through the hilum into the ureter.

The Ureters

Each ureter is a tubular organ about 25 cm long that carries urine from the kidney to the urinary bladder. The wall of the ureter is muscular, and peristaltic waves originating in the renal pelvis move the urine along its length. The flaplike fold of mucous membrane covering the opening to the bladder acts like a one-way valve, allowing urine to enter the bladder but not to leave it.

Kidney Stones

Kidney stones, or **calculi,** sometimes form in the renal pelvis. They may be composed of uric acid or magnesium phosphate, but most often, they are composed of calcium compounds such as calcium oxalate or calcium phosphate. If the stones pass into the ureter, they cause severe pain, typically beginning in the region of the kidney and radiating into the abdomen, pelvis, and legs. Kidney stones also may cause nausea and vomiting. The causes of kidney stone formation are diverse, including excess calcium intake, gout, and abnormal functioning of the parathyroid glands, which regulate calcium-phosphorus metabolism.

The Urinary Bladder

The urinary bladder is a hollow, expandable, muscular sac located behind the pubic symphysis and below the parietal peritoneum. The walls of the empty bladder have many folds that smooth out when the bladder is filled with urine, allowing it to swell to a capacity of several hundred milliliters.

Micturition, also called urination, is the voiding, or passing, of urine from the bladder through the urethra and out of the body. It is triggered by the micturition reflex center in the sacral region of the spinal cord. Although the bladder may hold as much as 600 mL, the desire to urinate usually is triggered when the bladder contains about 150 mL. In infants and small children, micturition is controlled by reflex. As individuals age and learn to control the need to urinate, it is accomplished by voluntary muscle tissue surrounding the urethra.

Urinary Tract Infections (UTIs)

Urinary tract infections (UTIs) are infections of the organs of the urinary tract system. Bladder infections are more common in women than in men. The urethra is shorter in women, allowing infectious agents like bacteria easier access to the bladder. Because the linings of the ureters and the bladder are continuous, infectious agents introduced to the bladder may enter the ureters. Inflammation of the bladder is called **cystitis,** and inflammation of the ureters is called **ureteritis.**

The Urethra

The urethra is a tube that carries urine from the bladder to the outside of the body. In males, the urethra also carries semen from the reproductive system. The wall of the urethra consists of a relatively thick layer of smooth muscle lined with mucous membrane. Numerous mucous glands, called urethral glands, secrete mucus into the urethral canal.

URINE FORMATION

Urine contains wastes, excess water, and excess electrolytes. It is formed in the nephrons in a three-stage process consisting of glomerular filtration, tubular reabsorption, and tubular secretion.

-Uria

-Uria is a suffix that denotes urine or urination.

Glomerular Filtration

The formation of urine begins when the plasma portion of the blood passes through the thin-walled membranes of the glomerular capillaries of the kidneys. If the entering, or afferent, arteriole is larger than the exiting, or efferent, arteriole, this will create a higher blood pressure than is found in most capillaries. The hydrostatic pressure forces water and other substances out of the blood. The resulting fluid, the **glomerular filtrate,** has about the same composition as tissue fluid elsewhere in the body. The concentrations of electrolytes, calcium, magnesium, sulfate, phosphate, glucose, urea, and uric acid, for example, are the same as in plasma. The glomerular filtrate lacks only the larger protein molecules.

Glomerulonephritis

Glomerulonephritis is a condition in which the glomerular capillaries are inflamed and become permeable to protein. Because protein appears in the glomerular filtrate and is excreted in the urine, the condition also is called **proteinuria.**

The glomerular filtration rate in both kidneys in the average adult is about 125 mL per minute, or some 180,000 mL in 24 hours. Loss of fluid from the body in urine is typically less than 1,500 mL per day. Obviously, most of the glomerular filtrate is reabsorbed by the plasma.

Blood Pressure and the Kidneys

People with high or low blood pressure are prone to kidney problems. This is because the rate of filtration goes up when blood pressure rises and down when blood pressure is lower.

Tubular Reabsorption

Much of the glomerular filtrate is reabsorbed in the renal tubules of the nephron. As a result, the fluid leaving the renal tubules as urine has a much different composition than does the glomerular filtrate entering them via Bowman's capsule membrane. The substances that remain in the renal tubules, like urea and uric acid, tend to become more and more concentrated as water is reabsorbed from the filtrate. Fluid absorption from the renal tubules is enhanced by the permeable wall and low pressure of the surrounding capillaries.

Reabsorption of most substances, including glucose and water, occurs in the proximal convoluted tubule. All of the glucose in the filtrate is reabsorbed in most people. Water reabsorption depends on the rate of absorption of sodium ions—as sodium reabsorption increases or decreases, so does the absorption of water. Almost all of the sodium in the glomerular filtrate is eventually reabsorbed. (See Table 7-1.)

Table 7-1   Composition of Glomerular Filtrate and Urine

	Glomerular Filtrate	Urine
Glucose concentration	100 mg/100 mL (or dL)	0
Urea concentration	26 mg/100 mL (or dL)	1820 mg/100 mL (or dL)
Uric acid concentration	4 mg/100 mL (or dL)	53 mg/100 mL (or dL)

When the blood concentration of a substance rises, it may reach its renal plasma threshold, or spillover point, the concentration above which the substance is not reabsorbed and remains in the urine for excretion.

The reabsorption of water from the tubule is regulated by antidiuretic hormone, ADH, which is produced by the hypothalamus. ADH inhibits the loss of water when there is danger of **dehydration.** Dehydration is the loss of body water in excess of intake, resulting in a net deficiency of water in the tissues. Dehydration is caused by either decreased intake or increased loss of water. ADH prevents dehydration by increasing the permeability of the tubule and collecting duct, causing rapid reabsorption of water.

Diabetes Insipidus

Diabetes insipidus is a metabolic disorder caused by a deficiency of ADH. Without ADH, nephron tubules fail to reabsorb water, causing the passage of large amounts of dilute urine, accompanied by excessive thirst.

Tubular Secretion

Some substances are secreted from the tubule into the urine, bypassing glomerular filtration. Penicillin and histamine, for example, are secreted into the proximal convoluted portion of the tubule, and hydrogen ions are secreted into both the proximal and distal segments.

VOLUME AND COMPOSITION OF URINE

The exact amount of urine formed in an individual depends on many factors, including fluid intake, diet, drugs, environmental temperature, relative humidity of the surrounding air, respiratory rate, body temperature, and emotional state. An output of less than 30 mL of urine per hour may indicate kidney failure.

The composition of urine varies considerably from time to time in the same individual because of changes in dietary intake and level of physical activity. In addition to being approximately 95 percent water, urine usually contains urea from the breakdown of amino acids and uric acid from the breakdown of nucleic acids. Urine also contains a variety of electrolytes such as sodium, potassium, chloride, and bicarbonates. The concentration of electrolytes tends to vary directly with their concentration in the diet.

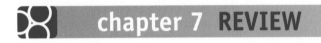

chapter 7 REVIEW

Review Questions

Physiology Review

Label the indicated parts in the following drawing

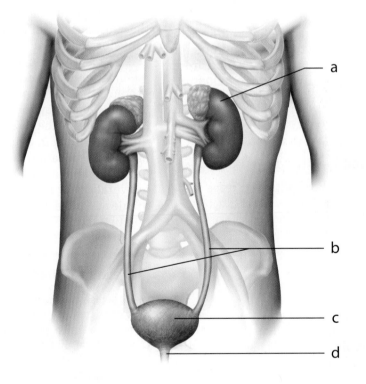

____**1.** Urethra
____**2.** Kidneys
____**3.** Ureters
____**4.** Bladder

Match the following terms.

____ **5.** Homeostasis

____ **6.** Electrolyte

____ **7.** pH

____ **8.** Renal threshold

a. when the concentration of a substance in the blood exceeds the level the kidney is capable of reabsorbing

b. degree of acidity or alkalinity of a solution

c. when the body is in a state of equilibrium

d. ion that is negatively or positively charged

Multiple Choice

Choose the best answer for the following questions.

9. The condition in which there is glucose in the urine is
   a. diabetes insipidus
   b. glucosuria
   c. pyelonephritis
   d. cystitis

10. Inflammation of the bladder occurs in which of the following conditions
    a. homeostasis
    b. cystitis
    c. glomerulonephritis
    d. glucosuria

11. Passing of urine from the body is
    a. glucosuria
    b. micturition
    c. homeostasis
    d. ureteritis

12. Which of the following correctly describes the flow of urine through the urinary tract system?
    a. bladder, ureters, kidneys, urethra
    b. kidneys, ureters, bladder, urethra
    c. urethra, kidneys, ureters, bladder
    d. ureters, bladder, urethra, kidneys

13. A condition in which the kidney no longer works is known as
    a. nephrosis
    b. nephrocystitis
    c. renal failure
    d. nephrotic syndrome

14. The structure through which various blood vessels, lymphatic vessels, and nerves enter the kidney is the
    a. hilum
    b. medulla
    c. cortex
    d. calyx

Acquiring Knowledge

Answer the following questions in the spaces provided.

15. Are men or women more prone to bladder infections? Why?

_____

_____

_____

16. What is the renal threshold?

_____

_____

_____

17. Mrs. Alvarez just called with regard to her new prescription. The doctor said that she had a bladder infection but the pharmacist mentioned cystitis. Now, Mrs. Alvarez is worried that she either has the wrong medication or she has a cyst instead of bladder infections. How would you straighten out this mix-up?

_____

_____

_____

18. A patient has a reading of 4+ urine glucose on the test strip. The normal range is "negative." What metabolic disorder might you suspect? Why is the glucose present in the urine?

_____

_____

_____

19. A patient's urine has a high level of protein. What condition does this suggest?

_____

_____

_____

20. What condition results when the body loses more water than it takes in?

_____

_____

_____

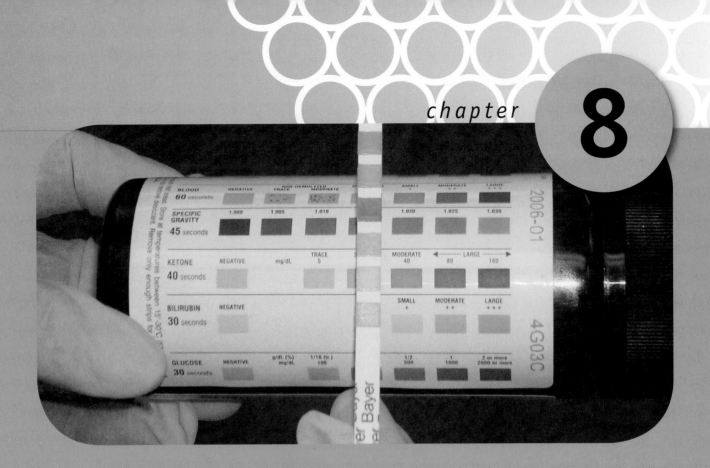

Urine Specimen Collection and Preservation

COGNITIVE OBJECTIVES

After studying this chapter, you should be able to

8.1 use each of the vocabulary terms appropriately.

8.2 describe the role of urinalysis and explain why urinalysis is used frequently in POLs to diagnose or screen for disease.

8.3 describe several different types of urine specimens and identify their diagnostic uses.

8.4 describe the different methods of urine collection and explain why each is used.

8.5 discuss what information must be communicated to patients to assure that urine specimens are collected correctly.

8.6 explain how to properly preserve the different types of urine specimens and the importance of specimen preservation in performing accurate urinalysis.

8.7 list the specimen labeling requirements for urine specimens.

8.8 identify the factors affecting urine volume.

PERFORMANCE OBJECTIVES

After studying this chapter, you should be able to

8.9 give instructions to a patient in the proper collection of a clean-catch, midstream specimen.

8.10 give instructions to a patient in the proper collection of a 24-hour urine specimen.

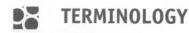

TERMINOLOGY

anuria: the complete absence of urine excretion.

casts, urinary: microscopic solid forms created from protein precipitates in the renal tubules and voided in the urine.

catheterization, urinary: the process of inserting a tube through the urethra into the urinary bladder to obtain a urine specimen.

clean-catch, midstream urine specimen: a urine specimen collected midstream after thoroughly cleaning the surrounding area to prevent contamination of the specimen; used when urine is to be cultured.

culture and sensitivity (C & S): microbiology testing used to determine the bacteria causing infection and make a determination regarding which antibiotics are effective.

diuretic: agent that increases urine production.

first morning urine specimen: also called eight-hour, overnight, early morning, or first morning specimen; a urine specimen collected as soon as the patient arises in the morning, consisting of urine that has collected and concentrated in the bladder during the night.

glucose tolerance test (GTT): a test of the ability to metabolize glucose, in which the patient is tested for blood and urine glucose at short intervals after consuming a known quantity of glucose in solution.

oliguria: the excretion of less than 400 mL of urine in 24 hours in adults. Oliguria is a life-threatening condition requiring immediate correction.

perineum: the outside area of the body immediately surrounding the rectum and urethra.

polyuria: the excretion of excessive amounts of nearly colorless urine. Polyuria is confirmed by a 24-hour urine volume greater than 2,000 mL.

postprandial urine specimen: an after-meal specimen; used most often to test for the presence of glucose in urine.

random urine specimen: a urine specimen that is taken at any time of day or night, usually during a visit to the physician's office.

timed urine specimens: urine specimens collected at timed intervals. Often used to diagnose diabetes or to assess the rate of renal clearance.

24-hour urine specimen: a collective specimen that includes the total urine output of a patient for a 24-hour period; usually collected by the patient at home and often used for quantitative analysis.

2-hour urine specimen: the total urine output of a patient for a 2-hour period.

urinalysis (UA): the clinical analysis of urine to determine its physical, chemical, and microscopic properties.

urinary sediments: solid substances found in standing urine specimen. Can include bacteria, red blood cells, white blood cells, urinary casts, etc.

urobilinogen: a colorless derivative of bilirubin; formed by the action of intestinal bacteria.

INTRODUCTION

Urine specimens can provide a great deal of information about the both the urinary tract system and other body systems. In order for the urine to provide diagnostic information, the urine specimen must be correctly collected and maintained. This chapter discusses the different types of urine specimens and their uses. Proper specimen handling for those specimens also will be discussed.

URINALYSIS

Urine may be analyzed for its physical, chemical, or microscopic properties. When all three types of analysis are made, this is referred to as complete, or routine, **urinalysis (UA).** On the other hand, only a few specific parameters of urine may be analyzed, such as the urine glucose level, which is measured in routine testing for diabetes and in monitoring

diabetic patients. Urinalysis is performed for three general reasons:

- Screening of large groups of people for disease, such as testing for urine glucose levels in diabetes screening.

- Diagnosis of suspected disease in individual patients, such as looking for the presence of bacteria in a suspected urinary tract infection.

- Monitoring the course of treatment to assess its effectiveness, such as checking the effect of an antibiotic on the bacteria count in a urinary tract infection or of a particular dosage or type of insulin on the glucose level in diabetes.

Urinalysis as a Diagnostic Tool

Diagnosis of disease is the main purpose of urinalysis in POLs. Urine may be abnormal because the kidneys are malfunctioning, or it may reflect problems in metabolism affecting other organs. Urinalysis in POLs can be used to detect kidney disease and many endocrine and metabolic disorders.

Detecting Kidney Disease. Patients with diseased kidneys may have abnormal urine because substances normally filtered out of the urine by the kidneys may appear in the urine. On the other hand, urine may be abnormal because patients have none or too little of a substance that is normally found in the urine. In either case, urinalysis can be an important diagnostic tool. The presence of protein in the urine, for example, may be indicative of glomerulonephritis.

Detecting Changes in Endocrine and Metabolic Function. Patients with endocrine or metabolic diseases, such as diabetes mellitus, may produce abnormal amounts of metabolic products such as ketones. These metabolic products often are excreted in the urine, where they may be detected through urinalysis. An abnormally high level of glucose in the urine, especially in a fasting patient, is a positive clinical sign of diabetes mellitus.

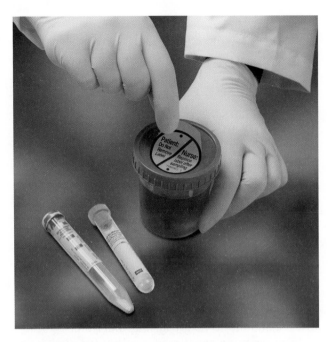

Figure 8-1 An example of a urine collection container.

Historical Note

The use of urine to diagnose disease dates back thousands of years. In 400 B.C., Hippocrates discovered that changes in the color and odor of urine often occur in patients with elevated temperatures. By the Middle Ages, the significance of urine in detecting disease was so widely recognized that the urine flask came to be an accepted symbol for physicians.

In 1827, an English physician named Richard Bright described the relationship between proteinuria, protein in the urine, and kidney disease. He made urine testing a regular part of medical examinations. By the middle of the 19th century, medical textbooks recommended that urinalysis be performed for every patient.

In the early part of the 20th century, the American physician Thomas Addis advanced the diagnostic use of urine when he discovered the diagnostic value of examining **urinary sediments,** solid substances found in standing urine.

SPECIMEN TYPES

The care that goes into collecting, handling, and preserving a urine specimen is the first stage of ensuring the accuracy of urinalysis. No degree of accuracy in performing subsequent tests on the urine in the lab can compensate for errors made in the process of getting the sample from the patient to the lab. Urine

must be collected at the correct time, in the right way, into an appropriate container, and then labeled and preserved correctly. (See Figure 8-1.) Only then is the analysis of the urine in the lab likely to be based on a reliable, representative specimen.

Random Urine Specimens

Random urine specimens are so named because they are collected randomly in terms of time. They may be collected at any time of the day or night and do not require any special patient preparation. They are convenient to collect in the physician's office restroom and require only a few simple instructions to the patient. Random specimens are most useful for qualitative assessment (positive or negative) of chemical and microscopic properties of urine. Semi-quantitative measurements also can be performed, but if precise quantitative measurements (determining the actual amount present) are required, other specimens should be collected. Random specimens are the most common urine specimen.

First Morning Urine Specimens

Also called overnight, early morning, or eight-hour specimens, **first morning urine specimens** are samples collected at the first urination upon arising in the morning. The concentration of urine varies during a 24-hour period, depending on fluid intake and activity level. Urine concentration is usually greatest in the first urination of the day, after the

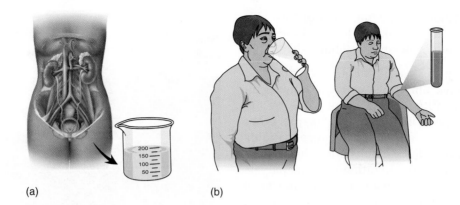

(a)   (b)

Figure 8-2 GTT example.

urine has collected undisturbed in the bladder throughout the night when there has been little, if any, fluid intake. Concentrations of bacteria in the urine also tend to be greatest at this time.

First morning specimens are best for nitrite and protein tests as well as for microscopic examination of the urine. The only drawback of the first morning urine specimen is that particles like red and white blood cells may decompose after standing in urine throughout the night, especially if the pH of the urine is high or the specific gravity is low. Furthermore, unless the patient is in the hospital with an on-site lab, there is generally a several-hour delay between collection and testing.

Timed Urine Specimens

Timed urine specimens are urine samples collected at specific intervals. Timed specimens often are collected during diabetic screening procedures. They also are used in renal clearance tests, which are performed to diagnose and evaluate kidney function.

Two-Hour Postprandial Urine Specimens. Post-prandial urine specimens, or after-meal specimens, often are collected to assess glucose metabolism. The patient is instructed to eat a meal high in carbohydrates. Two hours later, the urine specimen is collected. It is then analyzed for the presence of glucose.

Specimens for Glucose Tolerance Tests. The glucose tolerance test (GTT) uses blood and urine levels of glucose to screen and diagnose diabetes mellitus and gestational diabetes. The first urine specimen is collected after the patient has fasted. Then, the patient is given a known quantity of glucose in solution to drink, and urine and blood specimens are collected one-half hour, 1 hour, and 2 hours later. Sometimes, additional samples are collected after 2 hours if the patient is slow to metabolize

the glucose. When tested for using routine urinalysis strips, the result should be negative for normal, healthy patients. The presence of glucose in any amount is an abnormal finding. (See Figure 8-2.)

Volume Specimens

Volume specimens are cumulative specimens collected over a specified time interval, most often 2 or 24 hours. The entire volume of urine voided during the time interval is collected in one container and preserved for analysis at the end of the interval.

Two-Hour Volume Specimens. For **2-hour urine specimens,** urine is collected from the patient over a 2-hour period. This type of specimen usually is used to assess the level of **urobilinogen** in the urine. Urobilinogen is a colorless derivative of bilirubin that is formed by the action of intestinal bacteria.

24-Hour Volume Specimens. For **24-hour urine specimens,** urine is collected over a 24-hour interval. The large volume of urine can be used for quantitative analysis of the urine, which is usually performed in a reference lab, not the POL. (See Figure 8-3.)

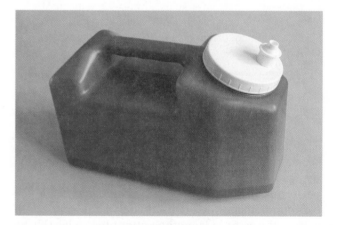

Figure 8-3 A 24-hour urine container.

A 24-hour specimen should be collected in the following manner:

- Empty the bladder into the toilet upon waking up in the morning. Do not save this sample but note the exact time at which urination occurred.
- Collect all urine samples throughout the next 24 hours and add each to the sample collection container, taking care to avoid spills or contaminating the inside of the container. Refrigerate the collection container, keep it on ice, or use a chemical preservative.
- If a chemical preservative is used, patients should be instructed on their health risks.
- At exactly the same time as noted on the first day, empty the bladder completely and add this sample to the collection container.

Safety Note

Some tests require a preservative be used to maintain the integrity of the specimen. Patients should be advised as to the presence of the preservative and that they should not discard the preservative. In addition, the patient should be informed that these preservatives can be toxic if they come into contact with the skin. Therefore, patients should collect their urine in a separate container and add each specimen to the 24-hour urine container, rather than urinating directly into the 24-hour urine container. If any specimens are missed or spilled, or if bed wetting occurs, a new 24-hour urine specimen must be collected at a later date.

VOLUME OF URINE

Urinary output may be affected by disease, so the measurement of urine volume during a timed interval, such as 24 hours, may be a valuable diagnostic aid. Diseases like diabetes mellitus, diabetes insipidus, and chronic renal disorders are characterized by **polyuria,** or the excretion of excessive amounts of urine. Polyuria is confirmed by a 24-hour urine volume greater than 2,000 mL. **Oliguria,** which is the excretion of less than 400 mL of urine in 24 hours, may result from dehydration, shock, edema, or acute kidney disease. **Anuria,** or the complete absence of urine excretion, may be due to acute renal failure, acute glomerulonephritis, or urinary tract obstruction. See Table 8-1 for normal urine volume ranges.

Table 8-1 Age and Sex Variation in Urine Volume Ranges

Age Group/Sex	Normal Volume
Newborn: 1–2 days	30–60 mL/day
Infant: 3–10 days 60–365 days	100–300 mL/day 400–500 mL/day
Child: 1–13 years 8–14 years	500–600 mL/day 800–1,400 mL/day
Middle-aged adult: Female Male	600–1,600 mL/day 800–1,800 mL/day
Elderly adult	250–2,400 mL/day

The Role of Drugs in Urine Volume

The volume of urine is increased with drugs that exert a **diuretic** effect. Diuretics are agents that increase urine production. Examples of some diuretic drugs are

- caffeine.
- alcohol.
- thiazides.
- oral hypoglycemic agents.

The volume of urine is decreased with drugs that cause nephrotoxicity, including

- analgesics (e.g., salicylates).
- antimicrobial agents (e.g., neomycin, streptomycin, and penicillin).

COLLECTING THE SAMPLE

The first step in patient testing in POLs is preparation of the patient to collect the specimen.

The Patient's Role

Collecting the urine specimen is usually up to the patient, who must be provided with the instructions and materials necessary to follow the collection procedure precisely. Instructions should first be given verbally, to allow the patient the opportunity to ask for clarification and to ask questions. The patient should then be given written instructions to refer to during the collection process. Patients who may need special assistance are the very weak, the extremely ill, the elderly, or very young children. Some patients who are not able to follow the urine collection procedures may require **urinary catherization,** which involves placing a tube called a catheter through the urethra into the bladder to obtain a urine specimen. This procedure is not performed by laboratory personnel.

Clean-Catch, Midstream Urine Specimens. Clean-catch, midstream urine specimens are the specimen of choice for patients with suspected infections in the urinary system. To reduce the risk of contamination from the urethra or **perineum,** which is the area outside of the body immediately surrounding the rectum and the urethra, ideally all urine specimens should be midstream specimens.

Clean-catch, midstream specimens are collected only after a strict cleansing procedure has been followed by the patient. This greatly minimizes the chance that the specimen will be contaminated with extraneous organisms during the collection procedure. This is required for all urine culture specimens to prevent extraneous organisms from proliferating in the culture medium and making the results meaningless.

Collecting clean-catch specimens requires that the patient be provided with careful, detailed instructions on the procedure, so it is virtually always done in the POL, not at home. Posting illustrated instructions in the POL patient bathroom is a good idea. The patient should be provided with an adequate supply of sterile towelettes saturated with cleansing solution and a sterile collection container. It is important to make sure you provide the patient with a sterile container for this procedure. The patient begins by voiding directly into the toilet. Then, he or she should collect about half a cup or 20 mL from the middle portion of the urination into the container. The remaining portion of the urination should go into the toilet. (See Figure 8-4.)

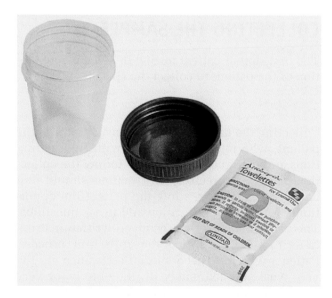

Figure 8-4 Example of a sterile container and towelettes needed for a clean-catch, midstream specimen.

Collecting Clean-Catch Specimens

For males:

- Wash and dry your hands before starting the collection procedure.
- If uncircumcised, retract your foreskin with a towelette.
- Clean the urethral opening three times: once on the left, once on the right, and directly over the urinary opening. Use a fresh towelette each time in a single wipe toward the glans.
- Start urinating into the toilet with the foreskin still retracted.
- Collect a midstream specimen of about 20 mL in the collection container. Do not touch the inside of the container or its lid!
- Void the rest of the urine into the toilet.
- Cap the container and take it to the lab.

For females:

- Wash and dry your hands before starting the collection procedure.
- Sit on the toilet seat with your legs spread apart as far as comfortable.
- If you are menstruating or have a heavy vaginal discharge, such as from a yeast infection, first insert a clean tampon.
- Spread the outer labia with your left hand (use your right hand if you are left handed).
- Clean both inner labia and the urethral opening, using a fresh towelette each time to wipe from front to back in a single stroke.
- Start urinating into the toilet with the outer labia still spread.
- Collect a midstream specimen of about 20 mL in the collection container. Do not touch the inside of the container or its lid!
- Void the rest of the urine into the toilet.
- Cap the container and take it to the lab.

Drug Screen Urine Collections

Urine drug screens may be done for a variety of reasons: some companies require them as part of pre-employment checks and life insurance companies routinely require them as part of the application for life insurance. At other times, they may be part of a criminal investigation to rule the use of drugs in or out.

The Drug Testing Custody and Control Form is the legal external chain-of-custody document used by the Department of Transportation (DOT) and industry (NON-DOT). The form identifies the urine sample and who has handled the sample from the time of collection until it is analyzed and released by the laboratory. Each company has specific forms and collection kits. These are typical collection procedure steps. (See Figure 8-5.)

1. Verify identification. Ask for a photo I.D. (e.g., driver's license) to properly identify the donor. If a photo I.D. is not available, an agent of the company may make a positive identification. Document on the form, "I.D. made by _____." Be sure to also examine proper I.D. of the agent. If the donor's identification cannot be established, *discontinue the collection procedure.*

2. Enter the donor's social security number and any other information requested at the top of the form.

3. Secure the restroom. Check the restroom for specimens that might have been left, that dye is present in the toilet bowl, and that faucets have been taped off with security tape.

4. Have the donor remove outer clothing such as a coat, sweater, or hat. These items, along with purses or parcels, and all contents of pockets are to remain outside the actual collection facility.

5. When the donor comes out of the restroom, check the specimen's temperature to make certain the temperature check is done within the required temperature limit. Temperature of the specimen must be between 90.5 and 99.0 degrees Fahrenheit. If the temperature is out of range, another specimen should be collected. If any difficulty occurs in collecting a new sample, the client/employer should be contacted for further instruction regarding what course of action to take.

6. The collector is now in receipt of the sample. Continue to fill out the custody form according to instructions on the form. Have the donor sign in the appropriate section.

7. Secure the specimen in a bag and the shipping container. Be sure to include the paperwork for the testing lab. Mail copies of the paperwork to the medical review officer (MRO) and the employer. Log the specimen in the drug screen log and call a courier for pickup.

Crossroads Medical Center
Newfield, New Jersey 07655-3213
201-555-4000

Drug Screen Consent Form

A urine drug test is required by_____ as part of your pre-employment screening. Please provide us with a list of all medications that you are presently taking.

_____

_____

_____

_____

I understand that my prospective or continued employment is contingent on a successful screening.

Date: _____   Signature: _____

Witness: _____

Figure 8-5 An example of a urine drug testing form.

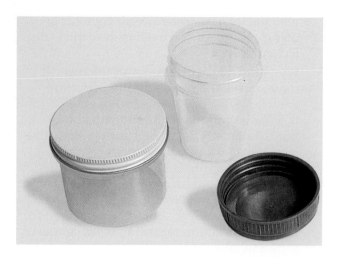

Figure 8-6 Examples of routine urine collection cups.

Specimen Collection Supplies

The preferred urine specimen container is a plastic urine container with a capacity of 50 to 100 mL and an opening at least 5 cm wide. Specimen containers must always be scrupulously clean and completely dry, but they need not be sterile unless the specimen will be cultured for microorganisms. This is also true for the container lids. (See Figure 8-6.)

Urine collection systems are available to help assure quality control in urine collection. Pediatric collection systems are available to collect urine specimens from infants and young children. The disposable collection apparatus consists of a plastic bag with an adhesive backing around the opening. This system can be worn under the child's diaper. Once the pediatric urine specimen has been collected, the urine is transferred from the collection bag to a urine container for testing. Urine collected from a diaper is not recommended for testing due to the contamination of the urine by the diaper material. (See Figure 8-7.)

LABELING AND PRESERVING THE SPECIMEN

It is important that the urine specimen be properly labeled and preserved to prevent spoilage.

Labeling

The label should be attached to the container, not the lid, which may become separated from the specimen. The label should include

- the patient's first and last name.
- the patient's identification number—usually the medical record or chart number.
- the date of specimen collection.

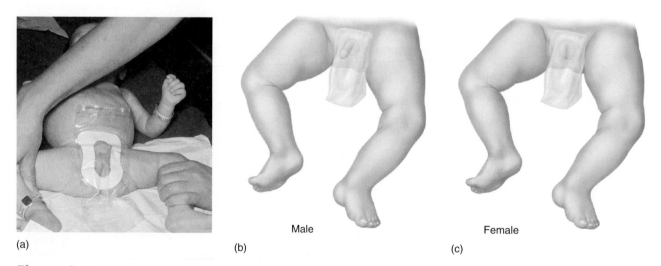

(a) (b) Male (c) Female

Figure 8-7 a) A pediatric collection unit consists of a clear plastic bag with adhesive for attaching to the child; b) A male collection unit; and c) A female collection unit.

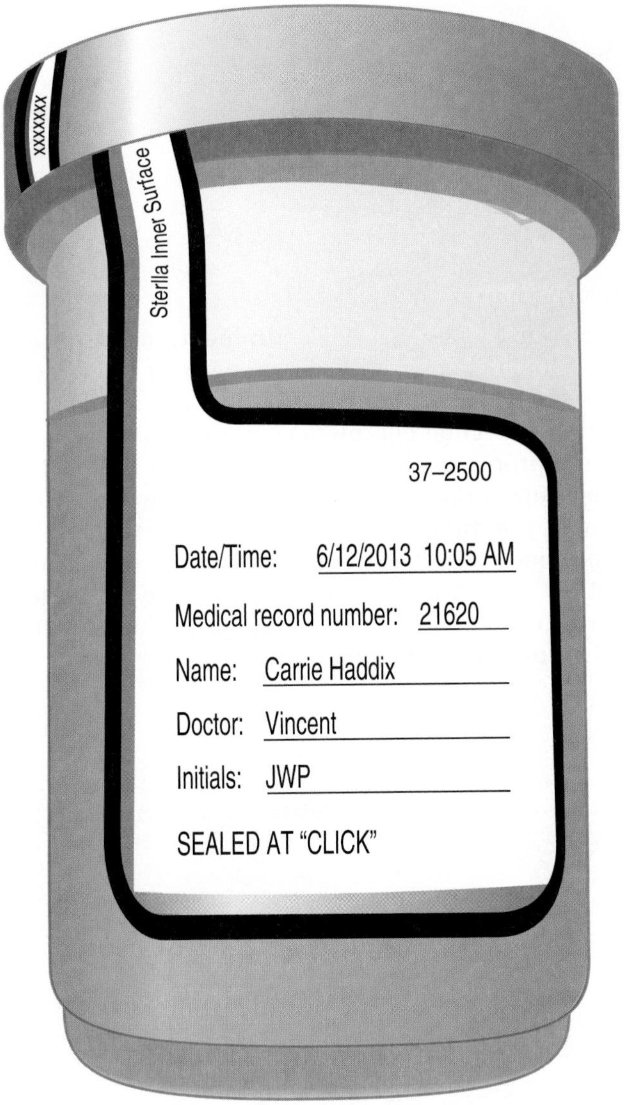

preservation, chemical preservatives may be used when a specimen cannot be refrigerated, such as when a patient transports a specimen from home to the POL or when the specimen is sent by mail to a reference laboratory. However, chemical preservation limits what tests can be performed as it will alter certain test results. Chemical preservation cannot be used for specimens that will undergo routine urinalysis testing.

Without proper preservation, decomposition and deterioration will occur. The following may characterize urine that has "gone bad" and should not be used for urinalysis testing:

- Glucose and ketones are reduced by bacterial consumption.
- Urea is converted to ammonia, making the urine alkaline.
- If the urine is alkaline or has low specific gravity, **urinary casts** (microscopic solid forms created from protein precipitates in the renal tubules and voided in the urine) and red blood cells decompose.
- Bilirubin is reduced due to light sensitivity.
- White blood cells can lyse.
- Urobilinogen is converted to urobilin, causing the urine to darken.
- Nitrite is produced by bacteria.
- The urine has a foul odor.

Figure 8-8 A properly labeled urine sample.

- the time of specimen collection.
- initials of the person who receives the specimen from the patient.

See Figure 8-8.

Preserving

A fresh urine sample should be used when a routine urinalysis is performed. If the specimen cannot be analyzed within one hour of collection, it should be refrigerated at a temperature of 4 to 6 degrees Celsius. Before being analyzed, the refrigerated specimen should be returned to room temperature and gently and thoroughly mixed. Although refrigeration is the preferred method of

Quality Assurance Note

Never discard a patient's urine sample until after the doctor sees the patient and the patient's urinalysis report. If the doctor decides that a urine culture should be done, you may have thrown out the only specimen that the patient can provide. Sometimes, physicians decide that he/she wants a **culture and sensitivity (C & S)** on a urine specimen that you might have thought was unremarkable. A second sample can be especially difficult to obtain from the pediatric patient or dehydrated patients.

Culture and sensitivity is a microbiology test used to determine the bacteria that are causing a patient's urinary infection. The sensitivity portion of the test determines which antibiotics will be effective in treating the infection. Therefore, it is important to maintain specimen sterility and integrity throughout the collection and testing process.

PROCEDURE 8-1

Instructing a Patient in the Collection of a Clean-Catch, Midstream Urine Specimen

Goal

To provide the necessary instructions to a patient so that he or she can successfully collect a clean-catch urine specimen.

Completion Time

20 minutes

Equipment and Supplies

- Lab coat
- Disposable gloves
- Hand sanitizer
- Premoistened towelettes
- Urine container
- Labels
- Pens

Instructions

Read through the list of equipment and supplies that you will need. Read the steps of the procedure. Be sure that you understand each step before you begin. Then complete each step correctly and in the proper order. If your completion time is too long; repeat the procedure until you increase your speed. For this procedure, you must work with a partner. One of you will assume the role of the patient; the other will assume the role of the lab personnel. After completing the procedure, switch roles and repeat the procedure.

Steps marked with (*) are critical and must have the maximum points to pass.

Performance Standards	Points Awarded	Maximum Points
1. Put on lab coat.		5
2. Disinfect hands; dry if necessary.		5
3. Put on gloves. Inspect for tears and replace if necessary.		5
4. Collect and prepare the appropriate equipment.		5
5. *Verify patient identity.		30
6. Using the instructions below, explain the procedure to the patient. If a chart illustrating the procedure is available, use it to clarify your explanation. Provide the patient with the opportunity to ask questions.	—	—
If the patient is a male:		
A. Wash and dry your hands.		5
B. If circumcised, retract your foreskin with a towelette.		5
C. Clean from the urethral opening to the base of the penis three (3) times, once on the left, once on the right, and once directly over the urinary opening. Use a fresh towelette each time in a single wipe.		5
D. Be sure not to touch the inside of the lid or the container throughout the procedure.		5
E. Start urinating into the toilet with your foreskin retracted.		5
F. Collect a midstream specimen of about 20 mL in the collection container.		5
G. Void the rest of the urine into the toilet.		5
H. Secure the lid on the container.		5
I. Return the specimen to the lab.		5

If the patient is a female:

A.	Wash and dry your hands.		5
B.	Sit on the toilet seat with your legs spread as far apart as comfortable.		5
C.	If your are menstruating or have a heavy vaginal discharge, such as from a yeast infection, insert a clean tampon.		5
D.	Spread the outer labia with your nondominant hand.		5
E.	Clean each side of the inner labia and the urethral opening, using a fresh towelette each time in a single wipe.		5
F.	Use a third clean, towelette to clean directly over the urethral opening.		5
G.	Be sure not to touch the inside of the lid or the container throughout the procedure.		5
H.	Begin urinating into the toilet with the outer labia still spread.		5
I.	Collect a midstream specimen of about 20 mL in the collection container.		5
J.	Void the rest of the urine into the toilet.		5
K.	Secure the lid on the container.		5
L.	Return the specimen to the lab.		5
7.	Receive the urine from the patient.		5
8.	Wipe the outside of the container with a tissue.		5
9.	Label the specimen with the patient's name, medical record number or date of birth, date and time of collection, and your initials.		10
10.	Be sure that the label is on the container, not the lid.		5
11.	Thank and release the patient.		10
12.	Discard disposable equipment.		10
	Total Points		**200**

Overall Procedural Evaluation

Student Name _____

Signature of Instructor _____ Date _____

Comments _____

_____

PROCEDURE 8-2

Instructing a Patient in the Collection of a 24-Hour Urine Specimen

Goal

To provide the necessary instructions to a patient so that he or she can successfully collect a 24-hour urine specimen.

Completion Time

20 minutes

Equipment and Supplies

- Lab coat
- Disposable gloves
- Hand sanitizer
- 24-hour urine container

- Labels
- Pens

Instructions

Read through the list of equipment and supplies that you will need. Read the steps of the procedure. Be sure that you understand each step before you begin. Then complete each step correctly and in the proper order. If your completion time is too long; repeat the procedure until you increase your speed. For this procedure, you must work with a partner. One of you will assume the role of the patient; the other will assume the role of the lab technician. After completing the procedure, switch roles, and repeat the procedure.

Steps marked with (*) are critical and must have the maximum points to pass.

Performance Standards	Point Awarded	Maximum Points
1. Put on lab coat.		5
2. Disinfect hands; dry if necessary.		5
3. Put on gloves. Inspect for tears and replace if necessary.		5
4. Collect and prepare the appropriate equipment.		5
5. *Verify patient identity.		30
6. Using the instructions below, explain the procedure to the patient. If a chart illustrating the procedure is available, use it to clarify your explanation. Provide the patient with the opportunity to ask questions.	—	—
A. On the first day of the procedure, upon waking up, urinate into the toilet.		5
B. Note the time of the first morning urination.		5
C. Collect every urine specimen over the next 24 hours.		5
D. Collect each urine into a routine urine container, then pour the urine into the 24-hour urine container.		5
E. If any urine is spilled or accidentally voided into the toilet, please notify the laboratory or physician office so that the procedure can be rescheduled.		5
F. Collect the last urine at the time previously noted the day before.		5
G. Secure the lid on the container throughout the procedure to prevent accidental spilling or evaporation.		5
H. Promptly return the urine to the laboratory for testing.		5
7. Describe any chemicals used in the procedure and instruct the patient with regard to their potential danger.		5
8. Receive the urine from the patient.		5
9. Wipe the outside of the container with a tissue.		
10. *Label the specimen with the patient's name, medical record number or date of birth, date and time of collection, your initials.		10
11. Be sure that the label is on the container, not the lid.		5
12. Thank and release the patient.		10
13. Discard disposable equipment.		10
Total Points		**135**

Overall Procedural Evaluation

Student Name _____

Signature of Instructor _____ Date _____

Comments _____

_____

chapter 8 REVIEW

Using Terminology

Supply the identifying term in the space provided.

1. The process of collecting urine by inserting a tube through the urethra into the bladder

   _____

2. The urine specimen collected as soon as the patient first arises in the morning

   _____

3. The urine specimen that requires the patient to clean the urethral area and collect the urine from the middle part of a single urination

   _____

4. The urine specimen taken after meals to check for glucose

   _____

5. The urine specimen collected as needed at any time of day or night

   _____

6. The area of the body immediately surrounding the rectum and urethra

   _____

7. The specimen collected at home by the patient over a 24-hour period

   _____

8. The urine test that requires a sterile container

   _____

9. The disease characterized by glucose and ketones in the urine

   _____

10. The container used to collect urine specimens from infants and young children

    _____

Match the term on the left with the most appropriate description on the right.

_____ **11.** oliguria

_____ **12.** anuria

_____ **13.** polyuria

_____ **14.** first morning urine

_____ **15.** culture and sensitivity

_____ **16.** random urine specimen

_____ **17.** 24-hour specimen

_____ **18.** timed specimen

a. urine collected immediately upon waking up in the morning

b. test performed to determine the bacteria responsible for causing an infection and which antibiotics will be effective in treating the infection

c. urine specimen collected at any time with no patient preparation

d. complete absence of urine excretion

e. collective specimen that includes all urine output over a 24-hour period

f. urine specimen collected at a specific time

g. excretion of less than 400 mL of urine within 24 hours in adults

h. production of more than 2,000 mL of urine in 24 hours

Multiple Choice

Choose the best answer for the following questions.

19. Which of the following is not a use of urine drug screens?
   a.   pre-employment requirement
   b.   as part of an application for life insurance
   c.   criminal investigations
   d.   routine pediatric screening

20. What is the preservation of choice for urine specimens?
   a.   left at room temperature
   b.   frozen
   c.   chemical
   d.   refrigerated

21. What information is included on a urine specimen label?
   a.   date of specimen collection
   b.   patient's name
   c.   patient's identification number
   d.   all of the above

22. Which of the following is a reason to perform a urinalysis?
   a.   test for a suspected disease
   b.   monitor a condition
   c.   screen for a disease
   d.   all of the above

Acquiring Knowledge

Answer the following questions in the spaces provided.

23. In general, why is a first morning urine specimen best for microscopic examination and for tests of nitrite and protein?

_____

_____

_____

24. Why are elaborate instructions given to patients for a clean-catch, midstream specimen?

_____

_____

_____

25. How soon after collection must urinalysis be completed without refrigeration of the specimen? Why?

_____

_____

_____

26. Why is a 24-hour urine specimen used for quantitative tests?

_____

_____

_____

27. Describe the preferred urine collection container.

_____

_____

_____

28. How is urine collected from infants?

_____

_____

_____

29. Describe how a urine container should be labeled.

_____

_____

_____

30. Describe the collection of a random urine specimen. What are their advantages?

_____

_____

_____

31. Why is the middle part of the urine stream the best for urinalysis?

_____

_____

_____

32. What special precautions should menstruating females take when collecting a urine specimen? Why?

_____

_____

_____

33. Describe a clean-catch, midstream urine specimen.

_____

_____

_____

34. Why does urine concentration vary during a 24-hour period?

_____

_____

_____

35. When collecting a clean-catch, midstream sample, how should the patient handle the container?

_____

_____

_____

36. What precautions are taken with the urine container to protect laboratory workers against disease?

_____

_____

_____

Applying Knowledge—On the Job

Answer the following questions in the spaces provides.

37. A 20-month-old toddler is in the doctor's office and needs a random urine specimen. How will you collect it?

_____

_____

38. A female patient is referred to the laboratory to collect a clean-catch, midstream urine specimen. What instructions should you give the patient to ensure that the urine specimen is not contaminated?

_____

_____

39. Two patients with urinalysis requisition slips come to the lab where you work. A sample is collected from each and the patients leave the office. When you go to do the urinalysis, you realize that the samples are unidentified, so you don't know which sample belongs to which patient. What should you do? What are some changes that should be made in the urine collection procedure in the lab?

_____

_____

40. A 24-hour urine specimen has been ordered for a patient. He has come to the laboratory for instructions. What instructions should you give the patient?

_____

_____

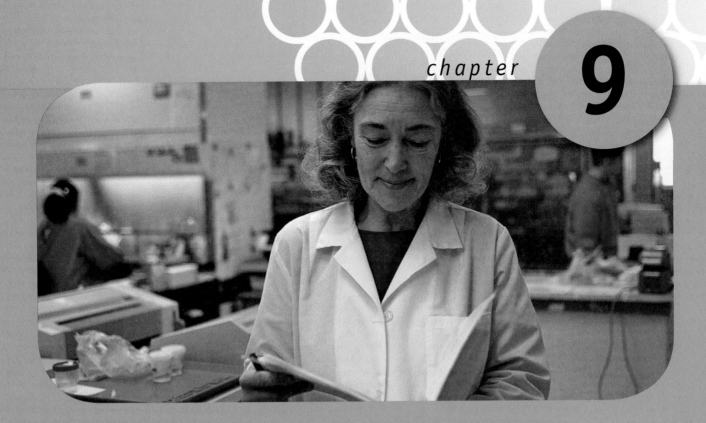

chapter **9**

Physical and Chemical Properties of Urinalysis

⚏ COGNITIVE OBJECTIVES

After studying this chapter, you should be able to

9.1   use each of the vocabulary terms appropriately.

9.2   list the three components of urinalysis.

9.3   describe quality assurance for urinalysis.

9.4   list the physical properties of urine.

9.5   describe the abnormal colors of urine and explain their clinical significance.

9.6   identify the different causes of turbidity in urine.

9.7   describe the relationship between urine odor and the patient's physiological state.

9.8   explain the general methodology of urinalysis strip tests.

9.9   distinguish between screening and confirmation tests in diagnosis and describe when it is appropriate to use each type of test.

9.10   describe laboratory safety related to urinalysis.

9.11   state the methodology for each analyte tested for in urinalysis.

9.12   identify the pathological conditions that each urinalysis analyte can detect.

9.13   state the normal ranges for each of the analytes of urinalysis.

9.14   define specific gravity and explain its relationship to urine concentration.

9.15   describe two methods used to measure specific gravity of urine.

133

9.16 identify the confirmation tests commonly used to follow urinalysis strip tests for reducing sugars, ketones, protein, bilirubin, and specific gravity.

9.17 discuss the advantages of automated urinalysis.

 PERFORMANCE OBJECTIVES

After studying this chapter, you should be able to

9.18 perform quality control testing for urinalysis strips.

9.19 perform a physical analysis of urine in order to determine the correct color and clarity of a urine specimen.

9.20 perform a chemical analysis of urine using urinalysis strips in order to correctly determine the concentration of glucose, pH, specific gravity, bilirubin, urobilinogen, ketones, protein, blood, leukocytes, and nitrite.

9.21 determine the specific gravity of a urine specimen using a refractometer.

9.22 use an ICTOTEST® to confirm the bilirubin concentration of a urine specimen.

9.23 perform a CLINITEST® analysis of a urine sample to assess the presence of reducing sugars.

9.24 perform quality control testing for urinalysis strips.

TERMINOLOGY

acidosis: abnormally low blood pH. The blood is more acidic than normal.

alkalosis: abnormally high blood pH. The blood is more alkaline than normal.

ascorbic acid: vitamin C.

bacteriuria: the presence of bacteria in the urine.

Bence Jones protein: an abnormal protein found in patients with multiple myeloma and other conditions. The urinalysis strip for urinary protein is not sensitive to it.

bilirubin: a product of the breakdown of red blood cells. A high serum level of bilirubin may result in excretion through the kidneys, in addition to the usual route of excretion through the intestines.

bilirubinemia: a high level of bilirubin in the blood.

bilirubinuria: the presence of bilirubin in the urine.

confirmation test: also known as a confirmatory test; a more precise and specific test used to confirm the results of a screening test. In urinalysis, the screening test is usually the urinalysis strips.

false negative: when the test result is negative and the patient has the disease or condition.

false positive: when the test result is positive, but the patient does not have the disease or condition.

foam test: a test to detect the presence of bilirubin in urine that appears yellow-orange.

galactose: a simple sugar formed from the breakdown of lactose (milk sugar).

galactosemia: the presence of galactose in the blood. Galactosemia is the condition in which galactose is not converted to glucose due to a lack of the enzyme galactase. If left undetected in children, it can lead to failure to thrive and ultimately can lead to death.

glucosuria: the condition in which there is glucose in the urine.

hematuria: the presence of erythrocytes (red blood cells) in urine. Hematuria can be caused by several different conditions and may be a sign of a serious clinical condition.

hemoglobinuria: the presence of hemoglobin in the urine.

hypersthenuria: the production of urine with high specific gravity. Hyperthenuria may be caused by several different diseases.

hyposthenuria: the production of urine with low specific gravity. Hypothenuria may be caused by several different diseases.

isosthenuria: the production of urine with consistently low specific gravity regardless of fluid intake. Isothenuria is a sign of marked impairment of renal function.

jaundice: yellowing of the eyes and skin caused by excess bilirubin in the blood. Urine may appear burnt-brown to orange.

ketoacidosis: an acid condition of the body marked by the presence of ketones.

ketone: an intermediary product of fat metabolism. Ketones can appear in the urine during periods of starvation, fever, and dieting.

ketonuria: the presence of ketones in the urine.

lipiduria: the presence of fat in the urine.

lyse: to break down a formed substance, such as red blood cells.

maple-syrup urine disease: a very rare inborn error of metabolism that is fatal if not treated. The urine of patients with this disorder has a maple-syrup odor.

myoglobinuria: the presence of myoglobin in the urine. Myoglobulin can appear in the urine during periods of muscle damage.

occult blood: blood that cannot be detected with the naked eye. It must be detected by chemical or microscopic analysis.

opalescence: the milky appearance in urine due to bacteria or lipids.

pH: the degree of acidity or alkalinity (basic) expressed in hydrogen ion concentration. It can range from 0 to 14.

phenylketonuria (PKU): an inborn error of protein metabolism that results in mental retardation if not treated. The urine of patients with PKU often has a distinctive mousy odor.

proteinuria: a condition in which protein appears in the urine.

pyuria: the presence of white blood cells in the urine.

qualitative tests: tests that produce a yes or no, positive or negative type result.

quantitative tests: tests that provide a numerical number to indicate an amount.

reduction test: also called Benedict's test. It tests for simple sugars such as lactose, galactose, fructose, and pentose, not just for glucose, in the urine.

refractometer: an instrument for measuring the refractive index, which is the ratio of the velocity of light in air to the velocity of light in a solution such as urine. It is used to determine the specific gravity of a liquid.

renal tubular acidosis: a condition in which the renal tubules are unable to excrete hydrogen ions that increase body acidity.

reticuloendothelial cell: cell of the spleen or bone marrow in which hemoglobin from lysed red blood cells is degraded to bilirubin.

screening tests: initial, noninvasive, inexpensive tests that can test large numbers of patients for health problems such as diabetes and kidney disease.

semiquantitative tests: tests that provide results that represent a range.

specific gravity (SG) of urine: the density of urine relative to the density of distilled water. The concentration of dissolved substances gives urine greater specific gravity because these substances give urine greater weight.

turbidity: cloudiness in a solution due to suspended particles that scatter light and produce the cloudy appearance.

urinalysis strips: also known as urine reagent strips and urine dipsticks; test strip impregnated with reagents that provide a quick and easy way to assess a variety of chemical characteristics of the urine. Strips can provide information about glucose, protein, ketones, and other analytes.

urine control: a pretested specimen, the result and value of which are known and can be used to test the variability of the POL's procedures, reagents, and equipment in performing urinalysis.

urobilinogenuria: excess urobilinogen in the urine.

urochrome: the yellow pigment that causes the characteristic yellow color of urine.

INTRODUCTION

Routine urinalysis examines the chemical, physical, and microscopic properties of urine. The findings from these examinations can provide a wealth of information about the patient's urinary health, as well as information about other body systems. This chapter examines the physical and chemical properties of urine and the methods employed to examine those properties.

QUALITY ASSURANCE IN URINALYSIS

Pretesting Guidelines

Before initiating urinalysis testing, observe the following guidelines to ensure that the testing is as accurate as possible.

- Make sure the urine was collected in a clean, dry container. The container should not contain any chemicals, as this will interfere with routine urinalysis testing.
- Urine containers should be covered by a lid to avoid possible contamination.
- Urine containers should be properly labeled. Be sure that the label is on the container, not just the lid, so as to avoid confusing patient specimens.
- Whenever possible, test the urine within one hour of collection. If this is not possible, urine can be stored in a refrigerator. However, the urine should be allowed to return to room temperature before you begin testing.
- Gently mix the urine well before you begin testing to ensure that all the chemical and physical substances are evenly distributed through the specimen.

- **Urinalysis strips** should be stored at room temperature, in a tightly capped container. Urinalysis strips are reagent strips impregnated with reagents that are exposed to a patient's urine to obtain information about the chemical characteristics of the specimen. Urinalysis strips are sensitive to light, heat, and moisture. Therefore, they should be stored in a cool, dark place that does not experience fluctuations in temperatures.

Quality Control in Urinalysis

There are two essential aspects of quality control in routine urinalysis: daily testing of quality control specimens and routine proficiency testing of unknown samples. Both are mandated by CLIA 1988, the federal law that governs certification and inspection of POLs.

Urine Controls

Urine controls are known value control specimens that are used to test the accuracy of the procedures, reagents, and equipment in performing urinalysis. They should be used every day that patient testing occurs to check all previously opened bottles of urinalysis strips as well as each new bottle of strips. New lab personnel also should run controls to check on the precision and accuracy of their performance. Results should be considered acceptable and the urinalysis strips okay to use if the results are within the manufacturer's control range or two standard deviations as established by the lab.

Many urine controls are manufactured to be ready to use. Others may need to be reconstituted just prior to use. Those urine controls must always be reconstituted with the appropriate diluting agent and exactly in accordance with the manufacturer's directions, which are included on the package insert. Each time a urinalysis strip is dipped into a control, some of the reagents from the strip leach out of the pads and contaminate the control. It is important, therefore, that controls be used only the specified number of times recommended by the manufacturer. A reconstitution date should be written on the QC bottles, along with the person's name that reconstituted them.

Some manufacturers give expected values for only one brand of urinalysis strips, while others give expected values for several different brands of urinalysis strips. Many also list the expected values for specific automated urine chemistry analyzers. Urine controls usually can be purchased with two levels of control for each parameter—a negative or normal level and a positive or abnormal level.

PHYSICAL EXAMINATION

The physical examination includes determining the color and clarity or appearance of the urine. While odor is not generally recorded, it may be noted as part of the physical examination. When performing testing on timed urine specimens, volume also may be included in the physical examination. (See Figure 9-1.)

THE APPEARANCE OF URINE

The appearance of urine depends on its color and its **turbidity,** or cloudiness.

Color

A freshly voided normal urine specimen may range in color from pale yellow to amber, depending on its concentration. (See Figure 9-2.) The yellow color comes from the pigment **urochrome,** which is more concentrated with increased metabolism. Patients with fever, starvation, or goiter (hyperthyroidism) have more urochrome and, thus, darker urine. The amount of fluids an individual drinks is also an important factor. In general, the more fluids a person drinks, the more dilute the urine that is produced. Other factors that may affect the color of urine include food pigments and dyes, some medications, and blood contamination of the specimen. Several pathological conditions also affect urine

Patient:			Collection date and time:		**URINALYSIS**	Medical record number:
Doctor:			Test date:			Test by:
VOID ☐	Color	Leuk	MICROSCOPIC			Other ....
CC ☐	pH	Blood	WBC	Bacteria		
CATH ☐	Sp. Gr.	Nitrite	RBC	Mucus		
TURBID ☐	Protein	Bilirubin				
HAZY ☐	Glucose	Urobili	Epith	Casts		
CLEAR ☐	Ketones	hCG	Crystals			

Figure 9-1 An example of a urinalysis form.

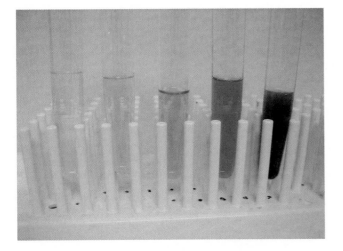

Figure 9-2 Examples of different urine colors, from left to right: straw, light yellow, yellow, red, and brown.

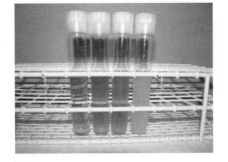

Figure 9-3 Examples of urine clarity including clear, hazy, cloudy, and turbid.

Turbidity/Clarity

A freshly voided normal urine specimen is clear to slightly hazy in appearance. A turbid urine specimen, one that has increased cloudiness, is due to the presence of solid substances in the urine. Solid substances that are found in urine include blood cells, protein, mucus, and so on. A cloudy urine specimen may be due to a number of nonpathological causes or to disease. (See Figure 9-3.)

Turbidity in Healthy Urine. Healthy urine specimens may appear cloudy due to sediment that precipitates when urine drops below body temperature.

color, so any unusual urine color should be noted in the patient's chart. Examples of abnormal urine color include red or reddish brown, which can indicate the presence of hemoglobin or red blood cells. Nonpathological causes of this color include eating certain foods or medications. Orange urine can be caused by bile pigments or certain drugs. Table 9-1 lists abnormal urine colors and some of their causes.

Table 9-1   Abnormal Urine Colors and Their Causes

	POSSIBLE CAUSES	
Color	**Pathological**	**Nonpathological**
Red or reddish brown	Hemoglobin Red blood cells Myoglobin Porphyrins	Beets, rhubarb Senna (cathartic) drugs and dyes Menstrual blood
Orange	Bile pigments	Drugs (e.g., pyridium and phenothiazine)
Yellow-orange or yellow-brown	Dehydration or fever Bilirubin	Carrots Riboflavin Nitrofurantoin (urinary antibiotic)
Green	Biliverdin (from oxidation of bilirubin) Bacteria (especially *Pseudomonas*)	Vitamin preparations Psychoactive drugs Proprietary diuretics
Blue or blue-green	None	Proprietary diuretics Methylene (urinary germicide)
Black or brownish black	Melanin Methemoglobins	Iron complexes Levodopa (anti-Parkinson drug)
Pale yellow	Diluted due to diabetes (mellitus or insipidus)	Diluted due to drinking large amounts of fluid

These sediment precipitates are known as urine precipitates. Acidic urines may have a white or pink haze due to urate precipitates. If the precipitates are so numerous that they interfere with the microscopic examination, they can be cleared by warming the urine to 60 degrees Celsius. Alkaline urines precipitate phosphates and carbonates. They can be cleared by adding dilute acetic acid. Both acidic and alkaline urines may collect precipitates as the urine stands in the patient's bladder.

Other substances also can increase urine turbidity. The presence of mucus can cause turbidity. Sperm and prostatic fluid also may cause turbidity in specimens from males. This turbidity will not clear when the sample is acidified or heated.

Sperm in Urine

MALE URINE

It is important to note when sperm is present in normal healthy males following sexual activity. When sperm is found in the urine and there was no recent sexual activity, sperm can be an indicator of disorders of the male reproductive system. Therefore, sperm in male urine also should be reported as part of the microscopic analysis so that the physician can do additional investigation.

FEMALE URINE

Sperm can be found in female urine as a vaginal contaminant following sexual intercourse. Unlike the male, in females it does not indicate a possible disorder in the urinary or reproductive system. Therefore, some labs choose not to report the presence of sperm in routine testing of female urine.

However, sperm should always be reported in known rape victims as it is additional proof of the rape. Sperm also should be reported in pediatric patients, as it can be a sign or proof of sexual abuse.

Turbidity Due to Disease. Cloudy or turbid urine samples that are pathologically significant are caused most often by white blood cells, red blood cells, or bacteria.

Leukocytes, white blood cells, may form a white cloud similar to that caused by phosphates, but it will not disappear when dilute acetic acid is added to the sample. Leukocytes may be detected microscopically. **Hematuria,** or the presence of erythrocytes, red blood cells, in urine, may give the sample a pink or red appearance. Red blood cells in the specimen may give a "smokey" appearance. Intact red blood cells also may be detected

microscopically, whereas hemolyzed red blood cells will not.

Large numbers of bacteria may appear in the urine specimens of patients with urinary tract infections. The presence of the bacteria themselves may cause a uniform **opalescence,** or milky appearance, that is not cleared when the sample is acidified. It also remains after filtration through paper. Increased alkalinity of the urine and high phosphate concentrations also contribute to cloudiness of urine when bacteria are present.

Fat globules also cause urine to appear opalescent. The presence of fat in urine is called **lipiduria.** It may be caused by degenerative nephron tubular disease.

THE ODOR OF URINE

Normal, freshly voided urine has a faint characteristic odor due to the presence of volatile acids. The odor is more marked in concentrated urine. Certain foods, such as asparagus, may produce a harmless but characteristic odor in the urine. Vitamins and some drugs also can cause a distinct odor in urine.

The odor of urine usually is not considered to be of special diagnostic significance. Therefore, odor is generally not documented by the lab or in the patient's chart. Nonetheless, urine with an abnormal smell should be investigated more closely. Several pathological states are characterized by urine with a marked odor. Some are very distinctive.

Bacteria in urine causes an odor of ammonia because bacteria split urea. Patients with **phenylketonuria (PKU)** produce urine with a distinctive "mousy" odor. Patients with **maple-syrup urine disease** produce urine that smells like maple syrup. The urine of patients with diabetes mellitus may have a sweet or fruity odor due to the presence of ketones. Malnutrition, vomiting, and diarrhea also can produce urine that smells sweet.

MEASURING THE VOLUME OF URINE

Measuring the volume of urine is generally associated with timed specimens, such as the 24-hour specimen. These specimens are usually collected in special containers that possess a measuring system on the outside of the container that allows the laboratory technician to measure the specimen while in the container. The results are recorded in mL as total volume (TV). If the container does not have measurements on the outside, a 1,000 mL graduated cylinder can be used for measuring the total volume.

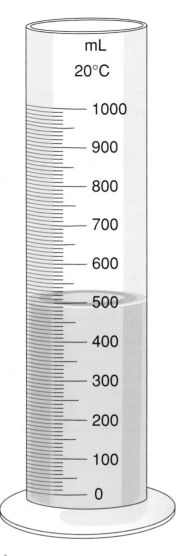

Figure 9-4 Urine volume measurement using a graduated cylinder.

It is important to save some of the measured sample in a smaller labeled container for further testing. (See Figure 9-4.)

CHEMICAL EXAMINATION

The diagnostic information provided by chemical analysis of urine is the reason that urinalysis is the most common laboratory test performed in POLs. Urinalysis is also one of the easiest and quickest tests performed in the POL due to the availability of urinalysis strips.

URINALYSIS STRIP TESTS

The most widely used technology in POLs for performing chemical analysis of urine is the urinalysis strip tests. The urinalysis strips are test strips

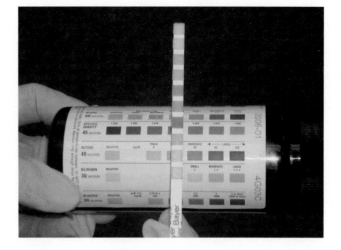

Figure 9-5 Bottle and urinalysis strip.

impregnated with reagents that change color when they come into contact with specific analytes. The degree of color change is directly related to the concentration of the tested analyte in the patient's urine. Urinalysis strips are popular because they are convenient to purchase, easy to use, and disposable. In addition, urinalysis strips are available for a variety of chemical tests including urinary pH, glucose, ketone, protein, and blood, among others. Most urinalysis strip systems allow you to test for multiple analytes simultaneously, allowing you to collect a lot of information quickly. An example of a urinalysis strip and bottle is shown in Figure 9-5.

The urinalysis strip results are qualitative in that color change indicates presence or absence of the analyte—as well as semiquantitative in that degree of color change indicates approximate concentration of the analyte. Urinalysis strips are used most often as **screening tests,** initial noninvasive, inexpensive tests that can test large numbers of patients for health problems such as diabetes and kidney disease. Those who test positive on the urinalysis strip test are often followed up with **confirmation tests,** which are more precise and specific diagnostic tools.

Materials and Procedure

The urinalysis strip consists of a firm plastic strip to which a pad or pads are attached. Each pad contains chemical reactants for a specific analyte, such as glucose or protein. When the pad comes into contact with urine containing the specific chemical or analyte, a chemical reaction occurs. This reaction is indicated by the change in the pad color. The color reaction produced on the pad is compared to a color chart provided by

Qualitative, Quantitative, and Semiquantitative

Laboratory tests are classified as qualitative, quantitative, or semiquantitative, depending on the type of result the test generates.

Qualitative tests are tests that produce a "yes" or "no," or a "positive" or "negative" type result. An example is urine pregnancy tests for home use. The result is either positive or negative. It does not indicate how much hCG (the hormone used to diagnose pregnancy) is present. Screening tests are often qualitative or semiquantitative.

Quantitative tests provide a numerical number to indicate an amount. For example, glucose testing is reported as a numerical amount such as 110. Confirmation tests are often quantitative.

Semiquantitative tests provide results that represent a range. For example, urinalysis strips report blood as a range of small, moderate, or large. Each result represents a possible range; small equals 5–8 red blood cells, moderate represents 10–15 red blood cells, and large represents greater than 20 red blood cells. Screening tests are often qualitative or semiquantitative.

Urinalysis strips are considered to be semiquantitative tests.

Urinalysis Safety

Urinalysis strip technology advances lab safety because it requires only minute amounts of reagents. However, urine, like all biological specimens, is potentially hazardous. Urine specimens should be kept covered in their containers as much as possible. Carefully discard contaminated testing equipment and emptied, used specimen containers into the biohazardous waste container according to your laboratory policy.

Urinalysis Strip Quality Control

It is important that you closely observe the timing as instructed by the manufacturer of the urinalysis strip. Failure to do so can result in false positive and false negative results.

instruction sheet inserted in the package. The general urinalysis strip procedure is illustrated in Figure 9-6.

the manufacturer. It is important to ensure that you are using the chart produced by the manufacturer for the specific strips that you are using. The color chart usually is placed on the label of the urinalysis strip container. Many urinalysis strips must be accurately timed for valid test results. The read time varies from 30 seconds to 2 minutes. The recommended read time for each test is printed on the manufacturer's

Storage

Always consult the manufacturer's instructions on the package insert for proper storage of urinalysis strips. Generally, the urinalysis strips should be stored at room temperature in tightly closed containers that protect them from heat, light, fumes, and moisture. Care must be taken to protect the urinalysis strips from other laboratory chemicals. Even detergents such as bleach may react with the strips if they are placed nearby.

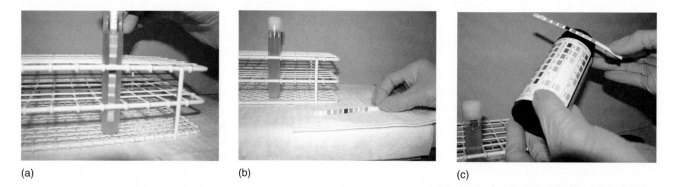

(a) (b) (c)

Figure 9-6 (a) Dip the urinalysis strip into the patient's urine. Be sure that all reagent pads come into contact with the urine specimen. Promptly remove the urinalysis strip. (b) Remove any excess urine from the urinalysis strip. (c) Using the chart provided by the manufacturer and following the timing requirements, compare the color of the reagent pad located on the urinalysis strip to the chart. Record all results.

URINALYSIS AUTOMATION

Until recently, chemical analysis of urine specimens was done manually. However, like other laboratory procedures, urinalysis is becoming more automated. Reacted urinalysis strips can be interpreted by instruments. Some laboratories have semi-automated bench-top analyzers that read urinalysis strips and print out the results. The saturated urinalysis strip is placed on a feed-load table and drawn into the instrument for reading. The specimen identification number and appearance can be entered and printed out along with the results of the chemical analysis.

THE NEED FOR AUTOMATION

Lab personnel variability and error can lead to loss of accuracy, precision, and reproducibility in routine urinalysis. The use of automation reduces variability and error and increases standardization. Specific advantages of automated urinalysis include the following:

- Instruments eliminate the variation in reading urinalysis strips that is due to individual differences in visual acuity and color blindness and also to differences in quality and quantity of light illuminating the urinalysis strip during the reading.
- Instruments eliminate timing errors in reading results. They are programmed to read each test at the optimal time.
- Instruments go through an automatic calibration cycle at each start-up. No extra calibration procedure is required.
- Specimen identification and test results are printed by the instrument, eliminating the possibility of transcription error.

Even though automation has replaced our need to read the urinalysis strips manually, lab personnel still need to know how to perform these vital tests if the instrument should happen to stop working. Lab personnel also need to know how to troubleshoot the instrument and be aware of the results the instrument reports prior to charting them.

CHEMICAL URINALYSIS

Perhaps the most diagnostically valuable portion of routine urinalysis is the chemical analysis of urine. The chemical portion of the test provides information regarding the presence or absence of several analytes including glucose, ketones, protein, and blood. In addition, specific gravity, pH, **bilirubin,** and urobilinogen also can be determined using the urinalysis strips. Many POLs also routinely measure leukocytes and nitrites to detect bacteria in the urine. Specific gravity and pH are not described as positive or negative, but as normal when results fall within the expected normal range. The remainder of the analytes should have a negative result. A positive test result indicates possible pathology. Test data can provide the physician with information on the patient's carbohydrate metabolism, kidney and liver function, infections of the urinary tract, and acid-base balance.

Medical Terms

The following terms describe abnormal urines:

- **bacteriuria:** the presence of bacteria in the urine.
- **bilirubinuria:** the presence of bilirubin in the urine.
- **glucosuria:** the presence of glucose in the urine.
- **hematuria:** the presence of red blood cells in the urine.
- **hemoglobinuria:** the presence of hemoglobin in the urine.
- **ketonuria:** the presence of ketones in the urine.
- **proteinuria:** the presence of proteins in the urine.
- **urobilinogenuria:** excess urobilinogen in the urine.

Urinary pH

A solution's **pH,** or concentration of hydrogen ions, can range from 0 to 14. (See Figure 9-7.) A pH reading of 7 is neutral; a reading above 7 is alkaline (basic); below 7 is acidic. The lower the reading, the more acidic; the higher the reading, the more alkaline.

Acid-Base Balance. The pH of the blood and other body tissues is referred to as the body's acid-base balance. Blood pH varies between 7.35 and 7.45 in normal individuals. This balance is regulated

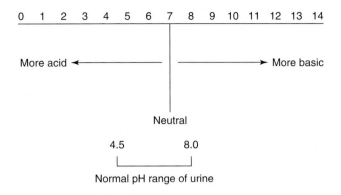

Figure 9-7 The pH scale.

by the kidneys and lungs, which excrete the waste products of body metabolism. The lungs excrete volatile wastes, predominantly carbon dioxide, and the kidneys excrete nonvolatile acid wastes, like uric acid. The kidneys help regulate blood pH by selectively secreting less acid when the blood is too alkaline or basic, **alkalosis,** or more acid when the blood is too acidic, **acidosis.**

Factors Affecting Urinary pH. Normal adult urine tends to be slightly acidic, at an average pH of 6.0. The normal adult range is from 4.5 to 8.0 pH. The following factors may decrease blood pH and result in urine that is more acidic:

- a high-protein diet
- uncontrolled diabetes mellitus
- starvation
- respiratory diseases involving carbon dioxide retention

The following factors may increase blood pH and result in urine that is more alkaline:

- diets high in vegetables, citrus fruits, or dairy products
- urinary tract infections
- bacterial contamination of the specimen
- respiratory diseases involving hyperventilation and loss of carbon dioxide
- sodium bicarbonate and potassium citrate, which are often used in conjunction with antibiotics in treating urinary tract infections

> ### Renal Tubular Acidosis
>
> **Renal tubular acidosis** is a condition in which the renal tubules are unable to excrete hydrogen ions that increase body acidity. Patients with renal tubular acidosis tend to have a neutral urine pH regardless of their body's acid level.

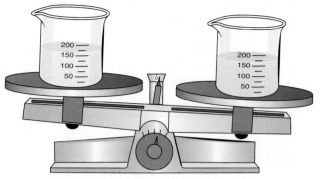

Figure 9-8 The distilled water on the left does not contain particles and therefore weighs less than the same volume of urine on the right, which does contain particles.

Measuring Urinary pH. The test strip is the primary method for determining urinary pH. Protein buffers from adjacent pads on the urinalysis strip should not be allowed to run over on the pH pad and alter its pH indicators.

Specific Gravity

Specific gravity (SG) is the density of a substance relative to the density of distilled (pure) water. (See Figure 9-8.) Assessing the specific gravity of urine is part of routine urinalysis. It is usually calculated as

$$SG = \frac{\text{Weight/Volume of urine}}{\text{Weight/Volume of water}}$$

In addition to water, urine contains minerals, salts, and organic compounds, which give it a density greater than that of distilled water and a specific gravity greater than 1.000. The specific gravity of normal urine ranges between 1.005 and 1.030, with most samples falling between 1.010 and 1.025. The specific gravity of urine varies throughout the day. It is generally highest (greater than 1.020) in the first morning specimen due to the urine concentrating overnight.

Testing for Specific Gravity. The most commonly used method of measuring specific gravity is the disposable colorimetric urinalysis strip. No special equipment is required.

Urines with a high specific gravity have high ion concentrations, and urines with low specific gravity have low ion concentrations. Changes in ion concentration affect pH, causing a color change in the urinalysis strip. This color change is compared to color blocks on the reagent vial to measure specific gravity.

The chemical nature of the urinalysis strip test may produce results that differ slightly from those of other methods when elevated amounts of protein and glucose are present. Highly buffered alkaline urines also may show low readings relative to other methods.

Causes of Abnormal Specific Gravity. Specific gravity of urine may be either abnormally low or abnormally high.

Low Specific Gravity. Production of urine with low specific gravity, **hyposthenuria,** characterizes patients with diabetes insipidus, in whom antidiuretic hormone (ADH) is lacking. Patients with glomerulonephritis and pyelonephritis also may have urine with low specific gravity because of tubular damage. The production of urine with a consistent low specific gravity (1.010), varying little from specimen to specimen regardless of fluid intake, is known as **isosthenuria.** It is a sign of marked impairment of renal function, occurring in patients with chronic renal disorders, whose kidneys are unable to concentrate or dilute urine. This urine has the same specific gravity as plasma filtrate.

High Specific Gravity. Production of urine with high specific gravity, **hypersthenuria,** occurs with diabetes mellitus, adrenal insufficiency, hepatic disease, and congestive cardiac failure. Patients who are dehydrated due to sweating, fever, vomiting, or diarrhea also may have urine with high specific gravity.

Glucose

Healthy individuals will have a negative urine glucose test if their blood glucose levels are 110 mg/dL or less. However, if blood glucose concentration rises as high as 180 mg/dL, which is the renal threshold for glucose, the reabsorption capacity of the kidneys is surpassed and glucose spills over into the urine. This condition may be benign due to emotional stress or ingestion of a large meal or pathological due to diabetes mellitus.

Diabetes Mellitus. Patients with diabetes mellitus have elevated blood glucose because they are unable to produce or use insulin, the pancreatic hormone that is needed to transport glucose across cell membranes. Measuring blood and urine glucose is important for screening and monitoring these patients.

Testing for Glucose. The glucose strip is specific for glucose. When the glucose in the urine reacts with the pad on the urinalysis strip, it changes the color of the pad. No other substance normally excreted in urine is known to give a positive result.

Even other sugars including lactose, galactose, and fructose do not cause a positive result with the urinalysis strip.

False positives may occur if the strip comes into contact with bleach. This may occur if the work area was recently disinfected with bleach and the pad is allowed to come into contact with the work area. False negatives can occur if (1) the urine has a high specific gravity, (2) the urine contains a large amount of **ascorbic acid** (vitamin C), or (3) the urine is not promptly tested and contains bacteria (some bacteria will digest the glucose as a food source).

False Positives and Negatives

Though most test results accurately reflect the patient's disease or condition, sometimes a test result is wrong. These are known as false positive or false negative results.

- **False negative**—when the test result is negative and the patient has the disease or condition.
- **False positive**—when the test result is positive, but the patient does not have the disease or condition.

Ketones

Glucose is the energy source usually utilized by the cells. However, when the patient's diet is inadequate in carbohydrates or the patient has a defect in carbohydrate metabolism or absorption, fat is used as the primary energy source. This results in incomplete metabolism of fatty acids and accumulation of intermediary products of fat metabolism, called **ketones.** Ketones include acetoacetic acid, acetone, and betahydroxybutyric acid.

Ketones appear in the urine before they increase significantly in the blood. When they are excreted in the urine, the condition is called ketonuria. Patients with ketonuria always excrete ketone bodies in the same proportions—20 percent acetoacetic acid, 2 percent acetone, and 78 percent betahydroxybutyric acid. Because ketones are excreted in combination with basic ions (Na, K, and Ca), ketonuria produces **ketoacidosis,** an acid condition of the body. Patients with ketoacidosis frequently have a fruity odor to their breath because acetone is highly volatile and is blown off in small amounts with air that is expelled from the lungs.

Causes of Ketonuria. The most important pathological condition that may produce ketonuria is diabetes mellitus. Ketonuria in a diabetic patient indicates the need for a change in insulin dosage or other aspect of treatment. Other conditions that may cause ketonuria include anorexia, starvation, vomiting, diarrhea, and fever. Other causes include a diet low in carbohydrates such as the Atkin's diet.

Testing for Ketones. The ketone urinalysis strip, which is based on a nitroprusside reaction, checks for the presence of acetoacetic acid, one of the three ketone bodies. The reaction occurs in the presence of a basic buffer. A positive result is indicated by a color change.

False positive results can occur in urine with strong colors. False negatives can occur when there are large amounts of vitamin C present or when there is a delay in testing due to the volatile nature of the ketones.

Proteins

Normally only small amounts of protein are excreted each day in the urine, ranging up to 150 mg/day or 20 mg/dL, because most of the protein filtered out of the blood into the kidneys is reabsorbed by the kidneys. Urine specimens normally test negative for protein. In several pathological conditions of the kidney, however, protein is detectable in the urine at relatively high concentrations, a condition called proteinuria. The degree of proteinuria is classified according to the amount of protein excreted per day.

The detection of protein in the urine is one of the most important indicators of renal disease in which there is glomerular or tubular damage.

Bence Jones Protein

Another type of protein that can produce proteinuria is **Bence Jones protein,** a globulin observed in the urine of over 50 percent of patients with multiple myeloma. It also is found in the urine of patients with macroglobulinemia and malignant lymphomas. The urinalysis strip for protein is not sensitive to Bence Jones protein. The urinalysis strip predominantly screens for albumin. It must be detected using a precipitation test or a coagulation test.

Usually, albumin is lost in greatest amounts in renal disease, making up 60 to 90 percent of protein excreted. Albumin normally makes up only about one-third of urinary protein. Other types of protein in normal urine are globulins and Tamm-Horsfall protein.

Degrees and Types of Proteinuria

- Marked proteinuria: over 4 grams of protein excreted per day. Causes: nephrotic syndrome, acute and chronic glomerulonephritis, nephrosclerosis, amyloid disease, systemic lupus erythematosus, and severe venous congestion of the kidney.
- Moderate proteinuria: between 0.5 and 4 grams of protein excreted per day. Causes: nephrotic syndrome, acute and chronic glomerulonephritis, nephrosclerosis, amyloid disease, systemic lupus erythematosus, severe venous congestion of the kidney, pyelonephritis, multiple myeloma, pre-eclampsia of pregnancy, toxic nephropathy, and inflammatory conditions of the lower urinary tract, including kidney and bladder stones.
- Minimal proteinuria: less than 0.5 gram of protein excreted per day. Causes: chronic pyelonephritis, polycystic kidney disease, various disorders of the lower urinary tract, and renal tubular diseases.
- Functional proteinuria: usually transient and benign; associated with fever, exposure to cold, emotional stress, or excessive exercise.
- Orthostatic proteinuria: increased protein levels in the urine when the patient is standing.

Testing for Protein. If protein is added to the urinalysis strip indicator, it changes color according to the concentration of protein. The reagent area is more sensitive to albumin than to globulins or other proteins.

Blood

A normal urine sample should not have any detectable blood even when the most sensitive tests are used. When urine contains blood, it may appear pink or red, but more often, blood is present in such minute quantities that it can be detected only by microscopic or chemical means. This blood, which cannot be seen by the naked eye, is called **occult blood.** Three different ways to detect blood in the urine are (1) chemically by means of urinalysis strips, (2) visually by observing the specimen, and (3) microscopically by examining the urine under magnification.

Blood in urine may be in the form of intact red blood cells, which is referred to as hematuria. Blood also may be in the form of free hemoglobin from **lysed** red blood cells that are also present, which is called hemoglobinuria. Finally, a positive test for occult blood may be detected in urine in which no red blood cells are present. This usually means that there is myoglobin in the urine. This is called **myoglobinuria.** Myoglobin is a hemoglobin-like molecule that stores oxygen in muscle tissue.

Causes of Blood in Urine. Detection of blood in urine indicates damage or disease of the kidney or urinary tract and, often, bleeding in the urinary tract. In infectious diseases like yellow fever, small-pox, and malaria, hemoglobin from lysed red blood cells is present in the urine, producing hemoglobinuria. Hemoglobinuria also occurs with renal disorders, kidney stones, and severe infections of the urinary tract. Myoglobinuria is usually a result of traumatic muscle injury. The only nonpathological reason for blood in urine is menstrual blood contamination, which can be ruled out if proper specimen collection procedures are followed.

Testing for Blood. The urinalysis strip test for blood is based on the oxidizing activity of hemoglobin,

which produces spots of color change if the blood consists of intact red blood cells and a uniform color change in the presence of free hemoglobin or myoglobin. The test can detect 5 to 20 intact red blood cells per microliter or 0.015 to 0.060 mg/dL of free hemoglobin. A positive urinalysis strip for blood should be followed up with a microscopic examination of urine sediment.

Bilirubin

Bilirubin is a yellow-orange bile-pigmented compound formed when red blood cells are lysed or ruptured.

The Formation and Excretion of Bilirubin. Figure 9-9 shows the process by which bilirubin normally is formed and excreted. Bilirubin forms when red blood cells reach the end of their life

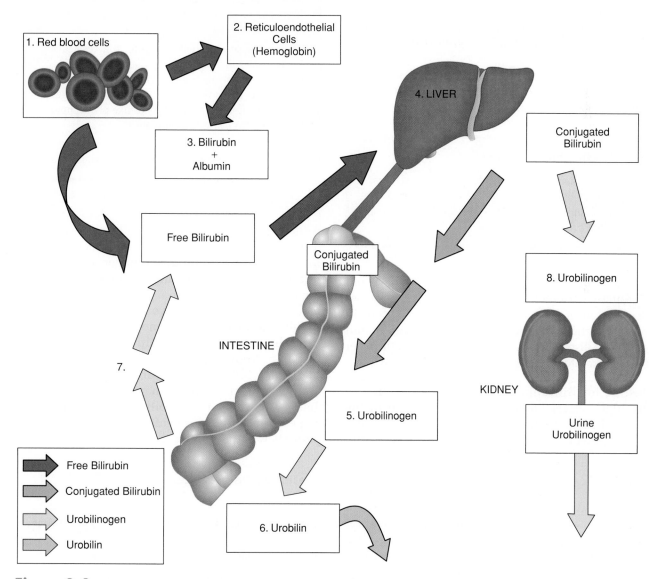

Figure 9-9 Normal bile pigment metabolism.

span, which averages 120 days. When old red cells lyse, hemoglobin is degraded to bilirubin in the **reticuloendothelial cells** of the spleen and bone marrow. The bilirubin then binds to albumin in the blood and is transported to the liver. This form of bilirubin, called free bilirubin, is not water soluble, so it cannot be excreted in the urine.

In the liver, Kupffer cells change free bilirubin to conjugated bilirubin, a soluble form. This is excreted into the small intestine through the bile duct and converted by bacterial action to urobilinogen, a colorless compound. Some of the urobilinogen thus formed is oxidized to brown-pigmented urobilin and excreted in the feces, where it gives color to fecal material. However, up to 50 percent of the urobilinogen formed in the intestine is reabsorbed into the blood, and a small amount of the reabsorbed urobilinogen is excreted in the urine.

When conjugated bilirubin levels are abnormally high, the conjugated bilirubin reenters the blood from the liver and a high level of bilirubin in the blood results. This condition is called **bilirubinemia.**

Excess bilirubin in the blood causes yellowing of the eyes and skin, a condition referred to as **jaundice.**

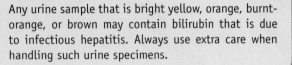

Watch Out for Hepatitis!

Any urine sample that is bright yellow, orange, burnt-orange, or brown may contain bilirubin that is due to infectious hepatitis. Always use extra care when handling such urine specimens.

There are two types of jaundice: hemolytic and obstructive. Hemolytic jaundice is due to excess destruction of red blood cells, which may occur in several forms of anemia, infectious hepatitis, and malaria. Obstructive jaundice occurs when the liver fails to excrete bile or the bile ducts are obstructed.

Testing for Bilirubin. If blood levels of bilirubin are high, excess amounts will be excreted in the urine. Bilirubin in the urine is called bilirubinuria. Bilirubin in the urine can be detected only

if the specimen is fresh because bilirubin decomposes rapidly in bright light. If the urine is allowed to stand, the bilirubin will be converted to biliverdin, a green compound not detected by the bilirubin urinalysis strip test. The bilirubin urinalysis strip test is based on the reaction of bilirubin with a diazonium salt in a strongly acid medium. This produces a color change that is proportional to the concentration of bilirubin in the sample. Normally, the amount of bilirubin in the urine is too small to be detected. False positives can occur in highly pigmented urine specimens. False negatives can occur when there is a delay in testing.

Detecting Bilirubin in the Urine

A **foam test** is sometimes performed to determine if bilirubin is present in a urine specimen that appears yellow-orange. Bilirubin is a product of the breakdown of red blood cells. The foam test procedure is as follows:

- Place a small volume of urine in a test tube. Cap the tube and shake it vigorously.
- If the foam on the top is white, bilirubin is absent. If the foam is orange, bilirubin is present. (Note: urinary analgesics like phenazopyridine also cause orange foam.)

In general, this method has been replaced by routine urinalysis strips and more sophisticated chemical assays.

Urobilinogen

As described, urobilinogen is a bile pigment formed directly from bilirubin by bacterial action in the intestine. Much of the urobilinogen is reabsorbed into the circulating blood, and some is filtered by the kidneys into the urine. Therefore, urine specimens normally test positive for urobilinogen.

Because urinary urobilinogen is higher whenever there is an increase in the production of bilirubin, knowing the concentration of both bile pigments, bilirubin and urobilinogen, may be more useful for diagnosis than knowing one alone. Table 9-2 gives urinary bilirubin and urobilinogen concentrations for healthy individuals and for patients with pathological liver conditions.

Table 9-2   Changes in Urobilinogen and Bilirubin Tests in Health and Disease States

	Normal	Hemolytic Disease	Hepatic Disease	Biliary Obstruction
Urine urobilinogen	Normal	Increased	Increased	Low or absent
Urine bilirubin	Negative	Negative	Positive or negative	Positive

Testing for Urobilinogen. The test for urobilinogen on the urinalysis strip involves the Ehrlich aldehyde reaction, which forms a red azo dye. The test must be performed using fresh urine because urobilinogen is unstable and breaks down to urobilin on standing. The test detects urobilinogen in concentrations of at least 0.1 mg/dL. The normal urobilinogen range obtained with this method is 0.2 to 1.0 mg/dL. A concentration of 2.0 mg/dL represents the transition from normal to abnormal, indicating that the patient needs further evaluation or that the test result should be confirmed with a follow-up test.

Nitrite

Nitrite in the urine is significant because it is an indicator of bacteriuria, or bacteria in the urine. Most of the common pathogens that cause bacteriuria (see Table 9-3) produce reductase enzymes, which reduce nitrate from the diet to nitrite while the urine is held in the bladder. (See Figure 9-10.) For the reduction reaction to occur, the bacteria must be held in the bladder for a minimum of four hours. First morning specimens are therefore the best samples to test. The urine has been held in the bladder for many hours and the number of bacteria is relatively large.

Testing for Nitrite. The nitrite test is based on the conversion of nitrate to nitrite by the action of gram negative bacteria in the urine. The nitrite will react with the acid pH of the reagent pad to produce a pink color. A negative nitrite result does not completely rule out bacteriuria, however. The pathogen may be one that does not reduce nitrate or there may be too few organisms present to produce nitrite at a detectable level. A positive nitrite

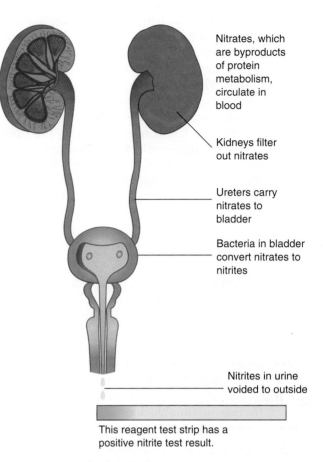

Nitrates, which are byproducts of protein metabolism, circulate in blood

Kidneys filter out nitrates

Ureters carry nitrates to bladder

Bacteria in bladder convert nitrates to nitrites

Nitrites in urine voided to outside

This reagent test strip has a positive nitrite test result.

Figure 9-10 Screening of bacterial infection using nitrite urinalysis results.

test result should be confirmed by microscopic findings of bacteria and leukocytes. Some POLs also perform cultures and smears with Gram stain. False positives can occur when poor collection techniques introduce bacteria into the specimen. False negatives can occur when there are large amounts of vitamin C present, the patient is on antibiotic therapy, the urine did not remain in the bladder for the minimum four hours, or the bacteria do not convert nitrate to nitrite.

Leukocytes

The presence of significant numbers of white blood cells in the urine, **pyuria,** usually indicates bacteriuria. It is associated with lesions of the urethra, ureters, bladder, and kidneys, and with urinary tract infections.

Testing for Leukocyte Esterase. Neutrophilic leukocytes contain granules that release esterases into the urine. These esterases can be detected by

Table 9-3 Common Causes of Bacteriuria

Type of Pathogen	Percent of All Urinary Tract Infections
E. coli	72%
Klebsiella/Enterobacter	16%
Proteus	5%
Staphylococcus	5%
Pseudomonas	1%
Streptococcus faecatis*	1%

*Does not reduce nitrate to nitrite.

chemical means using the leukocyte esterase urinalysis strip. The esterase splits an ester to form a pyrrole compound, which reacts with a diazo reagent to form a purple azo dye. The intensity of color is proportional to the amount of esterase in the urine and, indirectly, to the number of leukocytes present. The test can detect as few as 5 to 15 white blood cells per high-power microscope field. Zero to 2 cells per high-power field is normal. The leukocyte esterase test is not affected by the presence of a large number of erythrocytes or bacteria in the urine, but urinary tract antibiotics like cephalexin and tetracycline may affect the results, producing false negatives. False positives may occur with vaginal discharge in female patients.

CONFIRMATION TESTS

When the test results of a urinalysis strip test used in routine urinalysis are questionable, an additional testing method should be used to confirm the results. Confirmation tests generally are not used to screen patients because they are too time consuming and costly. Nor should they be run on every specimen just to confirm the accuracy of test results. Their use should be confined to cases in which there is reasonable doubt about a test result, such as when a test result seems illogical in light of other medical evidence. Repeating the urinalysis strip test on the same specimen or on a new specimen from the same patient may negate the need for a confirmation test.

Like all laboratory tests, quality control (QC) also must be performed on any confirmation test procedure using normal and abnormal control levels. These results also are documented in the quality control log book with date and person performing the quality control. Always follow the manufacturer's instructions for reconstituting, storage, and procedural information. Failure to perform quality control correctly will jeopardize accurate patient results, diagnosis, and treatment.

The five most often used confirmation tests in POLs are those for specific gravity, bilirubin, protein, reducing sugars, and ketones.

The Refractometer

When confirmation of the specific gravity determined by the reagent strip is needed, the **refractometer** can be used. It is also helpful when the specific gravity is above or below the range of the reagent strip. The refractometer measures the refractive index, which is the ratio of the velocity of light in air to the velocity of light in a solution such as urine. The ratio varies directly with the concentration of

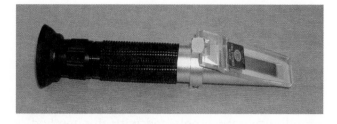

Figure 9-11 A refractometer is used for determining the specific gravity of urine.

dissolved particles in the solution because the light beam that enters the instrument is bent and slowed by the solutes in the specimen. This value is read on a scale, which is viewed through the ocular of the refractometer. It is important to read the scale of the instrument with the refractometer held toward a light source. The refractometer is accurate with samples in the temperature range of 16 to 38 degrees Celsius. (See Figure 9-11.)

The refractometer should be calibrated daily using distilled water and using the set screw to adjust the scale to read 1.000. The refractive index varies with, but is not identical to, the specific gravity of a urine sample, the refractive index usually being lower by about 0.002.

ICTOTEST® for Bilirubin

The ICTOTEST® is highly sensitive, and it is convenient for qualitative determination of bilirubinuria. This test can detect bilirubin concentrations as low as 0.05 mg/dL and as high as 0.10 mg/dL. Materials needed include an ICTOTEST™ reagent tablet, ICTOTEST™ mat, dropper, and distilled water. The reagent tablets must not be exposed to light, heat, or moisture, and they never should be used past the expiration date on the bottle. Deterioration of the tablets is indicated by a tan or brown discoloration.

Figure 9-12 illustrates the general procedure for ICTOTEST®. Remember always to check the instructions given in the manufacturer's package insert when you run the test.

Tests for Protein

There are three simple, yet sensitive, tests for protein in the urine: the acetic acid, sulfosalicylic acid, and concentrated nitric acid tests. These tests are performed on the supernatant, which is the top portion of a centrifuged sample. In all three, protein in the urine is coagulated and/or precipitated by the addition of acid or acid and heat. The acetic acid method uses acid and heat to test urine for protein. It is the most sensitive method for

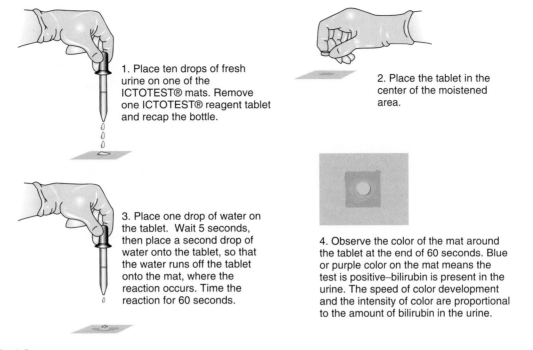

Figure 9-12 ICTOTEST procedure.

detecting protein at low concentrations—as low as 2 to 3 mg/dL, compared with 15 to 30 mg/dL for urinalysis strip tests.

Interpreting Protein Precipitation and Coagulation Test Results

The following factors will help you interpret protein precipitation and coagulation test results:

- no turbidity/clear—negative (no protein in the urine)
- faint precipitation when viewed against a black background—a trace
- a small degree of turbidity—one plus
- moderate turbidity—two plus
- heavy turbidity—three plus
- heavy flocculation (like cotton wool)—four plus

CLINITEST® for Reducing Sugars

The urinalysis strip test for urinary sugar detects only glucose. A **reduction test,** also called Benedict's test, is needed to detect other simple sugars such as lactose, galactose, fructose, and pentose. In POLs, the most frequently used reduction test is CLINITEST®.

These tests are used to test for lactase deficiency and galactosemia, among other disorders of carbohydrate metabolism. A color chart is used to determine if the result is positive or negative. A negative result means that no sugar is present in the urine. A positive result means that some type of sugar, although not necessarily glucose, is present in the urine.

Galactosemia

Galactose is a simple sugar formed from the breakdown of lactose, or milk sugar. Normal individuals do not test positive for galactose in the urine because they are able to convert galactose to glucose with the enzyme galactase. People who are born without the ability to manufacture the enzyme have an inborn error of metabolism called **galactosemia,** which is characterized by the presence of detectable levels of galactose in the urine. Galactosemia can be treated by eliminating sources of both galactose and lactose from the diet. Untreated infants with this disease deteriorate rapidly, both physically and mentally, and die at an early age, literally of starvation. A patient with galactosemia tests negative for sugar with the urinalysis strip tests but positive with CLINITEST®. Therefore, children should be tested by the urinalysis strip and the CLINITEST™ procedure. Both results should be reported to the physician. Continue this procedure and follow the POL policy to the age when the child no longer would be tested by both methods.

ACETEST® for Ketones

ACETEST® is a confirmation test for ketones. Like urinalysis strip tests, ACETEST® is based on a nitroprusside reaction, which detects both acetone and acetoacetic acid. Materials needed include an ACETEST® tablet, the ACETEST® color chart, and white paper. The procedure for ACETEST® is

- Remove an ACETEST® tablet from the bottle and recap the bottle.
- Place the tablet on a clean surface, preferably white paper.
- Put one drop of urine on the tablet.
- Time the reaction on the tablet for 30 seconds.
- Compare the color change on the tablet to the ACETEST® color chart at 30 seconds.

Testing Blood for Ketones

Serum, plasma, or whole blood also can be tested for ketones by substituting one drop of the fluid in place of one drop of urine. When using serum or plasma, take the reading at 2 minutes after applying the specimen to the tablet. When whole blood is added, wait 10 minutes before removing clotted blood from the tablet. Be sure to note which type of specimen was used for testing.

PROCEDURE 9-1

Physical Analysis of Urine

Goal

To determine the correct color and clarity of a urine specimen.

Completion Time

10 minutes

Equipment and Supplies

- Impermeable lab coat
- Disposable gloves
- Face shield or goggles
- Hand disinfectant
- Biohazard container
- Fresh urine sample
- Urine test tube
- Disinfectant wipes
- Pen
- Chart for recording results

Instructions

Read through the list of equipment and supplies that you will need and the steps of the procedure. Be sure that you understand each step before you begin. Then complete each step correctly and in the proper order. If your completion time is too long, repeat the procedure until you increase your speed.

Steps marked with (*) are critical and must have the maximum points to pass.

Performance Standards	Points Awarded	Maximum Points
1. Put on lab coat and face shield or goggles.		5
2. Disinfect hands; dry if necessary.		5
3. Put on gloves. Inspect for tears and replace if necessary.		5
4. Collect and prepare the appropriate equipment.		5
5. *Verify specimen identity.		30
6. Allow the urine to come to room temperature.		5
7. Mix the urine specimen by gently swirling the specimen.		5
8. Pour the urine into a urine test tube.		
9. Correctly identify color of the urine.		25

10. Document the color of the urine in the log book.		25
11. Correctly identify the clarity of the urine.		25
12. Dispose of the urine per lab policy.		10
13. Discard disposable equipment.		10
14. Clean and return all equipment to storage.		5
15. Wash hands.		5
Total Points		**165**

Overall Procedural Evaluation

Student Name _____

Signature of Instructor _____ Date _____

Comments _____

_____

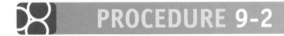 **PROCEDURE 9-2**

Chemical Analysis of Urine

Goal
To correctly perform the chemical analysis of a urine specimen.

Completion Time
20 minutes

Equipment and Supplies
- Impermeable lab coat
- Disposable gloves
- Face shield or goggles
- Hand disinfectant
- Biohazard container
- Fresh urine sample
- Urine test tube
- Disposable urinalysis strip
- Urinalysis strip color chart
- Watch with a second hand
- Paper towel
- Disinfectant
- Pen
- Chart for recording results

Instructions
Read through the list of equipment and supplies that you will need and the steps of the procedure. Be sure that you understand each step before you begin. Then complete each step correctly and in the proper order. If your completion time is too long, repeat the procedure until you increase your speed.

Steps marked with (*) are critical and must have the maximum points to pass.

Performance Standards	Points Awarded	Maximum Points
1. Put on lab coat and face shield or goggles.		5
2. Disinfect hands, dry if necessary.		5
3. Put on gloves. Inspect for tears and replace if necessary.		5
4. Collect and prepare the appropriate equipment.		5

—table continued

Performance Standards		Points Awarded	Maximum Points
5.	*Verify specimen identity.		30
6.	Allow the urine to come to room temperature.		5
7.	Mix the urine specimen by gently swirling the specimen.		5
8.	Pour the urine into a urine test tube.		5
9.	Remove one urinalysis strip from its container and replace the cover on the container.		5
10.	Note the time and quickly dip the urinalysis strip into the specimen, wetting all reagent pads. Do not immerse the urinalysis strip longer than one second.		10
11.	Remove excess urine from the strip by blotting the urinalysis strip on a paper towel. Hold the strip horizontally to prevent mixing chemicals from adjacent pads.		10
12.	At the appropriate time and in good light, hold the urinalysis strip next to the color chart. Be careful not to let the strip touch and contaminate the chart.		15
13.	Find the colors that best match the urinalysis strip pads and record the results for each test on the urinalysis report form.		5
14.	*Correctly record the results for each test in the log book.		30
15.	Dispose of the urine per lab policy.		10
16.	Discard disposable equipment.		10
17.	Clean and return all equipment to storage.		5
18.	Wash hands.		5
	Total Points		**170**

Overall Procedural Evaluation

Student Name _____

Signature of Instructor _____ Date _____

Comments _____

_____

PROCEDURE 9-3

Measuring the Specific Gravity of Urine Using a Refractometer

Goal

After successfully completing this procedure, you will be able to measure specific gravity with a refractometer.

Completion Time

20 minutes

Equipment and Supplies

- Impermeable jacket, gown, or apron
- Disposable gloves
- Face shield or goggles
- Hand disinfectant
- Surface disinfectant
- Paper towels and tissues
- Biohazard container
- Distilled water
- Refractometer
- Dropping pipette
- Urine report form and pen

Instructions

Read through the list of equipment and supplies that you will need and the steps of the procedure. Be sure that you understand each step before you begin. Then complete each step correctly and in the proper order. If your completion time is too long, repeat the procedure until you increase your speed.

Steps marked with (*) are critical and must have the maximum points to pass.

Performance Standards	Points Awarded	Maximum Points
1. Put on lab coat and face shield or goggles.		5
2. Disinfect hands; dry if necessary.		5
3. Put on gloves. Inspect for tears and replace if necessary.		5
4. Collect and prepare the appropriate equipment.		5
5. *Verify specimen identity.		30
6. Allow the urine to come to room temperature.		5
7. Mix the urine specimen by gently swirling the specimen.		5
8. Read the refractometer's manufacturer instructions.		5
9. With a pipette, place a drop of urine on the exposed area of the refractometer prism (glass plate) and close the cover plate completely.		5
10. Hold the refractometer toward the light.		5
11. Look through the ocular and, if necessary, rotate the eyepiece until the scale comes into view.		5
12. Read the specific gravity at the point on the scale where the dark area meets the light area.		20
13. *Record the result in the log book.		30
14. Wipe the prism clean with a tissue soaked in disinfectant.		5
15. Wipe the rest of the refractometer with disinfectant.		
16. Dispose of the urine per lab policy.		10
17. Discard disposable equipment.		10
18. Return all equipment to storage.		5
19. Wash hands.		5
Total Points		**165**

Overall Procedural Evaluation

Student Name _____

Signature of Instructor _____ Date _____

Comments _____

_____

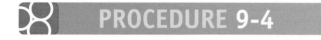

PROCEDURE 9-4

Determine the Glucose Level of a Urine Specimen Utilizing the CLINITEST™ Method

Goal

To correctly perform the chemical analysis of a urine specimen.

Completion Time

15 minutes

Equipment and Supplies

- Impermeable lab coat
- Disposable gloves
- Face shield or goggles
- Hand disinfectant
- Biohazard container
- Fresh urine sample
- CLINITEST™ tablet
- Small glass test tube (see note)
- Test tube rack
- Watch with a second hand
- Paper towel
- CLINITEST™ color chart
- Distilled water
- Pen
- Chart for recording results

> **Note**
>
> A plastic tube should NOT be used for this procedure. The reaction between the CLINITEST™ tablet, the distilled water, and the urine causes a very heated, boiling reaction. A plastic test tube could melt. Therefore, a glass test tube should always be used for this procedure.

Instructions

Read through the list of equipment and supplies that you will need and the steps of the procedure. Be sure that you understand each step before you begin. Then complete each step correctly and in the proper order. If your completion time is too long, repeat the procedure until you increase your speed.

Steps marked with (*) are critical and must have the maximum points to pass.

Performance Standards	Points Awarded	Maximum Points
1. Put on lab coat and face shield or goggles.		5
2. Disinfect hands; dry if necessary.		5
3. Put on gloves. Inspect for tears and replace if necessary.		5
4. Collect and prepare the appropriate equipment.		5
5. *Verify specimen identity.		30
6. Allow the urine to come to room temperature.		5
7. Mix the urine specimen by gently swirling the specimen.		5
8. Place a small glass test tube in a test tube rack.		5
9. Add five drops of urine to the glass test tube.		5
10. Add 10 drops of distilled water to the test tube.		5
11. Shake one CLINITEST™ tablet from the container onto the cap.		5
12. Close the cover on the bottle tightly.		5
13. Gently drop the CLINITEST™ tablet from the cap into the glass test tube. **Caution: Heat is produced from the chemical reaction that occurs as the tablet dissolves.**		5
14. Keep the glass tube balanced in the tube rack. Do not touch the tube or point it toward anyone.		10

	Points Awarded	Maximum Points
15. Observe the tube for a boiling reaction.		10
16. When the boiling has stopped, note the time.		10
17. Fifteen seconds after the boiling has stopped, compare the color of the reaction to the CLINITEST™ color chart.		10
18. *Record the result on the urinalysis report form, either as positive or negative.		30
19. Dispose of the urine and tablet per lab policy.		10
20. Discard disposable equipment.		10
21. Return all equipment to storage.		5
22. Wash hands.		5
Total Points		**190**

Overall Procedural Evaluation

Student Name _____

Signature of Instructor _____ Date _____

Comments _____

_____

PROCEDURE 9-5

Determine the Bilirubin Level of a Urine Specimen Utilizing the ICTOTEST™ Method

Goal
To correctly perform the chemical analysis of a urine specimen.

Completion Time
15 minutes

Equipment and Supplies
- Impermeable lab coat
- Disposable gloves
- Face shield or goggles
- Hand disinfectant
- Biohazard container
- Fresh urine sample
- ICTOTEST™ test mat
- Disposable pipette—choose size according to the manufacturer's instructions
- Distilled water
- Watch with a second hand
- Paper towel
- Pen
- Chart for recording results

Instructions
Read through the list of equipment and supplies that you will need and the steps of the procedure. Be sure that you understand each step before you begin. Then complete each step correctly and in the proper order. If your completion time is too long, repeat the procedure until you increase your speed.

Steps marked with (*) are critical and must have the maximum points to pass.

Performance Standards	Points Awarded	Maximum Points
1. Put on lab coat and face shield or goggles.		5
2. Disinfect hands; dry if necessary.		5

—table continued

Performance Standards	Points Awarded	Maximum Points
3. Put on gloves. Inspect for tears and replace if necessary.		5
4. Collect and prepare the appropriate equipment.		5
5. *Verify specimen identity.		30
6. Allow the urine to come to room temperature.		5
7. Mix the urine specimen by gently swirling the specimen.		5
8. Place 10 drops of urine on an ICTOTEST™ test mat.		5
9. Place an ICTOTEST™ reagent tablet on the center of the moistened area of the mat.		5
10. With a disposable pipette, drop two drops of distilled water over the tablet. Note the time.		5
11. Watch for 60 seconds. Follow the manufacturer's instructions for interpreting the test results.		5
12. *Record the result on the urinalysis report form.		30
13. Dispose of the urine and tablet per lab policy.		10
14. Discard disposable equipment.		10
15. Return all equipment to storage.		5
16. Wash hands.		5
Total Points		**140**

Overall Procedural Evaluation

Student Name _____

Signature of Instructor _____ Date _____

Comments _____

_____

PROCEDURE 9-6

Perform Urinalysis Quality Control Testing for Urinalysis Strips

Goal

To correctly perform urinalysis quality control testing for urinalysis strips.

Completion Time

15 minutes

Equipment and Supplies

- Impermeable lab coat
- Disposable gloves
- Face shield or goggles
- Hand disinfectant
- Biohazard container
- Urinalysis strips
- Urinalysis strip chart
- Urinalysis controls—high/low, normal/abnormal
- Manufacturer's control sheet
- Watch with a second hand
- Paper towel
- Urinalysis control report form
- Pen
- Chart for recording results

Instructions

Read through the list of equipment and supplies that you will need and the steps of the procedure. Be sure that you understand each step before you begin. Then complete each step correctly and in the proper order. If your completion time is too long, repeat the procedure until you increase your speed.

Steps marked with (*) are critical and must have the maximum points to pass.

Performance Standards	Points Awarded	Maximum Points
1. Put on lab coat and face shield or goggles.		5
2. Disinfect hands; dry if necessary.		5
3. Put on gloves. Inspect for tears and replace if necessary.		5
4. Collect and prepare the appropriate equipment.		5
5. Remove two urinalysis strips from the container.		10
6. Immediately recap the urinalysis strip bottle.		5
7. If necessary, reconstitute the urine control, carefully following the manufacturer's instructions.		5
8. Mix the urine controls by gently inverting the sealed control bottle 5–10 times.		5
9. Note the time, then dip the first urinalysis strip in one of the control vials, wetting all of the reagent pads. Immerse the strip no longer than one second.		10
10. Remove excess urine from the strip by blotting the urinalysis strip on a paper towel. Hold the strip horizontally to prevent mixing chemicals from adjacent pads.		5
11. At the appropriate time and in good light, hold the urinalysis strip next to the color chart. Be careful not to let the strip touch and contaminate the chart.		5
12. *Record the result on the urinalysis control form.		30
13. *Compare your results to the expected manufacturer results.		30
14. Determine which results, if any, need to be repeated.		30
15. *Troubleshoot any results outside the acceptable range per laboratory policy.		30
16. Repeat steps 9–15 with the second urinalysis control.		
17. Store the controls per lab policy.		10
18. Discard disposable equipment.		10
19. Return all equipment to storage.		5
20. Wash hands.		5
Total Points		**215**

Overall Procedural Evaluation

Student Name _____

Signature of Instructor _____ Date _____

Comments _____

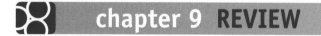

chapter 9 REVIEW

Using Terminology

Match the term on the left with the most appropriate description on the right.

____ 1. isosthenuria	a. urine containing blood
____ 2. lipiduria	b. production of urine with consistent low
____ 3. hypersthenuria	specific gravity, regardless of fluid intake
____ 4. hematuria	c. abnormally high blood pH
____ 5. acidosis	d. pus in the urine
____ 6. alkalosis	e. production of urine with high specific gravity
____ 7. pyuria	f. abnormally low blood pH
	g. presence of fat in urine

Match the confirmation test on the left with the substance on the right.

____ 8. refractometer	a. reducing sugars
____ 9. ICTOTEST®	b. ketones
____ 10. CLINITEST®	c. protein
____ 11. ACETEST®	d. specific gravity
____ 12. acetic test	e. bilirubin

Urinalysis strips are used to detect abnormal levels of each of the following. In the space provided, identify the clinical significance of each.

13. Glucose

_____

_____

_____

14. Ketones

_____

_____

_____

15. Protein

_____

_____

_____

16. Blood

_____

_____

_____

17. Bilirubin

_____

_____

_____

18. Urobilinogen

_____

_____

_____

19. Nitrite

_____

_____

_____

20. Leukocytes

_____

_____

_____

Multiple Choice

Choose the best answer for the following questions.

21. The presence of erythrocytes in blood is
   a. pyuria
   b. hematuria
   c. isosthenuria
   d. bilirubinuria

22. The term used to compare the density of a liquid relative to the density of distilled water is
   a. opalescence
   b. refractometer
   c. isothenuria
   d. specific gravity

23. A disease characterized by urine with a "mousy" odor is
   a. diabetes mellitus
   b. Bence Jones
   c. PKU
   d. jaundice

24. The foam test indicates the presence of which of the following?
   a. bilirubin
   b. leukocytes
   c. protein
   d. nitrates

25. Urine with a fruity odor indicates the presence of which of the following?
   a. bilirubin
   b. glucose
   c. protein
   d. nitrites

26. A positive nitrite test would indicate the presence of _____ in the urine.
   a. blood
   b. leukocytes
   c. bacteria
   d. glucose

27. What type of sugar is most commonly found in urine?
    a. glucose
    b. lactose
    c. fructose
    d. sucrose

28. How is the concentration of hydrogen ions in a solution expressed?
    a. specific gravity
    b. urobilinogen
    c. pH
    d. turbidity

29. An increase in which analyte in the urine is indicative of renal disease?
    a. pH
    b. bilirubin
    c. leukocytes
    d. protein

30. A diabetic who is not taking his insulin may have which of the following in his urine?
    a. ketones
    b. bilirubin
    c. nitrite
    d. protein

31. A patient with liver disease would have elevated levels of which of the following analytes in her urine?
    a. ketones
    b. bilirubin
    c. nitrite
    d. protein

32. Which of the following confirmation tests detects the presence of Bence Jones proteins?
    a. refractometer
    b. ICTOTEST®
    c. ACETEST®
    d. acetic test

33. A specimen of known value is referred to as
    a. proficiency testing
    b. control
    c. refractometer
    d. patient sample

34. A quantitative result is one that
    a. provides a numerical value
    b. provides a yes/no or positive/negative value
    c. provides a result that represents a range
    d. all of the above

Acquiring Knowledge

Answer the following questions in the spaces provided.

35. What end product of protein metabolism is secreted into the urine?

    _____

    _____

36. What three properties are examined in a routine urinalysis?

_____

_____

_____

37. What is the specific gravity of distilled water?

_____

_____

_____

38. Why is routine urinalysis one of the most commonly performed laboratory procedures?

_____

_____

_____

39. Name the analytes included in routine urinalysis.

_____

_____

_____

40. What is a screening test? When is it used?

_____

_____

_____

41. What is a confirmation test? When is it used?

_____

_____

_____

42. What type of testing is performed with urinalysis strips: screening or confirmation?

_____

_____

_____

43. What odor in urine may indicate a urinary infection?

_____

_____

_____

44. What visible clue may indicate that urine is concentrated?

_____

_____

_____

45. What sources of variation do urine chemistry analyzers eliminate?

_____

_____

_____

46. What differences among individual laboratorians may cause great variation in their interpretation of urinalysis strips?

_____

_____

_____

47. How are precision and accuracy affected by variation among laboratory personnel in the interpretation of urinalysis strips?

_____

_____

_____

Applying Knowledge—On the Job

Answer the following questions in the spaces provided.

48. Assume that you are employed in a clinical laboratory and that one of your duties is performing urinalysis. The urine specimens submitted for testing have a variety of appearances. Some are clear, others are cloudy, and there are variations in color. Some also have distinctive odors. Why is it important to make note of these physical characteristics of urine?

_____

_____

_____

49. A patient has just handed you a urine specimen with an intense orange-gold color. Yellow foam floats on top. What might be the cause of the abnormal appearance of the urine?

_____

_____

_____

50. Among the urine specimens this morning is one with a pungent odor of ammonia. What could this smell indicate?

_____

_____

_____

51. Assume that you perform the urinalysis in the POL where you work. What quality control will you employ to ensure that your specific gravity readings are accurate?

_____

_____

_____

_____

52. An infant's urine has been submitted to the laboratory with a request for a CLINITEST® along with routine urinalysis. Why would such a request be made?

_____

_____

_____

_____

53. In the lab where you work, several patients have tested positive for urinary protein. Classify each of the following protein levels as marked, moderate, or minimal, and list two possible causes of each

(a) 5 grams/day

_____

_____

_____

_____

(b) 2 grams/day

_____

_____

_____

(c) 0.2 gram/day

_____

_____

_____

_____

54. Mrs. Jones' urine specimen tests positive for nitrite and leukocyte esterase and is strongly alkaline (8.5). It also has an ammonia smell. What type of illness might she have?

_____

_____

_____

_____

55. Mr. Chan's urinalysis strip test for protein was negative, yet the physician has ordered a precipitation test for him, which you know also screens for protein. Why did the doctor order a confirmation test for an analyte when the screening test was negative?

_____

_____

_____

_____

56. Elaine's urine specimen appears normal, but the urinalysis strip test reveals occult blood. She does not understand how blood can be present without being obvious. The doctor has asked you to explain this to her. What do you say?

_____

_____

_____

_____

57. One of the urine specimens that you analyzed today tested positive for occult blood. What is the clinical significance of this finding?

_____

_____

_____

_____

58. Your student group is visiting a clinical laboratory. One of the students asks why both screening and confirmation tests are done for a single analyte. She thinks that it might be quicker and cheaper to do just confirmation tests in the first place and eliminate screening. Explain to her why the laboratory uses screening tests in addition to confirmation tests.

_____

_____

_____

_____

59. You are employed in a clinical laboratory where you perform a urinalysis that tests positive for bilirubin. With what infectious disease might this patient be infected?

_____

_____

_____

_____

60. As the clinical worker in charge of the urinalysis section, how will you maintain quality control of urine testing?

_____

_____

_____

_____

61. Jerry is having a busy day in the laboratory. He dips urinalysis strips into several different urine specimens at the same time and attempts to read several urinalysis strips simultaneously. What problem do you see in this scenario?

_____

_____

_____

_____

62. Clarisse has just received the printout from the new urine chemistry analyzer for the first batch of samples that she is testing using the new instrument. She cannot find anything on the printout about color or clarity of the samples and fears that the instrument is malfunctioning. What do you think might be the problem?

_____

_____

_____

_____

63. Juan has just one more urine sample to analyze before he is done with work for the day. There are no more urinalysis strips in the box, so he has to open a new one. The urine control has already been used the specified number of times. Juan decides just to test the urine sample and forgo quality control this one time. What should Juan have done? Why?

_____

_____

_____

_____

10 chapter

Microscopic Properties of Urinalysis

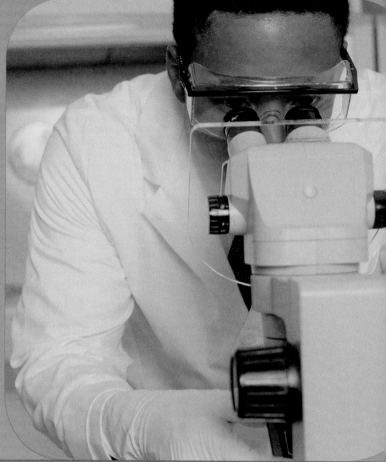

COGNITIVE OBJECTIVES

After studying this chapter, you should be able to

10.1 use each of the vocabulary terms appropriately.

10.2 explain the relationship between the microscopic examination of urine and the diagnosis and treatment of patients.

10.3 describe how to differentiate among the various elements found in urine under microscopic examination.

10.4 state the normal range of the commonly found elements in urinary sediment.

10.5 discuss the clinical significance of elements commonly found in urine sediment.

10.6 outline the technical procedure for obtaining precise and reproducible microscopic examinations of urine.

PERFORMANCE OBJECTIVES

After studying this chapter, you should be able to

10.7 prepare a urine specimen for microscopic examination of sediment.

10.8 identify and count casts, cellular elements, and crystals in a urine sediment slide.

TERMINOLOGY

balanitis: inflammation of the glans penis, most often due to *Trichomonas vaginalis, Herpes,* or *Chlamydia trachomatis.*

calculus: urinary stone. Also known as renal calculi.

crenated: usually used to refer to shrunken red blood cells that appear small and scalloped around the edges.

cylindruria: the condition characterized by large numbers of casts in the urine.

decantation: the process of pouring off fluid. In urinalysis, it usually refers to the pouring off of the liquid portion of urine after it has been centrifuged.

desquamation: the shedding of layers of cells or skin.

erythrocyte: a red blood cell.

fatty cast: renal cast that contains fat droplets because of chronic renal disease.

granular cast: fine- or coarse-grained dark renal cast that has degenerated from a hyaline or waxy cast. An increase in the number of granular casts may indicate pyelonephritis.

hyaline cast: the most common type of renal cast. Hyaline casts are colorless, homogeneous, and semitransparent. An increase in the number of hyaline casts indicates damage to the glomerular capillary membrane, permitting leakage of protein.

hypertonic urine: a concentrated urine with a specific gravity of 1.030 or greater.

hypotonic urine: a diluted urine with a specific gravity of 1.003 or less.

leukocyte: a white blood cell.

lymphocyte: a nongranular white blood cell with a single nucleus.

neutrophil: the most commonly found type of white blood cell in urine sediment; so named because it stains with neutral dyes.

orthostatic proteinuria: increased levels of protein in the urine when the patient is in a standing position.

phase microscopy: the type of microscopy in which differences in the refractive index are translated into differences in brightness; used to view unstained specimens.

prostatitis: inflammation of the prostate.

renal cast: the tube-shaped element in urine sediment, formed in the tubules of the kidney by the deposition of protein.

sperm: male reproductive cells.

supernatant: fluid remaining at the top of a specimen after centrifugation.

supravital stain: dye added to cells while they are living to make them easier to see.

urine sediment: the solid material that settles to the bottom of urine when it stands or is centrifuged.

waxy cast: the renal cast that is yellowish, with irregular broken ends.

INTRODUCTION

Microscopic examination of urine sediment is a valuable diagnostic procedure that can confirm some of the findings of the chemical analysis. It is a challenging and rewarding procedure that can provide the physician with valuable information. It is a procedure that requires a great deal of technical skill and clinical knowledge; therefore, it should only be performed by laboratory personnel that have the appropriate education and training. This chapter reviews the clinical significance of urine microscopy.

URINE SEDIMENT

Urine sediment, which is the solid material that settles to the bottom when it stands or is centrifuged, contains all of the insoluble materials that can be found in urine, including **erythrocytes** (red blood cells), **leukocytes** (white blood cells), casts, crystals, bacteria, fungi, parasites, mucous threads, and, in males, **sperm** (male reproductive cells). Next to actual biopsies of kidney tissue, microscopic findings are the best indicators of intrinsic renal disease. In fact, urine sediment analysis is sometimes referred to as "liquid biopsy" for this reason.

THE CONVENTIONAL METHOD OF MICROSCOPIC ANALYSIS

This section outlines the method of preparing and examining urine sediment that is most widely used in POLs today.

Preparation of the Specimen

Most urine specimens are centrifuged before microscopic examination of sediment to concentrate the formed elements. (See Figure 10-1.) The same specimen used for chemical testing should be used for microscopic analysis. The specimen should be fresh and thoroughly mixed prior to the physical and chemical analysis. (See Figure 10-2.) About 10 to 15 mL of urine are poured into a disposable conical-shaped urine tube. Lab personnel should first perform the physical examination of the urine. Once the physical examination is complete and the results recorded, the lab personnel should then perform the chemical examination of the urine, including performing any required confirmation tests. It is only after the physical and chemical examination are complete the lab personnel can begin preparing the specimen for microscopic examination. Specimen caps or

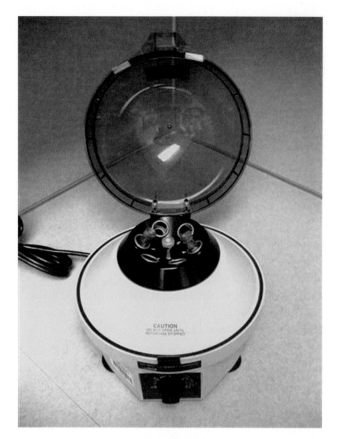

Figure 10-1 The six-tube capacity of the centrifuge is typical of those found in POLs.

covers should be placed on top to prevent spills and aerosol drops. Specimens are then centrifuged for five minutes at 1,500 to 2,000 rpm. After centrifuging, the **supernatant,** the fluid that floats on top, is poured off without disturbing the sediment. The amount of urine left with the sediment may vary from a few drops to 1 milliliter. (See Figure 10-3.)

The sediment is resuspended in the remaining urine and a drop is placed on a microscope glass slide using a pipette and covered with a 22-mm square cover slip. The cover slip performs three roles. It assures that the slide has a uniform

Order of Complete Urinalysis

Complete urinalysis should be performed in the following order:

1. physical analysis: color and clarity, volume if required
2. chemical analysis: urinalysis strips and any required confirmation tests
3. microscopic analysis

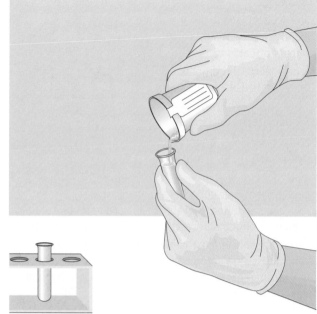

Figure 10-2 In order to prepare the specimen for microscopic analysis, pour 10–15 mL into a urine conical tube that can be centrifuged.

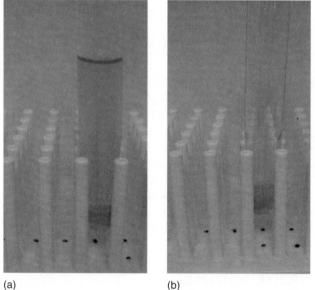

(a) (b)

Figure 10-3 (a) Centrifuged urine with sediment on the bottom. (b) Photo after urine supernatant has been decanted or poured off.

Quality Assurance Note

If protein confirmation testing is required, remember to save the supernatant for this procedure.

thickness, it helps keep the specimen still, and it protects the microscope objective from contamination with specimen material. To prevent the formation of bubbles when placing the cover slip on the drop of urine, let an edge of the cover slip touch the liquid first and then let the rest drop into place. If liquid runs out from under the cover slip or allows it to float, you have used too large a drop.

Staining. Sediment may be stained to improve refraction and to clarify the image at lower light intensities. Add one or two drops of stain to the sediment in the conical-shaped tube and thoroughly mix it before placing the sediment on the microscope slide. Avoid overstaining.

A number of different stains may be used for urine sediment. A toluidine blue stain is used to stain cells and casts. Sternheimer-Malbin (S-M) stain is most helpful in the identification of nucleated elements as well as casts, but some staining solutions require filtration before using because they form sediments that interfere with viewing.

A stabilized modification of S-M stain that does not require filtration is Clay Adams™ Sedi-Stain Concentrated Stain, distributed by Becton, Dickson & Company, that contains both crystal violet and safranine dyes, which are taken up in varying proportions depending on the chemical and physical properties of formed elements in the sediment. The results vary from pale pink to dark purple. (See Figure 10-4.)

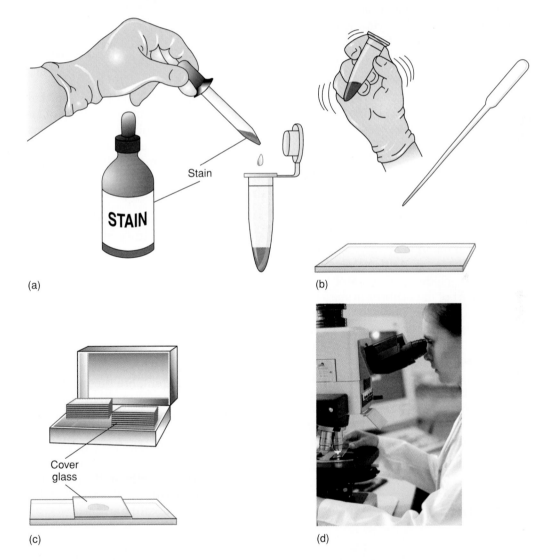

(a)

(b)

Cover glass

(c)

(d)

Figure 10-4 To stain urine sediment, follow these steps: (a) Add one drop of stain to approximately ½ mL of centrifuged urine sediment and mix together by shaking the tube. (b) Place one drop of stained urine sediment on the slide. (c) Place cover slip over drop on the slide. (d) View the slide under the microscope and count the formed elements in the sediment.

Scanning the Slide

After the slide is coverslipped, it is placed on the microscope stage for examination. Under low-power (10X) magnification and lower or subdued lighting (with the condenser lowered and/or the iris diaphragm partly closed), the entire slide is systematically scanned around all four sides of the cover slip. The fine focus adjustment knob should be used as needed to sharpen the image. This initial scan is necessary to locate the fields in which most of the formed elements are present.

Counting Formed Elements

Ten to 15 of the fields containing formed elements should be examined using high-power (45X) magnification and higher light intensity (with the condenser raised and/or the iris diaphragm opened). Under high power, the number of erythrocytes, leukocytes, and epithelial cells in the selected fields are counted and then the average number of each type of cell per field is calculated. The result is reported as the number per HPF, or high-power field. Casts should be identified as to type under high-power magnification and then counted in 10 to 15 fields using low-power magnification. The result is averaged and reported as the number per LPF, or low-power field.

Other elements observed in the slide may include crystals, mucus, bacteria, fungi, parasites, and sperm. These elements should be identified and quantified using the 45X objective. These should be reported but not reported as a numerical number. Instead, these elements are often reported as few, many, large, or other semiquantitative terms. Artifacts, extraneous materials such as hair, clothing fibers, and talcum powder that are not part of the urine or urinary tract, often are misinterpreted. For example, it is common to misinterpret clothing fibers as mucous threads. Take care to distinguish artifacts from any sediment elements that are to be identified and counted.

Phase microscopy, in which differences in refractive index are translated into differences in brightness, is used in some POLs to detect translucent elements in urine sediment. It is especially useful for detailing the outline of hyaline casts, mucous threads, and bacteria. Specimens are generally unstained.

CASTS AND THEIR CLINICAL SIGNIFICANCE

Renal casts (see Figure 10-5) are cylindrical bodies with parallel sides of varying diameter that form in the renal tubules and wash into the urine. The matrix of the cast is glycoprotein, Tamm-Horsfall

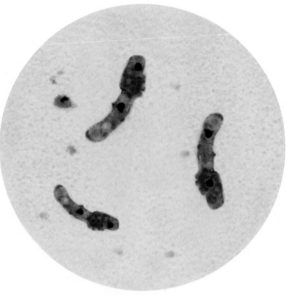

Renal Casts

Figure 10-5 Example of stained renal casts.

mucoprotein, produced by renal epithelial cells lining the ascending limb of the loop of Henle and the distal convoluted tubule of the kidneys.

The reference value for the number of casts in the normal urine specimen is 0 to 1 per LPF. An increased number of casts in the urine, which is called **cylindruria,** may be due to several factors including

- a decreased rate of tubular flow
- an increased acidity of urine
- a decreased volume of urine with increased protein or salt concentration.

The significance of an increased number of casts depends on their type.

Hyaline Casts

Hyaline casts, which are colorless, homogeneous, and semitransparent, are the most common type of cast (see Figure 10-6). An increase in their number indicates damage to the glomerular capillary membrane, permitting leakage of protein. This damage may be transient, resulting from fever, dehydration, emotional stress, strenuous exercise, or the effect of posture, **orthostatic proteinuria,** or permanent due to kidney disease. Hyaline casts usually dissolve in alkaline urine.

Granular Casts

Granular casts are casts that show the degree of degeneration that has occurred in the cellular inclusions. The granules may be fine or coarse grained. While an occasional granular cast is

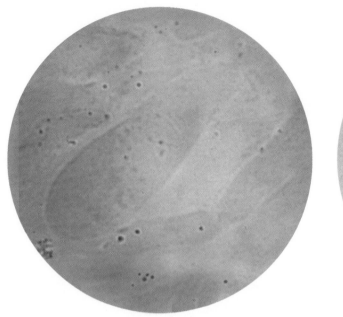

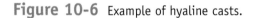

Figure 10-6 Example of hyaline casts.

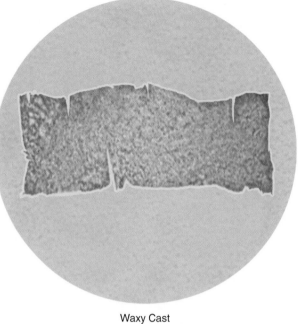

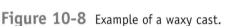

Figure 10-8 Example of a waxy cast.

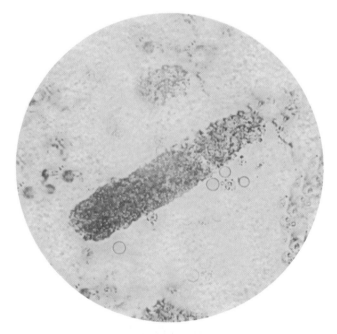

Figure 10-7 Example of granular casts.

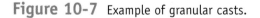

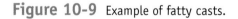

Figure 10-9 Example of fatty casts.

considered to be normal, an increase in number may indicate pyelonephritis. (See Figure 10-7.)

Waxy and Fatty Casts

Casts may be **waxy** and yellowish, with irregular, broken ends, or they may be **fatty,** that is,

containing fat droplets. Waxy casts form in the collecting tubules when the urine flow through them is reduced. Both waxy and fatty casts may be associated with the tubular inflammation and degeneration characteristic of chronic renal disease. These casts are always regarded as pathological. (See Figures 10-8 and 10-9.)

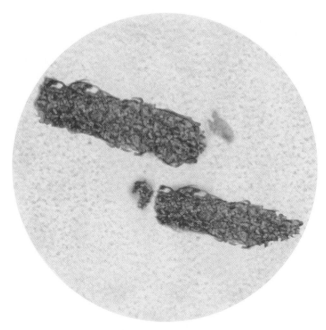

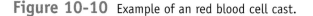
Red Blood Cell Cast

Figure 10-10 Example of an red blood cell cast.

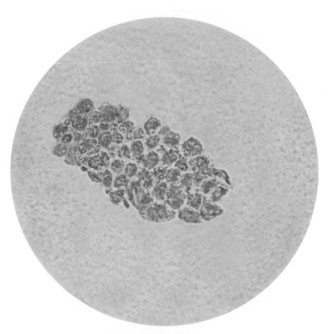

White Blood Cell Cast

Figure 10-11 Example of a white blood cell cast.

Red Blood Cell Casts

Red blood cell casts are casts that contain red blood cells in their matrix. Red blood cell casts indicate renal bleeding due to acute inflammatory or vascular disorders of the glomerulus. These casts should always be regarded as pathological. They may be the only symptom of acute glomerulonephritis, renal infarction, collagen disease, and kidney involvement in subacute bacterial endocarditis. (See Figure 10-10.)

White Blood Cell Casts

White blood cell casts are casts that include white blood cells in their matrix. White blood cell casts may be observed in the urine of patients with acute glomerulonephritis, nephrotic syndrome, or pyelonephritis. They are especially important in diagnosing pyelonephritis because this disease may remain completely asymptomatic while progressively destroying renal tissue. (See Figure 10-11.)

Epithelial Cell Casts

Epithelial cell casts are formed when epithelial cells are shed from the renal tubules and fuse together and are incorporated into the matrix of a cast. An increase in their number often indicates damage to the renal tubule epithelium, which may occur with nephrosis, eclampsia, amyloidosis, or toxic poisoning. (See Figure 10-12.)

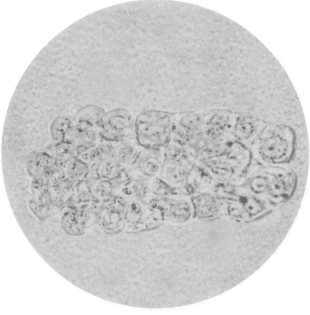

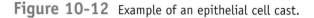
Epithelial Cell Cast

Figure 10-12 Example of an epithelial cell cast.

CELLULAR ELEMENTS AND THEIR CLINICAL SIGNIFICANCE

Three types of cells normally are found in urinary sediment (see Figure 10-13): red blood cells, white blood cells, and epithelial cells.

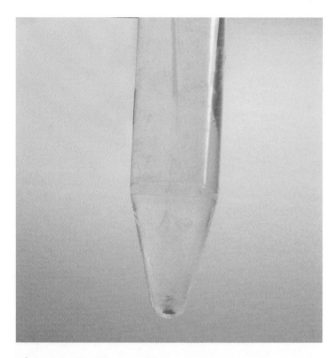

Figure 10-13 Example of urine sediment.

Table 10-1 Pathological Conditions Producing Hematuria

Renal Diseases	Calculus (stone)
Glomerulonephritis	Tumor
Lupus nephritis	Stricture (narrowing)
Calculus	**Extrarenal Diseases**
Tumor	Acute appendicitis
Acute infection	Diverticulitis
Tuberculosis	Tumors of the colon, rectum, pelvis
Renal vein thrombosis	
Renal trauma	**Drug Toxicity**
Polycystic kidney	Salicylates (aspirin)
Malignant nephrosclerosis	Anticoagulants
Infarction	
Lower Urinary Tract Diseases	
Acute and chronic infection	

Red Blood Cells

When viewed with high-power magnification, unstained red blood cells look like clear discs of slightly varying size. In **hypotonic urine,** red blood cells tend to lyse, and in **hypertonic urine,** they may shrink and become **crenated,** shrunken and notched or scalloped around the edges.

Normal concentrations of red blood cells on a urine sediment slide are one or two per HPF. More than three red blood cells per HPF are considered abnormal, unless due to contamination of the specimen by menstrual blood. Blood in the urine may result from a variety of renal or systemic disease. When an increase in red blood cells in urine is found in conjunction with red blood cell casts, it can be assumed that the bleeding is renal in origin. See Table 10-1.

White Blood Cells

When viewed under high-power magnification, white blood cells in urine look like round granular bodies, about twice as large as red blood cells. The type of white blood cell most often observed is the segmented **neutrophil,** so named because it stains with neutral dyes.

In normal urine sediment, only zero to five white blood cells per HPF are observed. Increased numbers of leukocytes in the urine are usually indicative of disease, although a temporary increase may follow strenuous exercise. Diseases associated with increased white blood cells in urine include calculi, cystitis, **prostatitis** (inflammation of the prostate), urethritis, and **balanitis** (inflammation of the glans penis). The presence of more than 50 leukocytes per HPF or of clumps of leukocytes is strongly suggestive of acute urinary tract infection. Gross pyuria may reflect the rupture of a renal or urinary tract abscess. When increased numbers of leukocytes are found together with leukocyte casts or mixed leukocyte-epithelial cell casts, they are most likely renal in origin, indicating renal disease such as glomerulonephritis, lupus nephritis, or pyelonephritis. Large numbers of mononucleated white cells, or **lymphocytes,** in the urine of a patient who has undergone kidney transplant surgery may be an early sign of tissue rejection.

Supravital stains such as those used to color living cells that have not been fixed or chemically treated usually are helpful in delineating the nuclear structure of leukocytes in urine sediment. However, in hypotonic (dilute) urine, neutrophils swell and are poorly stained with supravital stains. Then they are called glitter cells because their cytoplasmic granules exhibit Brownian movement, causing refraction. Leukocytes are rapidly lysed in hypotonic or alkaline urine. It is estimated that half are lost after urine stands at room temperature for 2 to 3 hours, underscoring the need to use fresh urine specimens in microscopic analysis.

> **Quality Control Note**
>
> "Fresh urine" is urine that is collected and tested within one hour or urine that is refrigerated upon collection. Remember that any urine specimen that is refrigerated must be allowed to return to room temperature prior to testing.

Epithelial Cells

Normal urine sediment may have an occasional epithelial cell or clump of epithelial cells because the renal tubules and their epithelium are always being renewed. However, renal epithelial cells that **desquamate,** or shed, at an excessive rate are indicative of disease damage to the renal tubular epithelium.

Renal epithelial cells are round, slightly larger than white blood cells, and have a single large nucleus. As the name implies, renal epithelial cells originate in the kidneys. Bladder epithelial cells are larger than renal cells but smaller than squamous epithelial cells. They originate in the bladder.

Squamous epithelial cells are large flat cells with a single small nucleus. They are often present in urine and originate in the urethra, vulva, or vagina. Their presence has little significance except when in sheets. If sheets of squamous cells are present, they should be reported as "sheets of squamous epithelial cells."

Fungi and Parasites

The type of fungus most commonly seen in the urine sediment is yeast. They are sometimes confused with red blood cells. However, a close examination of yeast will reveal them to be more ovoid than round. (See Figure 10-14.) They are

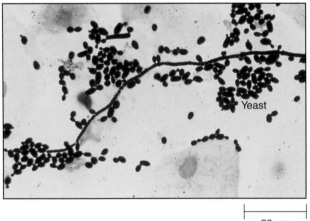

Figure 10-14 Example of *Candida albicans.*

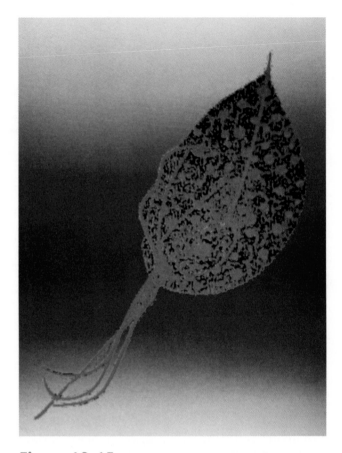

Figure 10-15 Example of *Trichomonas vaginalis.*

colorless and vary in size, and they may show budding. *Candida albicans* is the most common. It may be found in male or female urine samples with uncontrolled diabetes.

Trichomonas vaginalis is the parasite most frequently seen in urine. A unicellular organism with anterior flagellae, the parasites may resemble flattened, ovoid epithelial cells but are usually recognized by their swimming motion. This parasite must be moving in order to report its presence in the sample. Increasing the light source will stimulate the flagella to move. *Trichomonas vaginalis* may be found in female or male urine samples. (See Figure 10-15.)

CRYSTALS IN URINE SEDIMENT

Crystals commonly seen in normal urine sediment include phosphates, urates, and oxalates. Most are of limited clinical significance. However, a few crystals are clinically significant, so it is important to be able to recognize these crystals. (See Figure 10-16.) Urinary pH plays an important role in identifying crystals. See Table 10-2.

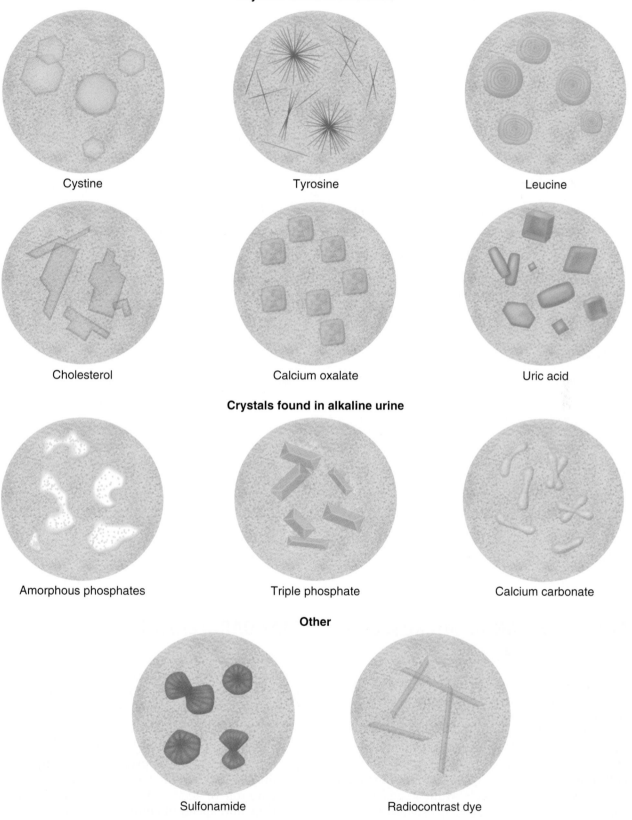

Figure 10-16 Examples of urinary crystals.

Table 10-2   Crystals Found in Urine

Normal Acid Urine (pH = 5–6)

- *Amorphous urates:* yellow-red granular precipitate that is soluble with heat and/or sodium hydroxide

- *Sodium acid urates:* brown spheres that revert to uric acid plates on acidification with acetic acid

- *Uric acid:* yellow or red-brown, irregularly shaped rhomboids that are soluble in sodium hydroxide when heated to 60 degrees Celsius

- *Calcium oxalate:* refractile, octahedral envelopes with very small to large crystals that are soluble in strong hydrochloric acid

Normal Alkaline Urine (pH = 7 or greater)

- *Amorphous phosphates:* fine, colorless, granular precipitate that is soluble in acetic acid

- *Triple phosphates:* colorless, three- to six-sided prisms, occasionally fern-leaf shaped, that are soluble in acids

- *Ammonium biurates:* yellow-brown, thorny spheres that are soluble in acetic acid

- *Calcium phosphate:* colorless, stellate, or rosette formation of individual crystals, shaped like slender prisms, which are readily soluble in acetic acid or ammonium carbonate solution

- *Calcium carbonate:* tiny colorless spheres or dumbbell shapes that are soluble in acetic acid and give off carbon dioxide gas

Abnormal Urine

- *Cystine:* colorless, refractile, hexagonal plates, found in congenital cystinosis, cystinuria, and cystine calculi

- *Tyrosine:* usually yellow, silky, fine needles arranged in sheaves or clumps, occasionally found (along with leucine crystals) in severe liver disease

- *Leucine:* yellow, oily-appearing spheres with radial, concentric markings, occasionally found, along with tyrosine crystals, in severe liver disease

- *Sulfonamides:* yellow-brown, asymmetrical, striated sheaves, or radially striated rounds, formed from sulfa drugs (not often seen with newer, more soluble sulfa drugs)

- *Renografin:* clear, colorless, flat rhombic plates, intersecting at 80 degrees, found briefly after urinary tract radiographs

- *Ampicillin:* long, fine, colorless crystals, formed at high dosages of the antibiotic ampicillin

CONFIRMATION OF MICROSCOPIC EXAMINATION

The results of microscopic examination of urinary sediment always should be verified against other results for the same sample. For example, if the microscopic examination reveals red blood cells, then the urinary strip test for blood in the urine should be positive, assuming that the red blood cells did not hemolyze. Furthermore, if the microscopic examination reveals white blood cells, then urinary strip tests for leukocyte esterase should be positive. Whenever there is disagreement among tests for the same sample, results should be held until retesting the same sample or a new sample produces confirmatory results.

STANDARDIZATION

Despite its great diagnostic value, microscopic examination of urine sediment is considered to be the most imprecise and inaccurate part of routine urinalysis. There are several reasons, including

- Variation in patient specimens.
- Variation in sample preparation. Samples may or may not be centrifuged, varying amounts of specimen may be centrifuged, time and speed of centrifuging may vary, and varying amounts of sample may be left in the centrifuge tube for resuspension after **decantation** (pouring off the top layer of liquid).

- Variation in the power of the microscopic field under which the sediment is examined.
- Lack of reference standards for urine sediments.

Standardization can help make microscopic examination of urine sediment more reliable for diagnosing and monitoring patients. Two methods of preparing urine sediments for examination have been developed to improve standardization—the KOVA® system and the volume quantitative method.

PROCEDURE 10-1

Microscopic Analysis of Urine

Goal

Determine and correctly identify and quantify the substances found in a urine specimen.

Completion Time

30 minutes

Equipment and Supplies

- Impermeable jacket, gown, or apron
- Face shield or goggles
- Disposable gloves
- Hand disinfectant
- Fresh urine specimen
- Biohazard container
- Surface disinfectant
- Paper towels and tissues
- Centrifuge
- Conical-shaped urine tubes
- Microscope
- Glass slides
- 22-mm plastic or glass coverslips
- Glass marking pen
- Tissues
- Disposable pipettes
- Urine specimen
- Urine tube cups
- Laboratory requisition form and pen

Instructions

Read through the list of equipment and supplies that you will need and the steps of the procedure. Be sure that you understand each step before you begin. Then complete each step correctly and in the proper order. If your completion time is too long, repeat the procedure until you increase your speed.

Steps marked with (*) are critical and must have the maximum points to pass.

Performance Standards	Points Awarded	Maximum Points
1. Put on lab coat and face shield or goggles.		5
2. Disinfect hands; dry if necessary.		5
3. Put on gloves. Inspect for tears and replace if necessary.		5
4. Collect and prepare the appropriate equipment.		5
5. *Verify specimen identity.		30
6. If the specimen has been refrigerated, allow the urine to come to room temperature.		5
7. Mix the urine specimen by gently swirling the specimen.		5
8. Pour the urine into a properly labeled conical-shaped urine tube and cap the specimen.		15
9. Centrifuge at 2,000 rpm for 5 minutes to concentrate the urine sediment.		15

—table continued

Performance Standards	Points Awarded	Maximum Points
10. Decant the urine into a properly designated sink, reserving 1.0 mL for mixing with the sediment.		15
11. Resuspend the sediment in the remaining urine by gently mixing the tube.		10
12. Place one drop of sediment onto a glass slide.		10
13. Cover the urine drop with a cover slip.		10
14. Using reduced lighting and low-power magnification (10X objective), scan the entire area of the cover slip. Note the presence of all formed elements: casts, epithelial cells, red blood cells, white blood cells, crystals, mucus, sperm, contaminants, and parasites.		10
15. View 10–15 low-power fields. Average the number of casts observed and record this number. Identify the cellular structure of the cast by going back and forth from low-power to high-power.		20
16. Rotate the microscope lens to the high-power (45X) objective.		10
17. Increase the microscope lighting.		10
18. Observe 10–15 representative fields.		10
19. Identify and enumerate the following significant formed elements: white blood cells, red blood cells, crystals.		10
20. Note the presence and quantify as appropriate: mucus, yeast, bacteria, parasites, epithelial cells, and sperm.		10
21. Dispose of the urine per lab policy.		10
22. Discard disposable equipment.		10
23. Clean and return all equipment to storage.		5
24. Wash hands.		5
Total Points		245

Overall Procedural Evaluation

Student Name _____

Signature of Instructor _____ Date _____

Comments _____

_____

chapter 10 REVIEW

Using Terminology

Match the term on the left with the most appropriate description on the right.

_____ **1.** supernatant

_____ **2.** desquamation

_____ **3.** calculus

_____ **4.** crenated

_____ **5.** cylindruria

a. shedding cells

b. shrunken red blood cell

c. urinary stone

d. large number of casts in the urine

e. fluid floating on top of the specimen after centrifugation

State whether the following crystals are found in acidic or alkaline urine.

6. Ammonium biurates _____

7. Amorphous phosphates _____

8. Sodium acid urates _____

9. Triple phosphates _____

10. Uric acid _____

11. Calcium phosphates _____

12. Calcium oxalate _____

13. Amorphous urates _____

In the space provided, identify the clinical significance of each urine sediment finding.

14. Hyaline cast

_____

_____

_____

15. White blood cells

_____

_____

_____

16. Red blood cells

_____

_____

_____

17. Waxy cast

_____

_____

_____

18. Epithelial cells

_____

_____

_____

Multiple Choice

Choose the best answer for the following questions.

19. When performing a microscopic examination of urine, you should begin with
    a. low-power objective (10X) and high lighting
    b. low-power objective (10X) and low lighting
    c. high-power objective (45X) and high lighting
    d. high-power objective (45X) and low lighting

20. When examining urine sediment for casts, you should use
   a. low-power objective (10X) and high lighting
   b. low-power objective (10X) and low lighting
   c. high-power objective (45X) and high lighting
   d. high-power objective (45X) and low lighting

21. When examining urine sediment for red blood cells, you should use
   a. low-power objective (10X) and high lighting
   b. low-power objective (10X) and low lighting
   c. high-power objective (45X) and high lighting
   d. high-power objective (45X) and low lighting

22. If the microscopic examination of urine sediment shows many white blood cells, what should the chemical analysis show?
   a. positive bilirubin
   b. positive leukocyte esterase
   c. positive protein
   d. positive nitrates

23. How many hyaline casts are likely to be found in a normal urine specimen?
   a. 0–1 per low-power field
   b. 2–5 per low-power field
   c. 8–10 per low-power field
   d. greater than 10 per low-power field

24. What happens to red blood cells in hypotonic (dilute) urine?
   a. they crenate
   b. they lyse
   c. they change color
   d. there is no change

25. What is the clinical significance of pyuria?
   a. bleeding
   b. infection
   c. increased protein breakdown
   d. poor renal function

26. What is the most commonly found white blood cell in urine?
   a. basophil
   b. lymphocyte
   c. eosinophil
   d. neutrophil

27. When performing urine microscopy, about how many fields should be scanned when quantifying urine sediment for the presence of mucus?
   a. 2–5 fields
   b. 5–8 fields
   c. 10–15 fields
   d. at least 20 fields

28. The presence of waxy casts in the urine indicates which of the following?
   a. bleeding
   b. infection
   c. increased protein breakdown
   d. renal disease

29. The presence of 10 red blood cells per high-power field indicates which of the following?
a. bleeding
b. infection
c. increased protein breakdown
d. renal disease

30. The purpose of centrifuging and decanting urine specimens before microscopic analysis is to
a. dilute the urine
b. concentrate the urine
c. this step is optional
d. remove any contaminants

Acquiring Knowledge

Answer the following questions in the spaces provided.

31. Why is microscopic examination of urine sediment considered to be the most difficult part of urinalysis to perform accurately and consistently?

_____

_____

_____

32. Why is microscopic analysis of urine sediment so useful diagnostically?

_____

_____

_____

33. Why is urine sediment analysis sometimes referred to as "liquid biopsy"?

_____

_____

_____

34. How is urine decanted after centrifuging?

_____

_____

_____

35. How are the numbers of red blood cells, white blood cells, and epithelial cells reported?

_____

_____

_____

36. What may cause an abnormal increase in the number of casts?

_____

_____

_____

37. When are epithelial cells clinically significant in urine sediment?

_____

_____

_____

38. List two medications that may produce crystals in the urine?

_____

_____

_____

39. How are red blood cells distinguished from white blood cells in microscopic analysis of urine sediment?

_____

_____

_____

40. How are casts formed?

_____

_____

_____

Applying Knowledge—On the Job

Answer the following questions in the spaces provided.

41. If several normal urines were examined microscopically in a day's work in the POL, what might they contain?

_____

_____

_____

42 What is wrong with the following scenario? A microscopic analysis of urine sediment revealed many white blood cells and bacteria. Chemical analysis of the same sample was negative for leukocyte esterase and nitrite.

_____

_____

_____

43. A laboratory personnel reported large numbers of red blood cells in the microscopic urine sediment with a negative occult blood from the urinalysis strip test. Do you think this is a correct report? How would you check the accuracy of the report?

_____

_____

_____

BLOOD COLLECTION

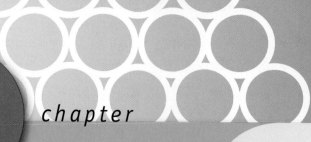
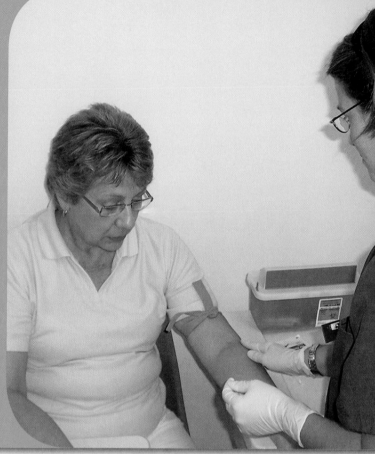

Routine Venipuncture

COGNITIVE OBJECTIVES

After studying the chapter, you should be able to:

11.1 use and spell each of the vocabulary terms appropriately.

11.2 describe the composition of blood and list its function.

11.3 state the three types of blood specimens and describe the method of collection for each.

11.4 describe the equipment needed for phlebotomy.

11.5 describe the primary and secondary venipuncture sites.

11.6 describe phlebotomy safety, including the supporting legislation.

11.7 list the basic uses for sterile, red, light blue, lavender, green, marble, and gray top tubes.

11.8 state the order of draw for routine venipuncture utilizing the evacuated tube system.

11.9 state the required blood to anticoagulant ratio for light blue top tubes.

11.10 list the acceptable criteria for verifying a patient's identity.

11.11 list the requirements for proper labeling of patient specimens.

11.12 compare whole blood, plasma, and serum.

11.13 explain how to centrifuge and store blood samples.

11.14 describe several different specimen collection requirements.

After studying the chapter, you should be able to:

11.15 perform venipuncture utilizing the evacuated tube system method.

██ TERMINOLOGY

aerobic: microorganisms that prefer or require an oxygen-rich environment for growth.

anaerobic: microorganisms that prefer or require a carbon-dioxide-rich environment for growth.

antecubital: in the inner arm at the bend of the elbow; the most common site for venipuncture.

anticoagulant: an agent that prevents the clotting of blood, such as oxalate, citrate, EDTA, or heparin.

bevel: sheared opening at the anterior end of the needle. Needles should enter the vein with the bevel side of the needle "up" or visible to the lab personnel.

coagulation studies: tests performed to see how fast and how well a patient is capable of forming a clot.

evacuated tube system: a vacuum tube system for drawing blood by venipuncture. It allows multiple samples to be drawn with a single puncture.

gauge: the diameter of the needle. The smaller the gauge, the larger the diameter.

hemoconcentration: the increased concentration of red blood cells due to decreased plasma volume.

hemoglobin (Hgb): the oxygen-carrying protein of red blood cells.

hemolysis: the breakdown of red blood cells, with the release of hemoglobin into the plasma or serum. In general, hemolyzed specimens are not acceptable for testing.

icteric: jaundiced; characterized by a high level of bilirubin. Icteric serum and plasma appear dark yellow or greenish.

lipemic: having an abnormally high level of fat. Specimens are cloudy or milky in appearance.

median cephalic vein: one of the major veins of the inner arm. It is used frequently in venipuncture.

median cubital vein: a short vein of the inner arm just below the elbow. It is used frequently in venipuncture.

needle holder: also known as hub or adapter; the plastic holder into which the posterior end of the needle is secured.

needlestick: the act of puncturing yourself with a used needle.

palpating: touching or feeling.

phlebotomy: blood collection by venipuncture.

plasma: the pale yellowish liquid part of whole blood.

platelet: a small round or oval disk-shaped fragment in human blood that assists in blood clotting.

quantity not sufficient (QNS): when the amount of specimen is not adequate and therefore testing cannot be performed.

serum: the yellow liquid portion of blood after the blood has been allowed to clot; it does not contain fibrinogen; the fibrinogen is in the clot.

tourniquet: a constrictor band used to distend veins to facilitate venipuncture.

venipuncture: the puncture of a vein for therapeutic purposes or for drawing blood.

INTRODUCTION

Every day, physicians and other advanced health care providers make decisions about how to treat a patient based on the patient's lab results. As a result, it is critical that a patient's lab results be as accurate as possible.

Blood specimens are one of the most commonly collected and tested specimens. Blood specimen types include venous, arterial, and capillary specimens. Arterial specimens are used for a limited number of tests, primarily arterial blood gases, which are used to assess a patient who is having respiratory difficulties. These specimens require special training to collect and a physician or a respiratory therapist generally does the procedure. Capillary specimens involve the use of a lancet to puncture the skin in order to collect a specimen. Venous specimens are the most commonly collected and tested. They are used for a variety of tests and require the use of a needle to remove blood from the patient's vein. This chapter reviews the information and techniques needed to collect a venous blood specimen utilizing routine venipuncture techniques.

BLOOD COMPOSITION AND FUNCTIONS

Proper technique in blood collection and handling requires knowledge of the composition and function of blood. While this will be covered in detail in subsequent chapters, the following provides a brief overview.

Blood is a body tissue made up of plasma and blood cells. **Plasma** is a pale yellowish liquid part of the whole blood. Plasma is composed of water and a variety of dissolved chemicals and proteins, including carbohydrates, lipids, electrolytes, enzymes, vitamins, trace metals, and hormones. Plasma also contains coagulation factors, which help form blood clots and stop bleeding. Plasma plays a major role in transporting nutrients to the various cells of the body, as well as assisting with the removal of waste.

The other major component of blood is the three different types of blood cells. Leukocytes, also known as white blood cells, are a major component of the immune system and help fight infection. Erythrocytes, also known as red blood cells, carry oxygen to the cells of the body and carbon dioxide back to the lungs, where it is removed from the body. Finally, thrombocytes, also known as **platelets,** play an active role in clot formation.

BLOOD COLLECTION METHODS

Blood samples can be collected by two different methods: capillary puncture or **venipuncture.** The method selected depends on the type of test that will be performed as well as the age and condition of the patient. Capillary puncture is the method of choice if only a small quantity of blood is needed. It is also the method most suitable for infants, and it may be preferable for elderly patients. Venipuncture has the advantage of drawing a larger quantity of blood, which may be required for some procedures or if a test must be repeated. Unlike capillary samples, venipuncture samples can be stored for later processing and testing. Although capillary and venous blood are not identical—capillary blood is more like arterial blood—they are close enough to be used interchangeably in most cases.

Both blood collection methods should be described in detail in the SOP manual of your POL. In addition, blood collection procedures may be outlined on a wall chart posted by the blood drawing station.

VENIPUNCTURE

The procedure of collecting blood by the venipuncture method, also called **phlebotomy,** takes blood directly from a vein, most commonly in the **antecubital** area of the arm, that is, the inner arm at the bend of the elbow. The veins used most often are the **median cephalic vein** and the **median cubital vein.** The basilic vein also may be used. Other sites sometimes used are the lower forearm, the back of the hand, and the wrist.

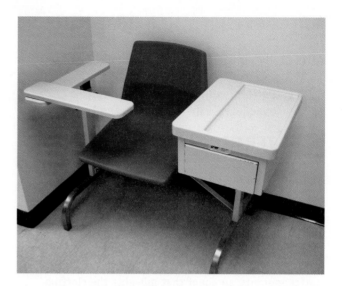

Figure 11-1 Phlebotomy chair.

Venipuncture Equipment

Phlebotomy Chair. For all blood collection procedures, the patient should either be lying down or seated in a phlebotomy chair. In the outpatient setting, venipuncture is generally performed in a phlebotomy chair. This is a special chair that supports a patient during the venipuncture procedure. The chair has an arm that locks into place once the patient is seated. This locking mechanism prevents the patient from falling out of the chair if the patient faints during the venipuncture procedure. In addition, the arm can be raised or lowered, allowing the phlebotomist to adjust the height of the arm to meet the comfort needs of the patient. It is critical to make the patient safe and comfortable during the procedure. A phlebotomy chair makes it easier to perform the phlebotomy and more comfortable for the patient. (See Figure 11-1.)

Personal Protective Equipment. Before beginning any procedure that includes the presence of blood, you should obtain the necessary personal protective equipment (PPE). PPE used during the venipuncture procedure includes gloves, lab coat, and face shield or goggles. A new pair of gloves must be used for each patient. Gloves can be made of latex, vinyl, or polyethylene. Latex gloves are commonly available and many individuals feel that latex provides "more feeling"—that is, it is easier to feel veins when compared to other types of gloves. However, in recent years, many individuals have developed a latex allergy. This condition can cause a life-threatening allergic reaction in some patients and practitioners. If you or your patients have a latex allergy, it is critical that latex gloves not be worn. Both vinyl and polyethylene avoid the latex allergy issue; however, they tend to rip more easily and it can be more difficult to feel for veins. Regardless of which type of glove is used, it is important that you check the gloves for tears prior to beginning the blood collection procedure. Tears are especially common in the fingertips, where fingernails can promote tears. If a tear is noted, the gloves should be discarded and a new pair obtained prior to beginning blood collection.

In addition to deciding which type of glove to use, gloves come with or without powder inside. Gloves that contain a powder inside are generally easier to put on, especially after cleaning your hands when a water residue can make glove application difficult. In addition, the powder can help keep your hands drier when wearing the gloves for long periods of time. However, many people are allergic to the powder or can develop skin irritations from the powder. In addition, for individuals with a latex allergy, the powder can carry the latex particles as an aerosol. This can be extremely dangerous for patients with a latex allergy. There have been instances where individuals with a latex allergy walk into a room where latex gloves with powder have been used and this can be enough to trigger an allergic reaction.

Phlebotomy Tray. In addition to the phlebotomy chair and personal protective equipment, a well-stocked phlebotomy tray is necessary to perform venipuncture. Included on the tray should be antiseptics, gauze pads, tape or bandages, tourniquets, needle holders, a variety of needles, and the different types of blood collection tubes. See Table 11-1.

Phlebotomy Supply Checklist

It is important that you remember to check the supplies in your phlebotomy tray every day to ensure that you have the items you need for each procedure. The following checklist should be used as a template. Modify as needed to meet the needs of your own POL, including maintaining minimums.

Antiseptics

In general, two different types of antiseptics are commonly used in the outpatient setting. The first is 70 percent isopropyl alcohol, the most commonly used antiseptic. Alcohol prevents the introduction of microorganisms into the body during the venipuncture. It is critical when using alcohol antiseptics to allow the alcohol to completely air dry. Failure to do so will result in increased pain

Table 11-1   Daily Checklist for Phlebotomy Tray

Item	Initials
All items are within expiration date. Rotate the stock so that expiring items are used first.	
Tubes are normal in appearance—no discolored anticoagulants, tubes are not cracked, rubber stopper appears intact.	
Hand sanitizer	
Alcohol preps	
Betadine preps	
Needles of various gauges	
Butterfly needles*	
Syringes (10 or 20 mL)*	
Straight needles*	
Needle holders	
Tourniquets	
Red top tubes	
Marble/tiger/speckled top tubes	
Lavender top tubes	
Light blue top tubes	
Green top tubes	
Gray top tubes	
Blood culture tubes (anaerobic and aerobic set)	
Latex or paper tape	
Gauze	
Bandage	
Biohazard container	
Transfer device*	
Lancet*	
Microcontainers*	

*These items are related to advanced phlebotomy procedures and will be discussed in detail in Chapter 12.

for the patient and possible hemolysis in the specimen. Betadine is the other antiseptic commonly used. It is most commonly used for blood alcohol levels, blood cultures, and blood donations. The advantage of betadine is that it does a better job of breaking down and removing skin contaminants. A disadvantage of betadine is that it is a dark,

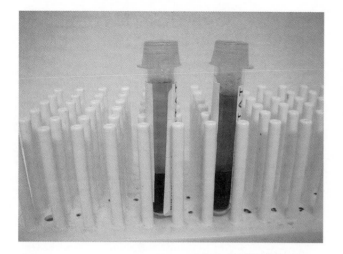

Figure 11-2 The specimen on the left is normal in appearance. The specimen on the right is hemolyzed.

viscous substance that will leave a film on the patient's skin. Besides being messy, it can make it difficult to visualize the patient's skin and veins. However, it is critical that the betadine be left in place and not be wiped away.

Hemolysis

Hemolysis releases red-pigmented **hemoglobin (Hgb)**, the oxygen-carrying molecule of red blood cells. The released hemoglobin can interfere with the optical reading of some chemistry tests. Because hemolysis changes the composition of the plasma or **serum**, it also prevents accurate results for many other tests, including the complete blood count, hemoglobin determination, hemotocrit, and tests for potassium, magnesium, lactic dehydrogenase, and aspartate aminotransferase. For this reason, hemolyzed blood samples generally are discarded. As a result, you should avoid anything that may cause hemolysis of the sample. (See Figure 11-2.)

Tourniquets

Tourniquets are used to help pool the blood in the veins, causing the veins to enlarge. This temporary enlargement allows for easier detection of the veins, facilitating the venipuncture procedure. In addition, the pooling of the veins makes it easier for the vein to tolerate the vacuum suction of the tubes withdrawing blood. Unlike a blood pressure cuff, tourniquets should not be applied so tightly that arterial blood is cut off.

Tourniquets come in two formats. The first is the elastic tourniquet. It is made of either latex or nonlatex, stretchable material that is about 15 inches in

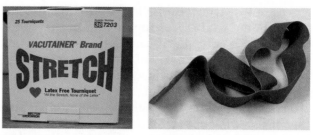

(a) Nonlatex tourniquet box   (b) Single tourniquet

Figure 11-3 An example of an elastic tourniquet.

length and 1 inch in width. These tourniquets are inexpensive and easy to use. Avoid the latex tourniquets if you or your patient is allergic to latex. Never use rubber tubing as a makeshift tourniquet and avoid the narrow strip tourniquets as they tend to be painful. In addition to the elastic tourniquets, there are plastic strip Velcro-type tourniquets that are similar to a blood pressure cuff. The Velcro-type tourniquets come in both adult and child sizes. These are more expensive and can be more difficult to use. In addition, they can be more difficult to disinfect. Both types of tourniquets should be disinfected with 70 percent alcohol after each use or discarded.

Venipuncture Tourniquets. Never leave a tourniquet on longer than 1 minute before drawing blood. This can result in **hemoconcentration,** the increased concentration of red blood cells. Stopping venous blood flow for more than 3 minutes will increase the cholesterol value by 5 percent compared to a 1 minute stoppage. If it is necessary to wait longer than 1 minute after putting on the tourniquet, remove the tourniquet and reapply it when ready. (See Figure 11-3.)

Quality Assurance Note

Release the tourniquet before removing the needle from the vein. Many laboratory personnel prefer to release the tourniquet as soon as the blood begins to flow into the syringe or vacutainer.

Needles and Barrels

Venipuncture needles come in a variety of lengths and gauges. (See Figure 11-4.) When referring to a needle, a **gauge** describes how wide the diameter of the needle is. Gauge size for venipuncture needles ranges from 16 (the largest) to 25 (the smallest). The average venipuncture needle is 21 or 22 gauge in size. Needle length varies from 1 inch to 1.5 inches. When selecting which needle is best for your patient, you should consider the following: (1) smaller gauge needles with bigger diameters may

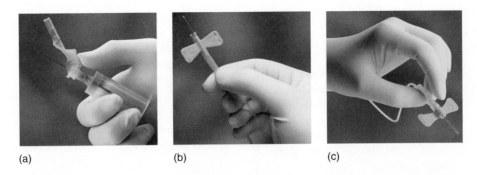

(a)   (b)   (c)

Figure 11-4 Various needles with safety mechanisms: (a) hinged cap; (b) protective shield; (c) retractable needle.

hurt more but are less likely to cause a hemolyzed specimen, thus requiring the specimen to be recollected; (2) larger gauge needles are less painful but tend to take longer to collect a specimen and are more likely to cause hemolysis in the specimen. Needles should be sterile—never use a needle in which someone other than you has broken the seal at the time of collection. Needles can only be used once and must be discarded in a biohazardous sharps container after they have been used. Never bend, break, or recap needles. In addition, the Needlestick Safety and Prevention Act signed by former President Clinton in 2000 requires that all needles have a safety mechanism to help avoid accidental **needlesticks.** Each manufacturer uses its own safety mechanism, so be sure to familiarize yourself with the mechanism *prior* to the use of the needle.

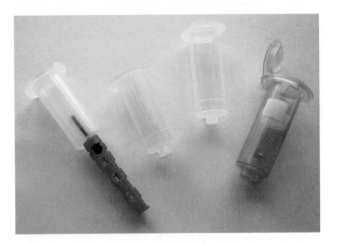

Figure 11-5 Examples of needle holders.

Needlestick Safety and Prevention Act

In November 2000, Congress passed the Needlestick Safety and Prevention Act, which was then signed into law by former President Clinton. In response to this legislation, OSHA revised the Bloodborne Pathogen Standard that all health facilities must observe. Together, these legislative changes require the following:

1. All needles must have a safety mechanism to prevent accidental sticks.
2. Employees must participate in the process of choosing the type of safety needle that they will use.
3. Employers must maintain a log of accidental needlesticks involving contaminated sharps.

It is important to note that depending on the manufacturer, each brand of safety needle has its own safety mechanism. It is advised that you practice with the safety mechanism with a clean needle before trying it on a contaminated needle.

For more information about the Needlestick Safety and Prevention Act, see http://www.osha.gov/SLTC/bloodbornepathogens/.

Bevel

Bevel is the sheared opening at the anterior portion of a needle. This part of the needle should be visible prior to puncturing the skin. This condition is known as "bevel up."

During routine venipuncture, needles are attached to a **needle holder** for additional support. The posterior portion of the needle screws into the holder. Needle holders are single use and must be disposed of with the needle when the venipuncture procedure is complete. (See Figure 11-5.)

Bandages

Gauze pads are used to cover the puncture site after the venipuncture is complete. Cotton balls should not be used as they have a tendency to stick to the venipuncture site and reintroduce bleeding when removed. Neither should it be used to dry the alcohol during the preparation of the site unless it is packaged as sterile. The most acceptable practice is to allow the alcohol to air dry.

What to Do in the Event of an Accidental Needlestick Injury

Despite the best practices, needlesticks can happen.

If you are accidentally stuck by a contaminated needle, you should follow the guidelines as outlined by your post–needlestick injury report policy. It is very important that all steps are completed to ensure minimal exposure with contaminants. Do not hide the injury in fear of punishment.

1. Wash the injured site immediately with an antimicrobial soap and warm water, which will increase circulation as you squeeze and massage blood out from the injured site. Be sure to have a glove on the hand that is performing the massaging and squeezing.
2. Notify your supervisor immediately and follow organization policy so that the incident can be documented.
3. Seek medical attention.

Place surgical tape over the gauze or other bandage once the patient has stopped bleeding. In general, latex tape does a better job of holding the gauze in place; however, it can be traumatic to the skin of geriatric patients. In addition, latex tape cannot be used on individuals with latex allergies. With both of these patient populations, paper tape is a better choice. Never use a bandage or tape on a child less than 2 years old as it can be a choking hazard.

Blood Collection Tubes

A variety of different tubes are required when performing venipuncture. Tubes vary in size, volume, and additives. Tubes are generally made of plastic or glass. The color of the rubber stopper located at the top of the tube indicates what additive is found in the tube. (See Figure 11-6.) Many tubes contain an **anticoagulant,** a chemical that interferes with the clotting process and prevents a clot from being formed in the tube. These tubes have a "vacuum"— a specified amount of air has been taken out by the

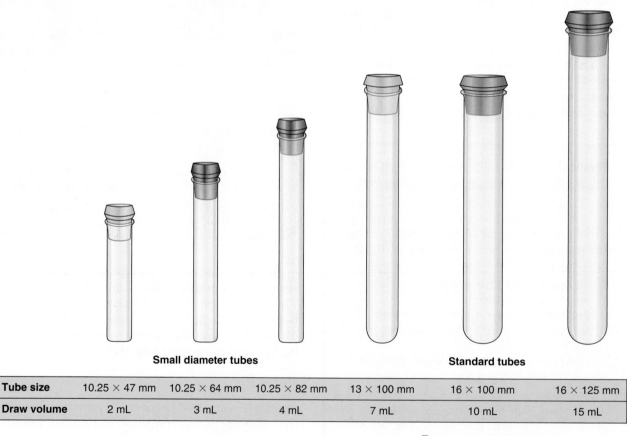

	Small diameter tubes			Standard tubes		
Tube size	10.25 × 47 mm	10.25 × 64 mm	10.25 × 82 mm	13 × 100 mm	16 × 100 mm	16 × 125 mm
Draw volume	2 mL	3 mL	4 mL	7 mL	10 mL	15 mL

Pediatric holder   Adult holder

Figure 11-6 Examples of different types of blood collection tubes and needle holders.

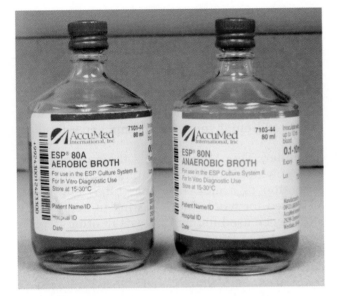

Figure 11-7 Aerobic and anaerobic blood culture bottles.

Blood Culture

Obtaining a good specimen for blood cultures is critical to the proper identification of the infecting microorganism.

1. Clean the first site with betadine for 1 minute. Betadine is used instead of alcohol because it has a stronger bacteria-killing action. Be aware that some patients are allergic to betadine, so another cleansing agent must be used.
2. Collect an anaerobic and an aerobic specimen, at the same time at the same site. Collect any other specimens required, observing the order of draw.
3. Label the specimens. Note the time of collection.
4. Thirty minutes later, return and repeat steps 1–3.

At the end of the process, you should have a total of four specimens—two aerobic and two anaerobic.

---

manufacturer so that when the tube is pierced by the needle, the tube will fill with a predetermined amount of blood. This ensures that only the proper amount of blood enters the tube. Allow the tubes to fill until the vacuum is exhausted and the blood flow ceases. This will ensure the correct ratio of blood to additive.

Sterile Blood Culture. A blood culture is a special collection technique used to determine if the patient has an infection of the blood, a condition that is very dangerous. This specimen is drawn as a pair of bottles, one for **anaerobic** specimens and one for **aerobic** specimens. Yellow top tubes containing SPS, sodium polyanethol sulfonate, also can be used. (See Figure 11-7.) Anaerobic microorganisms are those organisms that die in the presence of oxygen and prefer or require carbon dioxide. In contrast, aerobic microorganisms are those that require or prefer oxygen. Both types of organisms are capable of causing an infection of the blood. The first set of tubes is collected from one site; then, approximately a half an hour later, the second set is collected from a different site. The purpose of collecting from different sites at different times is twofold. The different sites help ensure that a positive specimen is due to an actual infection, rather than contamination. The difference in time is because some microorganisms are very temperature dependent. Ideally, the specimens should be collected during a febrile period, then a nonfebrile period. Separating the specimens allows for changes in body temperature that may be favorable to identifying the infecting microorganism.

Light Blue. This tube contains the anticoagulant sodium citrate 0.105M or 0.129M. Sodium citrate binds calcium, a factor required for clotting. It is extremely important that a 9:1 ratio of blood to anticoagulant be maintained. Failure to do so can alter the test results or the lab may reject the specimen as **quantity not sufficient (QNS).** This is the required specimen for PT, PTT, and other coagulation tests.

Former recommendations were that a red top tube must always be collected before a light blue top tube when performing **coagulation studies.** Coagulation studies are tests performed to see how fast and how well a patient is capable of forming a clot. It was believed that there was a release of coagulation factors at the site of the venipuncture that would alter the coagulation test results. Several studies have since proved this to be untrue and collecting a red top tube prior to collecting a light blue top tube is no longer recommended. However, when utilizing a winged infusion or butterfly set, a discard tube is recommended to "prime" the set and remove any excess air that might interfere with maintaining proper blood to anticoagulant ratios. Butterfly needles will be covered in detail in Chapter 12.

Plain Red. No additive or anticoagulant is used. This tube is generally used for a variety of serum chemistries and serology tests. It may be required for blood bank testing in some institutions.

Marble/Speckled/Tiger Top/SST Tube. This tube contains both a clot activator, thrombin, and a gel separator. The clot activator significantly reduces the amount of time required before a clot has formed in the specimen. This can be very beneficial in situations where a serum specimen is required in a short period of time. The gel separator is a waxy substance that physically separates the red blood cells from the serum after centrifugation. This can be very helpful in situations where the serum will not be tested for a long period of time. Red blood cells remain metabolically active in the tubes for several hours after collection. When in the tube, the red cells release additional carbon dioxide, leak potassium, and utilize glucose, thus affecting these results. By physically separating the red blood cells from the serum, you can ensure the accuracy of these test results. The disadvantage of this specimen is it cannot be used for any red blood cell testing.

Green. This tube contains one of three different anticoagulants: sodium heparin, lithium heparin, or ammonium heparin. The heparin component of the anticoagulant inhibits thrombin formation, thus preventing the formation of a clot. This plasma specimen is generally used for chemistry tests and is particularly helpful in those chemistry tests where fibrin interference is a factor. It is important to note that you cannot test for the substance found in the anticoagulant, as it would falsely elevate the result. For example, you cannot test for sodium if you use a sodium heparin tube.

Lavender. This tube contains the anticoagulant EDTA, which binds to calcium, preventing the formation of a clot. Lavender tubes are generally used for whole blood testing in hematology but may be used for certain tests in other departments also.

Gray. This tube contains two additives: sodium fluoride and potassium oxalate. Potassium oxalate binds with calcium to prevent clotting. Sodium fluoride prevents red blood cells from metabolizing glucose as a food source after collection. This specimen can be used for glucose testing, such as the glucose tolerance test.

See Table 11-2 for a summary of phlebotomy specimen tubes.

Table 11-2   Common Phlebotomy Specimen Tubes

Color	Additive(s)	Serum/Plasma/ Whole Blood	Test Examples	Special Consideration
Sterile	Broth to support growth of microorganisms	Whole blood	Microbiology	Need both anaerobic and aerobic in each set; generally drawn in sets of two
Light blue	Sodium citrate	Plasma	Coagulation studies, including PT/INR, PTT, and fibrinogen	9:1 anticoagulant ratio; no longer recommended to collect red top tube first
Red	None	Serum	Blood bank and serology	Prolonged contact between serum and red blood cells may alter some test results
Marble	Gel thrombin	Serum	Chemistry	Cannot be used for RBC testing. More accurate than a red top for glucose and potassium when there is a delay in testing
Green	Sodium heparin, lithium heparin, OR ammonium heparin	Plasma or whole blood	Chemistry tests	You cannot test for the analyte if the tube contains the additive of that being tested
Lavender	EDTA	Whole blood	Hematology tests, including CBC, ESR, reticulocyte count, etc. Other departments may use as well	
Gray	Sodium fluoride Potassium oxalate	Plasma or whole blood	Glucose	Used for glucose testing and stable for 5 hours

Order of Draw. The current standard for order of draw, or the order in which to collect blood, using an **evacuated tube system** is

1. Sterile/blood culture
2. Light blue
3. Red and/or marble
4. Green
5. Lavender
6. Gray

It is important to observe this order to ensure that the test results are accurate.

Routine Venipuncture Procedure

When performing venipuncture, the following steps must be completed:

1. Review paperwork.
2. Put on lab coat.
3. Identify yourself to the patient.
4. Verify patient identity.
5. Explain what you are going to do.
6. Confirm that the patient followed any pre-testing instructions, if required. For example: did the patient fast? Did the patient discontinue his or her medication as requested by the physician?
7. Wash your hands and don gloves.
8. Put on face shield or goggles.
9. Assemble equipment.
10. Reassure and position the patient.
11. Apply tourniquet.
12. Select and cleanse site.
13. Select needle based on vein size.
14. Uncap and inspect needle.
15. Perform the venipuncture:
     a. Insert the needle at 15- to 30-degree angle.
     b. Follow correct order of draw.
     c. Gently invert tubes as they are withdrawn from the needle to mix the specimen.
16. Release the tourniquet.
17. Remove the last tube.
18. Remove the needle and engage safety mechanism.
19. Cover puncture site with gauze and apply pressure.
20. Check the site for bleeding. When bleeding has stopped, apply a bandage.
21. Discard the entire blood collection set—needle and needle holder—into a biohazardous sharps container.
22. Label tubes before leaving the patient's side.
23. Thank and release the patient.

Review the Paperwork/Lab Requisition

It is always a good idea to review what tests the doctor ordered before calling in the patient to the phlebotomy station. This gives you the opportunity to determine what collection equipment is needed, which tubes need to be used, if any special specimen handling is required, or if any special patient preparation is required.

Identify Yourself

Always identify yourself to the patient. That includes stating your name and position or title. This is standard practice for any medical procedure. It is even more important for an invasive procedure like phlebotomy. This simple step establishes professionalism, a level of trust between you and the patient, and promotes the image of quality care. Most patients find it distasteful when health professionals perform procedures on them without ever identifying themselves to the patient. In addition, it is a great opportunity to educate patients about your profession.

Identify the Patient

Patient identification is the MOST critical step in any procedure or interaction with a patient. Properly identifying your patient before every interaction ensures that the right patient is getting the right treatment or procedure. Most medical errors, including laboratory errors, arise from failure to properly identify the patient.

When dealing with patients in the outpatient setting, the procedure for verifying a patient's identity is as follows:

*   Ask the patient for his or her first and last name.
*   Ask the patient to spell his or her first and last name.
*   Ask the patient for his or her date of birth, social security number, or other unique identifying number.
*   Some offices and laboratories require a patient's driver's license as a form of identification.

The above-listed information should be compared to the information printed on the laboratory requisition. If any information does not completely match, do not proceed with the procedure. This includes if even a single digit or letter is off. *All discrepancies, no matter how minor they may seem, must be resolved first.*

It is vitally important that you follow this procedure in this manner. It is not enough to simply ask a patient, "Are you Mr. Peter Smith?" Even if the patient answers, "yes," that does not confirm a patient's identity. Patients who are not mentally competent or patients with hearing difficulties may answer to a name other than their own.

Sometimes patients will be given an identification bracelet for the purpose of identification. The procedure for identifying a patient with a bracelet is similar to the verbal verification process. In this case, compare the lab requisition against the patient's wristband identification bracelet to ensure that the following information matches **EXACTLY**: (1) first and last name and (2) medical record number or birth date. Again, this information must match **EXACTLY**. *Any discrepancies must be resolved before beginning the phlebotomy procedure.*

Furthermore, it is critically important that you identify your patients **each and every** time that you interact with them. Health professionals sometimes become too relaxed when they are dealing with the same patients and believe it is no longer necessary to perform patient identification. Any lab professional can make an error in identifying a patient unless the steps of patient identification are all completed every time blood is collected. Patient identification must occur every time.

Legal and Ethical Considerations for Proper Patient Identification

The stringency of the patient identification process may initially seem overly inflexible and unnecessary. However, the process is the only way lab personnel can ensure that the patient they are working with is the right patient. Consequences for misidentifying a patient are severe, for both the patient and the lab personnel.

If the specimen is from the wrong patient, it is at best completely worthless and at worst potentially life threatening. For example, a diabetic patient may not get the insulin she needs if her specimen is incorrectly collected from a patient with normal blood sugar. In addition, when dealing with specimens that are used to prepare a patient for blood transfusion, an error could result in patient death. Consequences for the lab personnel can be equally damaging. Disciplinary action taken by the employer may include

- Being "written up," suspended, or terminated.
- Losing your license or certification.
- Having a malpractice suit brought by a patient who suffered a poor outcome due to your error.

Inpatient Identification Process

This text focuses on laboratory testing in the POL. However, there may be occasions where you need to collect blood from a patient in an in-patient setting such as a nursing home. In these circumstances, patient identification is achieved by comparing the patient information on the patient's identification bracelet against the information on the patient's laboratory requisition. You should compare the following information:

- Spelling of the patient's first and last name.
- Patient's medical record number or date of birth.

This information should match—perfectly. If even a single letter or number does not match, then you must resolve the discrepancy before collecting the patient's specimen.

What's Not Acceptable for Patient Identification?

Whether you ask the patient questions and compare the answers against a lab requisition or you use a bracelet to identify the patient, you should compare the first and last name and a unique identifier such as a medical record number or date of birth.

- If the name is spelled wrong by even one letter, it does NOT match.
- If the medical record number is off by one number, it does NOT match.
- If a bracelet is used, it must be on the patient. It cannot be attached to a bed or other device. Patients can be moved and the bracelet may remain on the bed.
- Name tags cannot be used either, for the same reason—they are not stationary.

Explain What You Are Going to Do

It is also important to explain what you are going to do to the patient, a simple phrase like, "I'm Chris and I am the medical assistant for Dr. Jones today. Dr. Jones has requested that I collect some blood samples from you. You're going to feel a little sting or pinch during the procedure. Do you have any questions before I begin?" This can also be done at the same time as your introduction. Remember, the procedure will go much more easily and quickly if the patient is relaxed and comfortable.

Confirm Patient Preparation

While most tests do not require any special patient preparation, some do. It is important to determine whether or not the patient has complied with any special instructions **prior** to beginning the procedure. This may include fasting, taking certain medications, or abstaining from a medication. If you are unsure if a particular test requires special patient preparation, refer to the laboratory directory.

Wash Your Hands and Apply Gloves

It is important for both the safety for your patients and for your own health that you disinfect your hands between each patient. Hand washing is the single most important step in preventing the spread of disease. This can be achieved through routine hand washing or through using a hand sanitizer. Currently, the Centers for Disease Control and Prevention (CDC) recommends using hand sanitizer over hand washing between patients. In addition, OSHA requires a new pair of gloves be used for each patient. These two actions are two of the most critical steps in breaking the chain of infection.

Assemble Equipment

Before beginning the venipuncture procedure, you should ensure that you have all of the equipment and supplies that you will need. Gather the necessary tubes, needles, needle holder, disinfectant, and gauze and make sure to have a bandage ready to use.

Reassure and Position the Patient

Many patients feel anxious about having their blood drawn. It is important to have confidence in your skills and to help the patient feel more relaxed about the procedure. Never tell the patient it won't hurt. There is a small degree of pain associated with the procedure. Being dishonest to the patient will damage the trust between you and the patient. It is particularly tempting to tell a small child who is anxious that it will not hurt. This may work to get the child to cooperate the first time, but it will make future procedures even more difficult.

The patient should be placed in a phlebotomy chair or allowed to lie on an exam table. Both of these situations help prevent the patient from getting injured should the patient faint during the procedure. Due to the risk of fainting, never allow patients to sit on a high stool or stand during a venipuncture procedure.

Apply Tourniquet

The tourniquet should be applied 3 to 4 inches above the intended site for venipuncture. Tourniquets should not be left on for longer than 1 minute. Leaving the tourniquet on for an excessive amount of time can result in pressure at the site, causing chemicals to leak out of the cells into the blood, altering test results. This is known as hemoconcentration.

In addition, tourniquets should not be applied over bruised, burned, or infected skin. Tourniquets should not be applied to an arm where a radical mastectomy has been performed or to an arm with a dialysis fistula.

Select and Cleanse the Site

The primary venipuncture collection sites are the three veins located in the antecubital fossa—the space on the inside part of the arm where

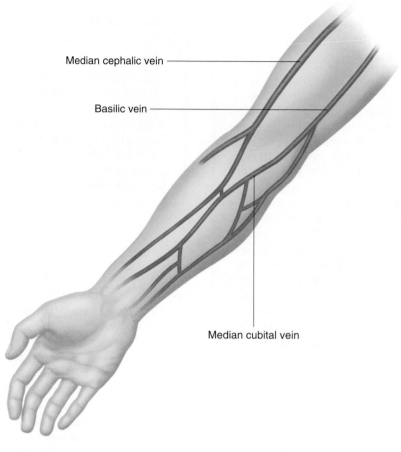

Median cephalic vein

Basilic vein

Median cubital vein

Figure 11-8 The antecubital fossa and veins.

the elbow is. Located here are the median cubital vein, the median cephalic vein, and the basilic vein. The median cubital vein is generally considered the best choice as it has a larger lumen, is usually well anchored, and has less of a tendency to roll than the other veins. It is also generally easy to locate and maintain visual site of. (See Figure 11-8.)

When it is not possible to draw from this site, other veins need to be located and utilized. Secondary venipuncture sites include the back of the hand, the thumb side of the wrist, and the forearm. (See Figure 11-9.) The feet and ankles should never be used as an alternative site as there is a greater risk of creating a clot or infection.

When selecting the site, it is often helpful to ask the patient to make a gentle fist. This helps to anchor and stabilize the vein. It is also helpful in make the veins more prominent. When selecting a vein, try to choose a larger vein. Also, choose a vein that is surrounded by tissue. You never want to select a vein that is located next to a bone or tendon.

Veins can be identified by **palpating** or by touch. They are often described as "bouncy," "spongy," "having resilience," or "springy." It is important

that you select a vein based on feel, as opposed to how it looks. You should never just select a blue line that looks like it might be a vein. Remember that prominent veins may not be the most suitable. They may have small lumens and roll because they are superficially attached.

It is always important to differentiate veins from arteries. ***Arteries should not be used for routine venipuncture.*** The distinguishing characteristic of arteries is the presence of a pulse.

When disinfecting the site, you can use either 70 percent isopropyl alcohol or Betadine. Clean the site using concentric circles, starting in the middle and moving away from the selected site. (See Figure 11-10.) Always allow the site to air dry. Never blow on the site or wave your hands over the site to make it dry faster. It is important to allow the site to completely dry before beginning the procedure, particularly when using alcohol. Failure to do so will result in increased patient pain and hemolysis of the red blood cells.

It is important to note that if it takes longer than 1 minute to complete this process when the tourniquet is in place, you must release the

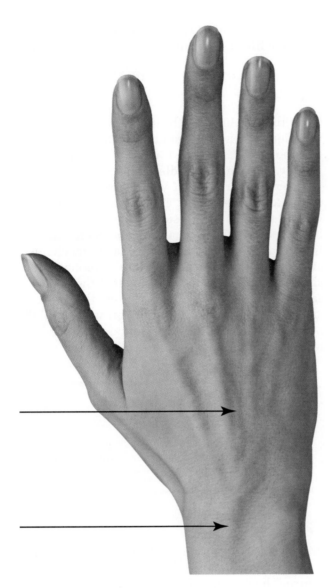

Figure 11-9 Alternate sites.

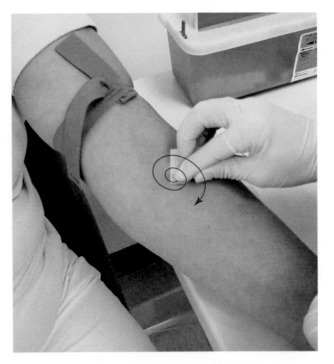

Figure 11-10 Cleansing the site using concentric circles.

tourniquet and allow normal blood flow to return to the site. If you again need to palpate the site to determine the vein location, you must clean the site again.

Uncap and Inspect the Needle

Before beginning any procedure utilizing needles, it is important to inspect the needle for defects such as a bent needle, spurs, or other defects. In addition, it is important to verify that the needle is sterile. Never use a needle for which someone other than you has broken the sterile seal. Once you have opened the needle and attached it to the needle holder, be sure not to touch the needle, as it must remain sterile. If you are unsure as to whether or not the needle is sterile, discard the needle and obtain a new one.

Finding a Vein

There are many circumstances where it is difficult to find a vein. Tricks for making veins more prominent include

- Hanging the arm down at the side for 2 to 3 minutes.
- Massaging the vein toward the trunk of the body.

Never attempt the venipuncture if you are uncertain of the exact location of the vein and never probe with the needle to find a vein.

Venipuncture Rule

Select the venipuncture site according to the feel of the vein, not its visibility.

Safety Note

When performing venipuncture, it is important to distinguish between an artery and a vein. Never use an artery because serious bleeding may occur. Veins are bluish, while arteries are pink or red. Arteries pulsate; veins do not.

Perform the Venipuncture

Begin by anchoring the vein using your non-dominant hand, using only your thumb. The skin should be pulled taut, but not so tight that it causes pain. (See Figure 11-11.) When the vein has been anchored, insert the needle at a 15- to 30-degree angle. (See Figure 11-12.) The needle should be inserted in one, quick, smooth movement. Once the needle is positioned in the vein, insert the first tube onto the anterior portion of the needle. The tube will begin to fill with blood and will continue until the vacuum is exhausted. Be sure not to overfill the tube. In addition, never fill the tubes by removing the stoppers. They will no longer be sterile nor will they have the correct vacuum.

Once the tube is full, remove the tube and gently invert the tube six to ten times, in accordance with the manufacturer's recommendations, to ensure that the additive is well mixed with the blood. Avoid shaking the tubes because this can hemolyze

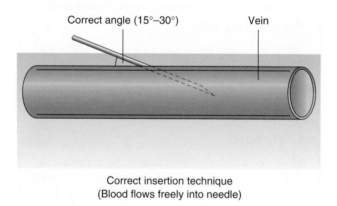

Figure 11-11 Anchoring the vein.

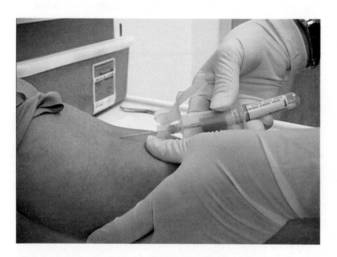

Correct insertion technique
(Blood flows freely into needle)

Figure 11-12 Needle inserted into a vein at a 15- to 30-degree angle.

the red blood cells. Observe the order of draw and continue filling tubes until the last tube is filled.

Release the Tourniquet and Remove the Needle

Once the last tube has been removed, release the tourniquet using one hand. Remember to release the tourniquet within 1 minute of application. Finally, remove the needle in one smooth motion. It is very important that you observe the removal of the tourniquet, tube, and needle in that order. Failure to do so may result in significant bruising for the patient. Once the needle has been removed, immediately engage the needle safety mechanism and dispose of the needle into a biohazardous sharps container. After ensuring that the needle is safely disposed of, apply pressure to the puncture site. It is important not to apply pressure until the needle has been withdrawn or you will cause significant pain for the patient.

Quality Assurance Note

Tourniquets can be removed at any point in the procedure, once blood collection has begun. The key is to ensure it is removed prior to removing the needle and within the time limit.

Apply Bandage

Pressure should be applied to the venipuncture site until the bleeding has stopped to prevent a bruise. The patient's arm should remain extended while the clot is forming and pressure is being applied to the site. If the patient has his or her arm bent during the clotting process, bleeding may be reinitiated when the patient moves his or her arm. In addition, women should be instructed not to carry their purses on the venipuncture side.

Once bleeding has completely stopped, apply a bandage over the site. Never apply a bandage to a child less than 2 years old as this can be a choking hazard. In addition, notify a physician if bleeding lasts longer than 5 minutes.

Label Tubes

Once you have properly disposed of the needle and verified that the patient is no longer bleeding, you should label the specimens. When labeling, be sure to use a pen with indelible ink or preprinted labels. You should always label specimens at the patient's side. Never label your specimens after

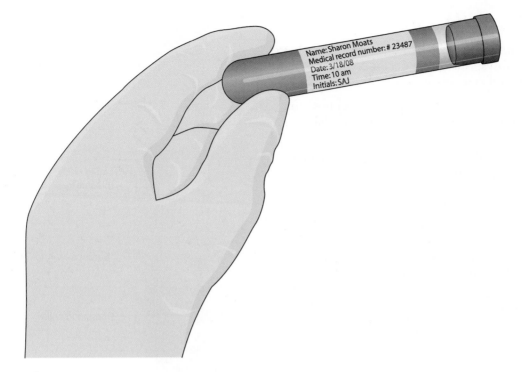

Figure 11-13 Properly label phlebotomy specimen.

leaving the patient. You should not label the tubes prior to collection either. Both of these practices can lead to mislabeled specimens. Information that must be on the tubes includes

- Patient's complete first and last name (no initials or shortened names)
- Medical record number or date of birth
- Date and time of collection
- Initials of the lab personnel who collected the specimen

Your institution or office may require additional information. (See Figure 11-13.)

In addition to properly labeling the specimen, it is important to make sure that the specimens are transported or tested in a timely manner. Finally, you should always end every patient interaction with some salutation, such as "Thank you, have a nice day. I hope you feel better."

Initialing Specimens

You should always label and initial your own specimens. You are the only person who can verify the identity of the specimens. Never ask another person to label them for you. Likewise, you should never label someone else's specimens, as you cannot verify the identity of those specimens.

HANDLING AND PREPARING BLOOD SAMPLES

Blood samples require proper handling and preparation to ensure lab personnel safety and accurate patient test results.

Failure to Collect the Blood Specimen

There are times when every lab staff "misses"—they are not able to collect blood. If you fail to collect blood, try again with another venipuncture site. If the second attempt also fails, ask another member of the lab staff to attempt to collect. If the second person is also unable to collect, STOP. Notify the physician of the difficulties. There are alternate methods of collection that should be employed by the physician.

Lab Safety

As always when working with body fluids, you should assume that all blood is contaminated and should follow the Standard Precautions. Disinfect all work surfaces and equipment and dispose of samples and used supplies appropriately.

Preserving Sample Integrity

Blood specimens must be handled appropriately to prevent hemolysis and other decomposition. When handling blood specimens, you should always

- Keep the specimen tube in a vertical position and handle it carefully to reduce the risk of spillage, agitation, and hemolysis.
- Try not to dislodge clots that stick to the top of the collecting tube. This can cause hemolysis.
- Avoid exposing the specimen to light, which decomposes bilirubin and other analytes. Cover clear containers with foil or use amber-colored containers.
- Refrigerate or freeze specimens per testing procedure if testing will not occur within 1 hour of collection. If serum or plasma is required for testing, be sure to centrifuge the specimen first. It may be necessary to separate the serum or plasma from the red cells prior to storage.

Clot Formation in Serum Samples

When a test requires a serum sample, the blood must be allowed to stand until a clot forms. If the collection tube has a marble stopper, serum separator gel has been added to the tube to separate the cells from the serum after centrifuging. If thrombin has been added, the tube will clot faster and centrifuging can be performed sooner. If the collection tube has a red stopper, no serum separator gel has been added, and the sample needs to stand for 20 to 30 minutes at room temperature to allow the clot to form. Patients taking anticoagulants such as Coumadin will take even longer to clot.

Centrifuging Blood Samples

Most centrifuge manufacturers recommend centrifuging blood samples for 5 to 15 minutes at 1,000 to 1,200 g, but you always should check the manufacturers' recommendations. Balance sample tubes before starting the centrifuge by placing tubes of equal weight opposite each other. The centrifuge lid must remain down until all spinning has stopped. Never try to stop the centrifuge by opening the lid and slowing it. This may cause spattering and mixing of tube contents, as well as possibly cause injury to you. Clean the centrifuge and disinfect it with a 10 percent bleach solution on a regular basis as well as immediately after spills.

Decanting and Storing Blood Samples

After centrifuging, serum samples that contain separator gel have a gel barrier between the blood cells at the bottom of the tube and the serum at the

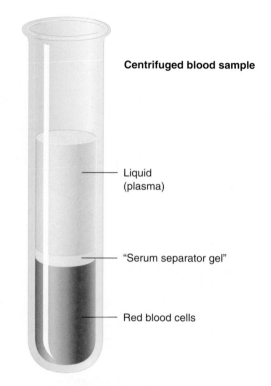

Centrifuged blood sample

Liquid (plasma)

"Serum separator gel"

Red blood cells

Figure 11-14 Centrifuged SST specimen.

top. (See Figure 11-14.) The serum can be stored in the refrigerator on the gel barrier for up to 48 hours with the tube stoppered. In samples without separator gel, plasma or serum should be pipetted into appropriately labeled tubes within 1 hour of centrifuging. Take care to avoid pipetting blood cells from the bottom of the tube.

After decanting, keep the tubes stoppered to reduce the risk of evaporation, spillage, and contamination. Use the samples for testing within 5 hours at room temperature or within 48 hours if they are refrigerated in a sealed container. If specimens must be kept longer than 48 hours, they should be frozen at -20 degrees Celsius in a freezer that does not have a self-defrost cycle.

Specimen Appearance

The normal appearance of serum or plasma is a clear, straw-colored liquid. If a sample has an abnormal appearance, note this on the lab report. **Lipemic** serum and plasma, for example, appear milky and turbid because they contain a high level of lipids. **Icteric** (jaundiced) serum and plasma look dark yellow or greenish because of a high level of bilirubin. The high level of bilirubin may be due to hepatitis. Icteric samples may be very contagious. All specimens, regardless of appearance, should be handled with great care.

Types of Venous Specimens

There are three major types of venous specimens.

Plasma. The specimen is placed in a centrifuge in order to separate the components based on their weights. After centrifugation, red blood cells settle to the bottom of the tube, the white blood cells and platelets form a thin buffy coat, and the liquid plasma portion of the blood remains on top. The plasma contains all of the dissolved components of the blood, including the coagulation factors. Since this specimen contains an anticoagulant, no clot has formed and fibrinogen will remain in solution.

Serum. Like the plasma specimen, the tube is placed in the centrifuge in order to separate the components based on their weights. Also similar to the plasma specimen, the red blood cells settle to the bottom. In this specimen, no anticoagulant is present, so a clot will form. During the formation of a clot, coagulation factors and platelets are used. As a result, the liquid portion of the blood lacks coagulation factors.

Whole blood. The specimen contains an anticoagulant to prevent clotting so that platelets and coagulation factors remain in solution. This specimen is well mixed so that the red blood cells, white blood cells, platelets, and plasma remain in solution together and is most similar to the blood found *in vivo.*

Some specimens specifically require plasma or serum. The liquid portion of the blood is identical in composition except for a few, significant differences. Plasma comes from an anticoagulated specimen in which there is no clotting *in vitro,* or inside of the tube. As a result, platelets remain free-floating and coagulation factors are not used and stay in the plasma. On the other hand, serum is derived from a specimen that does NOT contain an anticoagulant, so clotting does occur *in vitro,* or inside of the tube. Platelets clump together and coagulation factors are used up in the clot. These specimens cannot be used for platelet counting or coagulation studies. See Table 11-3.

Special Blood Collection Requirements

While many blood specimens do not require any special collection requirements, a number of specimens do. The following is an example of some of the more common collection requirements.

Table 11-3   Comparing Serum and Plasma

Characteristic	Plasma	Serum
Specimen contains anticoagulant?	Yes	No
Clotting occurs inside the tube?	No	Yes
Platelets clump inside specimen	No	Yes
Coagulation factors found in specimen	Yes	No
Can be used for platelet and/or coagulation studies	Yes	No
Tubes	Green, light blue, gray, lavender	Red or marble

Fasting. When a fasting specimen is required, a patient cannot eat or drink for 8 to 12 hours before the specimen is collected. In general, it is acceptable for the patient to drink water during this period. All other drinks, including teas, coffee, juice, and other beverages, are to be avoided. In addition, tobacco products should be avoided during the fasting and testing period. The purpose of a fasting specimen is to obtain a baseline for tests that may be affected by recent meals. Examples include glucose tolerance tests and lipid panels.

Timed Specimens. As the name implies, these are tests in which the time that the test is collected is important to the accuracy of the result. When collecting a timed specimen, it is important to label the specimen with the time it was collected.

Two special timed specimens are collected for therapeutic medication monitoring for certain drugs. Often, specimens are collected as a pair. The first specimen is a *peak specimen* that is collected when the medication tested is expected to be at its highest level in the bloodstream. Though it varies among medications, a peak specimen is usually drawn 15 to 60 minutes after administration of the drug, depending on the medication. The second specimen, called a *trough,* is collected when the lowest concentration of the medication can be found. This is usually a few minutes before the next dose is administered.

Iced Specimens. This requires that the specimen be placed immediately in an ice water bath.

The purpose of this is to stop the metabolic activity of the red blood cells. Failure to use water will result in uneven cooling of the specimen, leaving some spots for the red blood cells to remain metabolically active and alter test results. An example of specimens requiring this protocol is arterial blood gases.

Keep Warm. Some specimens must be kept at body temperature until they are tested. These specimens should be kept at or close to 37 degrees Celsius. This procedure is used to avoid reactions in the blood that only take place when the blood is cooled and does not reflect activity in the patient's body. Maintaining this temperature can be accomplished by placing the specimen in a warm water bath. An example of a specimen that needs to be handled in this manner is cold agglutinins.

Protect from Light. Some components of the blood break down when exposed to light. In order to avoid these reactions, these specimens should be wrapped in aluminum foil. Examples of specimens requiring this procedure include bilirubin from infants, vitamin B12, and carotene.

How Do I Know What the Special Collection Requirements Are?

When you first begin collecting patient specimens, all the different specimen requirements may seem overwhelming and it may seem like you will never be able to learn the various specimen requirements. Take comfort in knowing that in each POL, the doctors generally order a particular set of tests that you will quickly become familiar with. Until then, here are some helpful hints:

1. Check the requisition before you see the patient. This will give you the opportunity to make sure you have everything you need.
2. If you are unsure of the specimen requirements, refer to the Reference Manual for tests that will be sent to the reference lab. Refer to the package insert of specimen requirements for tests that are performed in house.
3. Be sure to review the package insert for specimen requirements whenever changing equipment or test kits. Many times different kits or equipment require different specimens.

PROCEDURE 11-1

Venipuncture Utilizing the Routine Evacuated Tube System

Goal

To successfully perform venipuncture using a routine evacuated tube system.

Completion Time

15 minutes

Equipment and Supplies

- Impermeable lab coat, gown, or apron
- Face shield or goggles
- Disposable gloves
- Hand disinfectant
- Biohazardous container
- Disinfectant, such as 70 percent isopropyl alcohol or prepackaged alcohol wipes

- Tourniquet
- Needle
- Needle holder
- Collection tubes
- Sterile gauze pads
- Bandage

Instructions

Read through the list of equipment and supplies that you will need. Read the steps of the procedure. Be sure that you understand each step before you begin. Then complete each step correctly and in the proper order. If your completion time is too long; repeat the procedure until you increase your speed.

Steps marked with (*) are critical and must have the maximum points to pass.

Performance Standards	Points Awarded	Maximum Points
1. Put on lab coat and face shield or goggles.		5
2. Disinfect hands; dry if necessary.		5
3. Put on gloves. Inspect for tears and replace if necessary.		5

4.	Collect and prepare the appropriate equipment.	5
5.	*Verify patient identity.	30
6.	Explain the venipuncture procedure and encourage the patient to relax.	5
7.	Remove the cover from the short end of the needle. Screw the short end into the needle holder and ensure that the needle is secure.	5
8.	Place the tourniquet around the patient's arm above the elbow. If you cannot feel a pulse at the wrist, loosen the tourniquet.	5
9.	Select a suitable vein by inspection and palpation. Determine the direction the vein is running and its depth.	10
10.	Clean the site with alcohol or betadine, using concentric circles.	5
11.	Tell the patient to make a gentle fist and to hold the arm straight. Rest the arm on the armrest of the phlebotomy chair or on a table or countertop for support.	5
12.	Place the evacuated tube in the needle holder until the short end of the needle touches the rubber stopper. Do not push the needle into the rubber stopper yet.	5
13.	Remove the cover from the long needle and inspect the needle.	5
14.	Grasp the evacuated tube needle holder with your dominant hand.	5
15.	Place your thumb below the puncture site, pulling the skin taut to anchor the vein.	5
16.	Hold the needle at a 15-degree angle with the bevel facing up.	5
17.	Insert the needle through the skin immediately adjacent to the vein to be punctured.	5
18.	Once you have penetrated the skin, push the tube all the way in to engage the tube's vacuum.	10
19.	Release the tourniquet.	5
20.	Tell the patient to relax his/her fist.	5
21.	After the tube has stopped filling, collect the remaining tubes while observing the order of draw.	10
22.	As each tube is removed from the needle, gently invert the tube several times.	10
23.	Remove the last tube from the needle and evacuated tube system.	5
24.	Cover the puncture site with gauze, without applying pressure.	5
25.	*Withdraw the needle and engage the safety mechanism.	30
26.	Apply pressure to the puncture site for 3–5 minutes, keeping the arm straight.	5
27.	Label each tube at the patient's side with the following information: patient's full name, identification number, the date, the time, and your initials.	15
28.	Check the puncture site to see if bleeding has stopped.	10
29.	When bleeding has stopped, apply a bandage. If bleeding does not stop within 5 minutes, notify the physician.	5
30.	Discard the needle and holder as a complete unit in the sharps container.	10
31.	Discard equipment properly, observing Standard Precautions.	10
32.	Disinfect your hands.	5
33.	Thank and release the patient.	10
	Total Points	**265**

Overall Procedural Evaluation

Student Name _____

Signature of Instructor _____ Date _____

Comments _____

_____

chapter 11 REVIEW

Using Terminology

Define the following terms.

1. Anticoagulant

_____

_____

_____

2. Antecubital

_____

_____

_____

3. Plasma

_____

_____

_____

4. Venipuncture

_____

_____

_____

Answer the following questions in the spaces provided.

5. How should needles and needle holders be disposed of?

_____

_____

6. What is the purpose of the tourniquet?

_____

_____

_____

Match the following.

_____ **7.** Lavender	a. blood cultures
_____ **8.** Light blue	b. plain/no additive
_____ **9.** Sterile	c. sodium fluoride
_____ **10.** Red	d. gel separator
_____ **11.** Green	e. sodium citrate
_____ **12.** Marble	f. EDTA
_____ **13.** Gray	g. sodium heparin

Match the following characteristic with serum or plasma.

14. contains platelets

_____

_____

_____

15. does not contain fibrinogen

_____

_____

_____

16. specimen contains anticoagulant

_____

_____

_____

17. specimen does not form a clot

_____

_____

_____

18. associated with green and light blue tubes

_____

_____

_____

19. can be used for coagulation studies

_____

_____

_____

20. clot forms in the tube

_____

_____

_____

Multiple Choice

Choose the best answer for the following questions.

21. At what point during the blood collection process should a specimen be labeled?
   a. prior to the procedure
   b. after you have finished the procedure, at the patient's side
   c. after you have left the patient
   d. when you are ready to begin testing

22. What is the preferred site for venipuncture?
   a. median cubital vein
   b. wrist vein
   c. brachial artery
   d. femoral artery

23. What information should be included on a blood specimen label?
   a. patient's full name
   b. unique identification number
   c. the date
   d. all of the above

24. Hematology requires a _____ top specimen.
   a. light blue
   b. sterile
   c. lavender
   d. marble

25. Coagulation studies require a _____ top specimen.
   a. light blue
   b. red
   c. lavender
   d. marble

Applying Knowledge

Answer the following questions in the spaces provided.

26. Why is a tourniquet used in venipuncture?

_____

_____

27. What does the color coding on the stoppers of blood collection tubes mean?

_____

_____

28. What is the order of draw using the routine evacuated tube system?

_____

_____

29. What is the preferred site for venipuncture?

_____

_____

30. At what point during blood collection should a specimen be labeled? Why?

_____

_____

31. What are the advantages of a phlebotomy chair?

_____

_____

32. Where should you place a venipuncture tourniquet? How long can you leave it on?

_____

_____

33. What information should you include on a blood specimen label?

_____

_____

34. When performing a venipuncture, when should you release the tourniquet? Why?

_____

_____

35. Why does hemolysis ruin a blood sample?

_____

_____

Applying Knowledge—On the Job

Answer the following questions in the spaces provided.

36. Assume a patient requires blood cultures. She wants to know why she needs to have her blood drawn twice during the same visit. Explain the procedure.

_____

_____

37. You need to draw three specimens—a lavender, blood culture, and marble. What is the correct order of draw?

_____

_____

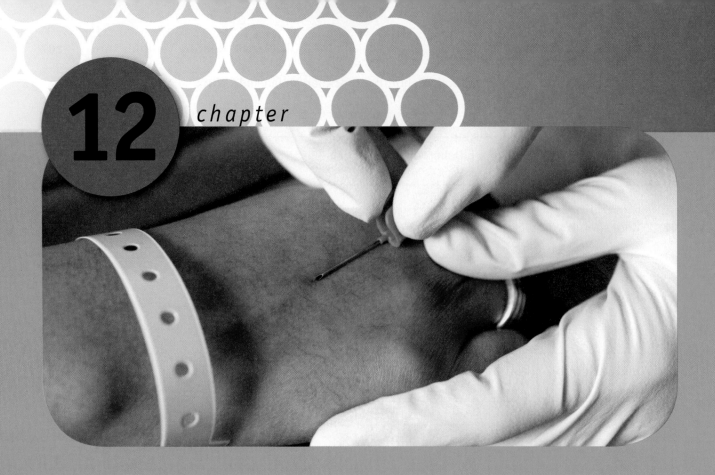

Advanced Venipuncture Techniques

COGNITIVE OBJECTIVES

After studying the chapter, you should be able to

12.1 use and spell each of the vocabulary terms appropriately.

12.2 describe the equipment used for capillary collection and the butterfly technique.

12.3 discuss the advantages and disadvantages of the capillary puncture collection method.

12.4 state the advantages and disadvantages of the butterfly method of collection.

12.5 discuss when it is best to use the routine evacuated tube method and syringe method of venipuncture.

12.6 describe several difficulties that may occur when performing venipuncture and how to avoid or correct these situations.

12.7 explain the special considerations needed for patients with mastectomies.

12.8 list several adverse reactions to blood collection and describe how to respond to each situation.

12.9 describe the circumstances in which you would perform a syringe or butterfly venipuncture, fingerstick, or heelstick.

12.10 state the correct site of a heelstick and fingerstick.

12.11 list the order of collection for syringe and capillary puncture procedure.

12.12 describe the difference between a capillary and a venous specimen.

PERFORMANCE OBJECTIVES

After studying the chapter, you should be able to

12.13 perform venipuncture using a butterfly system with evacuated tube system adapter.

12.14 perform venipuncture utilizing the syringe system, using either a butterfly or routine needle.

12.15 collect a capillary specimen.

TERMINOLOGY

butterfly needle: also known as a "winged infusion set." A modified venipuncture needle that is shorter in length, is held by its "butterfly wings," and has a tubing attached to the posterior portion of the needle that can be attached to a needle holder or syringe.

capillary: a small blood vessel that connects arterioles and venules. Contains a mixture of arterial and venous blood.

capillary puncture: the puncture of a capillary for the purpose of collecting a blood specimen.

fingerstick: puncturing the soft pad of the ring or middle finger in order to collect a blood specimen.

heelstick: puncturing the lateral portion of the heel in infants in order to collect a blood specimen. This may only be done on infants who have not yet begun to walk.

hematoma: a subcutaneous mass of blood at a venipuncture site. Also known as a bruise.

lancet: a sharp, piercing device used to puncture a finger or heel in order to obtain a capillary specimen.

microcontainer: a blood collection system used with capillary puncture.

point-of-care (POC) testing: laboratory tests that can be performed at the patient's bedside, rather than sending the specimen to the lab for testing. Requires a very small amount of specimen.

syringe: an instrument with a needle used for drawing blood from a vein.

transfer device: mechanical device used to assist in the transfer of blood from a syringe into the specimen tubes.

INTRODUCTION

Although routine venipuncture techniques will work in most situations when you need to obtain a blood specimen from a patient, it is not always possible or appropriate to obtain a sample this way. For example, it is more appropriate to obtain a small, capillary sample for a diabetic patient who needs their glucose checked. Likewise, it may be easier to obtain a venous specimen from the back of the hand utilizing a butterfly needle. This chapter will review the **butterfly needle** procedure and the **capillary puncture** and the various situations in which these procedures may be utilized.

BUTTERFLY WINGED INFUSION COLLECTION SET

The butterfly winged infusion device consists of a needle with plastic wings, plastic tubing, and an adapter. The easy-to-grasp, flexible wing design allows an entry angle that is almost parallel to the vein. The tubing is usually 5 to 12 inches in length. It can be attached to either a needle holder or a syringe, depending on the needs of the lab personnel. The needle itself is the same gauge as a routine venipuncture needle, usually 19 to 23 gauge. The length is generally shorter, ¾ of

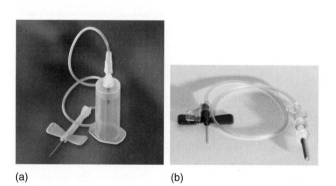

(a)   (b)

Figure 12-1 Butterfly needle. (a) Butterfly needle with luer adapter to needle holder. (b) Butterfly needle without needle holder.

an inch. (See Figure 12-1.) The purpose of the different type of needle is to allow the lab personnel to access veins that would be more difficult to draw from with a traditional needle. The shorter needle and tubing allow for greater flexibility and mobility. This can be especially helpful when collecting a specimen from a neonate, child, elderly, or severely traumatized patient.

Whether collecting the blood specimen with an evacuated tube system or a syringe, the principle is the same. The vacuum in the tube or the syringe pulls the blood out of the vein in which the needle has been inserted. In the case of the evacuated tube system, the amount of vacuum is predetermined. In the case of the syringe, the plunger of the syringe is pulled manually, thus creating a vacuum. The contents of the syringe must then be transferred to the tubes.

Coagulation Specimen Collection Note

When using a butterfly set to collect a coagulation specimen, a minor adjustment is required. If the blue top tube is the first specimen to be collected, draw a "discard" tube to ensure that any residual air is removed from the butterfly tubing. This will ensure that the proper blood to anticoagulant ratio is maintained. The discard tube should be a nonadditive or coagulation tube.

Procedure Note

When using a butterfly needle, you will know when the needle has entered the vein because you will observe a "flash" of blood in the shaft of the tubing.

Butterfly Utilizing Evacuated Tube System

When performing venipuncture utilizing a butterfly needle attached to the needle holder, the procedure is the same as routine venipuncture. The only significant difference is the needle should be inserted at a 10- to 15-degree angle, slightly lower than the standard needle insertion. In addition, grasping the needle is also different. Rather than holding onto the needle holder, you grasp the butterfly needle by its "wings."

Syringe Procedure

In general, the syringe procedure should only be utilized when no other options are available. In some cases, it is better to use a butterfly-syringe system for collecting blood from the patient. This is true whenever you suspect that a vein may be fragile and unable to tolerate the stress of the vacuum from a tube. Examples of these types of veins include veins in young children, veins in the elderly, some hand veins, and veins in very dehydrated patients. The syringe allows you to control the rate at which the blood is withdrawn from the vein, thus causing less stress to the vein.

Butterfly Venipuncture Procedure

1. Review paperwork.
2. Identify yourself to the patient.
3. Verify patient identity.
4. Explain the procedure.
5. Confirm patient preparation.
6. Wash your hands and put on personnel protective equipment.
7. Collect equipment.
8. Reassure and position the patient.
9. Apply tourniquet.
10. Select and cleanse site.
11. Uncap and inspect needle.
12. Perform the venipuncture:
    a. Insert the needle at a 10- to 15-degree angle.
    b. Follow correct order of draw.
    c. Gently invert tubes as they are withdrawn from the needle to mix the specimens.
13. Release the tourniquet.
14. Remove the last tube.
15. Place a piece of gauze over the puncture site but do not apply pressure.
16. Remove the needle and engage safety mechanism. Discard the entire blood collection set—butterfly needle and needle holder according to institutional policy.
17. Apply pressure to the gauze over the puncture site.
18. Check the site for bleeding. When bleeding has stopped, apply a bandage.
19. Label tubes before leaving the patient's bedside.
20. Thank and release the patient.

Patient Requests for Butterfly Needles

Occasionally, patients will request the butterfly needle. Because the length of the needle is shorter, patients believe the needle itself is smaller and therefore the procedure is less painful. Inform the patient that the gauge (diameter) of the needle is the same; therefore, there is no difference in pain between the two needles. Choose your needle based on the physical needs of the patient.

A **syringe** is a plastic barrel and plunger set that is manually pulled to control the flow of blood. Syringes come in a variety of sizes; 10 mL and 20 mL are the most commonly used in the venipuncture procedure. In general, you do not want to

Securing the Needle

When using a butterfly needle, it is important to ensure that the needle is secure throughout the procedure. While the tubing provides the advantage of greater flexibility and mobility, that same mobility makes an accidental needlestick more likely. Always keep your hand on the wings of the needle throughout the procedure. Be sure to immediately engage the safety mechanism upon withdrawal of the needle from the vein.

been collected in the syringe, the phlebotomist must engage the needle safety mechanism, remove the needle attached to the syringe, and replace it with a **transfer device** before transferring the blood to the tubes. This device reduces the risk of a

Procedure Note

When using a syringe, the order for draw remains the same.

use a syringe larger than 20 mL as it would be too cumbersome for the procedure. A syringe smaller than 10 mL may not collect enough specimen. The venipuncture needle is attached to the anterior end of the syringe, opposite from the plunger. Prior to attaching the needle, it is important to "prime" the syringe. Pull the plunger in and out of the syringe to ensure it moves smoothly. It is critical that the plunger be pushed back into place before beginning the phlebotomy procedure to avoid injecting air into the patient's vein.

A syringe can be attached to a butterfly needle or a regular straight needle. The procedure is the same for both types of needles. The procedure for collecting a venous specimen utilizing a syringe is similar to the other methods of venipuncture, with some necessary differences.

First, the *phlebotomist manually controls the rate at which the blood is being withdrawn.* The phlebotomist should observe the vein during the procedure and make adjustments to the rate of collection as needed. (See Figure 12-2.)

The second difference is *the transfer of blood from the syringe to the tubes.* Once the blood has

Venipuncture Utilizing Syringe System Procedure

1. Review paperwork.
2. Identify yourself to the patient.
3. Verify patient identity.
4. Explain what you are going to do.
5. Confirm patient preparation.
6. Wash your hands and put on personnel protective equipment.
7. Assemble equipment.
8. Reassure and position the patient.
9. Apply tourniquet.
10. Select and cleanse site.
11. Uncap and inspect needle.
12. Perform the venipuncture:
    a. Insert the needle at 10- to 15-degree angle with the bevel up.
    b. Pull on the plunger to withdraw blood. Continue until syringe is full or adequate blood amount has been collected.
13. Release the tourniquet.
14. Cover puncture site with gauze, without applying pressure.
15. Remove the needle and engage safety mechanism. Discard the original syringe needle following the institution's procedure.
16. Apply pressure to gauze covering the puncture site.
17. Check the site for bleeding. When bleeding has stopped, apply a bandage.
18. Replace syringe needle with a transfer device.
19. Insert each tube into the transfer device. Allow each tube to fill, carefully withdraw the transfer device, and insert it into the next tube.
20. When all tubes have been filled, discard the entire blood collection set, including the transfer device and syringe.
21. Gently invert tubes to mix specimen.
22. Label tubes before leaving the patient's bedside.
23. Thank and release the patient.

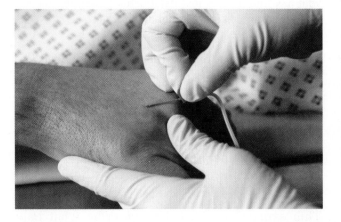

Figure 12-2 Lab personnel performing phlebotomy using butterfly needle and syringe.

needlestick when transferring blood into the tubes. This additional step must be performed carefully, to reduce the possibility of accidental needlestick. Insert each of the tubes into the transfer device. Allow the tubes to fill without applying pressure to the plunger. This increases the chance of hemolysis for the specimen. If a tube fails to fill, there is probably something wrong with the tube. Select another tube and try again. In addition, never fill tubes by removing the rubber stopper. The tubes will no longer be sterile nor will they have the correct vacuum to ensure proper blood to anticoagulant ratio.

Which Method to Use?

In general, the routine evacuated tube system method is usually preferable because it reduces the handling of the specimen, thus reducing the risk of occupational exposure. Furthermore, the routine evacuated tube system is less expensive due to the cheaper needles. On the other hand, the butterfly and syringe methods offer the advantage of greater flexibility and access to alternate venipuncture sites. The syringe method in particular allows the phlebotomist the ability to control the rate of blood flow, making vein collapse less likely. This is particularly helpful in geriatric and pediatric patients.

CHALLENGES IN VENIPUNCTURE

There are a variety of situations that may arise when you are attempting to collect a blood specimen that require special attention.

Failure to Draw Blood

Despite your best efforts and preparation, when you are performing a venipuncture procedure, you may not initially be able to collect the specimen. This may to due to a variety of reasons.

1. *The needle may be inserted too far* and has gone through the vein. This can be corrected by slowly backing the needle up until blood flows. (See Figure 12-3.)
2. *The needle is not inserted far enough.* In comparison, the needle may not be inserted far enough and the needle is resting above the vein. This can be corrected by pushing the needle until it penetrates the vein.
3. *The bevel of the needle is resting against the vein.* The bevel can be touching the top of the vein and therefore the blood can't get into the needle. This is similar to resting a straw against the side of a cup. This situation can be

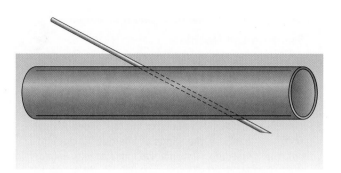

Figure 12-3 Needle inserted too far and the bevel is no longer in the vein.

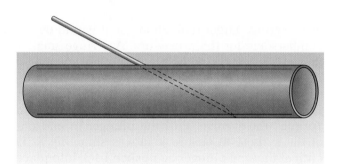

Figure 12-4 Needle into vein but bevel resting against the vein wall.

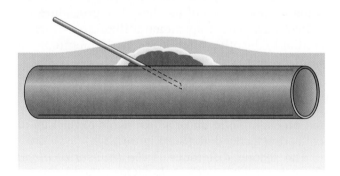

Figure 12-5 Needle is inserted into the vein. The vein has "blown" and lost its structural integrity. Blood has begun to leak into surrounding tissue.

avoided by adjusting the angle of the needle until the bevel is no longer against the vein wall. (See Figure 12-4.)
4. *The bevel of the needle isn't facing up.* In this situation, you must start over with a new needle and check that the bevel is up before beginning the procedure.

Vein "Blows"

This expression is used to describe what happens when a vein loses its structural integrity and begins leaking blood into the surrounding tissue.

It is often a visibly noticeable event as the skin begins to swell and has a blackish-bluish appearance. This usually happens in fragile veins that cannot tolerate the pressure of a venipuncture procedure. Once a vein "blows," there is nothing that can be done to save the site. You must withdraw the needle, select another site, and begin again. However, this can be avoided. If you suspect a vein is fragile and cannot withstand the stress of the procedure, use a syringe to control the rate of blood withdrawal and remove the blood slowly. (See Figure 12-5.)

Care for a Blown Vein

If you suspect a vein has lost its structural integrity, the following can be done to minimize bruising:

- Apply pressure to the site for an extended period (5 minutes).
- Apply ice for an extended period.

Collapsing Veins

Similar to veins that "blow," collapsing veins are veins that cave in on themselves due to the pressure from the vacuum in the tubes. Once the vein has collapsed, blood can no longer flow into the tube. This problem is associated with small veins or veins with thin walls. Once a vein has collapsed, in general, it is no longer usable for venipuncture until it has repaired itself. Select another site and begin again. Like the veins that "blow," collapsing veins can be avoided by using a syringe where the pressure can be controlled manually.

Tube Has a Faulty Vacuum

Occasionally, the tube you select will not have a proper vacuum and therefore will not withdraw blood from the vein. You will know this is happening because little or no blood will enter the tube. If you suspect that the tube has a faulty vacuum, simply remove the faulty tube and replace it with another tube. If the tube is the problem, you will begin collecting blood with no other changes. This is more likely to occur with expired tubes, which should never be used. Therefore, it is critical that you check the expiration dates of your tubes before you begin the procedure.

"Rolling" Veins

"Rolling" veins are those veins that move away from the needle when you puncture the skin. Depending on how much the vein has moved, it may be possible to redirect the needle. However, you should never blindly probe. It is often necessary to withdraw the needle, re-anchor the vein, and try again in another site with a new, sterile needle. To avoid "rolling" veins, use firm pressure to anchor the vein when the needle is inserted.

Hemoconcentration

Hemoconcentration is an increase of analytes in blood due to a shift in water balance. It can be due to prolonged tourniquet use or massaging. To prevent this problem, remove the tourniquet within 1 minute of application and do not have the patient excessively squeeze or pump his or her hand.

Hemolysis

The breakdown of red blood cells and the subsequent release of their internal chemicals can be avoided by observing the following:

1. Use the correct gauge needle. The smaller gauge needles that have the larger openings are less likely to cause hemolysis.
2. Gently mix the tubes to prevent trauma to the red blood cells.
3. Allow the alcohol to completely dry before starting the venipuncture.

Mastectomy

A mastectomy is the surgical removal of a breast. Sometimes, the axillary lymph nodes also are removed as part of the procedure. As a result, these patients are more susceptible to infection. Therefore, do NOT draw blood from the same side as the mastectomy. Furthermore, do NOT apply a tourniquet to the mastectomy side, as stasis is especially detrimental for these patients. Note that while mastectomies are more common in women, men also may require and undergo mastectomies.

Adverse Reactions

Drawing blood occasionally triggers adverse reactions in patients. Typical adverse reactions include fainting, nausea, vomiting, excessive bleeding, convulsions, and **hematomas,** which are subcutaneous masses of blood. If a patient shows signs of distress, notify the physician immediately and administer appropriate first aid treatment. Also make a written report of the incident. See Table 12-1 for additional adverse reactions and appropriate responses.

Table 12-1   How to Respond When an Adverse Reaction Occurs

Adverse Reaction	Response
Fainting/syncope	Immediately stop the procedure. Move the patient into a reclining position and elevate the patient's feet above his/her head. Once the patient is conscious, notify the physician. The physician will determine if it is safe to attempt the procedure again. Note, fainting is the loss of consciousness for 1–2 minutes. Loss of consciousness for a longer period indicates the problem is not fainting. Under these circumstances, EMS should be notified.
Nausea	Tell the patient to take deep breaths and to lower his/her head. Make the patient comfortable and place a cold cloth on the patient's forehead. Give the patient a basin, tissues, and a glass of water if vomiting occurs. Alert the physician to the patient's condition.
Excessive bleeding	If bleeding continues after the venipuncture, keep pressure over the venipuncture site with a clean gauze pad, adding additional pads as needed. Alert the physician if bleeding continues past 5 minutes.
Convulsions	Alert the physician immediately. Remove any objects from the area that could cause harm to the patient. Do not restrain the convulsing patient except to prevent self-injury. Do not insert anything into the patient's mouth.
Hematomas/bruises	These are usually harmless, but they may alarm the patient. They are less likely if the tourniquet is removed before the needle is withdrawn and if pressure is applied to the puncture site until bleeding has stopped.

CAPILLARY SPECIMEN COLLECTION

When it is not possible to collect blood from a vein or only a small amount of specimen is needed, the capillary specimen is a good choice for testing. It is often very difficult to collect specimens from patients undergoing chemotherapy, burn victims, patients with a lot of scarring, geriatric patients, and patients with fragile veins such as children. In these cases, capillary specimen collection may be the preferred method of obtaining a specimen. An example of testing that requires only a very small amount of specimen is **point-of-care (POC) testing** for glucose or hemoglobin. Again, the capillary specimen is the preferred choice.

Capillaries are small blood vessels that connect arterioles and venules. Therefore, the blood composition is different than blood obtained by venipuncture. Capillary specimens contain a combination of venous, arterial, and interstitial fluid. The amount of arterial blood is even higher if the area from which the specimen has been collected was prewarmed. Though the composition of capillary blood is similar to venous blood, it is different from venous blood; therefore, the specimen source should be noted on the lab requisition.

Sites used to collect capillary blood specimens include the heel of the foot for children under the age of 1 year who are not yet walking and the middle or ring finger for all others. The capillaries

are close to the surface in these locations. The incision should never exceed 2.0 mm in depth, as there is a risk you may puncture a bone. In infants and young children, a smaller lancet should be used to ensure you do not puncture the bone. Incisions should be perpendicular to the fingerprint or foot print, not parallel. This type of incision prevents the blood from pooling in the creases of the fingerprint, thus making the specimen easier to collect.

Safety Note—Lancets

Prior to the Needlestick Safety and Prevention Act, many **lancets** were pointed pieces of metal that lab personnel used to manually pierce the skin. Now, lancets are more sophisticated. The metal, piercing portion of the lancet is housed inside of a plastic compartment. There is generally a plastic plunger on top that the lab personnel depresses. Once this plastic trigger is pushed, the lancet is automatically activated to pierce the skin to a predetermined depth. Generally, the metal portion of the lancet is automatically retracted to prevent accidental needlestick. (See Figure 12-6.)

When performing a **fingerstick,** select a site on the central, fleshy portion of the ring or middle finger. The incision should be slightly off the middle of the finger and never too close to the nail

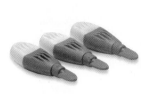
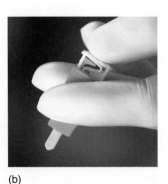

(a)   (b)

Figure 12-6 (a) Examples of safety lancets.
(b) Safety lancet held by lab personnel.

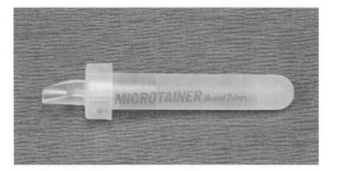

Figure 12-8 Microcontainer tube.

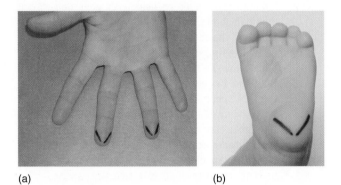

(a)   (b)

Figure 12-7 Sites for a capillary puncture:
(a) fingerstick sites; (b) heelstick site.

young children and infants, be sure not to overheat the washcloth as their skin is more sensitive. In addition, there are commercially available warmers that can be used.

Capillary specimens are collected in **microcontainers**—small plastic tubes specially designed to collect very small blood specimens. Similar to venous collection tubes, the microcontainers come in different colors to designate the different additives. (See Figure 12-8.)

After the specimen has been collected, check the site to make sure bleeding has stopped. When bleeding has stopped, you can apply a bandage. However, never apply a bandage to a child less than 2 years old, regardless of whether or not the incision was made on the finger or foot. Children at this age explore the world by putting things in their mouths and the bandage could become a choking hazard.

Order of Collection for Capillary Specimens

Due to the collection method, the order of collection is different for a capillary specimen. The order is as follows:

- Slide for blood smear (this may be done by the technologist—check with the lab)
- Lavender
- Other additive tubes
- Serum tubes

Though some point-of-care coagulation testing can be done, coagulation specimens cannot be collected with a fingerstick specimen due to the release of thromboplastin caused by the skin puncture and massaging of the site.

Blood cultures cannot be collected by capillary puncture due to the inability to properly disinfect the site and the inability to collect enough specimen.

bed. The index finger is not recommended as it contains a large number of nerves and therefore will be more painful for the patient. The little/fifth is not recommended due to its decreased tissue mass, which increases the risk of puncturing the bone. The thumb is not recommended because it is often calloused, thus making it harder to obtain a specimen. Furthermore, the thumb should not be used due to the presence of an artery, which could alter the composition of the specimen. (See Figure 12-7.)

When preparing the puncture site, cleanse the site with alcohol. Be sure to allow the alcohol to completely dry to prevent significant pain for the patient and decrease the risk of hemolyzing the specimen. Betadine should never be used to clean a fingerstick or heelstick site because betadine leaves residues that could contaminate the specimen and alter test results.

In order to facilitate collection, the puncture site should be prewarmed to increase blood flow up to seven times. Prewarming can be accomplished by using a warm, wet washcloth. When working with

Tips for Collecting a Quality Capillary Specimen

1. *Resuspend additives in the microcontainers.* The containers should be tapped to dislodge additives from the walls and the stopper prior to initiating collection. This is especially important for specimens with a powder additive that may be stuck to the sides or top of the container. This remixing process ensures that all of the specimen will come into equal contact with the additive, preventing microclots in anticoagulated specimens. The containers also should be tapped or gently shaken throughout the collection process to ensure mixing throughout the collection process.
2. *Wipe away the first drop of blood.* The first drop of blood contains a large amount of interstitial fluid, which could dilute the specimen. In addition, this step will remove any remaining residual alcohol.
3. *Avoid excessive squeezing of the puncture site.* Applying too much pressure to the puncture site can result in the introduction of excess interstitial fluid.
4. *Wipe the site between containers.* This action serves two purposes. First, it prevents any cross contamination that may occur since the finger does come into contact with each container. The second is that it helps to ensure additional bleeding through the collection process.

Skin Puncture Procedure

1. Review paperwork.
2. Identify yourself to the patient.
3. Verify patient identity.
4. Explain what you are going to do.
5. Confirm patient preparation.
6. Wash your hands and put on personnel protective equipment.
7. Assemble equipment.
8. Reassure and position the patient.
9. Puncture site should be prewarmed for at least 3 minutes.
10. Remix microcontainers with additives.
11. Clean the site with alcohol and allow it to air dry.
12. Support the finger or heel with your nondominant hand.
13. Puncture the selected site.
14. Allow the first drop of blood to form.
15. Wipe away the first drop of blood.
16. Hold the finger firmly and begin collecting the first specimen.
17. Wipe the site between specimens.
18. If microcontainers contain additive, tap tube several times during collection.
19. When all specimens have been collected, hold gauze on the puncture site.
20. Apply mild pressure and hold until bleeding stops.
21. When bleeding has completely stopped, apply bandage if appropriate.
22. Label specimen before leaving the patient's side.
23. Thank and release the patient.

Heelstick

Similar in procedure to the fingerstick, **heelsticks** are performed on newborns and infants who have not started to walk. The incision should be made on the side, fleshy portion of the heel. The center of the heel, the arch of the foot, and the toes are not acceptable for puncture. A puncture in one of these sites could result in damage to the nerves or tendons. Furthermore, there is the risk of puncturing the bone.

Maintaining Capillary Specimen Integrity

After the capillary specimen has been collected, there are some precautions that should be taken to ensure that the specimen integrity is preserved.

1. *Test the specimen as soon as possible.* Capillary blood samples should be tested as soon as possible after being drawn. Due to

Tips for Collecting a Heelstick Specimen

It can be incredibly stressful collecting a heelstick specimen from a baby. The baby cries because of the pain it feels from the incision and from being restrained during the procedure. While the crying and fussing can be very upsetting, remember the following:

1. Safely collecting a quality specimen is your number one responsibility. While you are causing the baby some distress, you are also performing a service to ensure that baby's well being.
2. Much of the crying is due to the baby being restrained. While the crying is upsetting, it can often promote blood flow, allowing the procedure to be completed more quickly.
3. Occasionally release the baby's foot and allow the baby to kick from time to time. This physical activity will help to increase the blood flow, allowing the specimen to be collected more quickly.

the very small size of the specimen, they are much more vulnerable to the environment. Lab personnel should adhere to specimen time constraints determined by the manufacturer of the test kit used in the office or by the reference lab to which the specimen will be sent. Note that the time constraints for a capillary specimen may be different than those of a venous specimen for the same test.

2. *Refrigerate specimens that will not be tested immediately.* When it is not possible to immediately test the specimen, be sure to store at 2 to 8 degrees Celsius.

3. *Keep specimen tubes capped at all times.* This should be done for safety reasons as well as specimen preservation.

4. *Avoid specimen agitation.* Capillary specimen red blood cells are more prone to hemolysis due to the collection technique. Hemolysis will occur when the specimen is agitated. Hemolyzed specimens are unacceptable for most chemistry and hematology procedures. Avoid shaking the specimen and always use gentle inversion to mix specimens.

Capillary Specimen Sources of Error

There are some specific sources of error that are related to the capillary specimen collection procedure.

1. *Abnormal fluid distribution caused by excessive squeezing.* Applying too much pressure to the puncture site when collecting the specimen can cause excess interstitial fluid to contaminate the specimen. This can significantly alter the test results by diluting the specimen.

2. *The presence of microclots.* Plasma or whole blood specimens that require anticoagulants should be free of clots. Anticoagulated specimens containing clots should be discarded. Note that the presence of clots, regardless of how small, requires the entire specimen must be discarded as constituency of the remaining blood is altered.

3. *Hemolysis.* Hemolysis may be caused by excessive squeezing or wet alcohol left at the puncture site.

4. *Altered chemistry results.* Serum and plasma in prolonged contact with the cells will result in changes in glucose, iron, LDH, and potassium levels.

SPECIAL PATIENTS

Some patients are more difficult to obtain a blood specimen from than others. Over time, as you gain experience, you will become more comfortable and proficient at obtaining samples from these individuals. During your learning period, take every opportunity to observe more experienced colleagues when they perform these procedures.

Patients Who Have Repeated Venipuncture Procedures

Veins can become hard and scarred from repeated use. Whenever possible, try to use a different site each time to avoid overuse of the same site. If the specimen requires only a small amount of blood, a capillary specimen may be a better choice.

Obese Patients

These patients can have especially deep veins that are difficult to find. Try the techniques listed in Chapter 11 to help find these veins. Again, if only a small specimen is required, capillary specimens may be an option.

Children

You should be especially patient when collecting a blood specimen from an infant or a child. Assistance is usually required. Parents can make the child feel more secure, but the parents may be uncomfortable with the procedure. When parents are unable to assist, seek help from another staff member. Infants must be held to prevent them from squirming and possibly rolling off the examination table while you are taking the sample.

When performing venipuncture on a child, explain the procedure as well as possible, given the child's age. In addition, be sure to give reassurance and praise. Tell older children that the procedure will hurt a little and that it is all right to cry. Never tell a child that it won't hurt. There is a minimal amount of pain associated with phlebotomy and telling the child it won't hurt is incorrect. It may work to gain the child's cooperation the first time, but it will make it harder to gain the child's trust in the future. It also may be useful to tell children that the blood is needed to help the doctor find out what is making them sick. Ask the child to try to hold still so the blood collection will be over more quickly and praise the child for any effort to cooperate.

Whenever the patient is an infant or a young child, the butterfly system is often easier to use due to the increased mobility of the system.

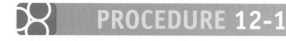

PROCEDURE 12-1

Venipuncture Using a Butterfly Needle and Evacuated Tube System

Goal

To successfully perform venipuncture using a butterfly needle and evacuated tube system.

Completion Time

15 minutes

Equipment and Supplies

- Impermeable lab coat, gown, or apron
- Face shield or goggles
- Disposable gloves
- Hand disinfectant
- Biohazardous container
- Sharps container
- 70 percent isopropyl alcohol or alcohol wipes
- Sterile gauze pads
- Tourniquets
- Evacuated tube holder
- Evacuated tubes
- Butterfly needle with adapter
- Bandage

Instructions

Read through the list of equipment and supplies that you will need. Read the steps of the procedure. Be sure that you understand each step before you begin. Then complete each step correctly and in the proper order. If your completion time is too long; repeat the procedure until you increase your speed.

Steps marked with (*) are critical and must have the maximum points to pass.

Performance Standards	Points Awarded	Maximum Points
1. Put on lab coat and face shield or goggles.		5
2. Disinfect hands; dry if necessary.		5
3. Put on gloves. Inspect for tears and replace if necessary.		5
4. Collect and prepare the appropriate equipment.		5
5. *Verify patient identity.		30
6. Explain the venipuncture procedure and encourage the patient to relax.		5
7. Remove the butterfly needle from its package. Screw the adapter end of the needle attached to the tubing into the needle holder and ensure that the needle is secure.		5
8. Place the tourniquet around the patient's arm above the elbow. If you cannot feel a pulse at the wrist, loosen the tourniquet.		5
9. Select a suitable vein by inspection and palpation. Determine the depth and direction the vein is running.		10
10. Clean the site with alcohol or betadine, using concentric circles, and allow the site to air dry.		5
11. Tell the patient to make a gentle fist and to hold the arm straight. Rest the arm on the armrest of the phlebotomy chair or on a table or countertop for support.		5
12. Place the evacuated tube in the needle holder until the short end of the needle touches the rubber stopper. Do not push the needle into the rubber stopper yet.		5

13.	Remove the cover from the butterfly needle.	5
14.	Grasp the butterfly needle by the "wings" with your dominant hand.	5
15.	Place your thumb below the puncture site, pulling the skin taut to anchor the vein.	5
16.	Hold the needle at a 10- to 15-degree angle with the bevel facing up.	5
17.	Insert the needle through the skin immediately adjacent to the vein to be punctured.	5
18.	Once you have penetrated the skin and vein, push the tube all the way into the back of the needle to engage the tube's vacuum.	10
19.	Release the tourniquet.	5
20.	Tell the patient to relax his/her hand.	5
21.	After the tube has stopped filling, collect the remaining tubes while observing the order of draw.	10
22.	As each tube is removed from the needle, gently invert the tube several times.	10
23.	Remove the last tube from the needle.	5
24.	Cover the puncture site with gauze, without applying pressure.	5
25.	*Withdraw the needle and engage the safety mechanism.	30
26.	Apply pressure to the puncture site for 3–5 minutes, keeping the patient's arm straight.	5
27.	Label each tube at the patient's side with the following information: patient's full name, identification number, the date, the time, and your initials.	15
28.	Check the puncture site to see if bleeding has stopped.	10
29.	When bleeding has stopped, apply a bandage. If bleeding does not stop within 5 minutes, notify the physician.	5
30.	Discard the needle and holder as a complete unit in the sharps container.	10
31.	Discard equipment properly, observing Standard Precautions.	10
32.	Disinfect your hands.	5
33.	Thank and release the patient.	10
	Total Points	**265**

Overall Procedural Evaluation

Student Name _____

Signature of Instructor _____ Date _____

Comments _____

_____

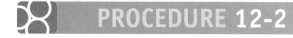

PROCEDURE 12-2

Venipuncture Using a Butterfly Needle and Syringe System

Goal

To successfully perform venipuncture using a butterfly needle and syringe system.

Completion Time

15 minutes

Equipment and Supplies

- Impermeable lab coat, gown, or apron
- Face shield or goggles
- Disposable gloves
- Hand disinfectant
- Biohazardous container
- Sharps container
- 70 percent isopropyl alcohol or alcohol wipes
- Sterile gauze pads
- Tourniquets
- Evacuated tubes
- Butterfly needle
- Transfer device
- 10- or 20-mL syringe
- Bandage

Instructions

Read through the list of equipment and supplies that you will need. Read the steps of the procedure. Be sure that you understand each step before you begin. Then complete each step correctly and in the proper order. If your completion time is too long, repeat the procedure until you increase your speed.

Steps marked with (*) are critical and must have the maximum points to pass.

Performance Standards	Points Awarded	Maximum Points
1. Put on lab coat and face shield or goggles.		5
2. Disinfect hands; dry if necessary.		5
3. Put on gloves. Inspect for tears and replace if necessary.		5
4. Collect and prepare the appropriate equipment.		5
5. *Verify patient identity.		30
6. Explain the venipuncture procedure and encourage the patient to relax.		5
7. Remove the butterfly needle from its package. Remove the cover from the short end of the needle. Screw the short end into the syringe and ensure that the needle is secure.		5
8. Remove the syringe from its wrapper and "prime" the syringe.		10
9. Place the evacuated tube in a tube rack, in the order of draw.		10
10. Place the tourniquet around the patient's arm above the elbow. If you cannot feel a pulse at the wrist, loosen the tourniquet.		5
11. Select a suitable vein by inspection and palpation. Determine the direction the vein is running and its depth.		10
12. Clean the site with alcohol or betadine, using concentric circles, allowing the site to air dry.		5
13. Tell the patient to make a gentle fist and to hold the arm straight. Rest the arm on the armrest of the phlebotomy chair or on a table or countertop for support.		5
14. Grasp the butterfly needle by the "wings" with your dominant hand.		5

15.	Place your thumb below the puncture site, pulling the skin taut to anchor the vein.	5
16.	Hold the needle at a 10- to 15-degree angle with the bevel facing up.	5
17.	Insert the needle through the skin immediately adjacent to the vein to be punctured.	5
18.	Once you have penetrated the skin, begin to slowly withdraw the blood by pulling on the plunger of the syringe.	10
19.	Release the tourniquet.	5
20.	Tell the patient to relax his or her hand.	5
21.	Continue pulling on the plunger until the syringe is full or you have collected enough blood.	10
22.	Cover the puncture site with gauze, without applying pressure.	5
23.	*Withdraw the needle and engage the safety mechanism.	30
24.	Ask the patient to apply pressure to the puncture site for 3–5 minutes, keeping the arm straight.	5
25.	*Remove and discard the syringe needle following the policy of your institute and replace with a transfer device.	30
26.	Pierce the first tube with the transfer device in the order of draw.	15
27.	Continue filling the tubes, allowing the tubes to fill on their own and not applying pressure to the plunger of the transfer device.	10
28.	As each tube is removed from the needle, gently invert the tube several times.	10
29.	Remove the last tube from the transfer device.	5
30.	Discard the syringe and transfer device as a unit.	15
31.	Label each tube at the patient's side with the following information: patient's full name, identification number, the date, the time, and your initials.	15
32.	Check the puncture site to see if bleeding has stopped.	5
33.	When bleeding has stopped, apply a bandage. If bleeding does not stop within 5 minutes, notify the physician.	5
34.	Discard equipment properly, observing Standard Precautions.	10
35.	Disinfect your hands.	5
36.	Thank and release the patient.	10
	Total Points	**330**

Overall Procedural Evaluation

Student Name _____

Signature of Instructor _____ Date _____

Comments _____

_____

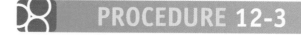

PROCEDURE 12-3

Capillary Puncture Method

Goal

To successfully perform a capillary puncture using a lancet.

Completion Time

15 minutes

Equipment and Supplies

- Impermeable lab coat, gown, or apron
- Face shield or goggles
- Disposable gloves
- Hand disinfectant
- Biohazardous container
- Sharps container
- 70 percent isopropyl alcohol or alcohol wipes
- Sterile gauze pads
- Microcontainers
- Lancet
- Bandage

Instructions

Read through the list of equipment and supplies that you will need. Read the steps of the procedure. Be sure that you understand each step before you begin. Then complete each step correctly and in the proper order. If your completion time is too long, repeat the procedure until you increase your speed.

Steps marked with (*) are critical and must have the maximum points to pass.

Performance Standards	Points Awarded	Maximum Points
1. Put on lab coat and face shield or goggles.		5
2. Disinfect hands; dry if necessary.		5
3. Put on gloves. Inspect for tears and replace if necessary.		5
4. Collect and prepare the appropriate equipment.		5
5. *Verify patient identity.		30
6. Explain the capillary puncture procedure and encourage the patient to relax.		5
7. Select an appropriate site.		10
8. Clean the site with alcohol, using concentric circles.		5
9. Allow the alcohol to completely dry.		5
10. Hold the patient's finger with your nondominant hand and gently apply pressure.		5
11. Quickly puncture the site with the lancet.		10
12. *Engage the lancet's safety mechanism if it is not automatic. Dispose of the lancet per institutional policy.		30
13. Wipe away the first drop of blood with dry gauze.		10
14. Collect the first specimen in the microcontainer, observing the order of draw. Apply gentle pressure, but avoid squeezing.		15
15. Continue collecting the microcontainers as needed.		10
16. As each microcontainer is filled, gently invert the tube several times.		10
17. When the last specimen has been collected, cover the puncture site with gauze and apply gentle pressure.		5

18.	Ask the patient to apply pressure to the puncture site for 3–5 minutes.	5
19.	Label each microcontainer at the patient's side with the following information: patient's full name, identification number, the date, the time, and your initials.	15
20.	Check the puncture site to see if bleeding has stopped.	5
21.	When bleeding has stopped, apply a bandage. If bleeding does not stop within 5 minutes, notify the physician.	5
22.	Discard equipment properly, observing Standard Precautions.	10
23.	Disinfect your hands.	5
24.	Thank and release the patient.	10
	Total Points	**225**

Overall Procedural Evaluation

Student Name _____

Signature of Instructor _____ Date _____

Comments _____

_____

chapter 12 REVIEW

Using Terminology

Define the following terms.

1. capillary

_____

_____

_____

2. point-of-care testing

_____

_____

_____

3. heelstick

_____

_____

_____

4. hematoma

_____

_____

_____

Match the following terms.

_____ **5.** lancet

_____ **6.** butterfly needle

_____ **7.** syringe

_____ **8.** microcontainer

_____ **9.** heelstick

_____ **10.** fingerstick

a. barrel and plunger

b. capillary puncture performed on an infant

c. small collection containers for capillary punctures

d. sharp, piercing object used for capillary punctures

e. capillary puncture performed on adults

f. needle with "wings"

11. List the order of draw for the *syringe* procedure

_____ a. lavender/EDTA

_____ b. blue/sodium citrate

_____ c. sterile/blood cultures

_____ d. red/no additive

_____ e. green/sodium heparin

_____ f. marble/gel separator

12. List the order of draw for the *capillary* procedure

_____ a. lavender/EDTA

_____ b. red/plain

_____ c. green/sodium heparin

_____ d. marble/gel separator

Multiple Choice

Choose the best answer for the following questions.

13. Which type of specimen cannot be collected by capillary puncture?

a. hematology

b. chemistry

c. blood cultures

d. serology

14. The angle of entry for a butterfly needle is

a. 3 degrees

b. 10 degrees

c. 20 degrees

d. 30 degrees

15. The advantage of utilizing a syringe in a venipuncture procedure is

a. It is a faster procedure

b. It decreases the risk of accidental needlestick

c. The phlebotomist controls the rate of blood withdrawal

d. There is less risk of a clot developing in an anticoagulated specimen

16. When performing a capillary puncture, you should

a. always use betadine disinfectant to prevent infection

b. cut with the grain of the fingerprint

c. cut against the grain of the fingerprint

d. perform fingerstick on newborns

17. When collecting blood from a patient with a mastectomy, you should
    a. never collect blood from a patient who has had a mastectomy
    b. not collect blood on the side on which the mastectomy was performed
    c. ask the patient on which side she prefers to have her blood drawn
    d. collect the specimen from her foot
18. When determining what type of phlebotomy technique you should use, the decision should be based on
    a. location of the selected site
    b. the physical condition of the patient
    c. amount of specimen needed
    d. all of the above

Acquiring Knowledge

Answer the following questions in the space provided.

19. How are capillary specimens different from venous specimens?

    _____

    _____

    _____

20. How should needles, lancets, and syringes be disposed of?

    _____

    _____

    _____

21. Why should you select a finger that is not calloused for a capillary puncture?

    _____

    _____

    _____

22. Why should you not excessively squeeze a capillary puncture site?

    _____

    _____

    _____

Acquiring Knowledge—On the Job

Answer the following questions in the space provided.

23. You are requested to obtain a small amount of blood from an infant. What blood collection technique should you use? Where and how do you make the incision?

    _____

    _____

    _____

24. Assume that you are employed by a POL as a phlebotomist. An elderly patient has returned after a recent phlebotomy with a large bruise at the puncture site. She is very alarmed. Explain to her why a hematoma may occur after a venipuncture. What steps should have been taken to minimize the chance of a hematoma?

_____

_____

_____

25. You have just completed a venipuncture. The patient begins to jerk uncontrollably. He appears to be having a seizure. What do you do?

_____

_____

_____

unit

IV

HEMATOLOGY

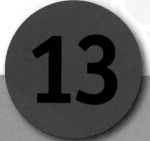

chapter

Hemoglobin and Hematocrit: Manual Procedures

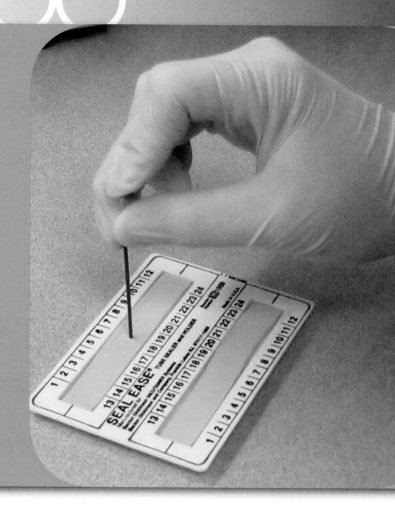

COGNITIVE OBJECTIVES

After studying this chapter, you should be able to

13.1 use each of the vocabulary terms appropriately.

13.2 list the blood tests performed as part of the complete blood count.

13.3 describe the structure, synthesis, and functions of normal hemoglobin.

13.4 identify three types of abnormal hemoglobin and describe the health problems caused by sickle-cell hemoglobin.

13.5 distinguish between hemoglobin concentration and hematocrit and give normal values for each.

13.6 explain how hemoglobin concentration and hematocrit values are used to assess the health of patients.

PERFORMANCE OBJECTIVES

After studying this chapter, you should be able to

13.7 determine the hemoglobin concentration from a blood specimen using a hemoglobinometer.

13.8 perform a microhematocrit by the manual method from a whole blood specimen.

TERMINOLOGY

adult hemoglobin: hemoglobin A.

anemia: the condition in which there is a deficiency in the amount of hemoglobin in the blood, thus reducing the oxygen-carrying capacity of the blood.

buffy coat: the 0.5- to 1.0-mm thick, whitish-tan layer of white blood cells and platelets that forms between the packed red blood cells and plasma when whole blood is centrifuged.

carotenemia: the presence of carotene in the blood.

complete blood count (CBC): a battery of hematological tests often requisitioned in POLs. It includes hemoglobin concentration, hematocrit, red and white blood cell counts, differential white blood cell count, and sometimes erythrocyte indices.

erythrocyte: a red blood cell.

erythropoiesis: the formation of red blood cells.

erythropoietin: the kidney hormone that triggers red blood cell formation. It is produced whenever hemoglobin concentration or oxygen saturation declines.

fetal hemoglobin: hemoglobin F.

hematocrit (Hct or "crit"): the volume of red blood cells packed by centrifugation in a given volume of blood. It is given as a percent.

hematology: the study of blood and blood-forming tissues.

hematology test: a blood test, including hematocrit, hemoglobin concentration, and red and white blood cell counts, among others.

hemoglobin A: the normal adult hemoglobin. It develops by 6 months of age to replace hemoglobin F, or fetal hemoglobin.

hemoglobin C: an abnormal hemoglobin that is more prevalent in African Americans. It causes chronic hemolytic anemia, splenomegaly, arthralgia, and abdominal pain.

hemoglobin E: an abnormal hemoglobin that is prevalent in India, Southeast Asia, and Southeast Asian immigrants in the United States. It causes a mild form of hemolytic anemia.

hemoglobin F: fetal hemoglobin. This hemoglobin is found in fetuses and infants until 6 months of age. It is replaced by hemoglobin A, or adult hemoglobin.

hemoglobin S: sickle-cell hemoglobin.

hemoglobin S-C disease: the disease in individuals heterozygous for hemoglobins S and C. The symptoms, which usually appear after age 40, include hematuria and pain in the bones, joints, abdomen, and chest.

hemoglobinopathy: any disease caused by abnormal hemoglobin.

hemolytic anemia: the anemia that is due to the breakdown of red blood cells.

hemolyze: the destruction of red blood cells, which releases the hemoglobin.

heterozygous: pertaining to the inheritance of different forms of a gene from each parent.

homozygous: pertaining to the inheritance of the same form of a gene from each parent.

hyperbilirubinemia: the presence of a high level of bilirubin in the blood.

iron-deficiency anemia: the anemia resulting from lack of or the inability to utilize available iron in the body.

leukemia: a disease characterized by unrestrained production of white blood cells.

lipemia: the presence of an abnormal amount of fat in the blood.

lyse: to break down a formed substance, such as red blood cells.

microhematocrit: a method of determining the hematocrit. It uses just two or three drops of blood collected in a capillary tube.

sickle-cell anemia: a life-threatening disease that occurs in individuals homozygous for the sickle-cell hemoglobin gene.

sickle-cell hemoglobin: the most common type of abnormal hemoglobin in the United States. It is found primarily in African Americans. Sickle-cell hemoglobin is so named because it causes red blood cells to become sickle shaped under conditions of low oxygen tension, thus producing sickle-cell anemia.

splenomegaly: the enlargement of the spleen. Splenomegaly is due to abnormal hemoglobin, among other possible causes.

INTRODUCTION

After urinalysis, **hematology** blood tests are the most frequently performed tests in the POLs. Hematology tests provide valuable information about the blood and blood-forming tissues in both healthy and disease states.

HEMATOLOGY PROCEDURES

The **hematology test** requested most often in the POL is the **CBC, complete blood count.** A CBC usually includes the following tests, which will be described in this and subsequent chapters:

- hemoglobin concentration—the weight of hemoglobin in grams per deciliter of whole blood

- hematocrit—the percent of red blood cells packed by centrifugation in a given volume of blood

- white blood cell count—the number of white blood cells per cubic millimeter of blood

- differential white blood cell count—the percent of each type of white blood cell seen on a stained blood smear

- red blood cell count—the number of red blood cells per cubic millimeter of blood
- red blood cell indices—indicators of size and hemoglobin content useful in diagnosis of anemias

All of the tests included in the CBC can be performed manually; however, most POLs have some type of automation that makes testing more efficient and time saving. CLIA waived testing as well as nonwaived testing will be included in the next chapters.

HEMOGLOBIN

A valuable diagnostic tool for the physician is the concentration of hemoglobin in a patient. To understand the tests and how to interpret them, it is important that you know more about this significant protein in the blood.

Normal Structure, Synthesis, and Function

Hemoglobin is the major component of red blood cells, or **erythrocytes,** comprising about 85 percent of their dry weight. Each hemoglobin molecule consists of four polypeptide chains, called globin chains, with a heme molecule attached to each chain, as Figure 13-1 shows. One oxygen molecule (O_2) can attach to each heme molecule. In the center of each heme molecule is an iron ion, so synthesis of each heme portion of the hemoglobin molecule requires iron. The source is dietary iron, which is absorbed in the duodenum of the small intestine.

Hemoglobin is produced by the endoplasmic reticula of red blood cells in the early stages of **erythropoiesis,** the formation of red blood cells. Figure 13-2 illustrates erythropoiesis. When new red blood cells are released from bone marrow into

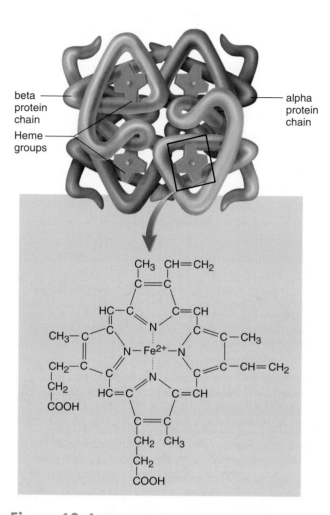

Figure 13-1 Normal hemoglobin molecule showing protein chains and heme.

the circulating blood, hemoglobin molecules are present and functioning.

The primary role of hemoglobin in the blood is to transport oxygen from the lungs to the cells. About 95 percent of the oxygen in the body is transported by the hemoglobin molecule. The remaining oxygen is dissolved in the plasma. Oxygen binds to the iron in the hemoglobin molecule, forming the molecule oxyhemoglobin, $HgbO_2$.

Hemoglobin is also responsible for transporting about 5 percent of the carbon dioxide, CO_2, from body

---

Erythropoiesis

Unlike nerve tissue or muscle tissue, blood is a tissue that continuously regenerates throughout life. As red blood cells die, new ones replace them in a process called erythropoiesis. Erythropoiesis is triggered by the kidney hormone **erythropoietin,** which is produced whenever hemoglobin concentration or oxygen saturation declines.

Erythropoiesis occurs almost entirely in the red bone marrow. The red bone marrow of basically all bones produces red blood cells from birth to about 5 years of age. Between the ages of 5 and 30, red bone marrow is limited to the flat bones of the ribs, sternum, vertebrae, and pelvis.

Carbon Monoxide Poisoning

The hemoglobin molecule has a greater affinity (attraction) for carbon monoxide than it does for oxygen and forms carboxyhemoglobin in carbon monoxide poisoning. Light to heavy cigarette smokers have 3 to 15 percent of carboxyhemoglobin levels in the blood, considered potentially significant.

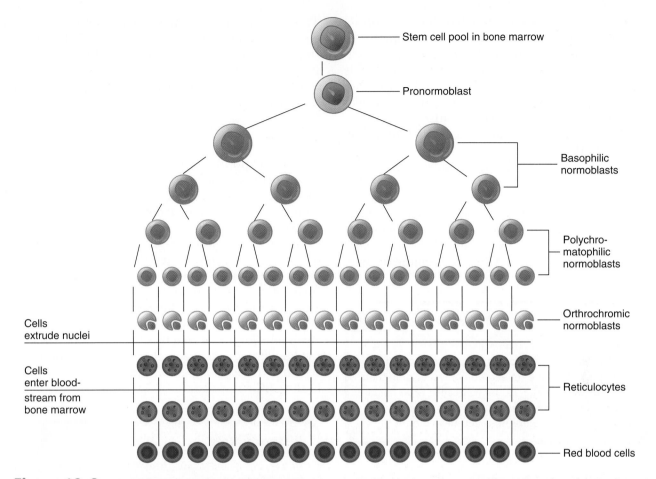

Figure 13-2 The stages of red blood cell formation, beginning in the bone marrow. The maturation time and life span for erythropoiesis are as follows: development from pronormoblast to release of reticulocyte from bone marrow = 72 hours; final development of reticulocyte in bloodstream = 1–2 days; life span of mature, circulating red blood cell = 120 days.

cells to the lungs, where it is expelled. The hemoglobin molecule combines with the carbon dioxide molecule to form carbaminohemoglobin, $HgbCO_2$.

A deficiency in circulating hemoglobin produces a condition called **anemia.** Anemia will result if any of the following occur:

* a reduction in the number of circulating red blood cells
* a decrease in the amount of hemoglobin per red blood cell
* a defect in the hemoglobin molecule

Anemia is not a disease in itself; it is a sign of underlying disease, just as a sore throat or a fever may be a sign of underlying viral infection. One cause of anemia is lack of available iron in the body. The amount of iron required varies from about 0.5 mg per day for adult males to 2 mg per day for menstruating females. Without adequate iron, hemoglobin production is hampered, and red blood cells have a lower-than-normal concentration of hemoglobin. The result is **iron-deficiency anemia.** It is usually treated with iron supplements.

Other factors that cause anemia include lack of erythropoietin, excessive or chronic bleeding, destruction of red blood cells, or malnutrition. Regardless of the cause, all patients with serious anemia are likely to be weak, easily fatigued, and prone to fainting because of reduced oxygen transport. They may be pale and have low blood pressure because of reduced blood volume. They may have heart palpitations or even congestive heart failure because of increased cardiac output.

Abnormal Hemoglobins

There are a number of relatively common forms of abnormal hemoglobin, including hemoglobins S, C, and E. All are inherited and controlled by codominant genes. Individuals who inherit two copies of one of these abnormal hemoglobin genes are said to be **homozygous.** They have only abnormal hemoglobin and suffer from **hemoglobinopathy,** or disease caused by abnormal hemoglobin. Invariably, they are anemic to some degree. Individuals with one abnormal gene and one normal gene are said to be **heterozygous.** They have enough normal hemoglobin to function without disease, but they are carriers of the abnormal gene, which they may pass on to their children.

Abnormal hemoglobins are most common in the parts of the world where the bloodborne disease malaria is prevalent. Heterozygous individuals tend to be partially resistant to malaria without suffering the harmful effects of abnormal hemoglobin. An increase in the frequency of these abnormal genes occurs in tropical Africa and Southeast Asia.

Screening for Abnormal Hemoglobin

Most screening for abnormal hemoglobin is postponed until after 6 months of age because fetuses and infants have a different form of hemoglobin than do older children and adults. It is called **fetal hemoglobin,** or **hemoglobin F.** It differs in structure from normal **adult hemoglobin,** called **hemoglobin A.**

Sickle-Cell Hemoglobin. Sickle-cell hemoglobin, or **hemoglobin S,** is the most common type of abnormal hemoglobin seen in the United States, occurring mainly in African Americans. Individuals homozygous for the gene for hemoglobin S have the life-threatening disease **sickle-cell anemia.** Hemoglobin S causes red blood cells to become sickle, or crescent, shaped when oxygen is taken up from the red blood cells by the surrounding tissues. This shape leads to obstruction of smaller blood vessels and destruction of the red blood cells by the body's own immune response. Severe **hemolytic anemia** results, that is, anemia due to the breakdown of red blood cells. Numerous other problems also result, including hyperplasia of bone marrow, impaired mental function, poor physical development, and damage to the heart, brain, joints, lungs, and kidneys.

Other Abnormal Hemoglobins. Another type of abnormal hemoglobin in African Americans is **hemoglobin C,** which causes chronic hemolytic anemia, **splenomegaly**—an enlarged spleen—joint pains, and abdominal pain. **Hemoglobin E** is prevalent in India and Southeast Asia, and in those of Southeast Asian descent in the United States. It causes a mild form of hemolytic anemia.

Some people inherit two different forms of abnormal hemoglobin, hemoglobin S and hemoglobin C.

This combination produces **hemoglobin S-C disease.** The symptoms, which are not life threatening, include hematuria, blood in the urine, and pain in the bones, joints, abdomen, and chest. Symptoms may not appear until the patient is in middle age.

Measuring Hemoglobin Concentration

The hemoglobin concentration is reported in grams per deciliter, g/dL, using whole blood and is measured routinely as part of the complete blood count. Hemoglobin concentration alone may be measured if anemia is suspected in the patient. There are several methods for determining the quantitative value of hemoglobin, most of which are performed by automated and semiautomated instruments. One common method used in POLs today is the handheld hemoglobinometer, which gives the physician quick and reliable results. Available for more extensive testing in POLs is the hematology analyzer, also called cell counters, which will test hemoglobin concentration as part of the CBC.

Historical Note

In the 1930s and 1940s, hemoglobin concentration was estimated by matching untreated blood samples to a color scale such as the Tallqvist and Dare methods. Another method, the Sahli-Hellige and Haden-Hausser method, used 1 percent hydrochloric acid solution to convert hemoglobin to hematin. Then, a hemoglobinometer was used to match the sample with a color standard. A later method converted hemoglobin to oxyhemoglobin by adding ammonium hydroxide. The resulting solution was read with a photoelectric colorimeter.

CLIA Waived Hemoglobinometer Test. The Hemo-Cue FIB 201® is one example of an instrument commonly used to measure hemoglobin. (See Figure 13-3.) Capillary blood or venous blood collected in EDTA can be used and is loaded in specially designed microcuvettes that contain the dried chemicals needed to **hemolyze** or **lyse** the red cells, thereby releasing the hemoglobin. Then the hemoglobin reacts further to form a compound called azidemethemoglobin, which is then automatically measured in the HemoCue photometer and the results are displayed on the digital readout. The system is calibrated by the factory and confirmed in the lab by running hemoglobin controls. The procedure for using a handheld hemoglobinometer, with performance standards, is at

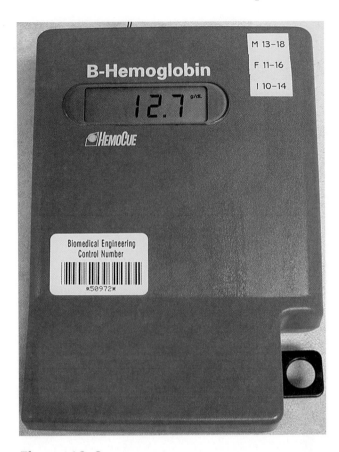

Figure 13-3 Hemoglobinometer used for measuring hemoglobin concentration from capillary or venous blood.

the end of this chapter. (See Figure 13-4.) Automated hematology, which includes the CBC, will be discussed and included in Chapter 16.

Cyanmethemoglobulin Test. This analysis converts hemoglobin to cyanmethemoglobin by the addition of a solution of potassium ferricyanide and sodium cyanide, commercially prepared and available in premeasured solutions. This reagent lyses the red cells, releasing the hemoglobin, and the reaction takes place. The solution is read photometrically using a spectrophotometer at a wavelength of 540 nm. This is the international reference method for the determination of hemoglobin concentration in blood and is used as a standard for other methods.

Limitations of Hemoglobin Determinations. Be aware that a number of blood conditions can sometimes cause falsely high hemoglobin readings. They include

- **hyperbilirubinemia**—the presence of a high level of bilirubin in the blood.
- **lipemia**—the presence of an abnormal amount of fat in the blood.
- **leukemia**—a disease characterized by unrestrained production of white blood cells.
- **carotenemia**—the presence of carotene in the blood.

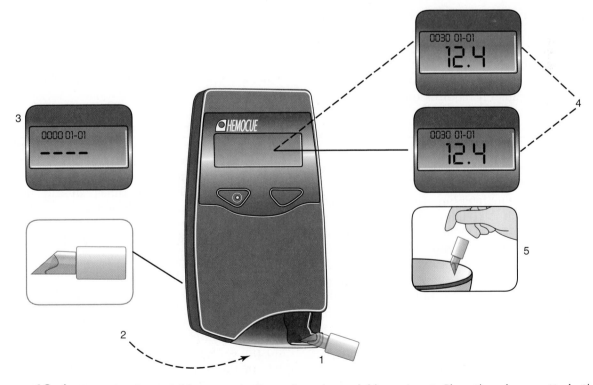

Figure 13-4 Measuring hemoglobin concentration using a hemoglobinometer: 1. Place the microcuvette in the holder. 2. Push the cuvette holder into the photometer measuring position. 3. Wait for the reading. 4. After 15–60 seconds the hemoglobin value will be displayed. 5. Dispose of biohazard properly.

Table 13-1 Normal Values for Hemoglobin Concentration

Age/Sex Group	Normal Hemoglobin Concentration (g/dL)
Adult males	14 to 18
Adult females	12 to 16
Newborns	17 to 23
Three-month-olds	9 to 14
Ten-year-olds	12 to 14.5

A high bilirubin value in neonatal jaundice, for example, can cause up to a 20 percent increase in the test result compared with the true value. Most manufacturers of hemoglobinometers use methods to compensate for turbidity in the blood sample.

Normal Values of Hemoglobin. Hemoglobin concentration values depend on the age and gender of the patient. Adult males and newborns have a higher normal value than adult females. The normal values for hemoglobin are included in Table 13-1.

THE HEMATOCRIT

The **hematocrit (Hct** or **"crit")** is a simple yet reliable test to measure the percent volume of red blood cells per volume of whole blood. Given as a percent, it is often used as an indirect measure of hemoglobin. In POLs, a **microhematocrit** method can be used because it requires only two or three drops of blood.

Cellular Layers

To measure the volume of red blood cells, you first must separate them from other blood components by high-speed centrifugation. During centrifugation, the red blood cells are packed at the bottom of the tube, as Figure 13-5 shows. Packed cell volume, or PCV, is another name for hematocrit. On top of the red blood cells are white blood cells and platelets, which form a 0.5 to 1.0 mm thick, whitish-tan layer called the **buffy coat.** Finally, plasma is at the top of the tube.

The Microhematocrit Method

Figure 13-6 illustrates the microhematocrit method. Either capillary puncture or venipuncture can be used to obtain microhematocrit blood samples.

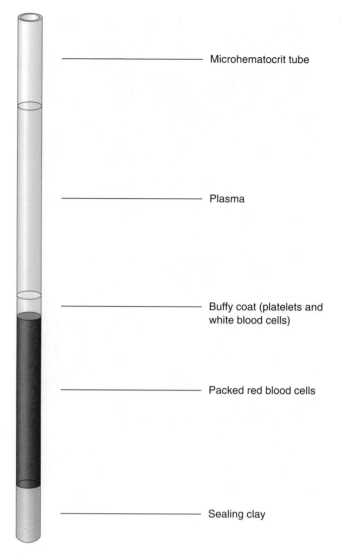

Microhematocrit tube

Plasma

Buffy coat (platelets and white blood cells)

Packed red blood cells

Sealing clay

Figure 13-5 The layers of centrifuged blood.

Duplicate samples always should be run as a quality control measure, and the results should be averaged. The two test results should agree within 2 percentage points.

Heparinized capillary tubes should be used when collecting capillary blood samples. They are filled about three-fourths full. If venous blood is used, it should be collected in an EDTA anticoagulant tube, lavender stopper. The venous blood is transferred to nonheparinized plain capillary tubes, which are filled about three-fourths full. The clean end of the tube is sealed with clay or a plastic cap. A gloved index finger should be placed over the open end to prevent blood from flowing into the sealing material. The seal must be complete or the test will give erroneously low results because red blood cells will be lost from the tube when it spins.

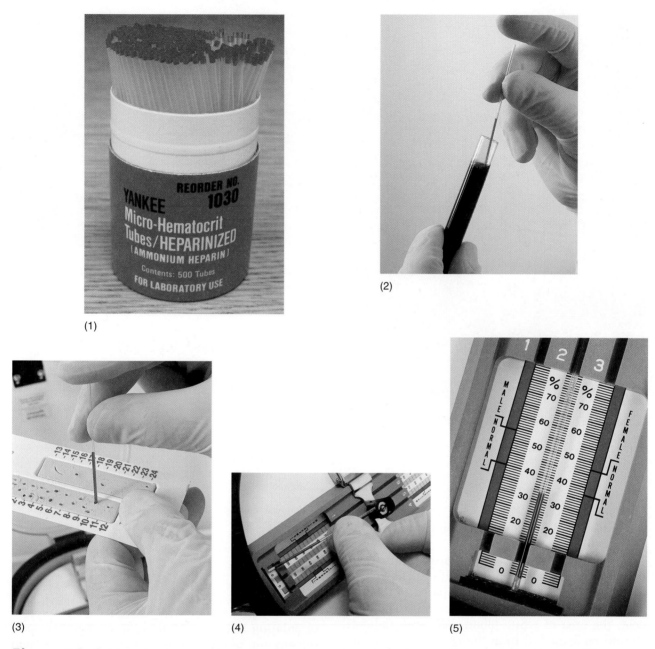

Figure 13-6 The microhematocrit method: (1) Collect the necessary supplies. Use heparinized capillary tubes for a capillary collection and nonheparinized tubes for venipuncture. (2) Collect the blood sample by either capillary puncture or venipuncture. (3) Seal the end of the capillary tube with clay or a plastic cap. (4) Place the sample in a microhematocrit centrifuge. Be sure to place the tubes in the centrifuge so that the sealed ends are pointing outward. (5) Compare the column of packed red blood cells in the microhematocrit tube with the hematocrit gauge to determine the hematocrit percentage and record the results.

The tubes are placed in the microhematocrit centrifuge with the sealed ends against the rubber gasket and the open ends pointing toward the center. The second tube is positioned opposite the first for balance. The cover is put on the centrifuge, and the centrifuge is spun according to the manufacturer's instructions, usually for 3 to 5 minutes. Some microhematocrit centrifuges have both an inside cover plus an outer lid, and others have only the outer lid cover. Centrifuging for too short a time produces falsely high readings because plasma is trapped among

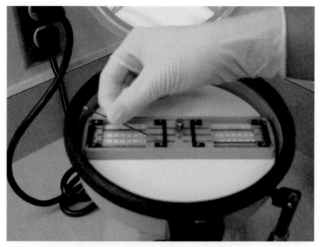

Figure 13-8 A microhematocrit with a built-in hematocrit reader.

Table 13-2 Normal Values for Hematocrit

Age/Sex Group	Normal Hematocrit Value (%)
Adult males	42 to 52
Adult females	36 to 46
Newborns	50 to 62
One-year-olds	31 to 39

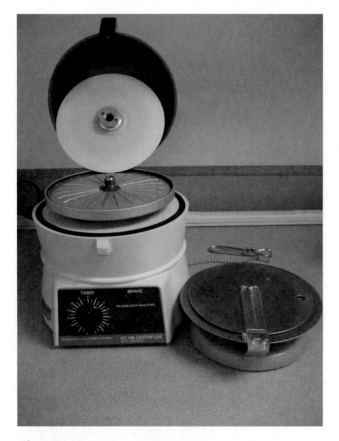

Figure 13-7 A microhematocrit centrifuge with a separate reader.

the red blood cells. This is especially likely in patients with hypochromic anemias and sickle-cell anemia.

As soon as the centrifuge stops spinning, the tubes are removed to prevent settling. The volume of packed red blood cells is compared to the total volume—the packed cells plus plasma. The buffy coat, the area of white blood cells and platelets, should be excluded from the reading. The hematocrit will be elevated if the buffy coat is included as part of the packed red blood cell volume. Some microhematocrit centrifuges have a separate reader (see Figure 13-7). Others have a built-in reader (see Figure 13-8), which allows laboratory personnel to determine the results while the tube is still in the centrifuge.

Quality control in hematocrit testing involves centrifuging control samples and comparing the results to the values given by the manufacturer of the controls. These usually are printed on the control bottle.

Normal Values for the Hematocrit

Normal values for the hematocrit vary by age and sex. See Table 13-2.

Interpreting Hematocrit Values

If the hematocrit is low, the number or volume of circulating red blood cells is low. In either case, the amount of circulating hemoglobin is less than normal and anemia results.

An elevated hematocrit can be caused by both normal physiological processes and disease states. For example, dehydration can cause an increase in hematocrit due to the decrease of body fluid, which affects the plasma level. The resulting hematocrit appears to have a greater number of RBCs, but, in fact, the RBC level is essentially the same as it was prior to the dehydration. Polycythemia vera, a chronic, usually fatal disease of the bone marrow, also can cause an increase in the hematocrit value. Iron deficiency anemia has a pattern of hematocrits that are higher than expected for the low hemoglobin reading. This is because the red blood cells lack hemoglobin due to the lack of dietary iron.

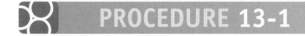

PROCEDURE 13-1

Measuring Hemoglobin Concentration

Goal

After successfully completing this procedure, you will be able to perform a hemoglobin concentration test using a hemoglobinometer.

Completion Time

20 minutes

Equipment and Supplies

- Disposable gloves
- Apron or lab coat
- Face shield
- Hand disinfectant
- Paper towels and tissues
- Biohazard waste container
- Hematology controls
- EDTA-anticoagulated blood specimen
- Hemoglobinometer
- Microcuvettes
- Paper and pen

Instructions

Read through the list of equipment and supplies that you will need and the steps of the procedure. Be sure that you understand each step before you begin. Then complete each step correctly, in the proper order, and within completion time.

*Steps marked with (*) are critical and must have the maximum points to pass.

Performance Standards	Points Awarded	Maximum Points
1. Wash your hands with disinfectant, dry them, and put on gloves, face shield, and apron or lab coat.		5
2. Follow standard precautions.		5
3. Assemble and prepare the appropriate equipment and supplies.		5
4. *Prepare the hemoglobinometer according to the manual supplied, checking calibration and/or optical self-test and hemoglobin controls.		15
5. *Inspect the EDTA-anticoagulated blood for proper labeling.		15
6. Mix the tube of EDTA-anticoagulated blood thoroughly.		5
7. Remove the cap from the tube of blood, using a tissue or cap remover; take care to avoid splattering blood.		5
8. *Load the microcuvettes, or other measuring device supplied or recommended by the manufacturer of the hemoglobinometer, with blood and wipe off any excess blood from the outside of the cuvette.		10
9. Load the cuvette into the holder of the photometric reader and push the measuring position.		5
10. Read the hemoglobin value from the display and record.		10
11. Discard all disposable materials in biohazard containers.		5
12. Disinfect the work area following standard precautions.		5
13. Remove and discard gloves and wash your hands.		5
14. Document procedure and record result in patient's chart.		10
Total Points		**105**

Overall Procedural Evaluation

Student Name _____

Signature of Instructor _____ Date _____

Comments _____

_____

PROCEDURE 13-2

Performing a Microhematocrit

Goal

After successfully completing this procedure, you will be able to perform a manual microhematocrit using centrifugation.

Completion Time

15 minutes

Equipment and Supplies

- Disposable gloves
- Apron or lab coat
- Face shield
- Hand disinfectant
- Surface disinfectant
- Paper towels and tissues
- Biohazard container
- EDTA-anticoagulated blood specimen
- Capillary tubes (plain)
- Sealing clay or plastic caps
- Microhematocrit centrifuge
- Hematocrit reader

Instructions

Read through the list of equipment and supplies that you will need and the steps of the procedure. Be sure that you understand each step before you begin. Then complete each step correctly, in the proper order, and within the completion time.

*Steps marked with (*) are critical and must have the maximum points to pass.

Performance Standards	Points Awarded	Maximum Points
1. Wash your hands with disinfectant, dry them, and put on gloves, face shield, and apron or lab coat.		5
2. Follow all standard precautions.		5
3. Collect and prepare the appropriate equipment and supplies.		10
4. *Inspect the EDTA-anticoagulant tube of blood for proper labeling.		15
5. Mix the tube of blood thoroughly.		5
6. Remove the cap from the tube of blood, using a tissue or cap remover; take care to avoid splattering the blood.		5
7. Tilting the tube so that the blood is near the opening, insert a plain capillary tube (nonheparinized) into the blood and allow it to fill by capillary action until about three-fourths full.		10
8. Remove the tube from the blood and wipe the outside of the capillary tube with a tissue to remove excess blood.		5
9. Using a gloved finger over one end of the tube, insert the other end of the capillary tube into a tray of sealing clay and seal the tube.		10
10. Repeat steps 7–9 for a second capillary tube of blood.		10

11.	Transfer the tubes to the centrifuge, recording the position number on the requisition or patient's chart. Make sure the centrifuge is balanced. The sealed end should be against the outside rubber gasket of the centrifuge.	10
12.	Secure the inner lid and clamp down the outer lid tightly.	5
13.	Centrifuge for the length of time recommended by the centrifuge manufacturer (usually 5 minutes).	5
14.	Allow the centrifuge to come to a complete stop before unlocking the lids.	5
15.	*Remove the tubes carefully to preserve their identity and place them in the hematocrit reader, first matching the total volume of the capillary tube to the 100 percent volume reading on the scale.	10
16.	Average the two readings and report this value as the patient's hematocrit. The readings have to agree within 2 percent. If not, repeat the procedure.	5
17.	Discard disposable equipment, specimens, and used supplies in the biohazardous waste container.	5
18.	Disinfect other equipment and return to storage.	5
19.	Clean the work area following standard precautions.	5
20.	Remove gloves and apron and wash your hands and dry them.	5
21.	Document the results in the patient's chart.	10
	Total Points	**150**

Overall Procedural Evaluation

Student Name _____

Signature of Instructor _____ Date _____

Comments _____

_____

chapter 13 REVIEW

Using Terminology

Match the term in the right column with the appropriate definition or description in the left column.

_____ **1.** a blood test measured in g/dL   a. erythrocyte

_____ **2.** a disease caused by abnormal hemoglobin   b. erythropoiesis

_____ **3.** having two copies of the same gene   c. hematocrit

_____ **4.** an oxygen-carrying molecule   d. hemoglobin test

_____ **5.** a red blood cell   e. hemoglobin

_____ **6.** red blood cell formation   f. hemoglobinopathy

_____ **7.** the volume of packed red blood cells   g. homozygous

Define the following terms in the spaces provided.

8. Buffy coat

_____

_____

_____

9. Hemolysis

_____

_____

_____

10. Microhematocrit

_____

_____

_____

11. Hemoglobin C

_____

_____

_____

12. Hemoglobin S

_____

_____

_____

13. Hemolytic anemia

_____

_____

_____

14. Hemoglobin E

_____

_____

_____

15. Complete blood count (CBC)

_____

_____

_____

16. Erythropoietin

_____

_____

_____

Multiple Choice

Choose the best answer for the following questions.

17. The normal range for hemoglobin concentration for a male includes
   a. 15.5 g/dL
   b. 18.5 g/dL
   c. 12.9 g/dL
   d. 11.8 g/dL

18. Which of the following gives the color to red blood cells

a. oxygen

b. plasma

c. hemoglobin

d. buffy coat

19. Normal adult hemoglobin is

a. Hgb A

b. Hgb F

c. Hgb C

d. Hgb N

20. Which of the following is not a part of a routine CBC?

a. hemoglobin

b. red blood cell count

c. hematocrit

d. plasma percentage

21. The major component of red blood cells, comprising about 85 percent of their dry weight, is

a. heme

b. oxygen

c. hemoglobin

d. iron

22. Erythropoiesis, the process of red cell production that takes place in the bone marrow, is triggered by the hormone erythropoietin, which is produced by the

a. liver

b. kidney

c. brain

d. bone marrow

23. A patient with sickle-cell disease would have which of the following types of hemoglobin?

a. Heterozygous hemoglobin AS

b. Homozygous hemoglobin S

c. Homozygous hemoglobin C

d. Heterozygous hemoglobin SC

24. The layers of blood in a microhematocrit after centrifugation include

a. plasma, buffy coat, red blood cells

b. serum, buffy coat, white cells, hemoglobin

c. plasma, white cells, platelets

d. hemoglobin, red cells, platelets

25. Which of the following is a normal hematocrit value for a newborn female?

a. 35%

b. 40%

c. 55%

d. 72%

26. Polycythemia vera, a disorder of the bone marrow, would cause the hematocrit to be

a. increased

b. decreased

c. normal

Acquiring Knowledge

Answer the following questions in the spaces provided.

27. Describe the functions of hemoglobin.

_____

_____

_____

28. List the hemoglobin concentration and hematocrit values for normal adult males, adult females, and newborns.

_____

_____

_____

29. Explain how red blood cell formation is regulated.

_____

_____

_____

30. How is hematocrit expressed?

_____

_____

_____

31. What tests usually are included in a complete blood count?

_____

_____

_____

32. What disease causes a low hemoglobin concentration and a normal hematocrit? Why?

_____

_____

_____

33. Describe the structure of the hemoglobin molecule.

_____

_____

_____

34. What are hemoglobinopathies?

_____

_____

_____

35. What is the most common abnormal hemoglobin in the U.S. population? What group is most often affected? Why?

_____

_____

_____

36. How did sickle-cell hemoglobin acquire its name?

_____

_____

_____

37. How do sickle-cell hemoglobin homozygous individuals differ from heterozygous individuals?

_____

_____

_____

38. What disease do physicians suspect when they order only a hemoglobin and a hematocrit?

_____

_____

_____

39. Name four conditions that could cause a falsely high hemoglobin reading.

_____

_____

_____

Applying Knowledge—On the Job

Answer the following questions in the spaces provided.

40. In the lab where Sonja works, an African-American husband and wife recently had their blood tested and were surprised to learn that each is heterozygous for sickle-cell hemoglobin. Because neither ever has had any symptoms of sickle-cell anemia nor known any close relatives to have sickle-cell anemia, they cannot understand how they could have a child with this life-threatening disease. What is the explanation for this?

_____

_____

_____

41. As part of a routine complete blood count, a 35-year-old female patient's hematocrit was determined to be 38 percent and her hemoglobin concentration was measured at 10 g/dL. What diagnosis is likely? Why?

_____

_____

_____

42. An apparently healthy male patient, age 44, has a hemoglobin concentration of 28 g/dL. Why should you suspect that this reading is incorrect? What might be the cause?

_____

_____

_____

43. Josh and Mark just started working in the same lab together, and they are having an argument about how to read hematocrits. Josh says that you should not include the "white part," while Mark says everything but the "watery part" should be included. Who is right? Why?

_____

_____

_____

44. When Alberto centrifuged two capillary tubes of blood from the same newborn patient for a hematocrit reading, one tube gave a result of 50 percent and the other gave a result of 56 percent. Should Alberto consider these results close enough to be in agreement? Why or why not?

_____

_____

_____

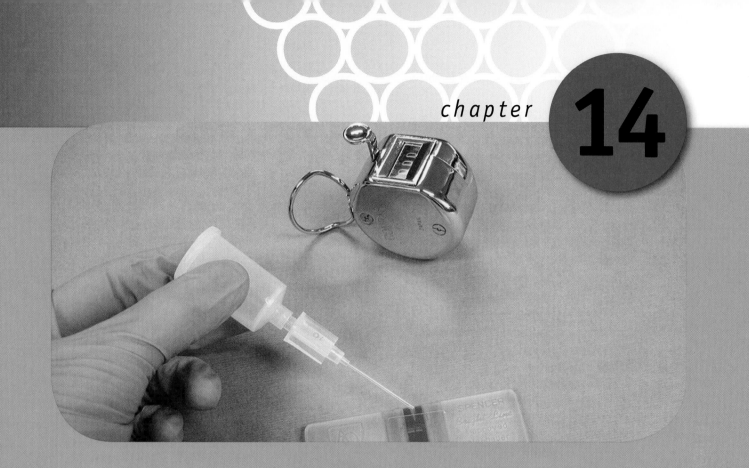

WBC and RBC Counts: Manual Procedures

COGNITIVE OBJECTIVES

After studying this chapter, you should be able to

14.1 use each vocabulary term appropriately.

14.2 list normal values for white and red blood cell counts by age and sex.

14.3 identify the ranges of abnormally low and high white and red blood cell counts and name at least one cause of each condition.

14.4 explain the components of the white and red blood cell count formulas.

14.5 discuss how the presence of nucleated red blood cells affects the white blood cell count and how to correct for this bias.

14.6 identify several sources of potential error in performing white blood cell and red blood cell counts.

PERFORMANCE OBJECTIVES

After studying this chapter, you should be able to

14.7 perform a manual white blood cell count with a Unopette kit and a hemacytometer and use the result to calculate the number of white blood cells per cubic millimeter.

14.8 perform a manual red blood cell count with a Unopette kit and a hemacytometer and use the result to calculate the number of red blood cells per cubic millimeter.

TERMINOLOGY

absolute polycythemia: erythrocytosis; an increase in the number of red blood cells because of increased red blood cell production.

agglutination: a clumping together, as of red blood cells.

anoxia: a deficiency of oxygen.

aplastic anemia: anemia caused by deficient red blood cell production, due to disorders of the bone marrow.

coverslip: small, thin glass used to cover liquid specimens on slides to protect the microscope and stabilize the specimen. A special coverslip is manufactured for use by the hemacytometer.

epinephrine: adrenaline; an adrenal gland hormone that stimulates the sympathetic nervous system.

erythremia: polycythemia vera.

erythrocyte count: red blood cell count.

erythrocytosis: absolute polycythemia.

hemacytometer: a counting device or counting chamber to count cells such as red or white blood cells.

hemolyze: the destruction of red blood cells, which releases the hemoglobin.

isotonic: having the same osmotic pressure. An isotonic solution with the same osmotic pressure as red blood cells is used to prepare blood for red blood cell counts.

leukocyte count: white blood cell count.

leukocytosis: an abnormally high white blood cell count.

leukopenia: an abnormally low white blood cell count, usually below 4,500/mm^3.

neoplasm: an abnormal growth of tissue, such as a tumor.

nucleated red blood cell (nRBC): a red blood cell that contains a nucleus. It resembles a white blood cell under low-power magnification and may erroneously inflate the white blood cell count.

pernicious anemia: a potentially fatal form of anemia that may be due to deficiency or malabsorption of vitamin B$_{12}$. Pernicious anemia is associated with an abnormally low white blood cell count.

polycythemia: an increase above normal in the number of red blood cells in circulation.

polycythemia vera: erythremia; a chronic, usually fatal disease of the bone marrow that results in greatly elevated red blood cell counts.

pseudoagglutination: the clumping together of red blood cells as in the formation of rouleaux but differing from true agglutination in that the clumped cells can be dispersed by shaking.

red blood cell (RBC) count: erythrocyte count; the number of red blood cells per cubic millimeter of blood; performed manually by counting red blood cells under high-power magnification on a hemacytometer. Whole blood is diluted with an isotonic solution that prevents lysing of red blood cells.

relative polycythemia: an increase in red blood cells relative to plasma volume. It occurs due to dehydration.

reticulocyte: an immature red blood cell that retains traces of endoplasmic reticula.

rouleaux: a clump of red blood cells that appear to be stacked like a roll of coins.

white blood cell (WBC) count: leukocyte count; the number of white blood cells per cubic millimeter of blood; counted manually under low-power magnification on a hemacytometer. Whole blood is diluted with a solution that lyses red blood cells.

INTRODUCTION

Both white and red blood cells frequently are counted in POLs to diagnose patient conditions, follow the progress of disease, or monitor patient treatment. In this chapter, you will learn how to count white and red blood cells and how to interpret the results.

THE WHITE BLOOD CELL COUNT

The **white blood cell (WBC) count,** or **leukocyte count,** is one of the tests included in a complete blood count. The WBC count measures the total number of white blood cells per cubic millimeter of whole blood. The chief functions of white blood cells are to fight infection and to provide immunity, so the WBC count is performed most often to diagnose infection in the body.

Normal Values for the WBC Count

Normal values for the WBC count vary by age (see Table 14-1). In general, the count declines as individuals get older. In healthy individuals, the WBC count varies throughout the day. It is lowest in the morning and gradually rises by about 2,000 cells/mm^3 through midafternoon, when it peaks. The WBC count also rises with meals, with strenuous exercise, with stress, with exposure to temperature extremes such as cold baths, and during pregnancy. The WBC count decreases when an individual is at rest.

Abnormal Values for the WBC Count

A WBC count may reveal either more or fewer white blood cells than normal due to a variety of pathological conditions (see Figure 14-1).

Table 14-1   Variation in WBC Count by Age

Age Group	WBC Count (cells/mm³)
Newborns	9,000 to 30,000
One-year-olds	8,000 to 14,000
Adults	4,500 to 12,000

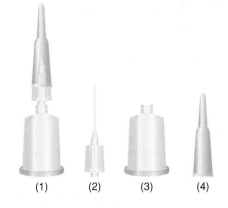

50,000 and above

Some cancers

Leukocytosis (elevated white blood cell count)		Bacterial infections Acute hemorrhage Stress Physiological factors
White blood cells Normal range for adults	12,000	Normal WBC count varies with age of patient, time of day, level of excercise, etc.
Leukopenia (depressed white blood cell count)	4,500	Viral infections, other causes
	1,000	Dangerous low limit

Figure 14-1 Normal and abnormal variation in the WBC count.

Abnormally High WBC Count. Leukocytosis refers to an abnormally high WBC count. Pathological conditions that may cause leukocytosis include, most commonly, bacterial infections and leukemia. Other causes include acute hemorrhage, sudden hemolysis of red blood cells, growing malignant **neoplasms** of the gastrointestinal tract or liver, epileptic seizures, **epinephrine** or adrenaline injections, pain, and **anoxia,** a deficiency of oxygen. The anoxia caused by cigarette smoking, for example, increases the WBC count by as much as 30 percent.

Abnormally Low WBC Count. Leukopenia refers to an abnormally low WBC count, usually below 4,500 cells/mm³. Conditions that may produce

leukopenia include viral infections such as flu and measles and exposure to radiation, lead, and mercury. Patients with **pernicious anemia,** a potentially fatal form of anemia that may be due to deficiency or malabsorption of vitamin B_{12}, also have an abnormally low WBC count. In pernicious anemia, the WBC count usually is in the range of 3,000 to 4,000 cells/mm³ and may fall below 2,000 cells/mm³. A WBC count of 1,000/mm³ or lower is considered to be dangerously low.

A Manual WBC Count

For a manual WBC count, a sample of whole blood is diluted with a solution that will **hemolyze** the red blood cells, leaving only the white blood cells intact. A solution of acetic acid is used to destroy the red blood cells and then the diluted sample is introduced into a **hemacytometer** counting chamber and the white blood cells are systematically counted under low-power magnification. In the POL, manual cell counts are most often performed because of an extremely low automated white blood cell count. The Unopette® system is the method most often used and the procedure will be described.

Manual WBC Count Using BD Unopette™ Kit. In this procedure, whole blood is added to a hemolyzing solution, mixed, and loaded in a hemacytometer and then the white blood cells are counted systematically. The Unopette kit consists of a prefilled disposable reservoir of 3 percent acetic acid as the diluting solution, a capillary pipette for measuring and mixing, and a pipette shield. A reservoir containing 0.475 mL of diluting solution is used with a 25 μL pipette of blood to yield a dilution of 1:20. A reservoir containing 1.98 mL of diluting solution is used with a 20 μL pipette of blood to yield a dilution of 1:100. The latter should be used when the WBC count is high. (See Figure 14-2.)

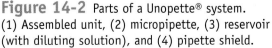

Figure 14-2 Parts of a Unopette® system. (1) Assembled unit, (2) micropipette, (3) reservoir (with diluting solution), and (4) pipette shield.

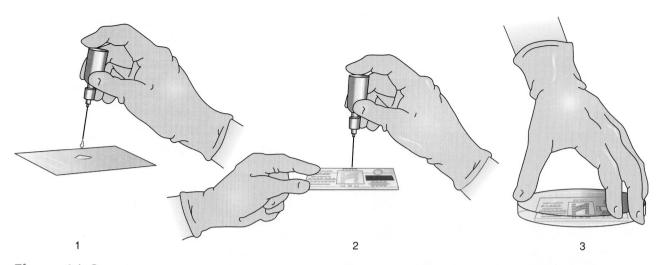

1

2

3

Figure 14-3 Charging a hemacytometer. (1) Expel two or three drops of fluid from the Unopette® pipette or blood cell pipette onto an absorbent tissue. (2) Let the fluid from the pipette fill the space between the coverslip and the hemacytometer. (3) Let the filled hemacytometer stand for 2 minutes before counting.

After mixing blood and diluting fluid in the reservoir, let the sample stand at least 10 minutes for the red blood cells to hemolyze before charging the hemacytometer. The sample may stand up to 3 hours at room temperature.

Charging the Hemacytometer. Clean the hemacytometer and **coverslip** with lens cleaner or alcohol and wipe dry. Position the coverslip over both sides of the hemacytometer. Using the dropper assembly of the Unopette reservoir and capillary pipette, discard a few drops of diluted blood. Gently squeeze the sides of the reservoir and fill the hemacytometer, allowing the sample to flow evenly under the coverslip and avoiding the depressed area, or moat, around the platform. Most hemacytometers have a V-shaped trough to help in the filling process. If the chamber overflows or if air bubbles form, clean the counting chamber, dry it, and refill it. After charging one side of the chamber, repeat the process on the other side. Then allow the filled chamber to stand 2 minutes in a moist covered dish, like a Petri dish, before counting to let the cells settle and stabilize. (Note: The moist Petri dish will also prevent excess evaporation and maintain proper dilution.) (See Figure 14-3.)

Counting the Sample. As Figure 14-4 shows, count the cells in the four corner squares, first on one side of the counting chamber and then on the other side. Use the average of the two sides in the WBC count formula. Each corner square measures 1 mm × 1 mm and is divided into 16 smaller squares.

Under low-power magnification, begin the count in the upper left corner and move through the 16 small squares systematically (see Figure 14-5).

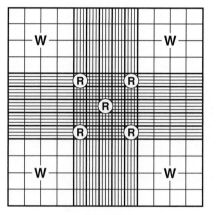

Figure 14-4 The ruled areas of a hemacytometer. Count the four corner squares labeled W for WBC count under the 10X objective. Count the five areas labeled R for an RBC count under the 45X objective.

Move horizontally across each row, starting at the top, and then go to the next adjacent row and repeat. Count the cells touching the border lines on just two sides of the corner square, omitting from the count cells that touch the border lines of the other two sides (see Figure 14-6). A hand tally counter is used when counting blood cells.

After counting all the cells in the upper left corner square in this way, repeat the process for the remaining three corner squares. If the counts for the four corner squares differ from one another by more than 10 cells, discard the count, clean the counting chamber, refill it, and start the counting process over again. Such an uneven distribution of cells usually is caused by a dirty hemacytometer or coverslip.

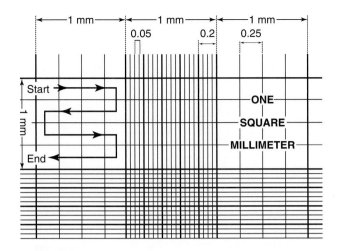

Figure 14-5 Counting the 16 small squares in each corner square. The direction followed in a WBC count through the 16 small squares must be consistent on each large square to prevent overlooking cells in the count.

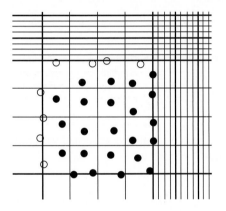

○ Skip these cells in the white blood cell count
● Count these cells in the white blood cell count

Figure 14-6 Count the cells that touch the borderlines on two sides of the corner square. Leave uncounted the cells that touch the borderlines of the other two sides of the square.

When Nucleated Red Blood Cells Are Present. Nucleated red blood cells (nRBC) resemble white blood cells when viewed under low-power magnification. Very few nucleated red blood cells normally are present in circulating blood, but they may reach significant numbers in cases of hemorrhage. Because nucleated red blood cells are not lysed by acetic acid, they may remain intact in the sample and inflate the WBC count. Nucleated red blood cells must be distinguished from white blood cells using 100X magnification on a stained blood smear, and their number per 100 white blood cells must be noted on the lab report. Their number per 100 white cells is used to correct the overall WBC count, as described below.

Calculating the WBC Count

The following formula is used to calculate the number of white blood cells per cubic millimeter of blood in the sample:

$$\text{WBC/mm}^3 = \frac{\text{Average number of cells counted} \times \text{Dilution factor} \times \text{Depth factor}}{\text{Area counted}}$$

Components of the WBC Count Formula. The number of cells counted in the WBC count formula is the average of the cells counted on both sides of the hemacytometer counting chamber, as described. The dilution factor is the ratio of blood to the total volume of blood plus diluting solution. In the WBC Unopette kit, the dilution factor is either 20 or 100, depending on which volume of diluent is used.

The depth factor in the formula is a constant, 10. It represents the depth of fluid between the counting chamber platform and the coverslip. The actual distance always is 0.1 mm, but the constant 10 is used so that the answer gives the number of cells present in 1 mm of depth (0.1 mm × 10 = 1.0 mm). The area counted is most often the four corners of the hemacytometer counting chamber, which cover a total of 4 mm². If the total area on each side of the counting chamber is counted instead of just the four corners, the area counted is 9 mm². The total area may be counted when the WBC count is low.

Whenever the dilution is 1:20 and just the four corners are counted, so the counting area is 4 mm², you can use this shorthand formula for calculating the WBC count:

$$\text{WBC/mm}^3 = \text{Number of cells counted} \times 50$$

because

$$\frac{\text{Dilution factor} \times \text{Depth factor}}{\text{Area counted}} = \frac{(20 \times 10)}{4} = \frac{200}{4} = 50$$

Using the Formula: A Worked Example. Assume that you have counted 28, 32, 33, and 26 white blood cells in the four corners of one side of the counting chamber and 31, 32, 25, and 33 white blood cells in the four corners of the other side. The total cells counted on the two sides are 119 and 121, for an average of 120 cells counted. Use your calculator to verify this. Also assume that the blood dilution is 1:20. Depth and area are the constants 10 and 4, respectively. Substituting into the formula, you get

$$\text{WBC/mm}^3 = \frac{120 \times 20 \times 10}{4} = 6,000$$

Correction for Nucleated Red Blood Cells. When significant numbers of nucleated red blood cells are present in a sample, the WBC count will be inflated unless their number per 100 white blood cells is known and used to correct the WBC count. The following two formulas are used:

$$nRBC/mm^3 = \frac{nRBC}{100 + \text{Number of nRBC}} \times WBC/mm^3$$

$$\begin{array}{c}WBC/mm^3 \\ \text{(corrected)}\end{array} = WBC/mm^3 - nRBC/mm^3$$

Consider the following example. Assume that the WBC count is 11,000 and a blood smear under 100X magnification shows 10 nucleated red blood cells per 100 white blood cells. The number of nucleated red blood cells/mm³ is calculated as

$$nRBC/mm^3 = \frac{10}{(100 + 10)} \times 11,000 = 1,000$$

The corrected WBC count is then

$$WBC/mm^3 \text{ (corrected)} = 11,000 - 1,000 = 10,000$$

THE RED BLOOD CELL COUNT

The **red blood cell (RBC) count,** or **erythrocyte count,** is another test included in the complete blood count. The RBC count determines the number of red blood cells per cubic millimeter of blood. Both mature red blood cells and immature red blood cells, called **reticulocytes,** are included in the count. The chief role of red blood cells is to transport oxygen to the tissues. A deficiency of red blood cells produces anemia, and diagnosing anemia is the most common reason for performing an RBC count. Normal values for an RBC count vary by age and sex (see Table 14-2).

Reticulocytes

Most red blood cells that are released from the bone marrow are in the reticulocyte stage. They retain traces of endoplasmic reticula that produce hemoglobin early in red blood cell formation. In circulating blood, reticulocytes mature into erythrocytes in 1 to 2 days. Normally, reticulocytes make up about 1 percent of the total RBC count.

Table 14-2   Normal Values for the RBC Count

Age/Sex Group	RBC Count (millions/mm³)
Newborns	5.0 to 6.5
One-year-olds	4.0 to 5.0
Adult females	4.0 to 5.5
Adult males	4.5 to 6.0

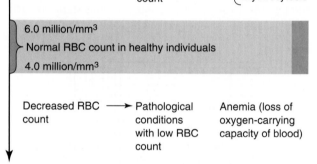

Figure 14-7 Normal and abnormal variation in the RBC count.

Abnormal Values for the RBC Count

An RBC count may reveal either more red blood cells or fewer red blood cells than normal due to a variety of pathological conditions (see Figure 14-7). Both conditions are stressful for the body.

An Abnormally High RBC Count. Polycythemia is an increase above normal in the number of red blood cells in circulation. There are two ways this may come about: through a decrease in blood fluid or through an increase in red blood cell production.

Relative polycythemia is the increase in red blood cells relative to plasma volume, which occurs with dehydration. This can be caused by a decrease in fluid intake or by loss of body fluids due to diarrhea or vomiting.

Absolute polycythemia, also known as **erythrocytosis,** is an increase in red blood cell production for any of a variety of reasons, including

- low oxygen tension in the blood due to high altitude or pulmonary diseases like emphysema.

- slowing of the circulation due to heart disease.
- defects in the hemoglobin molecule.

Polycythemia vera, also known as **erythremia,** is a type of absolute polycythemia in which RBC counts may be as high as 7 to 10 million cells/mm³. It is due to an unknown disorder of the bone marrow.

An Abnormally Low RBC Count. A low RBC count means that there are fewer than normal red blood cells per given volume of blood. With fewer red blood cells, there is less hemoglobin, and anemia results. Causes of abnormally low RBC counts include some therapeutic drugs and bone marrow disorders that reduce red blood cell production. The latter produce **aplastic anemia.**

Drugs and Anemia

Many different drugs may reduce red blood cell production or cause hemolysis of red blood cells, leading to a low RBC count. If your patient has a low RBC count, find out if it may be due to a drug such as the following:

- antineoplastic drugs such as azathioprine
- analgesics such as aspirin
- antimicrobials such as penicillin
- anticonvulsants such as primidone
- antimalarials such as chloroquine
- heavy metals such as gold compounds
- oral hypoglycemics such as rosiglitazone maleate
- psychotropics such as chlorpromazine
- diuretics such as furosemide

A Manual RBC Count

Performing a manual RBC count is very similar to performing a manual WBC count. A sample of whole blood is diluted, mixed, and introduced into a hemacytometer for counting. For RBC counts, however, the diluting solution is an isotonic solution, not an acid. The **isotonic** solution prevents hemolysis of the red blood cells because it has the same osmotic pressure as the red blood cells. Also for RBC counts, high-power magnification is used instead of low-power magnification for counting the cells.

Manual RBC Count Using BD Unopette™ Kit. The Unopette method for performing red blood cell counts is very similar to that described previously for the white blood cell manual counts. The red blood cell Unopette kit contains a disposable reservoir prefilled with 1.99 mL of 0.85 percent saline (sodium chloride) solution containing sodium azide as a preservative, a 10 μL capillary pipette, and pipette shield. The dilution is 1:200. After blood and diluting fluid are mixed in the Unopette reservoir, the sample can be kept at room temperature for up to 6 hours.

Charging the Hemacytometer. Charge the hemacytometer the same way as for a WBC count. Be sure that the counting chamber and coverslip are clean, and discard the first two or three drops from the Unopette capillary pipette dropper assembly (see Figure 14-2). Let the sample flow evenly under the coverslip. If any sample flows into the moat or if air bubbles form, clean the counting chamber and start over again. After filling both sides of the counting chamber, let the sample stand for 3 minutes before performing the count.

If the blood sample is too cold, it may cause **agglutination,** or clumping, of red blood cells on the hemacytometer. If you observe agglutination, dilute another specimen and warm it to body temperature before charging the hemacytometer. If warming does not eliminate the agglutination, it may be due to the presence of paraprotein in the sample, which is an indicator of multiple myeloma or other immunoglobulin disorder. Paraprotein produces **pseudoagglutination** of red blood cells, with the formation of **rouleaux,** clumps of red blood cells that appear to be stacked like rolls of coins. In pseudoagglutination, the red blood cells can be dispersed by shaking the sample.

Counting the Sample. It is at this stage of the procedure that the RBC count differs most from the WBC count. The RBC counting area on the hemacytometer is the 1 mm² square area located in the center of the counting chamber (see Figure 14-4). The five smaller squares labeled R in the figure are included in the count, making up a total of $\frac{1}{5}$ mm². Follow the same procedure that you used for the WBC count to systematically count the 16 smaller squares within each of the five squares labeled R:

- Begin counting in the upper left corner of each square and move horizontally across the row.
- After finishing one row, go on to the adjacent one until each row of the square has been counted.
- Count the cells that touch the border lines on just two sides of each square.

RBC counts are made under high-power magnification using the 40X objective (45X or 43X on some microscopes). First locate the field under low-power magnification and then change to high-power magnification following the procedure outlined in Chapter 2. If there is a difference greater than 25 cells among any of the five larger squares, discard the count, clean and refill the counting chamber, and start the counting process over again. Count cells on both sides of the counting chamber in this way and average the counts for the two sides.

Watch Out for Hydrazoic Acid!

The diluent used in the Unopette prefilled reservoir contains sodium azide. Under acidic conditions, sodium azide may produce hydrazoic acid, which is extremely toxic. Take great care to avoid contact with this compound. When discarding used diluent into the sink, dilute it with running water to avoid damage to the sink and pipes.

Calculating the RBC Count

The following formula is used to calculate the number of red blood cells per cubic millimeter of blood:

$$\text{RBC/mm}^3 = \text{Number of cells counted}$$
$$\times \text{Dilution factor} \times \text{Depth factor}$$
$$\times \text{Area counted}$$

Components of the RBC Count Formula. The components of the RBC count formula that differ from the WBC count formula are the area counted and the dilution factor. In the RBC count, the area counted is just $\frac{1}{5}$ mm^2. The value 5 is substituted into the formula in order to get the number of red blood cells in 1 mm^3 of blood. The dilution factor for the RBC count depends on how much blood was added to the red blood cell pipette. The dilution usually is 1:200, so the dilution factor is 200. The depth factor is the same as for the WBC count—the constant 10.

Whenever the dilution is 1:200, you can use this shorthand formula for calculating the RBC count:

$$\text{RBC/mm}^3 = \text{Number of cells counted} \times 10,000$$

because

$$\text{Dilution factor} \times \text{Depth factor} \times \text{Area counted}$$
$$= 200 \times 10 \times 5 = 10,000$$

Using the Formula: A Worked Example. Assume that you have counted 101, 92, 112, 95, and 104 red blood cells in the five squares on one side of the counting chamber and 99, 98, 100, 102, and 97 red blood cells in the five squares on the other side. The total cells counted on the two sides are 504 and 496, for an average of 500 cells counted. Verify this on your calculator. Substituting into the formula, you get

$$\text{RBC/mm}^3 = 500 \times 200 \times 10 \times 5 = 5,000,000$$

PROCEDURE 14-1

Determining a WBC Count by the Manual Method

Goal

After successfully completing this procedure, you will be able to dilute a blood sample in a Unopette kit, charge a hemacytometer, count white blood cells under low-power magnification, and calculate the WBC count.

Completion Time

30 minutes

Equipment and Supplies

- Disposable gloves
- Face shield
- Apron
- Hand disinfectant
- Surface disinfectant
- Paper towels and tissues
- Biohazard container
- WBC BD Unopette™ kit
- EDTA-anticoagulated blood
- Neubauer ruled hemacytometer and coverslip
- Lens paper
- 70% alcohol
- Microscope
- Hand tally counter
- Petri dish with moist filter paper disk
- Report form and pen

Instructions

Read through the list of equipment and supplies that you will need and the steps of the procedure. Be sure that you understand each step before you begin. Then complete each step correctly and in the proper order. If your completion time is too long, repeat the procedure until you increase your speed.

*Steps marked with (*) are critical and must have the maximum points to pass.

Performance Standards	Points Awarded	Maximum Points
1. Put on a protective apron, wash your hands with disinfectant, dry them, and put on gloves.		10
2. Follow standard precautions.		10
3. Collect and prepare the appropriate equipment.		5
4. *Mix the EDTA blood sample thoroughly and check for proper labeling.		15
5. Place the WBC Unopette reservoir on a flat surface and push the point of the pipette shield into the reservoir neck, puncturing the diaphragm. Rotate the shield to make sure there is an adequate opening and then remove the shield.		5
6. Remove the pipette from the shield with a twisting and pulling motion.		5
7. Holding the capillary pipette nearly horizontally in your dominant hand between your thumb and index finger and the tube of well-mixed blood in your other hand, tilt the tube slightly and insert the pipette tip into the blood. The blood will stop flowing in the pipette when it reaches the end.		10
8. Wipe the tip of the pipette with a clean tissue, making sure that none of the blood sample is wicked away.		5
9. Holding the pipette, pick up the reservoir and gently squeeze it to force some of the air from the reservoir.		5
10. Cover the overflow chamber with the end of your gloved finger, place the pipette tip into the diluent, and firmly seat the pipette into the reservoir neck. Remove your finger from the overflow chamber and release the pressure on the reservoir at the same time to draw the blood into the diluent.		5
11. Squeeze and release the reservoir gently to force the diluent-blood mixture up and into the pipette and back into the reservoir. This will rinse the blood from the pipette.		5
12. Allow the reservoir to set for 2–3 minutes.		5
13. After cleaning the hemacytometer and coverslip with 70% alcohol and drying them thoroughly with lens paper, align the coverslip on the hemacytometer plate.		5
14. Mix the WBC Unopette dilution again and prepare to charge the hemacytometer.		5
15. Remove the pipette from the reservoir, flip it over, and place the overflow chamber into the reservoir neck to make a dropper assembly.		5
16. Hold the reservoir and gently squeeze a few drops of diluted blood mixture into a tissue to clean the lumen of the pipette and steady the flow.		5
17. Charge the hemacytometer with the diluted blood by touching the pipette tip to the edge of the counting chamber–coverslip and squeezing the fluid into one side of the hemacytometer under the coverslip. It will fill by capillary action. Do not overfill.		10
18. Fill the other side of the hemacytometer in the same way.		5
19. Allow the charged hemacytometer to sit undisturbed for 2 minutes in a Petri dish containing a moistened pad to allow the cells to settle and equilibrate.		5

—table continued

Performance Standards	Points Awarded	Maximum Points
20. Place the filled hemacytometer carefully on the lowered stage of the microscope, secure it with the clamps, and center one side of the chamber under the low power objective.		5
21. Adjust the light and raise the microscope stage carefully while watching from the side until the hemacytometer is near but not touching the 10X objective.		5
22. Looking through the ocular, focus with the coarse-adjustment knob until the square of the hemacytometer comes into view.		5
23. Readjust with the fine-adjustment knob until you see the cells clearly.		5
24. *Count the white blood cells in the four large corner squares of the ruled area (each large square contains 16 small squares) using the hand tally counter to keep count. Refer to Figure 14-4 in the text. Follow the rules for counting the cells touching the sides.		15
25. When you have counted each corner square, record the number of cells counted, reset the tally to zero, and proceed to the next corner square until you have counted all four corner squares. If the counts differ by more than 10 cells, go back to step 14 and clean and recharge the hemacytometer.		10
26. Total the number of cells counted in all four corner squares.		10
27. Repeat the counting process on the opposite side of the hemacytometer.		5
28. Average the counts from the two sides.		5
29. Substitute the average number of cells counted into the WBC count formula and calculate the WBC count. Record the results as the WBC/mm^3.		15
30. Discard disposable supplies and equipment.		5
31. Disinfect other equipment and return to storage.		5
32. Clean the work area following the standard precautions.		5
33. Remove your PPE and gloves, and wash and dry your hands.		5
34. Record the results in appropriate records.		10
Total Points		**235**

Overall Procedural Evaluation

Student Name _____

Signature of Instructor _____ Date _____

Comments _____

_____

PROCEDURE 14-2

Determining an RBC Count by the Manual Method

Goal

After successfully completing this procedure, you will be able to dilute a blood sample in a Unopette kit, charge a hemacytometer, count red blood cells under high-power magnification, and calculate the RBC count.

Completion Time

30 minutes

Equipment and Supplies

- Disposable gloves
- Face shield

- Apron
- Hand disinfectant
- Surface disinfectant
- Paper towels and tissues
- Biohazard container
- RBC BD Unopette™ kit
- EDTA-anticoagulated blood
- Test tube rack
- Neubauer ruled hemacytometer and coverslip
- Lens paper
- 70% alcohol

- Microscope
- Hand tally counter
- Petri dish with moistened pad
- Report form and pen

Instructions

Read through the list of equipment and supplies that you will need and the steps of the procedure. Be sure that you understand each step before you begin. Then complete each step correctly and in the proper order. If your completion time is too long, repeat the procedure until you increase your speed.

*Steps marked with (*) are critical and must have the maximum points to pass.

Performance Standards	Points Awarded	Maximum Points
1. Put on a protective apron, wash your hands with disinfectant, dry them, and put on gloves.		10
2. Follow standard precautions.		10
3. Collect and prepare the appropriate equipment.		5
4. *Mix the EDTA blood sample thoroughly and check for proper labeling.		15
5. Place the RBC Unopette reservoir on a flat surface and push the point of the pipette shield into the reservoir neck, puncturing the diaphragm. Rotate the shield to make sure there is an adequate opening and then remove the shield.		5
6. Remove the pipette from the shield with a twisting and pulling motion.		5
7. Holding the capillary pipette nearly horizontally in your dominant hand between your thumb and index finger and the tube of well-mixed blood in your other hand, tilt the tube slightly and insert the pipette tip into the blood. The blood will stop flowing in the pipette when it reaches the end.		10
8. Wipe the tip of the pipette with a clean tissue, making sure that none of the blood sample is wicked away.		5
9. Holding the pipette, pick up the reservoir and gently squeeze it to force some of the air from the reservoir.		5
10. Cover the overflow chamber with the end of your gloved finger, place the pipette tip into the diluent, and firmly seat the pipette into the reservoir neck. Remove your finger from the overflow chamber and release the pressure on the reservoir at the same time to draw the blood into the diluent.		5
11. Squeeze and release the reservoir gently to force the diluent-blood mixture up and into the pipette and back into the reservoir. This will rinse the blood from the pipette.		5
12. Allow the reservoir to set for 2–3 minutes.		5
13. After cleaning the hemacytometer and coverslip with 70% alcohol and drying them thoroughly with lens paper, align the coverslip on the hemacytometer plate.		5
14. Mix the RBC Unopette dilution again and prepare to charge the hemacytometer.		5

—table continued

Performance Standards	Points Awarded	Maximum Points
15. Remove the pipette from the reservoir, flip it over, and place the overflow chamber into the reservoir neck to make a dropper assembly.		5
16. Hold the reservoir and gently squeeze a few drops of diluted blood mixture into a tissue to clean the lumen of the pipette and steady the flow.		5
17. Charge the hemacytometer with the diluted blood by touching the pipette tip to the edge of the counting chamber–coverslip and squeezing the fluid into one side of the hemacytometer under the coverslip. It will fill by capillary action. Do not overfill.		10
18. Fill the other side of the hemacytometer in the same way.		5
19. Allow the charged hemacytometer to sit undisturbed for 2 minutes in a Petri dish containing a moistened pad to allow the cells to settle and equilibrate.		5
20. Place the filled hemacytometer carefully on the lowered stage of the microscope, secure it with the clamps, and center one side of the chamber under the low power objective.		5
21. Adjust the light and raise the microscope stage carefully while watching from the side until the hemacytometer is near but not touching the 10X objective.		5
22. Looking through the ocular, focus with the coarse-adjustment knob until the large center square of the hemacytometer comes into view.		5
23. Switch to the high power (40X) objective and focus with the fine-adjustment knob, centering the small top right corner square from the large center square. (See Figure 14-4.)		5
24. *Count the red blood cells in the five small squares (the four corners and the one center square) within the large center square using the hand tally counter to keep count. Refer to Figure 14-4 in the text. Follow the rules for counting the cells touching the sides.		15
25. When you have counted each of the five squares, record the number of cells counted, reset the tally to zero, and proceed to the next square until you have counted all five squares. If the counts differ by more than 25 cells, go back to step 14 and clean and recharge the hemacytometer.		10
26. Total the number of cells counted in all five squares.		10
27. Repeat the counting process on the opposite side of the hemacytometer.		5
28. Average the counts from the two sides.		5
29. Substitute the average number of cells counted into the RBC count formula and calculate the RBC count. Record the results as the RBC/mm^3.		15
30. Discard disposable supplies and equipment.		5
31. Disinfect other equipment and return to storage.		5
32. Clean the work area following the standard precautions.		5
33. Remove your PPE and gloves, and wash and dry your hands.		5
34. Record the results in appropriate records.		10
Total Points		**235**

Overall Procedural Evaluation

Student Name _____

Signature of Instructor _____ Date _____

Comments _____

_____

chapter 14 REVIEW

Multiple Choice

Choose the best answer for the following questions.

1. The clumping together of red blood cells is referred to as
   a. leukocytosis
   b. erythremia
   c. agglutination
   d. anoxia

2. The RBC manual count is performed using which of the following?
   a. hemacytometer
   b. lancet
   c. centrifuge
   d. automated cell counter

3. An elevation of white blood cells is called
   a. polycythemia
   b. leukocytosis
   c. erythremia
   d. anemia

4. The last immature stage of a red blood cell, which makes up approximately 1 percent of the circulating red blood cells, is the
   a. reticulocyte
   b. leukocyte
   c. erythrocyte
   d. nucleated red blood cell

5. An abnormally low white blood cell count is common in patients with a potentially fatal form of anemia that could be caused by a deficiency of vitamin B_{12} called
   a. erythremia
   b. polycythemia vera
   c. aplastic anemia
   d. pernicious anemia

Using Terminology

Define the following terms in the spaces provided.

6. Isotonic

   _____

   _____

   _____

7. Leukocytosis

   _____

   _____

   _____

8. Leukopenia

_____

_____

_____

9. Polycythemia

_____

_____

_____

10. Erythrocytosis

_____

_____

_____

11. Nucleated red blood cell (nRBC)

_____

_____

_____

12. Rouleaux

_____

_____

_____

Match the term in the left column with the appropriate definition or description in the right column.

____ **13.** adrenaline	a. anoxia
____ **14.** bone marrow disorder	b. aplastic anemia
____ **15.** lack of oxygen	c. epinephrine
____ **16.** polycythemia vera	d. erythremia
____ **17.** WBC count	e. erythrocyte count
____ **18.** result of dehydration	f. leukocyte count
____ **19.** tumor	g. neoplasm
____ **20.** RBC count	h. relative polycythemia

Acquiring Knowledge

Answer the following questions in the spaces provided.

21. What functions do white blood cells serve in the body?

_____

_____

22. What does the WBC count measure? What is the most common reason it is performed?

_____

_____

23. How does the normal WBC count for newborns differ from that of adults?

_____

_____

_____

24. What are some causes of normal and abnormal variation in the WBC count?

_____

_____

_____

25. When performing a WBC count, why must you add acid to the blood before counting the white cells?

_____

_____

_____

26. Describe the area of the hemacytometer that is counted when performing a WBC count. What is the total area counted?

_____

_____

_____

27. How does the presence of nucleated red blood cells affect the WBC count? Why? What must be done to correct for this?

_____

_____

_____

28. Why is the depth factor in the WBC count formula 10 when the sample in the hemacytometer is only 0.1 mm deep?

_____

_____

_____

29. List some of the causes of normal and abnormal variation in the RBC count.

_____

_____

_____

30. When performing an RBC count, why is saline or a similar solution added to the blood before the count is made?

_____

_____

_____

31. Describe the area of the hemacytometer that is counted when performing an RBC count. What is the total area counted?

_____

_____

_____

32. When counting red or white blood cells, what is the rule for counting cells that fall on the borderlines between squares?

_____

_____

_____

33. What is the most common reason for performing an RBC count?

_____

_____

_____

Applying Knowledge—On the Job

Answer the following questions in the spaces provided.

34. If a patient is taking the drug primidone, how may his or her RBC count be affected? Why?

_____

_____

_____

35. Mrs. Potts just had a urinalysis and a complete blood count as part of a routine physical exam. Her WBC count was 16,000/mm^3 and the urinalysis revealed a small amount of blood in her urine. What diagnosis do you think the doctor will make? Why?

_____

_____

_____

36. In the POL where you work, you are responsible for doing blood counts. How would you respond to each of the following situations and why?

 a. In the first square you count on the hemacytometer, there are 30 white blood cells and in the second there are 45.

_____

_____

_____

 b. There appears to be an air bubble under one corner of the hemacytometer coverslip.

_____

_____

_____

c. The red blood cells appear to be clumped together in bunches on the hemacytometer.

_____

_____

_____

d. A blood sample was left at room temperature overnight because it was overlooked the day before, and the doctor wants to know what happened to the blood count that she ordered.

_____

_____

_____

37. It was nearing the end of Brad's shift, and he had just one more blood count to perform for the day. As soon as he flooded the hemacytometer, he focused the microscope and began counting red blood cells. To save time, he counted cells on only one side of the counting chamber. What errors did Brad make? What should he have done instead?

_____

_____

_____

38. Assume that you are performing an RBC count in the POL where you work using the Unopette kit for RBC. You count the red blood cells under high-power magnification and come up with these tallies for the five squares on one side of the hemacytometer counting chamber: 100, 99, 103, 94, and 105. For the other side of the counting chamber the numbers are 103, 105, 98, 97, and 101. Calculate the patient's RBC count, showing all of the steps.

_____

_____

_____

39. Before performing an RBC count for a patient, you notice on her chart that she is taking an anticonvulsant drug for epilepsy and a diuretic for high blood pressure. How will these medications affect her RBC count?

_____

_____

_____

40. You have just performed a WBC count, which turned out to be 990/mm^3. What should you do?

_____

_____

_____

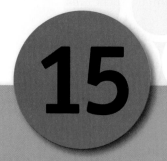

15 *chapter*

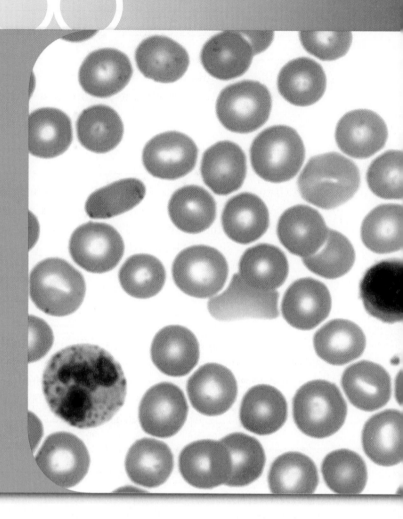

Differential WBC: Manual Procedure

COGNITIVE OBJECTIVES

After studying this chapter, you should be able to

15.1 use each vocabulary term appropriately.

15.2 list several potential reasons for examining a blood smear under 100X objective magnification (oil immersion).

15.3 describe the relative sizes and numbers of the formed elements in blood.

15.4 identify the regions of a properly prepared blood smear and explain why the body of the smear is the region examined under the microscope.

15.5 describe differences among the five types of white blood cells and list their identifying features on a differential blood smear.

15.6 define the normal range of adult values for differential white blood cell counts and list several causes of abnormal values.

15.7 discuss the relationship between staining and identification of formed elements in the blood.

PERFORMANCE OBJECTIVES

After studying this chapter, you should be able to

15.8 correctly prepare a differential blood smear slide.

15.9 stain a differential blood smear slide using the quick-stain method.

15.10 determine staining errors from the appearance of a differential blood smear slide.

15.11 perform a differential white blood cell count.

15.12 examine and describe the morphology and hemoglobin concentration of red blood cells on a differential blood smear slide.

15.13 estimate the number of platelets on a differential blood smear slide.

 # TERMINOLOGY

acute lymphocytic leukemia: predominantly a children's disease, in which the blood-forming tissues produce an excessive number of lymphocytes.

agranulocytes: the third of white blood cells, including both monocytes and lymphocytes, that have few, if any, visible granules.

agranulocytosis: an acute disorder characterized by severe sore throat, fever, complete exhaustion, and an extreme reduction in the number of neutrophils.

anisocytosis: the excessive variation in the size of cells, especially red blood cells.

basophil: the least common type of granular white blood cell, containing large cytoplasmic granules that stain blue-black with alkaline dyes.

brucellosis: a bacterial disease primarily of cattle, which leads to an increase in lymphocytes and a decrease in neutrophils.

cell counter: a manual counter for differential white blood cell counts with keys for each type of white cell.

chronic granulocytic leukemia: a type of chronic leukemia caused by a chromosomal abnormality, leading to an overproduction of immature granulocytes in the bone marrow.

differential white blood cell count: differential or "diff"; a determination of the percent of each type of white blood cell out of a total of 100 white blood cells observed under magnification by the oil immersion objective (100X) on a stained blood smear. Also can be calculated by automated CBC analyzer.

endocarditis: the inflammation of the lining of the heart. Endocarditis may be associated with an increase in the number of monocytes.

eosin: a red-orange acidic dye used to stain blood smears for microscopic examination.

eosinophil: a granular white blood cell with a bilobed nucleus and cytoplasmic granules that stain brilliant red-orange with eosin dye. Increased numbers of eosinophils are associated with allergies and internal parasitic infections.

granulocyte: a polymorphonuclear white blood cell that contains granules in its cytoplasm. This class includes neutrophils, eosinophils, and basophils.

hyperchromic: having excess hemoglobin; refers to red blood cells with excess hemoglobin that appear darker in color when stained with dye.

hypersegmented: having a nucleus with more than five segments, or lobes; used to describe certain neutrophils.

hypochromic: having too little hemoglobin; refers to red blood cells that appear lighter in color when stained with dye.

infectious lymphocytosis: a rare disorder, probably of viral origin, that leads to an increase in the number of small lymphocytes.

infectious mononucleosis: an acute infectious disease in which lymphocytes are both more numerous and larger than normal and often contain vacuoles, causing them to resemble monocytes—hence the name of the disease.

lymphocyte: the most common of all white blood cells in children; typically small and round with a nonsegmented nucleus and no cytoplasmic granules. Appears dark blue when stained.

macrocyte: a red blood cell that is unusually large (greater than 12 microns in diameter).

megakaryocyte: a large bone marrow cell with large or multiple nuclei. Megakaryocytes give rise to platelets, which are cytoplasmic fragments of megakaryocytes.

methylene blue: a blue alkaline dye used to stain blood smears for microscopic examination.

microcyte: a red blood cell that is unusually small (less than 6 microns in diameter).

monocyte: the largest type of cell in the blood; an agranulocyte that has gray-blue cytoplasm when stained with the appearance of ground glass.

monocytic leukemia: a form of acute leukemia in which abnormal monocytes proliferate and invade the blood, bone marrow, and other tissues.

mononuclear: having an undivided nucleus, such as lymphocytes and monocytes.

neutropenia: a decrease below normal in the number of neutrophils in the blood, due to certain drugs, some acute infections, radiation, or certain diseases of the spleen or bone marrow.

neutrophil: the most common type of white blood cell; a granulocyte with a multilobed nucleus and cytoplasm filled with fine pink granules when stained with dye.

normochromic: normal in color; used to describe red blood cells that have the normal amount of hemoglobin.

normocyte: an average-sized red blood cell, about 7.5 micrometers (μm) in diameter.

poikilocytosis: a condition in which many red blood cells have abnormal or multiple types of shapes.

polychromatic stain: a stain containing dyes of two or more colors, such as Wright's stain, which contains methylene blue and eosin.

polymorphonuclear: having a multilobed nucleus; used to describe cells such as granulocytes.

pyogenic: pus producing; includes organisms such as staphylococcus and streptococcus.

quick-stain method: a method of staining blood smears in which the smear is dipped sequentially in fixative, acidic stain, and alkaline stain; also called the three-step method.

vacuole: a clear space in cell cytoplasm that is filled with fluid or air.

Wright's stain: a polychromatic stain for fixing and staining blood smears. It contains eosin and methylene blue dyes in a methyl alcohol solution.

INTRODUCTION

Stained blood smears are examined under the highest power of magnification as part of the complete blood count. The main purpose is to count and assign percentages to the different types of white blood cells. Another reason for examining blood smears under the highest power of magnification is to identify abnormalities in white blood cells and in the other formed elements in the blood— the red blood cells and platelets. Microscopic examination of a blood smear also can provide an estimate of WBC and RBC counts, platelet count, and hemoglobin.

OVERVIEW OF THE FORMED ELEMENTS IN THE BLOOD

The most numerous formed elements in the blood observed on a differential slide are red blood cells. Each cubic millimeter of blood in the normal adult contains an average of 5,000,000 red blood cells. Red blood cells have no nuclei and are smaller than the average white blood cells. The average life span of mature red blood cells is 120 days, and new red blood cells are constantly being produced in the bone marrow to replace those that are worn out. Old red blood cells are removed from circulation by the spleen.

Unlike red blood cells, white blood cells are nucleated. They also are highly differentiated for their specialized functions, and they are larger than red blood cells. Normal adult blood contains an average of 7,000 white blood cells per cubic millimeter. Figure 15-1 shows types of blood cells found on a normal peripheral blood smear for an individual.

White blood cells fall into two general classes. One class is called **granulocytes** because they have granules in their cytoplasm that are visible after staining. Granulocytes also are called **polymorphonuclear** leukocytes because of their multilobed nuclei. There are three types of granulocytes— **neutrophils, eosinophils,** and **basophils**—with

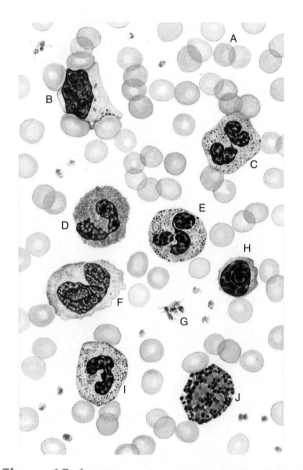

Figure 15-1 Cell types found in smears of peripheral blood from normal individuals. (A) Erythrocytes; (B) Large lymphocyte with azurophilic granules and deeply indented by adjacent erythrocytes; (C) Segmented neutrophil; (D) Eosinophil; (E) Segmented neutrophil; (F) Monocyte with blue-gray cytoplasm, coarse linear chromatin, and blunt pseudopods; (G) Thrombocytes; (H) Lymphocyte; (I) Neutrophilic band; (J) Basophil. (*Note:* Arrangement is arbitrary and the number of leukocytes in relation to erythrocytes and thrombocytes is greater than would occur in actual microscopic field.)

neutrophils being the most common. The average life span of granulocytes is about 9 to 10 days.

The other class of white blood cells is called **agranulocytes** because they have few, if any, visible granules after staining. There are two types: **monocytes** and **lymphocytes.** Monocytes are the largest cells in the blood, but they are relatively few in number. Lymphocytes, which are responsible for the formation of antibodies and cell-mediated immunity, are further subdivided by size into small and large lymphocytes. Small lymphocytes are just a little larger than red blood cells and make up the majority of lymphocytes. Next to neutrophils, they are the most common white blood cells. In children, lymphocytes are the most common white blood cells observed on a stained blood smear.

Platelets are the smallest formed elements in blood, being less than half as big as red blood cells. They are called platelets because of their plate-like flatness. They also are called thrombocytes for their role in clot, or thrombus, formation. Platelets are not cells but fragments of the cytoplasm of large cells called **megakaryocytes,** which remain in the bone marrow. Platelets average 250,000 per cubic millimeter of blood, making them more numerous than white blood cells but less numerous than red blood cells. Their average life span in the circulating blood is 8 to 10 days.

PREPARING AND STAINING BLOOD SMEARS

Blood smears are examined under the oil-immersion, 100X, objective of the microscope. Correct preparation and staining of the smear are crucial first steps in obtaining accurate results.

Preparing the Smear

The most common method of preparing a blood smear is the two-slide method. A glass slide, called the spreader, is used to spread a drop of whole blood on another glass slide, which holds the smear. Both slides must be free of dust, dirt, and oil, and they should be handled only by their edges to avoid smudges. Blood smears are often made in duplicate, so the second one can be referred to if the need arises.

> **Note**
>
> Blood used for a smear can be collected by either venipuncture or capillary puncture. A tube containing EDTA anticoagulant must be used for collecting the sample unless the smear is made before the blood has time to clot. Smears made with EDTA-anticoagulant blood should be made within 2 hours of collection.

Figure 15-2 illustrates how to make a blood smear. Place the smear slide on a flat surface and hold the spreader slide in the dominant hand. Place a single drop of blood about half an inch from the end of the smear slide—the right end for right-handed people, the left end for left-handed people. The drop of blood should be small, about twice the size of a pin head. Hold the spreader slide at a 35 to 40 degree angle and place it to the left of the

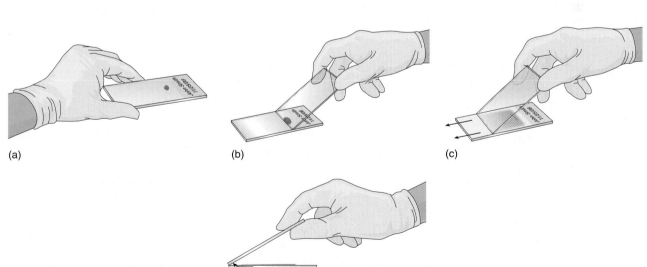

(a)   (b)   (c)

(d)

Figure 15-2 Making a peripheral blood smear. (a) Apply a drop of blood to the slide near the end of the slide. (b) Hold the spreader slide at a 35 to 40 degree angle. Pull the spreader slide until it touches the drop of blood. (c) Push the spreader slide across the bottom slide with a quick, even motion. (d) Pull the spreader slide up and away. Allow the smear to air dry. Do not blow on it.

drop of blood, or to the right for left-handed people. Back the spreader slide into the drop of blood until blood covers about three-fourths of its width. Then, push the spreader slide in the opposite direction in a quick, steady movement, reducing the angle as you go across the slide. Avoid jerky movements and pressure on the spreader slide.

The Significance of Size

If the angle of the spreader slide is too great when spreading the blood, the smear will be too thick. If the angle is too small, the smear will be too thin. The thickness of the smear, in turn, influences how large cells on the smear appear under the microscope. Cells appear larger in very thin films because the cells are flattened, leading to higher counts of large cells in thin smears and lower counts in thick ones. Because cells are differentiated, in part, on the basis of size, the thickness of the smear can influence the count of each type of cell.

After preparing and drying the slide, label it with a pencil on the frosted end where the blood drop was placed. The label should include the patient's name, the date, and the patient's identification number. If you cannot stain the slide immediately, preserve the cellular components by immersing the slide in methyl alcohol for 30 to 60 seconds and air drying again.

Preparing a blood smear is a skill that takes practice to perfect. If correctly done, a blood smear covers about two-thirds the length of the slide and coats the slide smoothly without grainy streaks or ridges. A correctly prepared smear is roughly the shape of a thumb print and has three different regions, as Figure 15-3 illustrates:

- *The heel:* the thick end of the smear, where the drop of blood was placed, which contains stacked red blood cells.
- *The feathered edge:* the end opposite the heel, which is the thinnest area of the smear, with spaces between the red blood cells.
- *The body:* the middle region of the slide, where the red blood cells barely touch one another and do not overlap.

Only the body of the blood smear is examined under the oil-immersion objective of the microscope. The cells are easiest to examine in this region because they are numerous yet arranged in a single layer, with minimal distortion from adjacent cells. Figure 15-4 shows a correct smear and some that would be difficult to read.

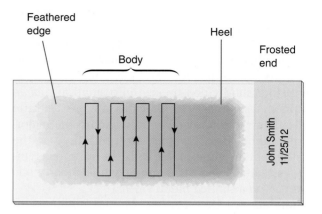

Figure 15-3 Representation of a correctly stained blood smear.

Staining the Smear

Before the slide is examined under the microscope, the smear must be stained. Staining heightens the contrast among the different types of cells and other structures and therefore differentiates them.

In today's POLs, a **polychromatic stain** is used most often. Polychromatic stains are multicolored, containing both an alkaline dye such as **methylene blue** and an acidic dye such as **eosin,** which is red-orange. Acidic structures in the blood such as cell nuclei appear blue after staining because they attract alkaline, or basic, dye. That is why they are called basophilic. Alkaline structures in the blood such as cytoplasm attract acidic dye, hence the name eosinophilic, or acidophilic. Structures that attract neutral dyes are termed neutrophilic. Both normal and abnormal formed elements in the blood are differentiated by their staining affinities.

Wright's Stain. Wright's stain is one of the most widely used polychromatic stains in the hematology lab. It is a solution of methyl alcohol, eosin, and a complex mixture of thiazines, including methyl blue. Because it contains methyl alcohol, Wright's solution both stains and fixes the smear in one operation.

To stain a slide with Wright's stain, place the air-dried slide on a rack, blood side up, and cover it with Wright's stain. Let the slide stand for 2 minutes and then cover it with an equal amount of buffer solution. Mix the stain and buffer by gently blowing on the mixture. Let the slide stand again, this time for 2 and a half to 5 minutes. A green metallic sheen should appear on the surface of the mixture, and the margins should show a reddish tint. Wash the slide with distilled water,

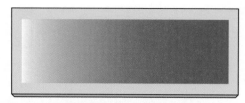

a. Ideal blood smear changes evenly from a thick area to a very thin area when spread from right to left.

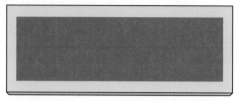

b. This smear has a thick, even layer of blood that does not permit viewing the individual cells' structures.

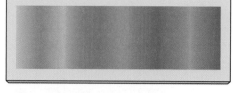

c. This smear was made with uneven pressure, so it does not permit accurate counts.

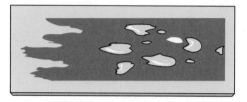

d. The slide this smear was made on was not clean; it probably had minute oil droplets on the surface.

Figure 15-4 Correct and incorrect types of slides.

first gently, then more vigorously using an overhead water bottle until all traces of excess stain are removed. Remove excess water by tilting the slide. Then leave the slide to dry in a tilted position.

An incorrectly prepared or incorrectly stained slide has a telltale appearance. Use the following guide to assess your technique:

If a slide appears too blue or too dark:
- The smear may be too thick.
- The stain may have been left on too long.
- The stain may have been washed off inadequately.
- The stain or buffer may be too alkaline.

If a slide appears too pink or too light:
- The staining time may have been too short.
- The stain may have been washed too long or too vigorously.
- The stain or buffer may be too acidic.

If a slide has precipitate on the blood film:
- The slide may be dirty.
- The slide may have dried during staining.
- The stain may have been washed off inadequately.
- The stain may have been filtered inadequately.

The Quick-Stain Method. The **quick-stain method,** also called the three-step method, is used widely in POLs because it is quicker and easier to use than is Wright's stain. The quick-stain method uses the same dyes as Wright's stain, but the two dyes, methylene blue and eosin, are in separate aqueous (water) solutions. Because the dyes are applied separately, there is more control over staining time with each dye (see Figure 15-5).

First, dip the air-dried, blood smear slide in a fixative solution five times, allowing 1 second for each dip. Wick away excess fixative from the slide by touching the edge of the slide to a paper towel. Next, dip the slide three to five times, allowing 1 second for each dip, in the eosin staining solution. Allow excess stain to drain away, but do not dry the slide. Finally, dip the slide three to five times in the methylene blue staining solution, again allowing 1 second for each dip and allowing the excess stain to drain. Follow this by a rinse with distilled or deionized water and air drying.

Caution!

The fixative solution used in the quick-stain method contains methyl alcohol in greater than 99 percent concentration. This solution can be fatal or cause blindness if ingested. Be certain that all supplies are closed tightly after use because evaporation can distort results and can cause chemical changes.

If a pale stain is desired, dip the slide just three times in each dye solution. Red tone may be intensified by increasing the number of dips in the first, acidic, stain solution. Blue tone may be intensified

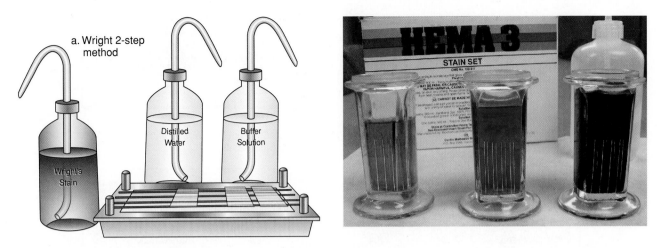

Figure 15-5 Two methods of staining blood smears. Both use a timed exposure to the stains. (a) The Wright's-stain method utilizes a rack, where the stains are added to the blood smear. (b) The quick-stain method is immersed in three solutions.

by increasing the number of dips in the second, alkaline, stain solution.

DIFFERENTIATING AND COUNTING WHITE BLOOD CELLS

The **differential white blood cell count,** also known as the differential or "diff," determines the percent of each type of white blood cell in a stained blood smear out of a total of at least 100 white blood cells. The white cells also are examined for abnormal morphology. The differential white blood cell count assists in the diagnosis and treatment of many diseases.

Differentiating White Blood Cells by Type

To perform a differential white blood cell count, you must be able to distinguish the different types of white cells in a stained blood smear. A good blood cell atlas such as Abbott Laboratories' *The Morphology of Human Blood Cells* is indispensable for this purpose.

Features that must be examined to differentiate the various types of white blood cells include

* the size of the cell
* the nuclear characteristics such as shape, size, structure, and color
* the cytoplasmic characteristics such as amount, color, and types of inclusions

Figure 15-6 shows characteristics of white blood cells.

Neutrophils. The neutrophil, also called a "seg" for segmented nucleus or "poly" for polymorphonuclear, is a granulocyte ranging from 10 to 15 micrometers in diameter. The nuclei of neutrophils usually have three to five lobes, each connected by an invisible, threadlike membrane. The arrangement of the lobes may resemble the letters *E, S,* or *Z.* The nuclear material is coarse and condensed and it stains deeply with blue.

The cytoplasm of neutrophils is abundant and stained light pink. Neutrophils are so named because the fine granules that fill their cytoplasm are stained by neutral stains. With Wright's stain they appear pink or lilac.

Band neutrophils, or "bands," are an immature form of neutrophil. They have the same diameter as the mature form, but the lobes of the nuclei are still connected by a wide strip of membrane that is clearly visible. The coarse-appearing nucleus is shaped like a link sausage or a band, and it stains deep purple-blue. The cytoplasm of band neutrophils is abundant and contains fine pale blue or pink granules.

Eosinophils. Eosinophil granulocytes have about the same diameter as neutrophils—10 to 15 micrometers—but the nucleus has just two lobes and stains less deeply. The cytoplasm has a faint sky-blue tinge or is colorless. The most distinguishing features of eosinophils are the large, coarse, spherical granules in the cytoplasm. These granules are uniform in size, are usually evenly distributed, and fill the cell without overlying the nucleus. The granules stain bright red with the acidic dye eosin.

	Segmented neutrophil 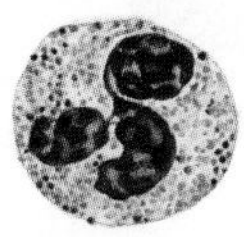	Neutrophilic band 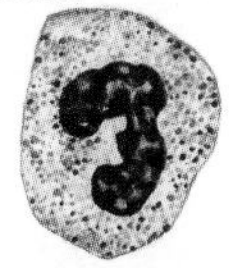	Eosinophil 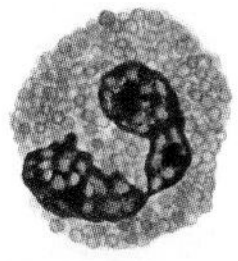	Basophil 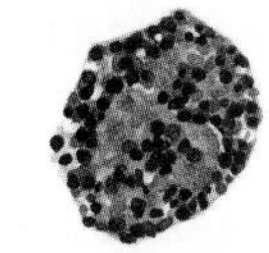	Lymphocyte 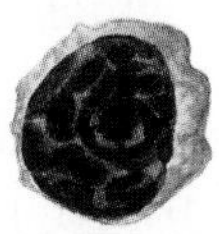	Monocyte 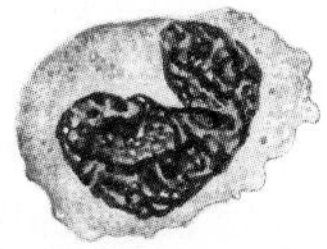
Cell Size	10–15 µm	10–15 µm	10–15 µm	10–15 µm	6–15 µm	14–20 µm
Nucleus Shape	2–5 lobes connected by slender filaments	Sausage or band shaped	Bilobed	Segmented	Usually round (oval)	Round or kidney-shaped
Structure	Coarse, condensed	Coarse	Coarse	Difficult to see; obscured by cytoplasmic granules	Lumpy or clumped, smudged (smoothly stained)	Folded, convoluted, may be deeply indented
Cytoplasm Amount	Abundant	Abundant	Abundant	Abundant	Scant	Abundant
Color	Pink to colorless or bright pink	Pink to tan	Pink to tan	Pink to tan	Clear to medium blue	Opaque, blue-gray
Inclusions	Small purple, lilac granules	Small lilac granules; fine pale blue or pink granules	Coarse, red or orange granules	Coarse, large, blue-back granules	Occasional granules, red-purple	Fine stain or ground-glass appearance, evenly cytoplasmic-distributed lilac granules
Normal % WBC Differential Adults	54–62	3–5	1–3	0–1	25–33	3–7

Figure 15-6 White blood cells (leukocytes) are identified by the individual characteristics of their nucleus and cytoplasm and according to size and color. Normal ranges are also given.

Is It a Neutrophil or a Basophil?

Neutrophils sometimes have large, darkly stained granules that resemble basophilic granules. When in doubt, it is usually safe to assume the cell is a neutrophil because basophils are far less numerous and are seldom seen on a blood differential slide. (Basophils average one-half or 0.5 percent or less of the total leukocytes.)

Basophils. Basophils average 10 micrometers in diameter. Like other polymorphonuclear leukocytes, they have a nucleus with lobes. Their distinguishing features are the large, irregularly shaped cytoplasmic granules, which stain blue-black with Wright's stain. In fact, the nucleus often is obscured by the cytoplasmic granules.

Lymphocytes. Lymphocytes are **mononuclear,** or single-nucleus, cells without visible cytoplasmic granules. Small lymphocytes range from 6 to 12 micrometers in diameter, being only slightly larger than red blood cells. Large lymphocytes range from 12 to 15 microns in diameter, comparable in size to granulocytes. Large lymphocytes are more common in the blood of children and generally are less mature cells, although size is not a reliable criterion for the age of lymphocytes. Small lymphocytes have less cytoplasm, perhaps because they shed cytoplasm as they supply antibodies. In any event, the size of lymphocytes usually is not relevant in diagnosis or treatment.

In the blood stream, lymphocytes are actively motile cells with irregular shapes. When a smear is prepared, the lymphocytes are exposed to air, chilled, brought into contact with glass surfaces, and dried. These disturbances give lymphocytes the spherical shape that they take on in a differential smear.

Lymphocytes have a single, sharply defined nucleus that contains heavy blocks of chromatin and stains a coarse dark blue or blue-black. The nucleus occupies a major portion of the cell in small lymphocytes, which may appear to have just a narrow rim of cytoplasm around it. The nucleus usually is round, but it may have an indentation at one side caused by the pressure of neighboring cells.

The cytoplasm of lymphocytes usually contains few granules, if any, and it stains a pale blue. However, about one-third of large lymphocytes have cytoplasmic granules that are large and round and stain red-purple. The granules are larger than the granules of neutrophils.

Monocytes. Monocytes are the largest cells normally found in circulating blood. They have a diameter of 14 to 20 micrometers, making them two to three times the size of the typical red blood cell. The nuclei of monocytes usually are round or kidney shaped, but they may be deeply indented or folded. Some monocytes have nuclei with superimposed lobes that look like convolutions of the brain.

The cytoplasm of monocytes is abundant. It stains gray-blue with Wright's stain and has a fine granular appearance, like ground glass. The cytoplasm also may contain fine lilac granules that are smaller and less distinct than are the granules of neutrophils. Cytoplasmic **vacuoles** are common in monocytes, and they may contain phagocytized red blood cells, leukocytes, cell fragments, or bacteria.

Is It a Lymphocyte or a Monocyte?

If you are having difficulty distinguishing monocytes and large lymphocytes from each other on differential smears, look closely at the chromatin. In lymphocytes, the chromatin is all in a clump. In monocytes, light spaces between the chromatin strands give the chromatin a coarse, linear appearance.

Remember

Refer abnormal cells to the laboratory director or other qualified personnel for identification.

Figure 15-7 shows the sequence of origin and maturation of myelocytic white blood cells. The stages of progressive maturation start with the myeloblast and end with the segmented cells. Only band and segmented forms of the cell on stained smears are considered to be normal. Classify any

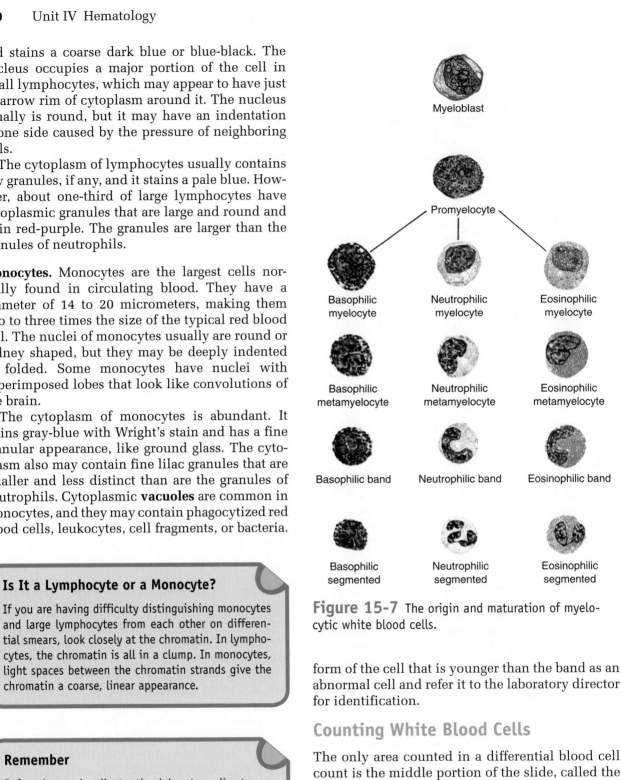

Figure 15-7 The origin and maturation of myelocytic white blood cells.

form of the cell that is younger than the band as an abnormal cell and refer it to the laboratory director for identification.

Counting White Blood Cells

The only area counted in a differential blood cell count is the middle portion of the slide, called the body, where the red blood cells are just one layer thick. First, locate the body of the smear under the low-power, 10X, objective. This also is a good time to identify cells that appear abnormal for closer examination under the oil-immersion objective. After locating the body of the slide under the low-power objective, perform the count using the oil-immersion objective. The light must be bright enough for the colors and small structures to be readily distinguishable.

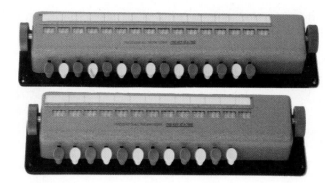

Figure 15-8 Cell counters make counting and classifying cells easier. The differential white blood cell counters can have keys labeled for each cell type.

Follow a definite pattern when counting cells on the slide, like the serpentine pattern shown in Figure 15-3, to avoid the possibility of counting the same area of the slide twice. A manual **cell counter** such as those shown in Figure 15-8 is used to tally the different types of white blood cells observed. Counters vary, but most can count up to six different types of cells per operation. When a total of 100 cells has been counted, the counter rings or locks. The counter can be reset if more than 100 cells are to be counted. The more cells counted, the greater the accuracy of the count. Error is on the order of ± 10 percent when 100 cells are counted and ± 7 percent when 200 cells are counted.

Estimating the WBC Count

You can estimate the total WBC count by counting the white blood cells in one field in the body portion of a blood smear under the low-power objective and then multiplying the count by 500. This method is much less accurate than the one described in Chapter 14 and should be used only as a screening check of the WBC count.

Express the number of each type of white blood cell as a percentage of the total number of white blood cells counted. See Figure 15-6 for normal adult values for each type of white cell.

Abnormal Values for the Differential White Blood Cell Count

A rise or fall in the number of white blood cells occurs in many pathological conditions. It usually leads to a change in the proportion of the various types of white blood cells. Changes in the proportions of the various types may be important in diagnosis.

An Increase in the Number of White Blood Cells. An increase in the number of white blood cells usually is due to an increase in the number of granulocytes, especially neutrophils. Increased numbers of neutrophils, in turn, are most often associated with infection by **pyogenic,** or pus-producing, organisms such as streptococcus, staphylococcus, gonococcus, pneumococcus, or meningococcus, which cause appendicitis, pneumonia, and other acute infections.

Hypersegmentation

When neutrophils have nuclei with six or more lobes, they are said to be **hypersegmented.** Hypersegmentation may indicate anemia, vitamin B12 deficiency, or folic acid deficiency. It is usually the last sign of the disease to disappear after therapy.

An increase in the number of neutrophils is usually accompanied by an increase in the "band" neutrophils, the immature form of a neutrophil. This increase in band forms is referred to as a "shift to the left" (Figure 15-7).

An increase in the percent of eosinophils is found in association with allergic reactions such as hay fever and skin disorders such as eczema. Parasitic infestations such as trichinosis and tapeworm also may be associated with elevated numbers of eosinophils. If basophils are elevated, it is most often related to an increase in granulocytes, as in **chronic granulocytic leukemia.**

An increase in the number of small lymphocytes is associated with whooping cough, tuberculosis, **brucellosis**—a bacterial disease primarily of cattle—and **infectious lymphocytosis,** a rare disorder that is probably of viral origin. In **infectious mononucleosis,** lymphocytes are both more numerous and larger than normal, and they often contain vacuoles, causing them to resemble monocytes—hence the name of the disease. A very high lymphocyte count also may indicate **acute lymphocytic leukemia,** predominantly a children's disease, in which there is excessive production of lymphocytes by the blood-forming tissues.

An increase in monocytes may be found in tuberculosis and acute **monocytic leukemia.** The latter is a form of acute leukemia in which abnormal monocytes proliferate and invade the blood, bone marrow, and other tissues. **Endocarditis,** inflammation of the lining of the heart, and ulcerative colitis also may be associated with an increased number of monocytes.

A Decrease in the Number of White Blood Cells. A decreased WBC count usually is due to **neutropenia,** or a decrease below normal in the number of neutrophils. Of itself, neutropenia causes no symptoms, but it may lead to frequent and severe bacterial infections. An extreme reduction in the number of neutrophils or even their complete disappearance from the blood is called **agranulocytosis.** It is an acute disorder characterized by severe sore throat, fever, and complete exhaustion.

A number of pharmaceutical drugs may cause neutropenia in sensitive people. These include pain relievers, antihistamines, tranquilizers, anticonvulsants, antimicrobial agents, sulfonamide derivatives, and antithyroid drugs. Neutropenia also is associated with some acute infections (such as typhoid fever, brucellosis, and measles), exposure to radiation, and certain diseases involving the spleen or bone marrow (such as aplastic anemia).

EXAMINING RED BLOOD CELLS

Red blood cells are easy to identify under the oil-immersion objective of the microscope. They stain light red or pinkish tan with Wright's stain and have no nuclei. They are examined under the oil-immersion objective for their size, shape, and hemoglobin content.

> **Technique Tip**
>
> Are the red blood cells on your slide blue or orange instead of red? Most likely, they were stained too dark or too light. See the guides on pages 266 and 267 on how to prepare a better blood smear slide.

Red blood cells normally range from 6 to 8 micrometers in diameter. Small lymphocytes are used as a point of reference to judge the size of red blood cells on the slide, as Figure 15-9 shows. A normal-sized red blood cell, a **normocyte,** has about two-thirds to three-fourths the diameter of a small lymphocyte. Small red blood cells, called **microcytes,** are half or less the diameter of small lymphocytes. They are common in patients with iron-deficiency anemia. Large red blood cells, called **macrocytes,** are equal to or larger than small lymphocytes. They are found in patients with vitamin B12 deficiency or folic acid deficiency. Occasional small or large red blood cells may be observed in normal individuals. A great deal of variation observed in the size of the red blood cells is referred to as **anisocytosis.**

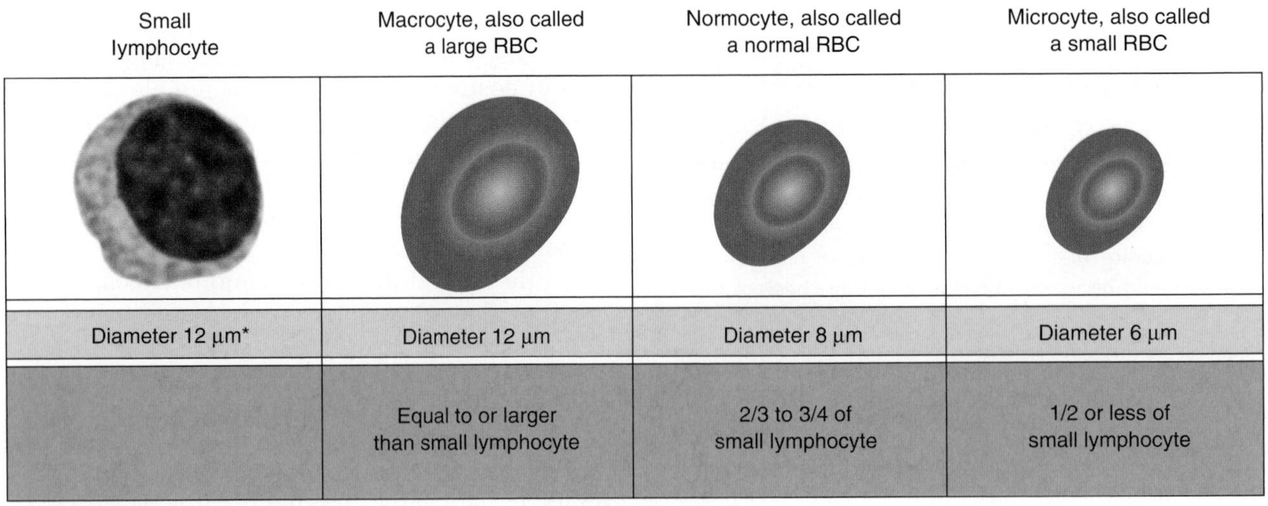

Small lymphocyte	Macrocyte, also called a large RBC	Normocyte, also called a normal RBC	Microcyte, also called a small RBC
Diameter 12 μm*	Diameter 12 μm	Diameter 8 μm	Diameter 6 μm
	Equal to or larger than small lymphocyte	2/3 to 3/4 of small lymphocyte	1/2 or less of small lymphocyte

*μm = a measure of the metric system
μm = micrometer
μm = 1/millionth of a meter
μm = 1/1000 of a millimeter

μm = .001 millimeter
μm = 10^{-3} mm
μm = micron

(all of the above are ways of expressing the same measurement)

Figure 15-9 Use small lymphocytes as a standard of reference to estimate the size of red blood cells on the stained differential blood smear.

What Is in a Shape?

Red blood cells develop in the bone marrow, where they contain a nucleus and have a spherical shape. Before a red blood cell is released into the circulating blood, it extrudes the nucleus, which causes the cell to collapse on both sides, giving it the biconcave disk shape that characterizes circulating red blood cells. This shape has more surface area per volume than does the spherical shape. The relatively greater surface area helps the hemoglobin in the cell function more effectively in transporting oxygen.

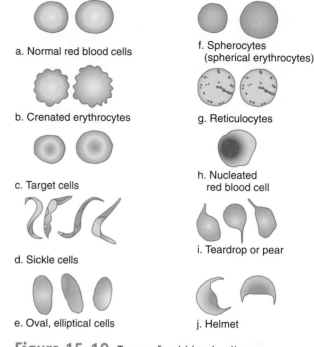

a. Normal red blood cells

b. Crenated erythrocytes

c. Target cells

d. Sickle cells

e. Oval, elliptical cells

f. Spherocytes (spherical erythrocytes)

g. Reticulocytes

h. Nucleated red blood cell

i. Teardrop or pear

j. Helmet

Figure 15-10 Types of red blood cells seen on stained blood smears (red blood cell morphology).

Normal red blood cells appear as circular, homogeneous disks that are concave on both sides, which gives them a pale center. (See Figure 15-10.) Occasional abnormally shaped cells are observed in normal individuals. The condition in which many red blood cells have abnormal shapes is **poikilocytosis.** Other abnormal cells may take on sickle, helmet, target, or pear shapes. Sickle-shaped red blood cells are due to the presence of hemoglobin S in the cells, as Chapter 13 describes.

Nucleated red blood cells (nRBCs), which are difficult to distinguish from white blood cells under low-power magnification, are easy to identify under the oil-immersion (100X) objective on a stained blood smear. Nucleated red blood cells, which are young red blood cells that have not expelled their nucleus, have the color and appearance of large erythrocytes containing a dense nucleus (see Figure 15-11).

The hemoglobin content of red blood cells is indicated by the depth of staining of the cells. The more hemoglobin present, the darker the stain. Red blood cells with normal hemoglobin content are

normochromic. Red blood cells with excess hemoglobin are **hyperchromic.** Red blood cells with too little hemoglobin are **hypochromic.** Hypochromic red blood cells may indicate a deficiency of iron, vitamin B12, or folic acid.

Another indicator of hypochromia is the size of the pale area in the center of the cell. Normal red blood cells have a central pale area, measuring about one-third the diameter of the cell, where the hemoglobin concentration is low. Hypochromic cells have larger pale areas, measuring about two-thirds the diameter of the cell. Borderline hypochromic cells have pale areas over about half the cell diameter (see Figure 15-12).

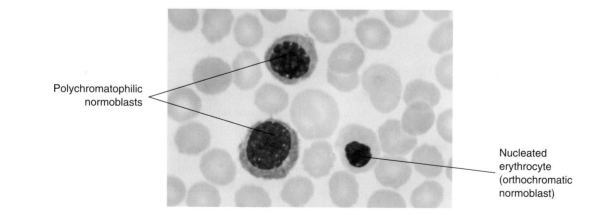

Polychromatophilic normoblasts

Nucleated erythrocyte (orthochromatic normoblast)

Figure 15-11 Nucleated red blood cells. Viewed under the oil-immersion (100X) objective of a stained smear, they have the distinctive coloring and appearance of large erythrocytes containing a dense nucleus.

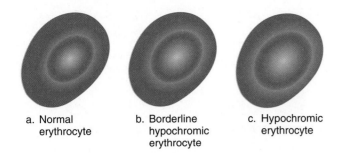

a. Normal
   erythrocyte

b. Borderline
   hypochromic
   erythrocyte

c. Hypochromic
   erythrocyte

Figure 15-12 Normal and hypochromic cells. The amount of hemoglobin present in red blood cells is estimated according to the intensity of color. (a) A normal erythrocyte shows a thick outer ring of darker color, approximately two-thirds the diameter of the cell, denoting hemoglobin. (b) A borderline hypochromic cell has a smaller outer ring of darker color, approximately one-half the diameter of the cell. (c) A hypochromic cell has only a thin ring of dark color, about one-third the diameter of the cell.

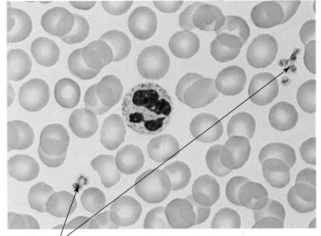

Platelets

Figure 15-13 The appearance of platelets with erythrocytes and white blood cell types on a stained blood cell differential smear.

COUNTING PLATELETS

Normal platelets, illustrated in Figure 15-13, vary in diameter from 1 to 4 microns. They may have round, oval, spindle, or disk shapes. Platelets usually have multiple tentacle-like protrusions, but some have smooth margins. The cytoplasm fragments of platelets stain light blue and contain variable numbers of small blue granules. The granules usually aggregate in the center of the cytoplasm, with the marginal zone being nongranular.

On a slide, platelets tend to adhere to each other. Both individual and clumps of platelets are more numerous at the feathered end of the blood smear. In the body portion of the smear, the number of platelets per oil-immersion field normally varies from 5 to 20, with about one platelet for every 10 to 30 red blood cells.

Estimate the platelets per cubic millimeter by counting the number of platelets in a few oil-immersion fields and multiplying the average by 20,000. For example, if you counted 10 platelets in one field, 20 in the next, and 15 in the next, for an average of 15 per high-power field, the platelet estimate would be 15 × 20,000, or 300,000 per cubic millimeter.

The normal range for the platelet count is 140,000 to 400,000 per cubic millimeter. A reduced platelet count occurs in acute bacterial infections, immunological disorders, certain hemorrhagic diseases, and anemias. An increased platelet count occurs after surgery, especially splenectomy; following strenuous exercise; and in inflammatory disorders.

PROCEDURE 15-1

Preparing, Staining, and Examining a Blood Smear Under High-Power Magnification

Goal

After successfully completing this procedure, you will be able to correctly prepare and quick stain a blood smear and examine the smear under the microscope, perform a white blood cell differential, note the red blood cell morphology, and estimate the number of platelets.

Completion Time

40 minutes

Equipment and Supplies

- Disposable gloves
- Goggles and apron
- Hand disinfectant
- Paper towels and tissues
- Biohazard container
- 70 percent alcohol
- Fresh EDTA-anticoagulated blood
- Capillary pipette

- Clean glass slides
- Quick stain with fixative
- Coplin jars or staining dishes
- Microscope
- Immersion oil
- Lens paper
- Differential cell counter or notepad and pen

Instructions

Read through the list of equipment and supplies that you will need and the steps of the procedure. Be sure that you understand each step before you begin. Then complete each step correctly, in the proper order, and in the time allowed.

*Steps marked with (*) are critical and must have the maximum points to pass.

Performance Standards	Points Awarded	Maximum Points
1. Put on a protective apron, wash your hands with disinfectant, dry them, and put on gloves.		10
2. Follow standard precautions.		10
3. Collect and prepare the appropriate equipment.		5
4. If slides are not precleaned, wash them, wipe them with alcohol, and dry them.		5
5. Mix the blood on a mechanical mixer for 2 minutes or invert several times to thoroughly mix the blood.		5
6. Lay a clean glass slide on the counter, holding by the edges with your nondominant hand.		5
7. Dispense a small drop of blood using a capillary pipette onto the slide about one-half inch from the end of the slide (the right end if you are right-handed, the left end if you are left-handed).		5
8. Holding another clean slide (the spreader slide) in your dominant hand, place it at a 35 to 40 degree angle in front of the drop of blood. Pull the slide back into the drop of blood, allowing the blood to spread along the width of the spreader slide.		5
9. Push the spreader slide forward with a smooth quick motion, maintaining the angle and allowing the blood to spread about three-quarters the length of the other slide. (Continue to hold the other slide with the nondominant hand to prevent it from moving.)		5
10. Gently but rapidly wave the slide to air dry the thin edge of the slide, then stand the slide with the thick end down to allow to dry completely.		5
11. Label the slide with the patient's name, date, and doctor on the thick end of the blood with a pencil.		5
12. Repeat steps 6–11 for a second blood slide.		5
13. Following manufacturer's instructions, transfer each of the three quick-stain solutions—the fixative, red stain (eosin), and blue (methylene blue) stain—to Coplin or other staining jars.		5
14. Dip one of the dried blood smear slides into the fixative solution for 1 second. Allow any excess to drain by blotting the end of the slide on paper towels. Do not allow to dry.		5
15. Dip the slide three to five times (1 second each dip) into solution #1, the eosin stain. Allow any excess to drain.		5
16. Dip the slide three to five times (1 second each dip) into solution #2 (methylene blue). Allow the slide to drain but do not dry.		5

—*table continued*

Performance Standards	Points Awarded	Maximum Points
17. Carefully rinse the slide with deionized water using a steady stream of water. Wipe the back of the slide with a tissue to remove the excess stain.		5
18. Allow the slide to air dry by standing it on its end.		2
19. Place the stained, dried blood smear slide on the mechanical stage of the microscope and secure the slide with the clamp.		2
20. Focus with the low-power (10X) objective, adjusting the light as needed.		5
21. Scan the slide to find the body region of the slide, the area where the cells barely touch one another, and observe the smear for normal staining characteristics.		5
22. Rotate the objective with the nosepiece out of place so the oil will not touch the objective and place a drop of immersion oil on the slide and carefully rotate the oil-immersion objective (100X) into place while watching from the side of the microscope.		5
23. Adjust the fine-focus adjustment knob until you focus the details of the cells clearly. Adjust the lighting to the correct level. If you lose the focus, return to 10X and begin focusing again.		5
24. Check the quality of staining on the slide, using the following criteria:		5
a. red blood cells—pinkish tan		
b. nuclei of lymphocytes—purple		
c. platelets—purple		
d. eosinophil granules—red/orange		
25. *Scan the slide systematically as Figure 15-3 shows. Count 100 consecutive white blood cells and record the types of cells observed with a differential cell counter, if available, or with a notepad and pen. Also record any unusual findings or questionable cells.		15
26. *Using systematic movement again, examine the appearance of red blood cells in at least 10 fields, noting		10
a. color—normochromic or hypochromic		
b. size—normocytic, microcytic, or macrocytic		
c. shape—description of any abnormal shapes present		
d. inclusions—description of any inclusions present		
27. Systematically observe the platelets in at least 10 fields, noting		5
a. if they are clumped or single		
b. the approximate number in each field (5–15 per field = adequate; fewer than 4 per field = decreased; more than 15 = increased)		
28. Rotate the 10X objective into place and remove the slide from the microscope stage.		5
29. Clean all lenses—beginning with the 10X and finishing with the 100X objective—gently with lens paper to remove any debris or oil. Clean the microscope stage of any oil or debris.		5
30. Discard disposable supplies and equipment.		5
31. Disinfect other equipment and return to storage.		5

32.	Clean the work area following the standard precautions.		5
33.	Remove your PPE and gloves, and wash and dry your hands.		5
34.	Record the results in appropriate records.		10
	Total Points		**194**

Overall Procedural Evaluation

Student Name _____

Signature of Instructor _____ Date _____

Comments _____

_____

chapter 15 REVIEW

Using Terminology

Write a brief definition of each of the following terms in the spaces provided.

1. Anisocytosis

_____

_____

_____

2. Eosin

_____

_____

_____

3. Hypersegmented

_____

_____

_____

4. Infectious mononucleosis

_____

_____

_____

5. Megakaryocyte

_____

_____

_____

6. Methylene blue

_____

_____

_____

7. Neutropenia

_____

_____

_____

8. Poikilocytosis

_____

_____

_____

9. Polychromatic stain

_____

_____

_____

10. Polymorphonuclear

_____

_____

_____

11. Quick-stain method

_____

_____

_____

12. Wright's stain

_____

_____

_____

13. Monocytic leukemia

_____

_____

_____

14. Acute lymphocytic leukemia

_____

_____

_____

15. Endocarditis

_____

_____

_____

Compare and contrast each of the following sets of terms by listing their similarities and differences in the spaces provided.

16. Granulocyte, agranulocyte

_____

_____

_____

17. Neutrophil, eosinophil, basophil

_____

_____

_____

18. Normochromic, hyperchromic, hypochromic

_____

_____

_____

19. Lymphocyte, monocyte

_____

_____

_____

20. Macrocyte, microcyte

_____

_____

_____

Multiple Choice

Choose the best answer for the following questions.

21. The most common white blood cell seen on a WBC differential is the
   a. lymphocyte
   b. segmented neutrophil
   c. basophil
   d. monocyte

22. In a patient with infectious mononucleosis, the white blood cell that is both more numerous and larger than the normal cell is the
   a. monocyte
   b. lymphocyte
   c. basophil
   d. eosinophil

23. Blood smears can be made from venous blood collected with which of the following anticoagulants?
    a. EDTA
    b. heparin
    c. sodium citrate
    d. warfarin

24. Platelets are not cells but fragments of the cytoplasm of large cells in the bone marrow called
    a. myeloblasts
    b. thromboblasts
    c. megakaryocytes
    d. neutrophils

25. A patient diagnosed with allergies could possibly have an increased percentage of which of the following WBCs?
    a. eosinophils
    b. basophils
    c. bands
    d. monocytes

26. The stain specific for blood smears and used most often in the medical office laboratory is
    a. gram stain
    b. Wright's stain
    c. quick stain
    d. EDTA

27. An increase in the absolute number of lymphocytes in an adult blood smear would most likely indicate which of these disorders?
    a. viral infection
    b. parasitic infection
    c. allergic reaction
    d. bacterial infection

28. A stained white blood cell that has a multilobed nucleus and cytoplasm filled with fine pink granules is a/an
    a. neutrophil
    b. basophil
    c. eosinophil
    d. monocyte

29. Red blood cells on a stained blood smear appear to have varied abnormal shapes. This would be referred to as
    a. anisocytosis
    b. erythropenia
    c. normal
    d. poikilocytosis

30. Which of the following WBC counts would be considered the most normal count for an adult female?
    a. 15, 000 WBC/mm^3
    b. 1,500 WBC/mm^3
    c. 7,500 WBC/mm^3
    d. 5,000 WBC/mm^3

Acquiring Knowledge

Answer the following questions in the spaces provided.

31. How do red blood cells differ from most other cells?

_____

_____

_____

32. How many formed elements of each type normally are found in one cubic millimeter of blood? What are the size relationships among the different types of formed elements?

_____

_____

_____

33. Why is it important that a blood smear not be too thick or too thin? How is thickness of the smear related to the manner in which the spreader slide is held?

_____

_____

_____

34. Describe the characteristics of a properly prepared blood smear slide.

_____

_____

_____

35. What region of a blood smear slide is examined under the microscope in a differential count? Why?

_____

_____

_____

36. What may cause a stained blood smear to appear too blue? Too pink?

_____

_____

_____

37. What features must be examined to differentiate among the various types of white blood cells?

_____

_____

_____

38. How can you tell if an agranulocyte is a lymphocyte or a monocyte?

_____

_____

_____

39. Explain how white blood cells are counted on a differential blood smear slide.

_____

_____

_____

40. What are some causes of an abnormally high or low neutrophil count in a differential blood smear?

_____

_____

_____

41. What disorders may lead to an increase in the number of small lymphocytes?

_____

_____

_____

42. Which features of red blood cells are examined in a differential blood smear slide?

_____

_____

_____

43. Explain how hemoglobin concentration can be assessed from examination of a differential blood smear slide.

_____

_____

_____

44. What are the origin and function of platelets?

_____

_____

_____

45. What factors may lead to a reduced platelet count? an increased platelet count?

_____

_____

_____

Applying Knowledge—On the Job

Answer the following questions in the spaces provided.

46. Assume that you have been instructed by your lab supervisor to help a new lab worker identify stained white blood cells in a differential blood smear slide. What characteristics of stained white cells would you point out as most useful in distinguishing the different types?

_____

_____

_____

47. Assume that you just got a platelet count of 30,000 using the automated hematology machine in your POL. How can you confirm the low platelet count by examining the patient's stained blood smear slide?

_____

_____

_____

48. You have a stained differential blood smear slide for a 9-month-old infant showing small red cells with very little color. The pale center is larger than in a normal red cell. What condition does this child have? What is the child's hemoglobin concentration likely to be?

_____

_____

_____

49. A patient's differential blood smear slide, which was stained using the quick-stain method, is too dark for good viewing. What is the problem and how can it be corrected?

_____

_____

_____

50. A differential blood smear slide that you are examining has dark blue and purple sediment scattered over it, which interferes with a clear view of the formed elements. What is the problem and how can it be corrected?

_____

_____

_____

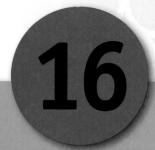

16 *chapter*

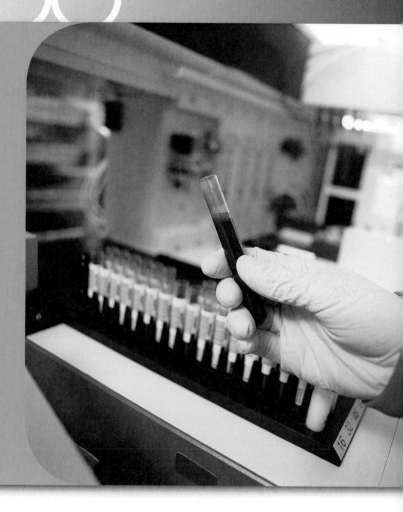

Automated Hematology and Quality Control

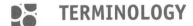

TERMINOLOGY

aperture: an opening, as in the probe of an electrical impedance or electron-optical cell counter, through which blood cells and other formed elements in diluting solution pass in single file.

cyanmethemoglobin: a very stable cyanide and hemoglobin compound that results when a solution of potassium ferrocyanide and potassium cyanide is added to blood, lysing the red blood cells and releasing their hemoglobin content.

electrical impedance cell counter: an automated hematology instrument, such as the Beckman Coulter and Abbot Cell Dyn instruments, that analyzes formed elements in the blood on the basis of their impedance of an electrical current.

electrical impedance method: the method of studying the formed elements in the blood that depends on their resistance to the flow of an electrical current.

flow cytometry: a technique that analyzes cells as they are forced through a detector system; this system could be an electric current, a light or laser beam, or fluorescent dyes.

hematology calibrator: a hematology control that is certified to be highly stable over its entire life;

used to set the electronics of automated hematology instruments.

hematology control: an artificial blood, containing both human and animal cells, that is used to check the stability of electronic settings of automated hematology instruments.

histogram: a graph derived from sampling showing frequency distributions.

light-scattering (optical counting) method: the method of studying formed elements in the blood that depends on their interruption of a beam of light from a laser lamp.

optical counting method: light-scattering method.

QBC (quantitative buffy coat) calibration check tube: the tube used with a QBC instrument to perform a daily quality control check. It gives a set of expected values and acceptable deviation values for each parameter.

QBC (quantitative buffy coat) instrument: an automated hematology instrument that centrifuges nondiluted blood samples and estimates blood parameters such as hemoglobin, hematocrit, platelet counts, and WBC counts on the basis of differences in density and fluorescence.

INTRODUCTION

Some form of automated hematology instrument is widely used in medical laboratories because of the greater accuracy and speed of automated methods over manual methods. These hematology analyzers have become the cornerstone of clinical laboratories, including the POLs that can perform more detailed complete blood counts.

AN OVERVIEW OF AUTOMATED HEMATOLOGY INSTRUMENTS

Innovations in automated hematology instruments from the simple low-volume compact analyzers to the high-volume complicated analyzers have made it possible for even the smallest laboratories to perform complete blood counts more efficiently and accurately. CBCs routinely include automated WBC differential counts and now can include further classification of abnormal cells or immature cells and platelet counts. More sophisticated instruments enable the use of auto-sampling, barcode sample identification, reticulocyte counts,

nucleated red blood cell counts, and quality control data management. We will discuss some of the methods of counting and differentiating blood cells used in some of the hematology analyzers on the market.

Hematology analyzers can be divided into two major types: one that dilutes the EDTA blood in buffered isotonic suspensions before counting and measuring and the other that uses an undiluted blood sample, separating the formed elements by centrifugation.

The type of instrument best suited for a particular laboratory depends on several considerations, including

- the hematology tests most commonly performed
- the degree of automation required
- the cost of the instrument and maintenance
- the amount of laboratory space available
- the number of staff and their qualifications
- the level of CLIA certification of the laboratory

HEMATOLOGY INSTRUMENTS REQUIRING DILUTED SAMPLES

The basic principle of most automated hematology instruments involves a method known as **flow cytometry.** This is a technique in which particles (cells) are measured and analyzed using electrical current, a light beam (usually laser), or fluorescent dyes. Blood cells and platelets can be counted and differentiated automatically and the results recorded on a printout. Flow cytometry is possible when the particles are diluted in a suspension of fluid. Two of these procedures will be discussed below.

Instruments Using Electrical Impedance

The hematology analyzers used most commonly in labs count blood cells and platelets by counting electrical impulses generated when blood cells impede an electrical current. This is called the **electrical impedance method** and has been used since the earliest cell counters were built by the Coulter company. A few examples of these instruments frequently found in low-volume hematology laboratories include Beckman Coulter® AcT Diff™ Hematology Analyzer (Beckman Coulter, Fullerton, California) and CELL-DYN® 1800 (Abbott Laboratories, Abbott Park, Illinois). (See Figure 16-1.)

In this method, a volume of diluted blood is drawn through a small (78–100 μm) **aperture,** or opening, in the probe of the **electrical impedance cell counter.** A constant current is passed across the aperture from one side to the other. When a particle (cell) passes through the aperture, it causes a change in resistance, which in turn causes a voltage pulse. The number of pulses indicates the number of particles that pass through the aperture. This gives the blood cell counts. (See Figure 16-2.)

The size of the pulse is proportional to the size of the cell passing through the aperture; the larger the cell, the greater the pulse. Pulse magnitude can be used to measure cell volume as well as to differentiate the type of cells by size. Figure 16-3

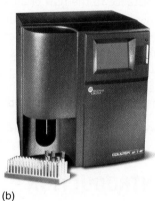
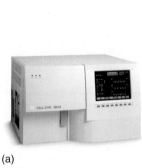

(a)   (b)

Figure 16-1 Examples of instruments frequently found in low-volume hematology laboratories. (a) Abbott CELL-DYN® 1800 Hematology analyzer (b) Coulter AcT Diff® Hematology analyzer.

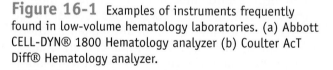
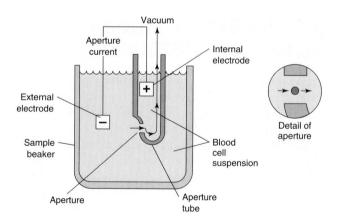

Figure 16-2 A schematic of an electrical impedance counter.
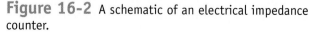

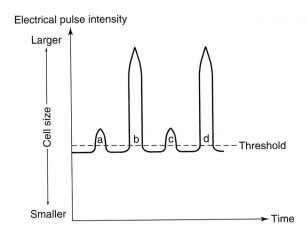

Figure 16-3 Electrical pulses from cells of different sizes.

Table 16-1   Normal Volume of Blood Cells and Platelets

Type of Blood Cell or Platelet	Range in Volume (in cubic microns)
White blood cells	120 to 1,000
Red blood cells	85 to 95
Platelets	3 to 30

shows how cells of two different sizes generate pulses of different magnitudes. If the pulses labeled *a* and *c* were produced by platelets, those labeled *b* and *d* would have been produced by red blood cells, which are considerably larger. See Table 16-1.

Most hematology instruments operate with very similar methods, varying in the reagents or dilution volumes. Generally speaking, to perform a complete blood count, the analyzer aspirates a small volume of whole blood from a well-mixed EDTA tube, usually in the range of 18 to 30 μL. This is mixed with reagent and the primary dilution is made, 1:250. This dilution sample is then divided into two samples; one is diluted further for the red blood cell count and platelet count. The remainder of the dilution is mixed with lysing reagent that ruptures the red cells, allowing the white blood cells to be counted without the interference of the red blood cells. Rupturing the red cells also causes the release of hemoglobin, which can now be measured using light absorption. The results of each parameter of the complete blood count are printed. (See Figure 16-4.)

WBC Counts. WBC counts are performed using a dilution of approximately 1:250 with the lysing reagent added. The cells are counted as they pass through the aperture of the WBC counting chamber using electrical impedance, as previously discussed. Differential white blood cell counts also are done at this stage of the process by the differences in pulse amplitude. The size or amplitude of the pulses is used to distinguish the different types of WBCs. Most instruments can determine three WBC subpopulations: small-cell population (lymphocytes), midrange cells (monocytes, basophils, eosinophils), and large cells (granulocytes), creating a three-part differential. More advanced instruments can determine a five-part differential.

RBC and Platelet Counts. RBC counts are performed using a larger dilution than white cells, approximately 1:30,000. The dilutions depend on the particular analyzer. After the dilution is prepared, the red blood cells and platelets are counted as they pass through the aperture in the RBC/PLT counting chamber. The sizes of these particles determine the counts. Platelets are much smaller than RBCs, so they can be distinguished from red cells and counted at the same time as the red blood cells. Red blood cells are counted and sorted according to size and a **histogram** is produced.

MCV. The mean cell volume (MCV) is the average volume of individual RBCs. After the red blood cells have been sized, an average can be extracted from the RBC histogram. (See Figure 16-5.)

Hematocrits. Hematocrits, the percent of whole blood volume that is composed of red blood cells, can be calculated using the analyzer's RBC and MCV measurements.

Hemoglobin Determinations. Hemoglobin measurements made with an electrical impedance type instrument use an optical absorbance across the white blood cell counting chamber. Hemoglobin is converted to **cyanmethemoglobin** in a colorimetric reaction and absorbs green light of wavelength 540 nm in a ratio compared to a zero blank reference of solution. (See Figure 16-6.) The analyzer determines the hemoglobin and prints out values in grams per deciliter.

Instruments Using Laser Light Scattering

Some hematology analyzers use flow principles to count elements in blood. This is a technique of analyzing individual cells and can be done using a light beam, usually a laser, and is called

ANY CLINIC LABORATORY

Sample No.:   John Doe   Rack: 9   Tube: 9   01/24/2010   15:24:26
Patient ID: Ward: Dr.:
Name: Birth: Sex:
Comments: Inst.ID: XS-1000ix11690

Any Clinic Laboratory

101 Line Drive
Russellville, AR 72801
555-123-4567   **Adult Reference Values**

WBC	6.35	[10^3/μL]				4.1 – 10.9	[10^3/μL]
NEUT	3.61	[10^3/μL]	56.8		[%]	1.56 – 6.13	[10^3/μL]
LYMPH	1.79	[10^3/μL]	28.2		[%]	1.18 – 3.74	[10^3/μL]
MONO	0.75	[10^3/μL]	11.8	+	[%]	0.24 – 0.82	[10^3/μL]
EO	0.15	[10^3/μL]	2.4		[%]	0.04 – 0.54	[10^3/μL]
BASO	0.05	[10^3/μL]	0.8		[%]	0.01 – 0.08	[10^3/μL]

RBC	4.69	[10^6/μL]	4.2 – 6.3
HGB	13.4	[g/dL]	12.0 – 18.0
HCT	39.2	[%]	37.0 – 51.0
MCV	83.6	[fL]	80.0 – 97.0
MCH	28.6	[pg]	26.0 – 32.0
MCHC	34.2	[g/dL]	31.0 – 36.0
RDW-CV	14.3	[%]	11.6 – 14.4
PLT	220	[10^3/μL]	140 – 440

Manual Diff Results

NEUT	_____	50 – 70	[%]
BAND	_____	0 – 3.5	[%]
LYMPH	_____	25 – 40	[%]
MONO	_____	3 – 7	[%]
EO	_____	1 – 3	[%]
BASO	_____	0 – 1.0	[%]
META	_____	0 – 1	[%]
MYELO	_____	0	[%]
PRO	_____	0	[%]
BLAST	_____	0	[%]
OTHER	_____	0	[%]
COMMENTS:			

Figure 16-4 Complete blood count report.

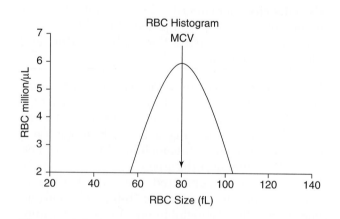

Figure 16-5 RBC histogram.

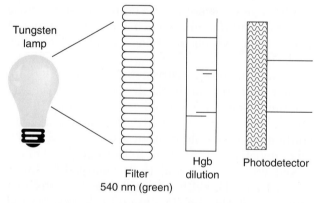

Figure 16-6 The hemoglobin colorimetric measurement method.

light scattering or **optical counting.** These instruments are designed to handle large volumes of blood samples and are not commonly used in POLs.

As with electrical impedance counters, optical counters use blood samples diluted in a known solution to ensure the separation of cells so that they can be conducted in single file past the counting point. The dilutions are usually lower than those used for the electrical impedance method. This makes it possible to count a larger number of cells in a given volume of diluted sample. (See Figure 16-7.)

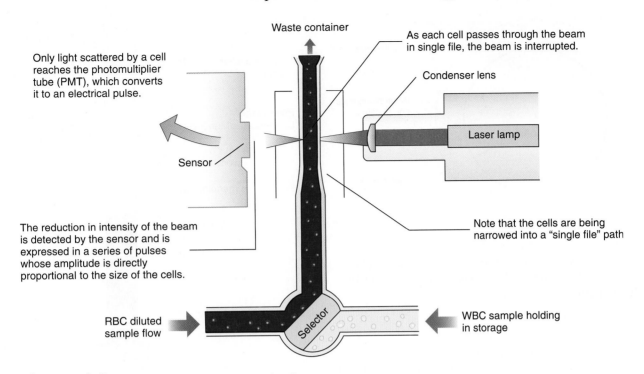

Figure 16-7 The flow of cells in an optical cell counter.

Optical cell counters use a laser lamp that has an extremely sharp focus of discrete, monochromatic light. This allows the beam to be focused to a point that approaches the total diameter of the aperture through which the cells pass. The intensity of the beam is a known specific value at this point. As each blood cell in the flow cell passes through the beam, it interrupts the beam, reduces the intensity of the beam by a degree proportional to the size of the cell, and results in light-scattering patterns characteristic for the particle.

HEMATOLOGY INSTRUMENTS REQUIRING UNDILUTED SAMPLES

QBC Diagnostics, Inc., State College, Pennsylvania, manufactures hematology instruments, one of which is called the QBC Autoread System, shown in Figure 16-8. This is an analyzer that uses an undiluted blood sample. The **QBC (quantitative buffy coat) instrument** is a centrifugal system that uses dry hematology reagents and can be used to perform the following nine hematology parameters:

- hemoglobin
- hematocrit
- platelet count
- total WBC count
- total granulocyte count
- percent granulocytes

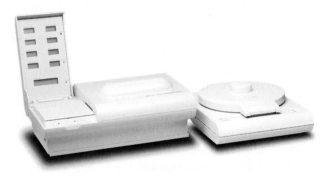

Figure 16-8 QBC Autoread System.

- total lymphocytes/monocytes count
- percent lymphocytes/monocytes
- mean cell hemoglobin concentration (MCHC)

In the QBC instrument, a sample of whole blood, which is collected by either finger puncture or venipuncture, is drawn into a very precise microhematocrit-type capillary tube.

> **Note**
>
> The QBC instrument does not perform an RBC count. It cannot be used to calculate mean cell volume (MCV) or the mean cell hemoglobin (MCH), two of the red blood cell indices described in the next chapter. The QBC instrument does calculate a mean cell hemoglobin concentration (MCHC).

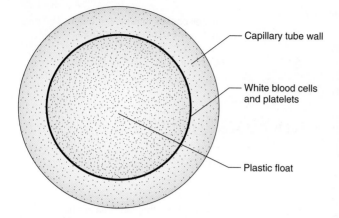

Figure 16-9 A cross-section of a capillary tube in the buffy coat area. Expansion of the buffy coat (platelets and white blood cells) is seen between the plastic float and the capillary wall.

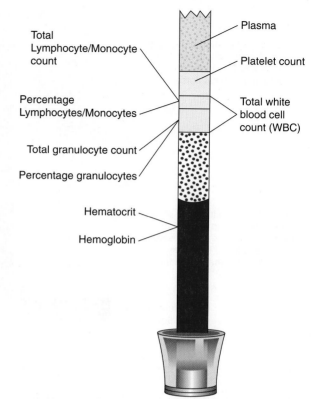

Figure 16-10 A spun capillary tube. Centrifugation of the tube separates the formed elements of the blood into distinct layers.

A cap is placed on the end of the capillary tube. The tube is treated on the inside with a special stain, which is picked up by the nuclei of the white blood cells. The capillary tube is fitted with a precisely sized plastic float, which has a somewhat lower density than red blood cells, causing it to float on top of the red blood cells. The float is slightly smaller in diameter than the diameter of the capillary tube. This forces the buffy coat, which is on top of the red cells, to be expanded between the float and the wall of the capillary tube, as Figure 16-9 shows.

First, blood is centrifuged in the capillary tube for 5 minutes at 12,000 rpm. Then the capillary tube is placed in a reader that contains a fluorescent microscope and a micrometer. In the older QBC instruments, the tube is moved manually, by turning the transport knob to advance the tube in the reader. In an automated reader (QBC Autoread or QBC Hescan), it is moved automatically until it comes to a distinct interface in the buffy column. Chemical and physical differences among the cells cause them to fluoresce different colors. The different layers of the buffy coat represent different types of white cells and platelets in the column, as Figure 16-10 shows.

Hemoglobin concentration is indicated by the height of the plastic float in the red blood cell column. Red blood cells that contain large amounts of hemoglobin are more dense and cause the float to ride high. Red blood cells that are low in hemoglobin have a lower density, causing the float to sink in the column when it is centrifuged.

QUALITY CONTROL

As is true with all other instruments used in POLs, automated hematology instruments require a good system of quality control to test their accuracy and precision. Quality control must be an ongoing process and not just part of the initial installation. Quality control testing involves the use of controls and calibrators to test the accuracy and precision of the instrument, the procedure, and the operator. Some automated hematology instruments store test results in their computers and provide a monthly printout that can be mailed to the manufacturer of the controls and calibrators to verify the accuracy of the instrument. Required reagents also must be checked daily for quality.

Some POLs use split samples in their quality control program. Part of a sample is analyzed in the POL and part is sent to an outside reference laboratory for comparison. Split-specimen testing is useful for detecting inaccurate or imprecise test results caused by improper calibrations, mechanical problems, and operator errors.

Controls

A **hematology control** is artificial blood that is used to check the stability of electronic settings of automated hematology instruments. Most hematology controls include both human and animal cells. Human red blood cells are used, but instead of human leukocytes, bird red blood cells are substituted. They have the same volume as human leukocytes but are more stable. Bird RBCs have nuclei and are very similar in size to human WBCs, and they have very long life spans. Swine platelets are also used in hematology controls.

Hematology controls normally are available in three levels: abnormal low values, normal values, and abnormal high values. The manufacturers provide the expected values and the allowable deviation for each level of the control for a given instrument using the stated reagent systems. Thus, the values stated for one instrument will not be the same as those for a different instrument. Most manufacturers also list expected values for manual determinations.

Controls for a test must be run before you perform that test on a patient's specimen. CLIA 1988 requires performing two levels of controls. Controls are usually performed at the beginning of each workday or whenever an instrument has been shut down for 4 hours or more. CLIA 1988 also requires POLs with extended hours to run controls for some automated hematology tests at 8-hour intervals. Quality control checks on the QBC instrument are performed daily using a **QBC calibration check tube**. This gives a set of expected values and acceptable deviations for each parameter.

Calibrators

A **hematology calibrator** normally is a control that is certified to be highly stable over its entire life. Calibrators are used to set the electronics of the instrument, while controls are used to check the stability of these settings. Calibrators are specially prepared for specific instruments, as listed on the insert sheet that comes with each set of calibrators, and they must be used with the reagent system on which the expected values have been determined.

> **Caution—Biohazard!**
>
> Because hematology controls and calibrators contain human blood, you must handle them with the same caution as with other blood samples.

Automated electronic hematology instruments should be calibrated as scheduled by the manufacturer or whenever controls give erroneous results. CLIA 1988 requires that calibration of automated hematology instruments be performed at 3-month intervals and that the POL enroll in a proficiency testing program for the automated hematology instrument.

Reagents

In addition to checking the instrument daily with controls, it is also necessary to check all reagents. For example, a background check must be run on the isotonic diluent each day to be sure that yeast or mold is not growing in the solution. Yeast and mold would be counted as blood cells and would give falsely high readings.

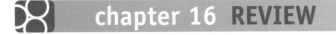

chapter 16 REVIEW

Using Terminology

Write a brief definition of each of the following terms in the spaces provided.

1. Cyanmethemoglobin

_____

_____

_____

2. Electrical impedance method

_____

_____

_____

3. Light-scattering method

_____

_____

_____

4. Hematology calibrator

_____

_____

_____

5. QBC (quantitative buffy coat) instrument

_____

_____

_____

6. Aperture

_____

_____

_____

7. Electrical impedance cell counter

_____

_____

_____

Multiple Choice

Choose the best answer for the following questions.

8. A technique in which hematology analyzers force blood cells through a measuring detector system such as a laser beam or an electric current is known as
   a. centrifugation
   b. flow cytometry
   c. color measurement
   d. buffy coat analysis

9. A graph that is generated and printed by a hematology analyzer showing the size and frequency distributions of cell populations is called a
   a. print-out
   b. calibrator cycle
   c. histogram
   d. electrogram

10. The best advantage of using a hematology analyzer in a POL would be which of the following?
   a. improved efficiency of reporting results to the physician
   b. improvement in quality control
   c. more profit for the clinic
   d. less staffing needed

11. Using an electrical impedance analyzer, which feature is used to differentiate the white blood cell populations?
   a. the number of electrical pulses
   b. the sizes of the electrical pulses
   c. the color of the white cells counted
   d. the brand of instrument used

12. Which of the following formed elements found in whole blood would generate the largest electrical pulse in the electrical impedance analyzer?
   a. platelet
   b. erythrocyte
   c. nucleated red blood cell
   d. leukocyte

Acquiring Knowledge

Answer the following questions in the spaces provided.

13. What are the main advantages of using automated hematology instruments over using manual methods?

_____

_____

_____

14. What are the main purposes of automated hematology instruments?

_____

_____

_____

15. What are some of the parameters that automated hematology instruments perform?

_____

_____

_____

16. List several factors that should be considered when selecting an automated hematology instrument for a particular POL.

_____

_____

_____

17. Briefly state how an electrical impedance cell counter works.

_____

_____

_____

18. How does the electrical impedance cell counter differentiate cells on the basis of size?

_____

_____

_____

19. Why is it necessary to dilute blood samples when performing tests with some automated hematology instruments?

_____

_____

_____

20. Explain why two different dilutions are necessary when using electrical impedance cell counters. When is each dilution used?

_____

_____

_____

21. Why must a lysing agent be added to the blood sample for WBC counts and hemoglobin determinations when using an electrical impedance cell counter?

_____

_____

_____

22. What method is used to determine hemoglobin concentration with an automated cell counter? How does it work?

_____

_____

_____

23. How are different types of blood cells distinguished with a QBC instrument?

_____

_____

_____

24. Describe how hemoglobin concentration is estimated with a QBC instrument.

_____

_____

_____

25. What is the role of quality control in the use of automated hematology instruments? What are some ways in which quality control is achieved?

_____

_____

_____

26. List the hematology parameters that can be estimated with a QBC instrument.

_____

_____

_____

Applying Knowledge—On the Job

Answer the following questions in the spaces provided.

27. The physician you work for has ordered a manual differential white blood cell count in addition to the one furnished by the QBC instrument. What additional information can be obtained from a manual differential?

_____

_____

_____

28. One of your duties in the POL is to operate an automated hematology instrument. What precautions should you take when handling the artificial blood used as a control?

_____

_____

_____

29. The laboratory where you are employed is required to calculate erythrocyte indices. What type of automated hematology instrument should be purchased for this purpose? Why?

_____

_____

_____

30. The business manager of the physician's office where you are employed has asked you to compose a list of factors you feel are important in selecting a new hematology analyzer to replace the one currently being used. What would you include in your list?

_____

_____

_____

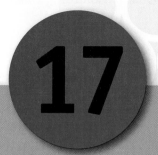

17 chapter

chapter

Advanced Hematology Procedures

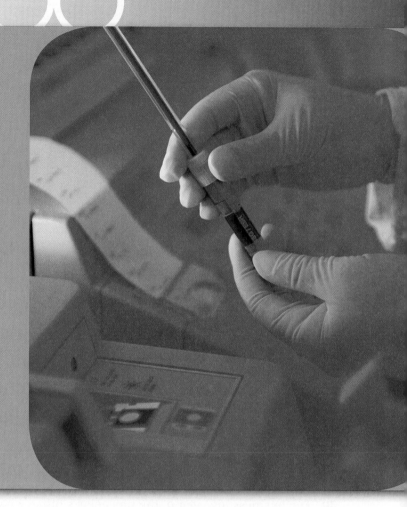

COGNITIVE OBJECTIVES

After studying this chapter, you should be able to

17.1   use each of the vocabulary terms appropriately.

17.2   differentiate the three important erythrocyte indices.

17.3   explain what high and low values for each erythrocyte index mean.

17.4   differentiate the direct and indirect methods of counting platelets.

17.5   list potential sources of error in performing platelet counts.

17.6   identify the three stages of erythrocyte sedimentation.

17.7   list potential sources of error in measuring the erythrocyte sedimentation rate.

17.8   discuss the factors that influence the erythrocyte sedimentation rate.

17.9   explain how the erythrocyte sedimentation rate is used as a diagnostic tool.

17.10   list potential sources of error in performing reticulocyte counts.

17.11   explain why the reticulocyte count is a valuable indicator of erythropoiesis.

17.12   describe the clinical applications of the reticulocyte count.

PERFORMANCE OBJECTIVES

After studying this chapter, you should be able to

17.13   calculate and interpret erythrocyte indices.

17.14   count platelets using direct and indirect methods.

17.15 calculate the platelet count.

17.16 use the Westergren method to determine erythrocyte sedimentation rates.

17.17 prepare a smear and count reticulocytes.

17.18 calculate the percent and absolute number of reticulocytes.

░ TERMINOLOGY

erythrocyte indices: three indicators of the size or hemoglobin content of the red blood cells that are used in the diagnosis of anemia. They include the mean cell volume (MCV), the mean cell hemoglobin (MCH), and the mean cell hemoglobin concentration (MCHC).

erythrocyte sedimentation rate (ESR or sed rate): the rate at which red blood cells settle out of plasma when placed in a vertical tube.

mean cell hemoglobin (MCH): the average weight of hemoglobin in red blood cells in a sample (also called mean corpuscular hemoglobin).

mean cell hemoglobin concentration (MCHC): average concentration of hemoglobin in a given volume of packed red blood cells in a sample (also called mean corpuscular hemoglobin concentration).

mean cell volume (MCV): the average volume of red blood cells in a sample (also called mean corpuscular volume).

reticulocytopenia: the lowering of the number of circulating reticulocytes; usually found in patients with pernicious anemia, aplastic anemia, or bone marrow failure.

spherocytosis: a condition in which red blood cells assume a spherical shape.

supravital stain: a stain that stains only living cells, not dried blood smears.

INTRODUCTION

This chapter describes the following advanced hematology indices and procedures that may be performed in POLs:

- erythrocyte indices
- platelet counts
- the erythrocyte sedimentation rate
- reticulocyte counts

ERYTHROCYTE INDICES

Three **erythrocyte indices** were introduced by Dr. Maxwell Wintrobe:

- the mean cell volume (MCV)
- the mean cell hemoglobin (MCH)
- the mean cell hemoglobin concentration (MCHC)

The indices are indicators of the size and hemoglobin content of the average red blood cell in a given sample of blood. They are used primarily for diagnosing anemia.

Calculating the Indices

Each index is calculated from two of the following three blood parameters: RBC count, hemoglobin, and hematocrit. The validity of the indices depends on the accuracy of these three blood parameters. For this reason, the indices became a routine part of the complete blood count only

Table 17-1 A Review of Metric Units

Unit	Symbol	Equivalent
Deciliter	dL	0.1 liter
Femtoliter	fL	10^{-15} liter
Micrometer	μm	10^{-6} meter
Picogram	pg	10^{-12} gram
Micromicrogram	$\mu\mu$g	10^{-12} gram

when automated methods increased the accuracy of the RBC count. The validity of the erythrocyte indices can be checked against the appearance of the red blood cells on a stained differential blood smear slide.

Erythrocyte indices are expressed in very small units, some of which were defined in Chapter 3. See Table 17-1.

The Mean Cell Volume. Mean cell volume (MCV) is the average volume of a red blood cell in the sample. It is expressed in femtoliters (fL), or their equivalent cubic micrometers (μm^3), and reported to the nearest whole number.

MCV is calculated from the RBC count and the hematocrit (Hct) using the formula

$$MCV = \frac{Hct\ (\%) \times 10}{RBC\ (millions)}$$

The Mean Cell Hemoglobin Concentration. The **mean cell hemoglobin concentration (MCHC)** is the average concentration of hemoglobin in a given volume of packed red blood cells in the sample. It is expressed in percent (%), or grams per deciliter (g/dL), and reported to the nearest tenth. The ratio of the weight of hemoglobin to the volume of red blood cells, the MCHC is calculated from the hemoglobin concentration (Hgb) and hematocrit (Hct) using the formula

$$MCHC = \frac{Hgb\ (g/dL) \times 100}{Hct\ (\%)}$$

The Mean Cell Hemoglobin. The **mean cell hemoglobin (MCH)** is the average weight of hemoglobin in a red blood cell in the sample. It is expressed in picograms (pg) or micromicrograms ($\mu\mu$g) and is reported to the nearest tenth.

MCH is directly proportional to the amount of hemoglobin and the size of the red blood cell. It is calculated from the hemoglobin concentration (Hgb) and the RBC count using the formula

$$MCH = \frac{Hgb\ (g/dL) \times 10}{RBC\ (millions)}$$

Interpreting the Indices

In healthy adults, the erythrocyte indices show little variation from the normal ranges (see Table 17-2). A deviation of more than one unit from the normal range usually indicates some type of anemia.

The Mean Cell Volume. The MCV indicates the size of the red blood cells. Cells in the normal range of 82 to 102 fL are considered normocytic. Cells with MCV less than 80 fL are considered microcytic. Those over 102 fL are considered macrocytic. The greater the deviation of MCV from the normal range, the more the cells differ from normal size.

MCV is higher than normal in anemia caused by vitamin B12 deficiency and in pernicious anemia. These conditions are referred to as macrocytic anemias. In macrocytosis with many oval macrocytes, MCV is usually in the range of 120 to 140 fL. MCV is decreased in iron-deficiency anemia, which is characteristically microcytic.

The Mean Cell Hemoglobin Concentration. The MCHC indicates whether the red blood cells are normochromic, meaning that they have normal color and hemoglobin content, or hypochromic, meaning that they are pale and low in hemoglobin. MCHC values below 32 percent indicate hypochromia, which is associated with iron-deficiency anemia. In macrocytic anemias, MCHC is normal or slightly reduced. MCHC values above 38 percent only occur with **spherocytosis,** a condition in which erythrocytes assume a spheroid shape. It is characteristic of certain hemolytic anemias.

Interpretation Tips

- When the MCHC is above 40 percent and other blood parameters are normal, the automated hematology instrument should be checked for malfunction.
- When all three indices are markedly elevated, the cause may be autoagglutination of the red blood cells or rouleaux formation. Figure 17-1 illustrates rouleaux.

Table 17-2 Normal Adult Values for Erythrocyte Indices

Index	Normal Adult* Range
MCV	82 to 102 fL or μm^3
MCH	27.0 to 33.0 pg or $\mu\mu$g
MCHC	33.0 to 38.0% or g/dL

*MCV and MCH values are higher at birth and lower at 1 year of age than they are in adulthood. Both rise to adult values by puberty.

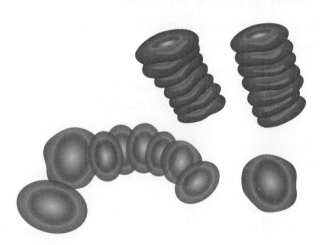

Figure 17-1 Erythrocytes in rouleaux formation resemble a stack of coins. Because they fit together in less space, rouleaux cells have a higher sedimentation rate than do normal cells. Rouleaux formation results from pathologic changes in the blood.

Table 17-3   Patient Data for Erythrocyte Indices Example

Patient	RBC (millions/mm³)	Hgb (g/dL)	Hct (%)
Patient A	4.2	6.5	24
Patient B	2.2	9.0	27

The Mean Cell Hemoglobin. The MCH indicates the weight of hemoglobin in the average red blood cell. Elevated MCH values are present in macrocytic anemia. The cells contain more hemoglobin because they are large, although the concentration of hemoglobin per unit volume of the cell (MCHC) may be normal or even slightly reduced. Lower-than-normal MCH values are found in microcytic anemia, unless the red blood cells also are spherocytic. MCH also is lower than normal in normocytic cells that are hypochromic. If the cells are both microcytic and hypochromic, the MCH value is even lower.

Calculating Erythrocyte Indices: Two Worked Examples

The following two worked examples show how to calculate and interpret the erythrocyte indices. See Table 17-3 for patient data.

Patient A.

$$MCV = \frac{Hct\ (\%) \times 10}{RBC\ (million)} = \frac{24 \times 10}{4.2} = 57\ fL$$

$$MCH = \frac{Hgb\ (g/dL) \times 10}{RBC\ (million)} = \frac{6.5 \times 10}{4.2} = 15.5\ pg$$

$$MCHC = \frac{Hgb\ (g/dL) \times 100}{Hct\ (\%)} = \frac{6.5 \times 100}{24}$$
$$= 27.1\ g/dL$$

Compared with normal values, Patient A has low values for all three indices. This means that the patient's red blood cells are both microcytic and hypochromic, which is characteristic of iron-deficiency anemia.

Patient B.

$$MCV = \frac{HCT\ (\%) \times 10}{RBC\ (million)} = \frac{27 \times 10}{2.2} = 123\ fL$$

$$MCH = \frac{Hgb\ (g/dL) \times 10}{RBC\ (million)} = \frac{9.0 \times 10}{2.2} = 40.9\ pg$$

$$MCHC = \frac{Hgb\ (g/dL) \times 100}{Hct\ (\%)} = \frac{9.0 \times 100}{27}$$
$$= 33.3 g/dL$$

Compared with normal values, Patient B has elevated MCV and MCH values but a normal MCHC value. This means that the patient has macrocytic normochromic red blood cells, which are characteristic of pernicious anemia.

PLATELET COUNTS

Platelets can be counted directly using the Unopette system and a hemacytometer or with an automated hematology instrument. They are counted indirectly using a stained blood smear slide and an oil-immersion objective.

The Direct Method

Using the Unopette System. The most common direct method of counting platelets involves using the Unopette kit that contains a 20 µL capillary pipette and a disposable prefilled reservoir containing 1.98 mL of reagent giving a dilution of 1:100. The reagent is ammonium oxalate to which a phosphate buffer has been added to maintain pH. The blood sample is collected by capillary puncture or by venipuncture using EDTA anticoagulant.

In the Unopette method, first puncture the diaphragm of the reservoir with the protective shield on the capillary pipette (see Figure 17-2). Then fill the capillary pipette with capillary blood or with well-mixed whole blood and transfer it to the reservoir. Let stand at least 10 minutes to allow RBCs to completely lyse. The erythrocytes are lysed, leaving intact the platelets and white blood cells.

> **Note**
>
> Capillary blood may be used instead of venous blood for a platelet count. Be aware, however, that blood collected by capillary puncture usually is lower in platelets than is blood collected by venipuncture. Because the function of platelets is to adhere to wounds and skin punctures, there is inevitably a loss of platelets during the collection process.

Charging the Hemacytometer. Mix the diluted sample thoroughly by inverting the reservoir to resuspend the cells. Remove the capillary pipette and convert it to the dropper assembly. Expel the air in the pipette and discard the first two drops of

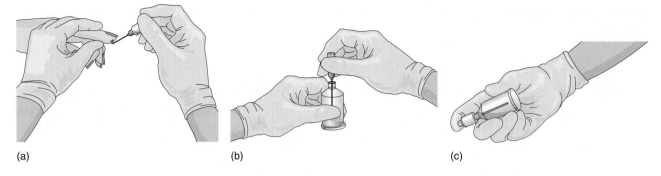

(a)   (b)   (c)

Figure 17-2 The Unopette system for counting platelets requires puncturing the diaphragm of the reservoir, which contains Thimerosol, with the pipette shield. (a) Collect the specimen with the Unopette pipette. (b) Transfer the blood specimen to the reservoir. (c) Place a finger over the reservoir and mix by inversion.

dilution to ensure the sample used is from the reservoir and not from the pipette. Charge both sides of the well-cleaned counting chamber as described in Chapter 14. Place the charged hemacytometer in a covered Petri dish that is lined with a disk of moist filter paper to prevent evaporation of the sample. Allow the sample to stand undisturbed for 10 minutes so that the platelets can settle.

Counting the Platelets. The area of the hemacytometer counted is the central ruled area of 1 square millimeter. If you use a light microscope, the condenser must be well down to view the platelets, which appear as small round or oval bodies with a pink or purple sheen under the high power objective (40X). White blood cells in the sample are unaffected by the lysing reagent and are readily visible. However, because they are so much larger than the platelets, they are unlikely to be confused with them during the count.

Calculating the Platelet Count. Use the number of platelets observed to calculate the platelet count using the formula for hemacytometer counts:

$$\text{Platelet count} = \text{Number of platelets counted} \\ \times \text{Dilution} \times \text{Depth factor} \\ \times \text{Area counted}$$

where,

Dilution = 100
Depth factor = the constant 10
Area counted = 1 mm^3

Assume, for example, that you counted 160 platelets in the central counting area of the hemacytometer. Then:

$$\text{Platelet count} = 160 \times 100 \times 10 \times 1 \\ = 160,000 \text{ platelets/mm}^3$$

Whenever the dilution is 1:100, you may use this shorthand formula:

$$\text{Platelet count} = \text{Number of platelets counted} \\ \times 1,000$$

Sources of Error. There are several potential sources of error in performing manual platelet counts using the direct method. Take care to avoid these causes of erroneous results:

- improper dilution of the sample
- contaminated or cloudy reagent in reservoir
- clots in the blood sample or clumping of platelets (EDTA prevents clotting)
- overfilling or underfilling of the hemacytometer
- the inclusion of red blood cells or dust particles in the count
- incorrect calculations

To reduce errors in reporting the platelet count, always check it against an estimate of the platelet count made from examination of a stained blood smear slide. The direct count and the estimate from the slide should agree. The slide also has the advantage of showing morphological characteristics of individual platelets.

The Indirect Method

The indirect method for counting platelets determines the number of platelets per 1,000 red blood cells on a stained blood smear slide using an oil-immersion objective and then multiplies that number by the RBC count.

To perform a platelet count using the indirect method, follow this procedure:

- Make a blood-smear slide using either venous blood collected in an EDTA tube or blood from a freely flowing capillary puncture.

- Allow the slide to air dry and stain it with Wright's stain or quick stain.
- Using the oil-immersion objective, count the number of platelets per 1,000 red blood cells.
- Perform an RBC count on an EDTA-anticoagulated blood sample.
- Calculate the platelet count using the formula

$$\text{Platelet count} = \frac{P \times RBC}{1,000}$$

where,

P = number of platelets counted per 1,000 red blood cells

RBC = RBC count

Assume, for example, that 60 platelets per 1,000 red blood cells were counted on a stained blood smear slide. For the same sample, the RBC count was found to be 5,000,000 per cubic millimeter. Then:

$$\begin{aligned}\text{Platelet count} &= \frac{60 \times 5,000,000}{1,000}\\ &= 300,000 \text{ platelets/mm}^3\end{aligned}$$

THE ERYTHROCYTE SEDIMENTATION RATE (ESR)

The **erythrocyte sedimentation rate (ESR** or **sed rate)** is the rate at which red blood cells settle out of plasma when placed in a vertical tube. The ESR is calculated by measuring the distance the red blood cells travel through the plasma during a given interval of time.

Stages of Erythrocyte Sedimentation

Three stages can be observed in the fall of red blood cells through the plasma column when an ESR test is performed:

- *Initial period of aggregation:* the first 10 minutes, during which rouleaux form and relatively slow sedimentation of red cells occurs.
- *Period of rapid settling:* the next half hour to 2 hours (depending on the length of the tube), during which sedimentation occurs at a fairly constant rate.
- *Third stage:* the final stage, during which sedimentation slows as the sedimented red blood cells are packed at the bottom of the column.

The second stage, the period of rapid settling, is the most significant for the ESR.

Methods Used to Measure the ESR

Manual methods of measuring the ESR include the Wintrobe and the Westergren and are CLIA waived procedures. The Wintrobe method is the least sensitive and the Westergren method or a variation of the Westergren sed rate method is usually performed. Modified Westergren kits are available and provide a safe, closed system that will be described later in this chapter. These methods use blood samples collected by venipuncture in EDTA tubes.

> ### Blood Sample Storage
>
> The ESR test must be set up within 2 hours for blood left at room temperature. The sample can be refrigerated at 4 degrees Celsius up to a maximum time of 12 hours before testing. Refrigerated blood must always be brought to room temperature before testing. Always refer to the manufacturer's instructions for sample storage.

Automated ESR analyzing systems are also available and provide a safe and convenient method for performing erythrocyte sedimentation rates. These automated ESR procedures are categorized as CLIA nonwaived testing. The Ves-Matic™ Automated ESR System (Diesse Inc., 1690 West 38 Place, Unit B1, Hialeah, Florida) is one example of an instrument for ESR measurement. Specialized tubes included with the system serve as both collection tubes and testing cuvettes. Blood samples are collected in these Vacu Tec testing tubes containing sodium citrate and then the samples are inserted into the instrument, which mixes the samples and reads the ESR value after 20 minutes using photometric infrared method. The patient samples are stable in the Vacu Tec tubes for 4 hours at room temperature and 12 hours in the refrigerator.

The Polymedco Sedimat Automated ESR™ (Polymedco, Inc., 510 Furnace Dock Road, Cortlandt Manor, New York) is another "walk away" procedure for automated erythrocyte sedimentation rates that uses the Sediplast tubes and provides ESR results in 15 minutes. The results are read on an LCD display and can be stored in memory for access later or they can be automatically printed at the end of the test. The Sediten Analyzer™ is another ESR system by Polymedco, Inc., that uses special collection tubes and reads results directly from these tubes. (See Figure 17-3.)

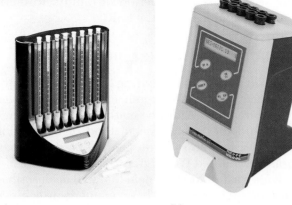

(a)   (b)

Figure 17-3 Examples of automated methods for performing ESR. (a) Polymedco Sedimat Automated ESR™ Reader using Sediplast Westergren tubes; (b) Ves-Matic™ Automated ESR System Analyzer.

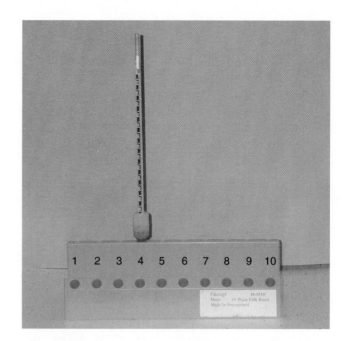

Figure 17-4 The Sediplast ESR system for the Westergren erythrocyte sedimentation rate is a completely closed system that protects against risks associated with blood handling.

The Westergren Method. Mix trisodium citrate anticoagulant with the blood sample in a ratio of four volumes of blood to one volume of anticoagulant. Draw the blood-citrate mixture up to the zero mark of a Westergren ESR tube, which is graduated from 0 to 200 millimeters and has a bore of 2.55 millimeters.

Place the filled tube in its rack on a level surface at room temperature and note the time. In exactly 1 hour, read the distance from the plasma meniscus to the top of the column of sedimented red cells. Report the ESR in millimeters per hour. Figure 17-4 shows the Westergren system.

Using a Sediplast Westergren System. As Figure 17-5 illustrates, a disposable Westergren system uses a disposable tube, called the autozero Westergren tube, for the ESR reading. The tube is inserted in a vial, called the Sedivial, that contains the diluted blood sample. Blood rises in the tube to the zero mark, and the excess blood flows into a reservoir compartment.

Pasteur pipette to fill the Sedivial to the fill line with blood (about 0.8 mL is needed). Thoroughly mix the blood and diluent by replacing the cap and gently inverting. Blood and diluent are automatically added to the pipette tube when it is inserted into the Sedivial. After 1 hour at room temperature, read the distance between the top of the plasma and the top of the sedimented red blood cells directly from the vertical scale on the tube. Report the result in millimeters per hour (see Figure 17-6).

For Safety's Sake

The Sediplast Westergren ESR kit has the following safety features:

- The autozero Westergren tube has a vented cap that prevents squirting of the blood sample from the top of the tube, thus reducing the risk of accidental exposure to biohazardous materials.
- The entire Sediplast system is disposable, thus reducing the need for cleaning and handling of biohazardous materials.

Technique Tip

Insert the autozero Westergren tube into the Sedivial with a slight, gentle twisting motion. The tube must completely touch the bottom of the Sedivial to ensure proper results.

The Sedivial can be purchased prefilled with diluent, which is 3.8% sodium citrate. Use a

Sources of Error in ESR Testing. There are several potential sources of error in ESR testing.

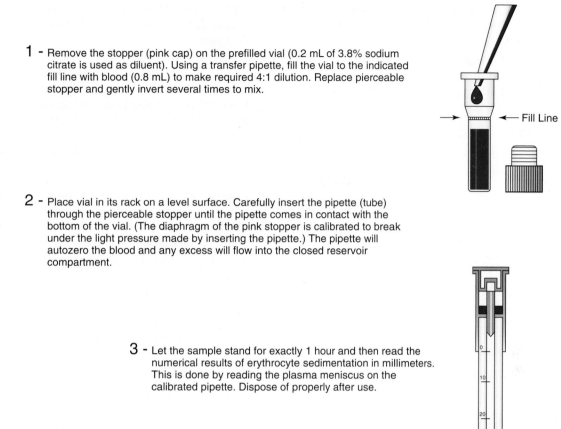

1 - Remove the stopper (pink cap) on the prefilled vial (0.2 mL of 3.8% sodium citrate is used as diluent). Using a transfer pipette, fill the vial to the indicated fill line with blood (0.8 mL) to make required 4:1 dilution. Replace pierceable stopper and gently invert several times to mix.

← Fill Line

2 - Place vial in its rack on a level surface. Carefully insert the pipette (tube) through the pierceable stopper until the pipette comes in contact with the bottom of the vial. (The diaphragm of the pink stopper is calibrated to break under the light pressure made by inserting the pipette.) The pipette will autozero the blood and any excess will flow into the closed reservoir compartment.

3 - Let the sample stand for exactly 1 hour and then read the numerical results of erythrocyte sedimentation in millimeters. This is done by reading the plasma meniscus on the calibrated pipette. Dispose of properly after use.

Figure 17-5 Instructions from the Sediplast ESR system explain how to use the Westergren procedure.

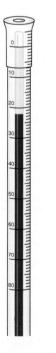

Figure 17-6 This is an example of erythrocyte sedimentation. The reading at the bottom of the meniscus after 1 hour is 22 millimeters.

Whenever you perform an ESR test, avoid the following pitfalls:

- *Tilting:* tilting the ESR tube even slightly away from vertical accelerates the ESR; an angle of 3 degrees from vertical may accelerate the ESR by as much as 30 percent.
- *Vibrations:* vibrations to the tube, such as those caused by nearby centrifuges, increase the ESR.
- *Temperature:* deviation of room temperature from a constant 20 to 25 degrees Celsius, or placement of the ESR rack in a draft or sunlight, may affect the ESR.
- *Heparin used as anticoagulant:* heparin alters the charge on the red blood cells and changes the ESR.
- *Testing time:* blood that has stood longer than 2 hours at room temperature after being drawn may have a falsely low ESR because the red blood cells have become spherical and less inclined to form rouleaux.

- *Reading time:* the ESR may be decreased if reading time is less than 1 hour and increased if reading time is over 1 hour.
- *Clots or air bubbles:* clots and air bubbles in the sample interfere with sedimentation of cells and affect the ESR.

Table 17-4   Normal Reference Values for the ESR

Method	Sex	Age	ESR (mm/hr)
Westergren	Males	<50	0 to 16
	Males	>50	0 to 20
	Females	<50	0 to 20
	Females	>50	0 to 30

Normal Values for the ESR

Normal values for the ESR vary with age, sex, and test method. See Table 17-4.

Factors Influencing the ESR

The speed at which red blood cells settle in the column of plasma is influenced by two general categories of factors: red blood cell factors and plasma factors.

Red Blood Cell Factors. Red blood cells settle in plasma because they are more dense than is the plasma; that is, they have more weight, or mass, per unit of volume. The rate at which the red blood cells settle is directly proportional to their density. If they clump together in aggregates, such as rouleaux, they tend to settle faster, leading to a higher sedimentation rate.

Countering the tendency of red blood cells to settle in the plasma column is their buoyancy, which is their tendency to float because of the upward force exerted by the plasma. The buoyancy of the red blood cells is directly proportional to their surface area-to-volume ratio—the greater their surface area relative to their volume, the more buoyant they are and the slower the rate at which they settle. Large cells have a smaller surface area in relation to volume than do small cells. Therefore, macrocytes have a relatively high sedimentation rate, and microcytes have a relatively low one.

Red blood cells in rouleaux formation have a decreased surface area-to-volume ratio relative to individual red blood cells, another reason for their greater sedimentation rate. Because red blood cells with abnormal shapes are less likely to form rouleaux, they have a slower-than-normal sedimentation rate.

Red blood cell concentration also affects the rate at which the cells settle. Decreased red blood cell concentration, as in some anemias, reduces the erythrocyte-to-plasma ratio, thus favoring rouleaux formation. An elevated rate of sedimentation results. Increased red blood cell concentration, as in polycythemia, has the opposite effect and results in a lowered sedimentation rate.

Plasma Factors. Three proteins in the plasma affect the rate at which red blood cells settle: fibrinogen, globulin, and albumin. Increases in the levels of fibrinogen and globulin decrease the negative charge on the surface of the red blood cells. As a consequence, the red blood cells repel each other less, promoting the formation of rouleaux and a faster rate of sedimentation. Increases in the level of albumin, on the other hand, retard the rate of sedimentation of the red blood cells.

ESR as a Diagnostic Tool

Many disease processes and some normal physiological states result in an elevation of the ESR, and a few diseases lead to a decrease. As a result, the ESR is used worldwide as an index of the presence of active diseases of many different types, especially inflammatory disorders.

The ESR is elevated in patients with tissue breakdown, such as occurs in acute infectious diseases. In most acute infections, globulins and fibrinogen are increased, while albumin is somewhat reduced. This combination increases the rate at which red blood cells settle. The ESR is particularly useful as an indicator of the presence of obscure active infections such as tuberculosis, subacute bacterial endocarditis, and systemic lupus erythematosus. The ESR may remain elevated for some time after recovery from infectious disease.

In nephrosis, a disease of the kidney, and cirrhosis, a disease of the liver, globulins are increased and albumin is decreased, resulting in an elevated sedimentation rate. The ESR also is increased in patients with nephritis and acute attacks of gout as well as heavy metal poisoning. Although the ESR is not elevated in malignancy, it is generally rapid when metastases, or the breakdown and inflammation of tumors, occur. The ESR increases after the 12th week of pregnancy and following abortion at any time.

The ESR is slower than normal in patients with hemolytic jaundice and sickle-cell anemia due to changes in shape of the red blood cells that reduce rouleaux formation.

RETICULOCYTE COUNTS

Reticulocytes are immature red blood cells that are present in small numbers in circulating blood. They are counted in POLs as a valuable index of red blood cell production.

Background

Erythropoiesis, or blood cell production, was described in Chapter 13 and the reticulocyte stage of red blood cell development was described in Chapter 14. This section reviews and expands upon that material to illustrate why the number of circulating reticulocytes can be used as an index of erythropoiesis.

Erythropoiesis. The major factor that controls the rate of erythropoiesis is the oxygen content of the blood. Low blood oxygen stimulates production of the kidney hormone erythropoietin, which acts directly on the bone marrow to increase red blood cell production. Low blood oxygen may be due to several conditions, including anemia, cardiovascular disease, and low atmospheric oxygen, which is due, for example, to high altitude.

Erythropoiesis occurs in several stages. Stem cells in the bone marrow first differentiate into pronormoblasts, which mature into basophilic normoblasts. Polychromatophilic normoblasts, the last stage capable of mitosis, develop into orthochromic normoblasts, also known as nucleated red blood cells, which are seen occasionally on blood smears. Orthochromic normoblasts, in turn, extrude their nuclei, giving rise to reticulocytes. Each pronormoblast gives rise to 16 reticulocytes, and the entire process takes 3 to 5 days.

Reticulocytes. After their formation from normoblasts, reticulocytes normally remain in the bone marrow for 1 day before being sent out into the circulating blood. There they remain as reticulocytes for another 1 to 2 days before developing into mature red blood cells. Reticulocytes are slightly larger than mature red blood cells, and they retain aggregates of ribosomal RNA. The role of the RNA is to synthesize hemoglobin, which is needed by mature red blood cells for oxygen transport.

The maturation time of reticulocytes in the circulating blood depends on the body's demand for hemoglobin. When hemoglobin is low, the maturation time is longer, allowing more hemoglobin production by the ribosomal RNA in the reticulocytes. Not surprisingly, maturation time is correlated inversely with hematocrit (see Table 17-5.)

The amount of ribosomal RNA is greatest when reticulocytes are first formed. It declines as they age.

Table 17-5   The Correlation between Hematocrit and the Maturation Time of Reticulocytes

Hematocrit (%)	Maturation Time of Reticulocytes (days)
45	1.0
35	1.5
25	2.0
15	2.5

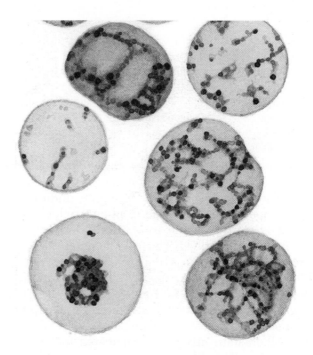

Figure 17-7 Stained reticulocytes.

Generally, the younger the reticulocyte, the more diffuse and marked is the network of RNA. Ribosomal RNA is completely absent from mature red blood cells. As Figure 17-7 shows, the ribosomal RNA is seen as dense blue granules or filaments when reticulocytes are stained with brilliant cresyl blue, new methylene blue, or Nile blue sulfate. These are called **supravital stains** because they stain only living cells, not dried blood smears. The incubation time will vary according to the type of supravital stain used.

Reticulocyte Count Procedures

Reticulocytes are counted on stained blood smears under the oil-immersion objective.

Preparing the Smear. Using new methylene blue stain and a small test tube, place three drops of stain and three drops of capillary blood or

EDTA-anticoagulated venous blood into the tube. If capillary blood is used, increase the number of drops of stain to prevent the blood from clotting. Venous blood stored at 4 degrees Celsius for up to 24 hours produces satisfactory reticulocyte preparation. Incubate the mixture for 15 minutes at room temperature, and then prepare a blood smear using the procedure described in Chapter 15 and allow it to air dry. The smear should be thin, and it should not be counterstained with a polychromatic stain such as Wright's stain or quick stain.

> **Note**
>
> Particles of stain adhering to the surface of mature red blood cells may be a serious source of error in reticulocyte counts. You must observe strictly the recommended incubation time for the blood-stain mixture. The longer you allow the mixture to stand beyond this recommended time limit, the greater the possibility of stain adhering to mature blood cells and causing erroneous counts.

Using a Unopette Kit. The principle underlying the Unopette method for performing a reticulocyte count is similar to the principle underlying the method just described. The test kit contains a 7 mL dropper bottle of supravital stain (new methylene blue N) and a 25 µL capacity Unopette capillary pipette. The supravital stain is stable until the expiration date if the dropper bottle is recapped after each use and stored below 30 degrees Celsius. The blood-stain mixture is incubated for exactly 10 minutes. Thin blood smears are prepared in the same manner as was followed in the previous new methylene blue stain method.

Counting Reticulocytes. Examine the slide under the oil-immersion objective in the body region of the smear. Both mature erythrocytes and reticulocytes have a light greenish-blue background in a correctly prepared smear. You can distinguish the reticulocytes from the erythrocytes by their deep blue granules and filaments of ribosomal RNA. Count a total of 1,000 red blood cells including both reticulocytes and mature erythrocytes. You may use one slide for the entire count, or you may use two slides by counting 500 red blood cells on each slide.

Sources of Error in the Procedure. There are several potential sources of error in performing a reticulocyte count. Avoid these pitfalls when you perform the procedure:

- *Overincubation of the blood-stain mixture:* too much staining makes viewing difficult

and may result in mature red blood cells being counted as reticulocytes.

- *Unfiltered stains:* without frequent filtering, stains form precipitations on the smears that may be confused with reticula and bias the count upward.
- *Undercounting reticulocytes:* overlooking reticulocytes with small amounts of cellular reticular material in the count biases the count downward.
- *Too few cells counted:* counting too few cells can lead to a count that is unrepresentative of the sample.
- *Nonsystematic counting of the cells in the counting area:* unless a systematic pattern of counting the cells is followed, some cells may be counted twice and others may be overlooked, producing a miscount.
- *Artifacts counted as reticula:* numerous cell artifacts may be confused with reticula and may bias the count upward.

> **Note**
>
> The following cell features may be confused with reticular material:
> - *Howell-Jolly bodies,* which are composed of nuclear fragments.
> - *Heinz bodies,* which are composed of denatured hemoglobin.
> - *Stippling,* or *spotting,* which occurs in basophilic red blood cells in some types of anemia.

Calculations

The number of reticulocytes may be reported in two ways: as the percent of reticulocytes of all red blood cells counted or as the absolute number of reticulocytes counted.

The Percent of Reticulocytes. The percent of reticulocytes of all red blood cells counted is calculated as

$$\text{Percent of reticulocytes} = \frac{\text{number of reticulocytes counted} \times 100}{\text{number of erythrocytes counted}}$$

Whenever 1,000 erythrocytes are counted, the following shorthand formula may be used:

$$\text{Percent of reticulocytes} = \frac{\text{number of reticulocytes counted}}{10}$$

Assume, for example, that 40 reticulocytes were observed out of 1,000 erythrocytes counted on a smear. The calculation is

$$\text{Percent of reticulocytes} = \frac{40 \times 100}{1{,}000}$$

$$= 4 \text{ percent reticulocytes}$$

The Absolute Number of Reticulocytes. The absolute number of reticulocytes counted is equal to the percentage of reticulocytes times the RBC count:

Absolute number of reticulocytes
= Percent of reticulocytes × RBC count

Assume, for example, that the RBC count is 4,000,000 per cubic millimeter and that reticulocytes make up 2 percent of the red blood cells. The calculation is

Absolute number of reticulocytes
$= 2\% \times 4{,}000{,}000 \text{ reticulocytes/mm}^3$
$= 80{,}000 \text{ reticulocytes/mm}^3$

Which Calculation Should You Use?

The absolute number of reticulocytes can be used directly to assess bone marrow response to anemia. It has more clinical significance than the percent of reticulocytes, which must be correlated with other hematological parameters to be useful clinically. Many POLs report the reticulocytes only as a percentage. Some report both the percentage and the absolute number. The latter is the recommended format.

The Normal Values for Reticulocyte Counts

To interpret individual patient test results for the reticulocyte count, you need to be familiar with normal values for both the percent and the absolute number of reticulocytes.

The Percent of Reticulocytes. Normal values for the percent of reticulocytes vary by age and sex. See Table 17-6.

The higher value for females is due to replacement of blood lost during menstruation. The newborn value drops to the adult value by 2 to 5 days after birth.

The Absolute Number of Reticulocytes. The average for the absolute count is 60,000 reticulocytes per cubic millimeter. This is the basal value. The maximum response under appropriate circumstances is considered to be seven times the basal rate.

Table 17-6 Normal Values for the Percent of Reticulocytes

Age/Sex	Percent Reticulocytes
Adult males	0.5 to 1.5
Adult females	0.5 to 2.5
Newborns	2.0 to 6.0

Clinical Applications

Reticulocytopenia, which is a lowering of the number of circulating reticulocytes, usually is found in patients with pernicious anemia, aplastic anemia, or bone marrow failure. A satisfactory response to therapy in these conditions is a rise in the reticulocyte count, which is used as an index of red blood cell production. In patients with pernicious anemia, for example, an increase in reticulocytes usually is seen by the fourth day following specific therapy, and the maximal response generally is reached by the eighth to tenth day. This is followed by a gradual decline in reticulocytes coupled with a steady increase in the erythrocyte count and hemoglobin level until normal values are reached.

If anemia is known to exist and the bone marrow is not responding as indicated by an increase in reticulocytes, the cause must be investigated. Possibilities include vitamin B12 deficiency, folate deficiency, and invasion of the bone marrow by malignant cells.

In patients with low hematocrits, the percent of reticulocytes may appear to be elevated even if an unchanging number of reticulocytes are produced each day and the absolute number of reticulocytes is normal. This apparent reticulocytosis is due to the relatively small number of red blood cells, not to an increase in the number of reticulocytes. The lower the hematocrit, the greater the degree of apparent reticulocytosis. If the hematocrit is half of the normal value, for example, erythrocyte production can be assumed to be increased only if the percent of reticulocytes is consistently greater than twice normal, say, in the range of 5 to 6%. By comparison, in nonanemic patients, erythrocyte production is considered to be increased if the reticulocyte count is consistently greater than 2.5 to 3.0%.

Occasionally, the percentage of reticulocytes may be increased by factors other than an increased rate of erythropoiesis. For example, there may be premature release of reticulocytes from the bone marrow. This occurs acutely in response to massive hemorrhage.

PROCEDURE 17-1

The Sediplast Disposable Westergren Erythrocyte Sedimentation Rate

Goal

After successfully completing this procedure, you will be able to set up an erythrocyte sedimentation rate using the Sediplast Westergren system and read the result at the end of 1 hour.

Completion Time

1 hour, 10 minutes

Equipment and Supplies

- Impermeable jacket, gown or apron, and eye shields
- Disposable gloves
- Hand disinfectant
- Surface disinfectant
- Paper towels and tissues
- Biohazard container
- EDTA-anticoagulated venous blood
- Disposable transfer pipette
- Sediplast kit (disposable Westergren sedimentation tube, diluent, Sedivial, and rack)
- 1-hour timer with alarm
- Report form and pen

Instructions

Read through the list of equipment and supplies that you will need and the steps of the procedure. Be sure that you understand each step before you begin. Then complete each step correctly and in the proper order. If your completion time is too long, repeat the procedure until you increase your speed.

*Steps marked with (*) are critical and must have the maximum points to pass.

Performance Standards	Points Awarded	Maximum Points
1. Put on a jacket, gown, or apron; wash your hands with disinfectant, dry them, and put on gloves.		10
2. Follow the standard precautions.		10
3. Collect and prepare the appropriate equipment.		5
4. *Verify identification of the blood specimen and label the container.		15
5. Mix the blood sample gently and well.		5
6. Remove the cap on the Sedivial, which is prefilled with 3.8% sodium citrate.		5
7. Using a transfer pipette, fill the Sedivial to the indicated fill line with 0.8 mL of blood.		10
8. Mix the blood and sodium citrate solution together by replacing the stopper in the Sedivial and gently invert several times.		5
9. Place the sample in the rack in a level position away from vibrations, sunlight, and temperature extremes.		5
10. With a slight twisting motion, gently insert the Westergren sedimentation tube into the Sedivial of blood. Be sure that the tube is inserted all the way to the bottom of the Sedivial to ensure an accurate reading (blood will rise to the top of the sedimentation tube and excess will overflow into the reservoir compartment at the top of the tube).		10
11. Set the timer for 1 hour.		10
12. *In exactly 1 hour, read the length of the plasma column on the sedimentation tube.		10

	Performance Standards		Maximum Points
13.	Report the result in millimeters per hour on the report form and turn in to your instructor.		10
14.	Discard disposable equipment.		5
15.	Disinfect other equipment and return it to storage.		5
16.	Clean the work area following the Universal Precautions.		5
17.	Remove the jacket, gown, or apron, and gloves; wash your hands with disinfectant, and dry them.		5
	Total Points		**130**

Overall Procedural Evaluation

Student Name _____

Signature of Instructor _____ Date _____

Comments _____

_____

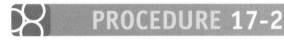

PROCEDURE 17-2

Reticulocyte Determination Using New Methylene Blue

Goal

After successfully completing this procedure, you will be able to prepare a reticulocyte stain, count the reticulocytes present, and report the results.

Completion Time

40 minutes

Equipment and Supplies

- Impermeable jacket, gown or apron, and eye shields
- Disposable gloves
- Hand disinfectant
- Surface disinfectant
- Paper towels and tissues
- Biohazard container
- Disposable transfer pipettes
- Clean small test tube
- Glass slides
- Fresh capillary blood or venous blood collected in EDTA anticoagulant
- Methylene blue N stain
- Immersion oil
- Microscope with oil-immersion objective
- Report form and pen

Instructions

Read through the list of equipment and supplies that you will need and the steps of the procedure. Be sure that you understand each step before you begin. Then complete each step correctly and in the proper order. If your completion time is too long, repeat the procedure until you increase your speed.

*Steps marked with (*) are critical and must have the maximum points to pass.

Performance Standards	Points Awarded	Maximum Points
1. Put on a jacket, gown, or apron; wash your hands with disinfectant, dry them, and put on gloves.		10
2. Follow the standard precautions.		10

—*table continued*

Performance Standards	Points Awarded	Maximum Points
3. Collect and prepare the appropriate equipment.		5
4. *Identify the correct specimen and mix thoroughly.		15
5. Using a disposable transfer pipette, place 3 drops of well-mixed whole blood in a clean small test tube.		5
6. Using another disposable transfer pipette, add 3 drops (equal amounts) of new methylene blue stain to the blood and mix gently and thoroughly. (Be sure the stain is free of debris by filtering.)		10
7. Allow the blood-stain mixture to incubate at room temperature for 10 minutes.		5
8. After 10 minutes, prepare two thin blood-stain smears in the same manner as preparing whole blood smears. Allow the slides to air dry.		10
9. Place a slide on the stage of the microscope and focus using low-power objective to locate counting areas.		5
10. Put a drop of immersion oil on the slide and carefully focus using the oil-immersion objective.		5
11. *Count 1,000 erythrocytes by counting all the red blood cells in one field after another until you reach 1,000 (include the reticulocytes in the 1,000 count).		15
12. Record the number of reticulocytes counted in the 1,000 erythrocytes. Repeat steps 9–11 with the second slide until counts agree within 10 percent.		10
13. Average the reticulocyte counts in both slides and calculate the percent of reticulocytes using the following formula: $$\text{Percent of reticulocytes} = \frac{\text{Number of reticulocytes} \times 100}{1{,}000}$$		15
14. Record the results on the report form.		5
15. Discard disposable supplies and equipment.		5
16. Disinfect other equipment and return to storage.		5
17. Clean the work area following all standard precautions.		5
18. Remove gloves and wash your hands with disinfectant and dry.		5
Total Points		145

Overall Procedural Evaluation

Student Name _____

Signature of Instructor _____ Date _____

Comments _____

_____

chapter 17 REVIEW

Using Terminology

Match the term in the right column with the appropriate definition or description in the left column.

_____ 1. condition with spherical red blood cells

_____ 2. large cell

_____ 3. low in hemoglobin

_____ 4. low number of reticulocytes

_____ 5. mean cell hemoglobin

_____ 6. mean cell hemoglobin concentration

_____ 7. mean cell volume

_____ 8. normal in hemoglobin

_____ 9. sedimentation rate

_____ 10. stains living cells

a. ESR

b. hypochromic

c. macrocyte

d. MCH

e. MCHC

f. MCV

g. reticulocytopenia

h. normochromic

i. supravital

j. spherocytosis

Define the following terms in the spaces provided.

11. Erythrocyte indices

_____

_____

_____

12. Erythrocyte sedimentation rate (ESR or sed rate)

_____

_____

_____

13. Mean cell volume (MCV)

_____

_____

_____

14. Mean cell hemoglobin (MCH)

_____

_____

_____

15. Mean cell hemoglobin concentration (MCHC)

_____

_____

_____

Multiple Choice

Choose the best answer for the following questions.

16. If the MCV is greater than 102 fL, you would expect the red blood cells to appear
    a. microcytic
    b. macrocytic
    c. normocytic
    d. normochromic

17. The hemoglobin and hematocrit are needed to calculate which of the following indices?
    a. MCV
    b. MCH
    c. MCHC
    d. HCT

18. MCHC values below 32% indicate hypochromia, which is associated with which of the following?
    a. iron-deficiency anemia
    b. pernicious anemia
    c. spherocytosis
    d. ovalocytosis

19. On a stained blood smear, 80 platelets were counted per 1,000 red blood cells in a sample of blood in which the RBC count was found to be 4,500,000 per cubic millimeter. Calculate the indirect platelet count.
    a. 250,000 platelets/mm^3
    b. 360,000 platelets/mm^3
    c. 450,000 platelets/mm^3
    d. 560,000 platelets/mm^3

20. The most significant stage of the erythrocyte sedimentation rate is the
    a. initial period of aggregation
    b. second period of rapid settling
    c. final stage of settling
    d. stage of rouleaux formation

Acquiring Knowledge

Answer the following questions in the spaces provided.

21. What are the normal adult ranges for the erythrocyte indices?

_____

_____

_____

22. What does a deviation of more than one unit from the normal range of an erythrocyte index usually mean?

_____

_____

_____

23. What conditions lead to an increase over normal in the value of MCV? To a decrease?

_____

_____

_____

24. When is the value of MCH likely to be greater than normal?

_____

_____

_____

25. List several potential sources of error in performing manual platelet counts using the direct method.

_____

_____

_____

26. How can you check the validity of a platelet count?

_____

_____

_____

27. Describe the three stages of erythrocyte sedimentation. Which stage is the most significant for the ESR?

_____

_____

_____

28. What sources of error should be avoided in performing an ESR test?

_____

_____

_____

29. What red blood cell factors influence the sed rate?

_____

_____

_____

30. What plasma factors influence erythrocyte sedimentation? How do they respond to acute infections?

_____

_____

_____

31. Name several potential sources of error in performing reticulocyte counts.

_____

_____

_____

32. Explain why the reticulocyte count is a valuable indicator of erythropoiesis.

_____

_____

_____

33. Describe the clinical applications of the reticulocyte count.

_____

_____

_____

Applying Knowledge—On the Job

Answer the following questions in the spaces provided.

34. A patient has just reported to the laboratory for a reticulocyte count. Both the absolute number and the percentage of reticulocytes have been requested. What will the physician learn directly from these reports?

_____

_____

_____

35. You have just received a request for a Westergren sed rate. What equipment and reagents will you need? How long will it take? What units are the results reported in?

_____

_____

_____

36. A patient in the clinic where you work has the following blood parameters: RBC of 4.1 million/mm^3; Hgb of 6.4 g/dL; and Hct of 25 percent. Calculate the erythrocyte indices for this patient and make a tentative diagnosis.

_____

_____

_____

37. The physician has requested a platelet count for a patient. You counted 162 platelets using the direct method (dilution = 1:100). What platelet count will you report to the physician?

_____

_____

_____

38. You just performed a reticulocyte count for a patient who has an RBC count of 3,500,000. You observed 43 reticulocytes out of 1,000 erythrocytes on the smear. What is the percent of reticulocytes? What is the absolute number of reticulocytes?

_____

_____

_____

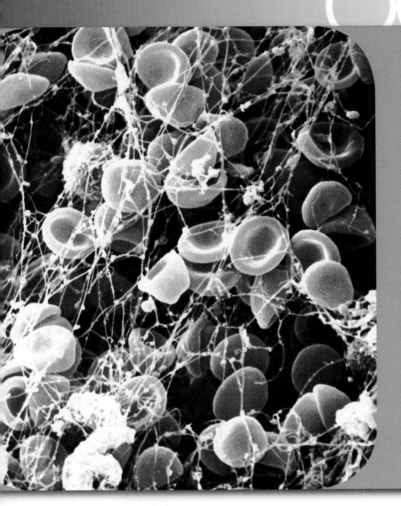

chapter **18**

Blood Coagulation

COGNITIVE OBJECTIVES

After studying this chapter, you should be able to

18.1 use each of the vocabulary terms appropriately.

18.2 explain the role of hemostasis as an aspect of homeostasis.

18.3 name the three mechanisms by which hemostasis comes about.

18.4 identify the intravascular, vascular, and extravascular phenomena of hemostasis.

18.5 describe the two pathways through which coagulation is initiated.

18.6 explain how blood clots form.

18.7 list several diseases of coagulation and explain their causes.

18.8 discuss the management of coagulation diseases.

18.9 discuss the differences among bleeding time, prothrombin time, and activated partial thromboplastin time.

PERFORMANCE OBJECTIVE

After studying this chapter, you should be able to

18.10 perform a prothrombin time determination.

TERMINOLOGY

activated partial thromboplastin time (aPTT): a coagulation procedure that tests for coagulation factors II, V, VIII, IX, X, XI, and XII, all of which are involved in the intrinsic pathway of coagulation. It is used to evaluate the effect of the administration of anticoagulant drugs.

bleeding time: the time it takes a small, standardized incision to stop bleeding.

cerebrovascular accident: stroke. A cerebrovascular accident is characterized by the sudden loss of consciousness followed by possible paralysis. Cerebrovascular accidents may be caused by an embolus or thrombus that occludes a cerebral artery, among other causes.

clotting disorder: a coagulation disease in which clots form in the blood spontaneously.

coagulation: the process of clotting, which depends on the presence of several coagulation factors, including prothrombin, thrombin, thromboplastin, fibrinogen, and calcium.

coagulation factor: one of 12 compounds required for the coagulation process. Coagulation factors must be present in appropriate amounts for clotting to occur effectively.

coumarin: a group of drugs, including warfarin, used to prevent and treat clotting disorders. Coumarin drugs act in the liver, where they interfere with the synthesis of vitamin K–dependent coagulation factors (II, VII, IX, and X).

embolism: the sudden obstruction of a blood vessel by an embolus.

embolus: an undissolved mass in a blood or lymphatic vessel. It is usually a blood clot but may consist of fat globules, bacteria, or other debris. About 75 percent of emboli arise in the deep veins of the legs.

fibrin: the whitish, filamentous protein formed by the action of thrombin on fibrinogen. Other formed elements in the blood become entangled in the interlacing filaments of fibrin, thus forming a blood clot.

fibrinogen: coagulation factor I; a compound in plasma that is converted to fibrin by thrombin in the presence of calcium.

hemophilia: one of a group of diseases in which excessive bleeding occurs because of inherited deficiencies in blood coagulation factors; characterized by uncontrolled hemorrhaging, possibly even from the slightest injury.

hemophilia A: classic hemophilia; the most common type of hemophilia, caused by a recessive sex-linked gene that leads to the inability to synthesize coagulation factor VIII, antihemophilic factor (AHF).

hemophilia B: Christmas disease; the second most common type of hemophilia, caused by a recessive sex-linked gene that leads to the inability to synthesize coagulation factor IX, plasma thromboplastin component (PTC).

hemophilia C: a relatively uncommon type of hemophilia, caused by a dominant autosomal gene, that leads to the inability to synthesize factor XI, plasma thromboplastin antecedent (PTA).

hemorrhagic disease: any of several diseases in which excessive bleeding occurs because blood fails to clot.

hemorrhagic disease of the newborn: a bleeding disease due to lack of vitamin K–producing intestinal flora in less than 1 percent of newborns, occurring between the second and seventh day after birth. Hemorrhagic disease of the newborn is treated by administration of vitamin K. Vitamin K is necessary to the formation of several clotting factors, including prothrombin.

hemostasis: the arrest of bleeding.

heparin sodium: a widely used anticoagulant drug for the management of clotting disorders. It works by inhibiting the conversion of prothrombin to thrombin.

international normalized ratio (INR): a method of reporting PT results for patients on oral anticoagulant therapy.

myocardial infarction: an infarct, or area of necrosis (tissue death), in the myocardium. Myocardial infarction is usually due to occlusion of a coronary artery and is associated with pain, shock, cardiac failure, and frequently death.

myocardium: the middle, muscular layer of the walls of the heart.

platelet plug: a clump of platelets that adhere to an injured vessel to help stop bleeding; often sufficient to stop the flow of blood in capillary wounds.

prothrombin: coagulation factor II; a compound in circulating blood that is converted to thrombin by the action of thromboplastin.

prothrombin time (PT): a coagulation procedure that tests for coagulation factors I, II, VII, and X, all of which are involved in the extrinsic pathway of coagulation. Prothrombin time is used to evaluate the effect of the administration of anticoagulant drugs.

serotonin: a potent vasoconstrictor that is released by platelets adhering to a wounded blood vessel.

template method (Ivy bleeding time): a method of testing bleeding time. The template method standardizes the size and depth of the incision.

thrombin: an enzyme formed from the conversion of prothrombin by thromboplastin and other coagulation factors. Thrombin joins soluble fibrinogen molecules into long, hairlike molecules of insoluble fibrin.

thrombocytopenia: a hemorrhagic disease due to a deficiency of platelets, which results in many small hemorrhages.

thrombophlebitis: the inflammation of a vein due to a blood clot. Thrombophlebitis is a common problem in elderly, immobile patients.

thromboplastin: coagulation factor III; the immediate initiator of the blood-clotting mechanism.

Thromboplastin interacts with other coagulation factors to convert prothrombin to thrombin.

thrombosis: the formation of a blood clot, or thrombus, within the vascular system. Thrombosis is treated with anticoagulants.

thrombus: a blood clot within the vascular system.

vascular phenomenon: one of three major components of hemostasis. The term *vascular phenomenon* refers

to the vascular response to bleeding, which is vasoconstriction.

vasoconstriction: the constricting, or narrowing, of a blood vessel.

warfarin: one of the coumarin group of anticoagulants used to prevent and treat clotting disorders. Warfarin also is used as a rodent poison.

INTRODUCTION

This chapter describes the processes of **hemostasis,** or the arrest of bleeding, and blood **coagulation,** or clot formation. It also describes diseases that affect coagulation and laboratory tests of coagulation.

HEMOSTASIS AND BLOOD COAGULATION

Hemostasis is part of the process of homeostasis, the dynamic balance, or equilibrium, of the internal body environment that is maintained by feedback and regulation. The balance that must be maintained in hemostasis is between fluid blood, which must circulate, and coagulated blood, which prevents blood loss. Death can occur when either bleeding or clotting is uncontrolled.

Blood coagulation is one of three mechanisms by which hemostasis comes about. The other two mechanisms are **vasoconstriction,** which is a narrowing of the injured blood vessel, and the formation of a **platelet plug,** which is a clump of platelets that adhere to the site of injury.

Components of Hemostasis

The process of hemostasis, which Figure 18-1 shows, can be divided into three types of phenomena: vascular, extravascular, and intravascular.

The Vascular Phenomenon. The **vascular phenomenon** is the reaction of the injured blood vessel itself. The injured vessel undergoes vasoconstriction, an immediate response that decreases blood loss until clotting can occur. It is enhanced and prolonged by **serotonin,** a potent vasoconstrictor that is released by platelets adhering to the wounded blood vessel.

The Extravascular Phenomena. The extravascular phenomena are those that occur outside the injured blood vessel. They consist of physical and biochemical reactions of the surrounding tissues,

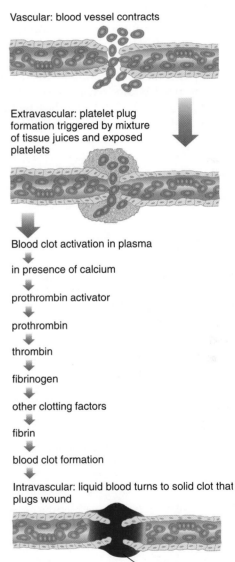

Vascular: blood vessel contracts

Extravascular: platelet plug formation triggered by mixture of tissue juices and exposed platelets

Blood clot activation in plasma
↓
in presence of calcium
↓
prothrombin activator
↓
prothrombin
↓
thrombin
↓
fibrinogen
↓
other clotting factors
↓
fibrin
↓
blood clot formation
↓
Intravascular: liquid blood turns to solid clot that plugs wound

solid clot

Figure 18-1 The process of hemostasis.

including release of **thromboplastin,** a compound that triggers coagulation. The tissue reactions activate other vascular and intravascular phenomena of hemostasis.

The Intravascular Phenomena. The intravascular phenomena are the processes that occur within the blood vessel. First, platelets adhere to the damaged site and accumulate to form a platelet plug. The platelet plug may be sufficient to stop the bleeding if the site of bleeding is very small. If not, coagulation occurs next, through an extremely complex pathway of biochemical changes that transform liquid hemorrhaging blood into a solid clot around the platelet plug. Coagulation normally seals the injured vessel and stops the bleeding.

The process of coagulation requires 12 different compounds, called **coagulation factors,** that must be present in appropriate amounts for clotting to occur effectively (see Table 18-1). Most of these clotting factors are enzyme proteins and numbered with Roman numerals I–XIII. Factor VI stopped being used when it was discovered to be an activated form of factor V. The last factors are produced by platelets and abbreviated PF.

Coagulation

The initiation of coagulation occurs by one of two pathways: the extrinsic or the intrinsic. The

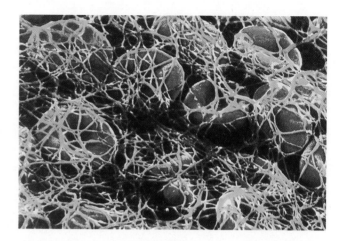

Figure 18-2 Scanning electron micrograph of a blood clot. Yellow fibrin threads are covering red blood cells.

extrinsic pathway is followed when blood comes into contact with traumatized tissues. The intrinsic pathway is followed when there is trauma to the blood itself, due, for example, to slow circulation, bacterial endotoxins, or vascular diseases. Each pathway has several steps and both pathways end with formation of factor X.

At this point the rest of the coagulation pathway is the same for both pathways. Factor X then combines with factors III, V, IV, and PF to produce an enzyme called prothrombin activator. A clot is formed as follows:

* Prothrombin activator converts **prothrombin** to **thrombin.**
* Thrombin joins soluble **fibrinogen** molecules into long, hairlike molecules of insoluble **fibrin.**
* Fibrin filaments form a meshlike network of strands, trapping cells and small amounts of serum, thus forming the clot (see Figure 18-2) .

DISEASES AFFECTING COAGULATION

Diseases that affect coagulation fall into two opposing categories: **hemorrhagic diseases** and **clotting disorders.** In hemorrhagic diseases, there is failure of the blood to clot. In clotting disorders, on the other hand, blood clots form spontaneously. Either extreme may be life threatening. Some blood coagulation diseases are inherited, while others are acquired later in life. In general, the inherited disorders are more easily studied and better understood.

Table 18-1 Coagulation Factors

Factor	Synonym
Factor I	Fibrinogen
Factor II	Prothrombin
Factor III	Thromboplastin
Factor IV	Calcium
Factor V	Labile factor (proaccelerin)
Factor VI	—*
Factor VII	Serum prothrombin conversion accelerator (SPCA)
Factor VIII	Antihemophilic factor (AHF)
Factor IX	Plasma thromboplastin component (PTC)
Factor X	Stuart-Prower factor
Factor XI	Plasma thromboplastin antecedent (PTA)
Factor XII	Hageman factor (contact factor)
Factor XIII	Fibrin stabilizing factor
Platelet factor	Cephalin

*Factor VI is no longer considered a separate entity, but a form of factor V.

Diseases and Hemostasis

Given the complexity of the process, it is not surprising that hemostasis is affected by diseases of several different organs and tissues; for example:

- *Bone marrow diseases* may reduce bone marrow production of platelets so that fewer are available for platelet plug formation.
- *Connective tissue diseases* may encourage hemorrhaging due to weakness and ease of trauma to blood vessels and other tissues.
- *Circulatory diseases* may impair circulation and encourage clot formation.
- *Liver diseases* may adversely affect coagulation because the liver synthesizes blood-coagulation factors, including prothrombin and fibrinogen.
- *High blood pressure* may lead to hemorrhaging.
- *Infections* may lead to tissue damage and bleeding.

Hemorrhagic Diseases

The category of hemorrhagic diseases includes the hemophilias and several other disorders in which excessive bleeding occurs.

The Hemophilias. The **hemophilias** are a group of diseases in which excessive bleeding occurs because of inherited deficiencies in blood coagulation factors. They are characterized by uncontrolled hemorrhaging, possibly even from the slightest injury.

Most cases of hemophilia are sex linked; that is, they are caused by a defective gene on the X chromosome, which is one of two sex chromosomes, X and Y. Females have two X chromosomes and males have one X chromosome and one Y chromosome. Males with a defective gene on their one X chromosome have the disease hemophilia. Because the hemophiliac gene is recessive, only females with defective hemophiliac genes on both of their X chromosomes are affected by the disease. Females with one normal and one defective X chromosome, on the other hand, do not have the disease. Instead, they are carriers of hemophilia because they can pass the defective gene on to their children. Because males need only one hemophilia gene to be affected by the disease, while females need two, the sex-linked forms of the disease affect males far more frequently than they do females. This is why female hemophiliacs are extremely rare. One in 10,000 males is born with hemophilia.

There are several types of hemophilia, each associated with the absence of a different clotting factor. Eighty percent of cases are **hemophilia A,** or classic hemophilia, in which a recessive sex-linked gene leads to the inability to synthesize factor VIII, antihemophilic factor (AHF). Another 15 percent of cases are **hemophilia B,** or Christmas disease, in which a recessive sex-linked gene leads to the inability to synthesize factor IX, plasma thromboplastin component (PTC). The remaining 5 percent of cases are due to deficiency of other coagulation factors. **Hemophilia C,** for example, is due to an autosomal (nonsex chromosome) dominant gene that leads to the inability to synthesize factor XI, plasma thromboplastin antecedent (PTA).

The adverse effects of hemorrhaging associated with hemophilia are numerous. Bleeding into the soft tissues, the gastrointestinal tract, kidneys, and joints can have grave consequences. Bleeding into a joint, for example, can cause swelling, stiffening, and permanent crippling of the joint. The leading cause of death in hemophiliacs is intracranial bleeding.

Hemophiliacs need constant protection from injuries and blood loss. Whenever they receive injections, for example, small-gauge needles should be used, and pressure should be applied to the injection site afterward. The injection site should be monitored until all danger of hemorrhaging is past. Even small cuts are potentially life threatening and require medical attention. Hemophilia is much better controlled today than it was in the past due to the availability of clotting factors derived from donated whole blood. Severe bleeding may require transfusion of normal fresh plasma or of the missing clotting factor.

Other Hemorrhagic Diseases. Vitamin K is important because it stimulates liver cells to synthesize prothrombin and several other clotting factors. It is stored in the liver. Vitamin K deficiency leads to the lack of prothrombin, which in turn results in prolonged blood-clotting time and increased hemorrhaging. Lack of vitamin K, which is essential to formation of factors II, VII, IX, and X, also causes **hemorrhagic disease of the newborn,** which occurs in less than 1 percent of newborns between the second and seventh day after birth. Administration of vitamin K corrects this condition until vitamin K–producing bacterial flora become established in the newborn.

Hypofibrinogenemia is a hemorrhagic disease caused by a deficiency of clotting factor I (fibrinogen). It may be inherited or acquired after severe liver damage. Generally, it is a mild disorder. **Thrombocytopenia** is a hemorrhagic disease due to a deficiency of platelets, which are also called thrombocytes for their role in clot formation. Without platelets to form platelet plugs, many small hemorrhages result.

Drugs and Blood Clotting

The process of blood coagulation is adversely affected by a variety of drugs such as aspirin, other analgesics, and antihistamines. Aspirin, for example, prevents platelets from adhering to one another. Patients with hemophilia should be especially careful when using drugs such as these.

Clotting Disorders

In clotting disorders, clots form in the blood spontaneously. A clot that obstructs blood flow creates a serious condition and can result in death.

Thrombus Formation. Thrombosis refers to the formation of a blood clot, or **thrombus,** in the vascular system. A thrombus may arise spontaneously in the blood for a variety of reasons, including slowed blood flow and roughened or injured inner linings of blood vessels. Increased platelet activity or an elevated concentration of procoagulants also may be involved in the spontaneous formation of blood clots. If a clot arises within a major blood vessel or in the brain, death may occur because blood flow—and hence oxygen and nutrients—are blocked from vital areas.

The body has some natural defenses against thrombosis. They include phagocytic cells, which may engulf a clot, and inhibitors of the coagulation factors such as antithrombin, a substance that opposes the action of thrombin.

Embolisms. Embolism refers to the sudden obstruction of a blood vessel by an **embolus,** which is usually a blood clot but may be fat globules, bacteria, or other undissolved matter. About three-fourths of emboli arise in the deep veins of the legs, where they may cause **thrombophlebitis,** or inflammation of the vein due to the clot. This is a common problem in elderly, immobile patients. Emboli that obstruct blood flow in the extremities may result ultimately in necrosis and gangrene.

Often, emboli tear loose and move through the circulatory system, lodging in vital organs such as the lungs, heart, or brain. In the heart, they may cause **myocardial infarction,** which is an infarct, or area of necrosis, in the **myocardium** (middle wall of the heart) due to cessation of blood supply. Myocardial infarction is usually caused by occlusion of a coronary artery. It is associated with pain, shock, cardiac failure, and frequently death. In the brain, an embolus may cause a **cerebrovascular accident,** or stroke, which is accompanied by sudden loss of consciousness followed by paralysis.

Anticoagulant Drugs. Anticoagulants are drugs that prevent coagulation. They are used in the management of patients with a history of clotting disorders such as thrombosis, thrombophlebitis, pulmonary embolism, acute myocardial infarction, and stroke.

Heparin sodium occurs naturally in the body and is obtained from domestic animals for use as a therapeutic drug. It interferes with coagulation by forming an antithrombin compound and preventing platelets from releasing thromboplastin, thus inhibiting conversion of prothrombin to thrombin.

The **coumarin** group of drugs, including **warfarin,** are ingested orally, absorbed from the gastrointestinal tract, and then carried to the liver. Here, they interfere with the synthesis of vitamin K–dependent coagulation factors (II, VII, IX, and X).

The effectiveness of anticoagulants may be increased by drugs such as aspirin and decreased by others such as barbiturates. Alcohol intake and physiological processes also may affect their efficacy. Underdosage of anticoagulant drugs may lead to a life-threatening blood clot, while overdosage can cause a fatal hemorrhage. For these reasons, patients taking anticoagulant drugs require routine monitoring with laboratory tests.

Antidote for Warfarin Poisoning

Warfarin is used as not only an anticoagulant but also a rodent poison. In this form, it has been ingested accidentally by children. Overdosage of warfarin anticoagulant also sometimes occurs. The antidote in both cases, and for coumarin overdose in general, is administration of vitamin K.

LABORATORY TESTS OF COAGULATON

Several different types of laboratory tests are available to monitor hemostasis, including tests of **bleeding time** and tests for specific coagulation factors. In the POL most tests performed are to monitor anticoagulant therapy, specifically the prothrombin time. Most bleeding and clotting disorders are investigated in hospital laboratories, as well as screening for presurgical patients. In this section we will look at some of the most common tests performed.

General Tests of Bleeding Time

The bleeding time test is used to test the body's ability to stop bleeding after an incision is made. The bleeding time test is sometimes used to evaluate recurrent bleeding, screen patients with family history of bleeding disorders, and screen presurgical patients. This test includes several factors causing failure of hemostasis, but it cannot distinguish among the possible causes. In general a test of platelet function has replaced the bleeding time test in many laboratories.

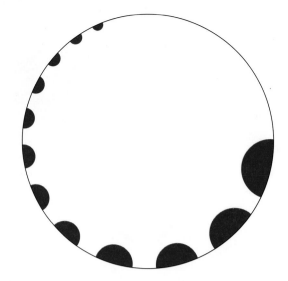

Figure 18-3 As clotting proceeds, the circles of blood on the filter paper become smaller.

Aspirin Advisory

Because aspirin ingestion may increase bleeding time, you should advise patients not to ingest aspirin or related analgesics for several days before a test of bleeding time.

For a general test of bleeding time, capillaries are punctured with a small, clean incision to produce bleeding. After the incision begins to bleed, the time is noted, and welling blood around the cut is removed every 15 to 30 seconds with filter paper, taking care not to disturb the platelet plug. As clotting proceeds, the circles of blood on the filter paper become smaller, until no fluid blood is left on the paper, marking the end of bleeding (see Figure 18-3). The interval between the beginning and end of bleeding is reported as the bleeding time.

Note

In order for bleeding time to be normal, the platelet count must be over 80,000, with platelets showing normal adherence and aggregation.

General bleeding times tend to be imprecise because of variations in lab personnel technique, external conditions, and the site of incision. For this reason, more standardized methods have been developed, including the template method and Duke's bleeding time.

The Template Method. The **template method,** also known as the Ivy bleeding time, standardizes the size and depth of the incision by using a template device, which is shown in Figure 18-4. One example is the Triplett® Bleeding Time device (Helena Laboratories, Beaumont, Texas). The incision is made in the forearm above the wrist in an area cleaned with 70 percent alcohol. The area should be free of skin disease and obvious veins. In order to stabilize capillary pressure, a blood pressure cuff is placed above the elbow, inflated to 40 mm, and maintained in place throughout the procedure. With the first appearance of blood from the incision, a stop watch is started. Then, every 30 seconds, blood from the cut is blotted onto a round of filter paper in a circular, rotating pattern. The time is noted when the blood flow stops. Bleeding time is the interval required for the bleeding to stop.

Duke's Bleeding Time. The Duke's bleeding time test is less standardized and less precise than the template method, but it may be used with children. Bleeding times usually are not done on children because hairline scars and keloid formations may occur at incision sites. The incision site for this test is the earlobe. The lobe of the ear is warmed by gentle rubbing with a cotton ball, cleansed with 70 percent alcohol, and punctured with a device that gives a standardized wound. The same technique of blotting with filter paper is used that was described for the template method. Again, bleeding time is the interval required for bleeding to stop.

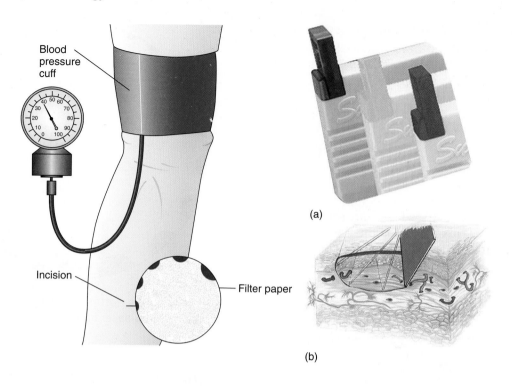

(a)

(b)

Figure 18-4 (a) Ivy bleeding times are performed on adults by making an incision with a Triplett device, (b) which standardizes the depth and length of the incision. Pressure in the cuff remains at 40 mm throughout the procedure. Normal range is 2.3 to 9.5 minutes.

Specific Tests of Coagulation Factors

Laboratory tests of specific elements of the coagulation process that are simple enough to be performed in POLs include the prothrombin time (PT) and the activated partial thromboplastin time (aPTT). Results from these two tests, when correlated with the results of other tests such as platelet counts, help determine the cause of coagulation problems. Both tests also are used routinely to monitor the coagulation status of patients on heparin and coumarin therapy.

Prothrombin Time. A **prothrombin time** (protime or **PT**) tests coagulation factors I, II, VII, and X, all of which are involved in the extrinsic pathway of coagulation. One example of testing uses a decalcified sample of blood plasma (citrated anticoagulant) that is added to a solution of calcium and tissue extract from animal brain that contains thromboplastin. Prothrombin time is measured as the time required for clot formation. Normal PT is 11 to 13 seconds. Protime results are more commonly reported in a number called **INR (international normalized ratio)**. The INR was developed to eliminate interlab variations of the protime results of those patients taking coumarin therapy.

Each lab compares its protime results to an international standard using a mathematical formula supplied by the manufacturer of the reagents. This product is reported as the INR, with therapeutic range of 2–3.

Activated Partial Thromboplastin Time. **Activated partial thromboplastin time (aPTT)** tests coagulation factors II, V, VIII, IX, X, XI, and XII, all of which are involved in the intrinsic pathway of coagulation. A solution of calcium, a platelet substitute, and an activator are added to a plasma sample. The time needed for fibrin clot formation is measured as the activated partial thromboplastin time.

Methods. There are special analyzers and special blood collection techniques that are used for performing prothrombin times and activated partial thromboplastin times. Prothrombin time, or protime, can be measured using various FDA-approved CLIA-waived instruments that can use whole blood from fingerstick or venous anticoagulant-free blood. One such device is the ProTime Microcoagulation System (International Technidyne Corporation [ITC], Edison, New Jersey). This portable instrument uses a blood collection device and a specialized disposable test cuvette. The cuvette has channels for the test assay and also for two levels of controls. A precise volume of blood is drawn into the test channel of the cuvette, which contains the thromboplastin and other reagents. The blood sample and reagent mixtures are moved through the instrument channel until the instrument detects a clot; the results displayed are represented by both PT seconds and INR.

The CoaguChek S System (Roche Diagnostics, Indianapolis, Indiana) is another model of a CLIA-waived monitoring test for prothrombin time. This device uses test strips, very similar to the commonly used glucose testing strips, that are inserted into the monitor and then a drop of fresh whole blood is placed on the strip. The blood is drawn into the reaction chamber and mixed with reagents that cause coagulation to begin. In the test strip, tiny iron particles are mixed with the sample and magnetic fields cause the particles to move. The endpoint is reached when the blood stops the iron particles from moving and the PT results in seconds or INR are displayed by the monitor. This system has two levels of both liquid controls and electronic controls that are tested according to CLIA regulations to ensure the performance of the strips and the device (see Figure 18-5).

An example of a fully automated CLIA non-waived instrument that can perform numerous clotting factor assays, including the PT and the aPTT, is the ACL 100 Coagulation Analyzer (Beckman Coulter, Fullerton, California). (See Figure 18-6.) It can process and analyze up to 110 samples per hour and uses an automatic robotic sampling arm

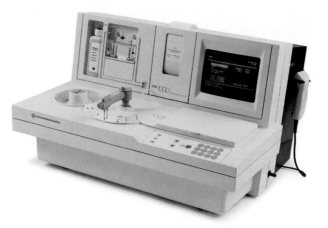

Figure 18-6 Fully automated coagulation analyzer, ACL 100 (Beckman Coulter), used in higher volume laboratories.

to pipette citrated plasma and thromboplastin into an optically clear cuvette that passes through a fixed beam of light as the cuvette rotates. The instrument measures light scattered from the fibrin strands as the fibrin clot is formed. The results are displayed and reported.

Correct specimen collection is critical. For most coagulation studies, citrated plasma is obtained through venipuncture. Blood is collected using sodium citrate as the anticoagulant in the light blue stopper tube. The plasma must be separated from the red blood cells using centrifugation. After centrifuging, the plasma is carefully extracted, avoiding any buffy coat or red cells. If testing is delayed, plasma must be frozen to −20 degrees Celsius or lower.

Quality Control and Safety

As with all laboratory procedures, careful attention to sample collection and handling is necessary to maintain quality control. Standardization, such as the use of the template device for bleeding time, also helps maintain quality control. For prothrombin time testing, CLIA requires two levels of daily control test results. Additional quality control is required when a new box or new lot number of test strips or reagents is used, if improper storage or handling of reagent strips is suspected, or if the instrument has been dropped or mishandled.

Whenever performing coagulation studies, keep in mind that patient specimens, some control specimens, and used test cuvettes and strips should be considered biohazardous and potentially infectious. They should be handled with care and disposed of in accordance with regulations. Always follow standard precautions.

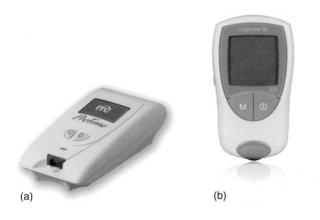

(a)   (b)

Figure 18-5 Examples of diagnostic devices.
(a) ITC ProTime3 Microcoagulation System is a CLIA-waived prothrombin time instrument that detects fibrin clot formation. (ITC, Edison, NJ); (b) CoaguChek S System is a CLIA-waived prothrombin time instrument. (Roche Diagnostics, Indianapolis, IN).

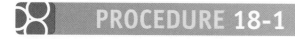

PROCEDURE 18-1

Prothrombin Time Determination

Goal

After successfully completing this procedure, you will be able to perform a prothrombin time using a CLIA-waived microcoagulation instrument and the supplies listed below.

Completion Time

15 minutes

Equipment and Supplies

- Disposable gloves
- Goggles and apron
- Hand disinfectant
- Paper towels and tissues
- Biohazard container
- 70 percent alcohol
- ITC ProTime3 Microcoagulation System (or a similar device)
- Tenderlett® lancet and cuvette
- Coagulation controls

Instructions

Read through the list of equipment and supplies that you will need and the steps of the procedure. Be sure that you understand each step before you begin. Then complete each step correctly, in the proper order, and in the time allowed.

*Steps marked with (*) are critical and must have the maximum points to pass.

Performance Standards	Points Awarded	Maximum Points
1. Wash your hands with disinfectant, dry them, and put on gloves and apron.		10
2. Follow standard precautions.		10
3. Collect and prepare the appropriate equipment. The ITC ProTime3 is precalibrated and does not need additional calibration. Allow the instrument to warm up and self-check. Watch the screen and follow the prompts.		5
4. *Identify the proper patient.		20
5. At the prompt insert the cuvette properly and allow to warm up (1–3 minutes).		5
6. Prepare the finger for blood collection by cleansing with alcohol and drying with gauze.		5
7. Place the Tenderlett Plus device firmly against the side of the finger. Press the red trigger to puncture the finger.		10
8. Wipe away the first drop of blood and form a large drop of blood.		5
9. Touch the drop of blood to the collection cup and collect blood to the proper level.		5
10. Place the front end of the device into the slot in the instrument and click in place. Controls are run in the same cuvette simultaneously with the patient.		5
11. Press the start button. Wait for the prompt and immediately remove the Tenderlett Plus from the instrument in allowed time.		5
12. *Read results and document in proper charts and control logs.		10
13. Discard disposable equipment and supplies.		5
14. Disinfect equipment and clean the work area following standard precautions.		5
15. Remove your gloves and apron; wash your hands with disinfectant and dry them.		5
Total Points		**110**

Overall Procedural Evaluation

Student Name _____

Signature of Instructor _____Date _____

Comments _____

_____

chapter 18 REVIEW

Using Terminology

Define the following terms in the spaces provided.

1. Coagulation

   _____

   _____

   _____

2. Cerebrovascular accident

   _____

   _____

   _____

3. Clotting disorder

   _____

   _____

   _____

4. Coagulation factor

   _____

   _____

   _____

5. Coumarin

   _____

   _____

   _____

6. Hemorrhagic disease

   _____

   _____

   _____

7. Platelet plug

_____

_____

_____

8. Prothrombin

_____

_____

_____

9. Serotonin

_____

_____

_____

10. Template method (Ivy bleeding time)

_____

_____

_____

11. Thromboplastin

_____

_____

_____

12. Thrombus

_____

_____

_____

13. Warfarin

_____

_____

_____

Match the term in the right column with the appropriate definition or description in the left column.

____ **14.** arrest of bleeding   a. hemophilia

____ **15.** narrowing of blood vessels   b. bleeding time

____ **16.** bleeding disorder   c. thrombocytopenia

____ **17.** deficiency of platelets   d. fibrin

____ **18.** obstruction of blood vessel   e. hemostasis

____ **19.** test for bleeding disorder   f. fibrinogen

____ **20.** end product of clotting   g. vasoconstriction

____ **21.** coagulation factor I   h. embolism

Multiple Choice

Choose the best answer for the following questions.

22. The Ivy bleeding time uses a standardized incision made on the forearm and a blood pressure cuff inflated to
    a. 40 mm
    b. 80 mm
    c. 100 mm
    d. 120 mm

23. The coagulation lab test that is performed to monitor patients on coumarin therapy is
    a. Duke bleeding time
    b. prothrombin time
    c. ivy bleeding time
    d. partial thromboplastin time

24. The activated partial thromboplastin time (aPTT) measures which of the coagulation pathways?
    a. intrinsic
    b. extrinsic
    c. common pathway

25. Normal values of prothombin time (PT) on a patient NOT on anticoagulant therapy is
    a. 11–13 seconds
    b. 12–14 seconds
    c. 14–16 seconds
    d. 18–20 seconds

Acquiring Knowledge

Mark each of the following statements as true or false, and rewrite the false statements to make them true.

26. The mechanisms by which hemostasis comes about are coagulation, vasoconstriction, and erythropoiesis.

    _____

    _____

    _____

27. The process of hemostasis can be divided into three types of phenomena: intravascular, vascular, and extrinsic.

    _____

    _____

    _____

28. Thromboplastin interacts with other coagulation factors to convert prothrombin to fibrinogen.

    _____

    _____

    _____

29. Thrombin joins insoluble fibrinogen molecules into long, hairlike molecules of soluble fibrin.

_____

_____

_____

30. Diseases that affect coagulation fall into two opposing categories: hemorrhagic diseases and bleeding diseases.

_____

_____

_____

31. Most cases of hemophilia are acquired.

_____

_____

_____

32. Female hemophiliacs are extremely rare because the female sex hormone, estrogen, protects females from this disease.

_____

_____

_____

33. Vitamin D, an antihemorrhagic factor normally present in blood, aids in blood coagulation and is necessary for the formation of thromboplastin.

_____

_____

_____

34. Thrombocytopenia is a hemorrhagic disease due to a deficiency of platelets.

_____

_____

_____

Answer the following questions in the spaces provided.

35. What is thrombosis and how is it treated?

_____

_____

_____

36. How are myocardial infarction and cerebrovascular accident similar?

_____

_____

_____

37. How do the drugs heparin and warfarin work to prevent clot formation?

_____

_____

_____

38. Name two general tests of bleeding time and two specific tests of coagulation factors.

_____

_____

_____

39. How is quality control maintained in blood coagulation testing?

_____

_____

_____

Applying Knowledge—On the Job

Answer the following questions in the spaces provided.

40. A patient has come into the lab where you work for a bleeding time test, which was just ordered by the physician. The patient mentions that his arthritis has been acting up, so he has been taking aspirin for a few days. How does this information relate to the patient's test? What should you do?

_____

_____

_____

41. An elderly patient has been told to come to the lab routinely for blood tests to monitor his medication. The patient has a history of thrombosis and recently suffered a mild stroke. What type of medication is the patient most likely taking? What test or tests will the physician probably routinely order on this patient's blood?

_____

_____

_____

42. A patient in the clinic where you work is scheduled for major surgery tomorrow, so the physician has ordered screening tests to see if she has a hemorrhaging tendency. What tests are likely to be checked off on the requisition form for this patient? What further test might be requisitioned if the platelet scan appears abnormal?

_____

_____

_____

BLOOD CHEMISTRY

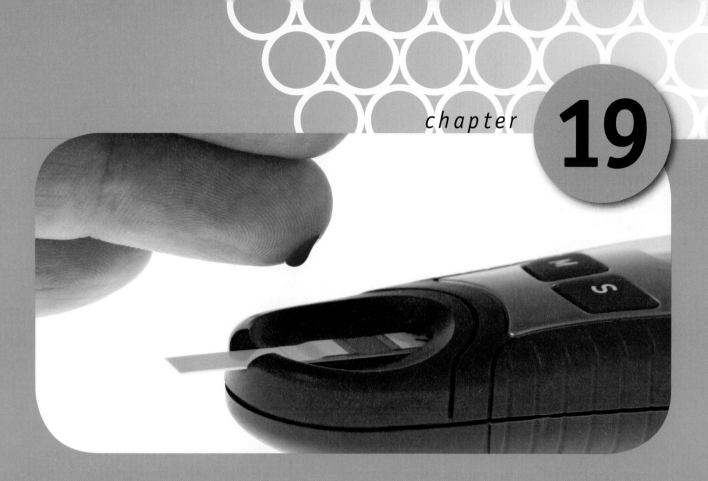

Blood Glucose:
Measuring and Monitoring

COGNITIVE OBJECTIVES

After studying this chapter, you should be able to

19.1   use each of the vocabulary terms appropriately.

19.2   describe how glucose is metabolized and stored.

19.3   identify the normal range of blood glucose for nonfasting and fasting samples.

19.4   list causes of abnormally low and high blood glucose levels.

19.5   explain the cause of diabetes mellitus.

19.6   distinguish between type 1 and type 2 diabetes mellitus.

19.7   list several clinical and biochemical characteristics of type 1 diabetes mellitus.

19.8   compare and contrast blood glucose tests performed in POLs.

19.9   describe how to care for a glucose meter and blood glucose reagent strips.

19.10   explain the role of patient monitoring of blood glucose in the management of type 1 diabetes mellitus.

PERFORMANCE OBJECTIVE

After studying this chapter, you should be able to

19.11   perform a quality control test and a whole blood glucose test using a glucose meter.

acidosis: abnormally low blood pH. The blood is more acidic than normal.

diabetes mellitus (DM): a syndrome caused by inadequate production or utilization of insulin, leading to impaired carbohydrate, protein, and fat metabolism. Diabetes mellitus occurs in two major forms. Type 1 was formerly known as insulin-dependent or juvenile-onset. Type 2 was formerly known as noninsulin-dependent or adult-onset. A third form, gestational diabetes, only occurs in pregnant women.

fasting blood sugar (FBS) test: the blood glucose test performed on a specimen collected after the patient has fasted for 8 to 12 hours. The FBS test is usually scheduled for early morning, before the first meal of the day.

fructose: a simple, six-carbon sugar in fruit and honey.

galactose: a simple, six-carbon sugar derived from lactose, or milk sugar.

gestational diabetes: a transient form of diabetes that develops in response to the metabolic and hormonal changes of pregnancy in previously asymptomatic women. Gestational diabetes generally resolves after delivery.

glucagon: the hormone produced by the alpha cells in the islets of Langerhans of the pancreas; called the fasting hormone because it increases when blood glucose levels are low and stimulates the liver to break down stored glycogen.

glucose: a simple, six-carbon sugar found in many foods. Glucose metabolism provides most of the energy needed for normal growth and functioning.

glucose meter (glucometer): an instrument to measure blood glucose "at the patient's bedside," allowing patients to monitor their glucose levels at home.

glucose tolerance test (GTT): see standard oral glucose tolerance test.

glycogen: a carbohydrate formed from excess glucose that is stored in liver and muscle cells. Glycogen serves as a source of stored energy for the body.

glycogenolysis: the process for breaking down stored glycogen into glucose. Glycogenolysis occurs in the liver when stimulated by the hormone glucagon.

glycosuria: the presence of glucose in the urine.

glycosylated hemoglobin (G-hemoglobin, G-Hgb): hemoglobin with an attached glucose residue.

hemoglobin A_1C test (glycosylated hemoglobin test): a recently developed blood glucose test based on the amount of glycosylated hemoglobin in the blood. The glycosylated hemoglobin test detects hyperglycemia that may be missed in type 1 patients who have wide swings in their blood glucose levels. There is a direct correlation between the amount of hemoglobin A_1C and the average glucose level in the patient's blood over the last 3 months.

hyperglycemia: an abnormally high blood glucose level, most commonly caused by diabetes mellitus.

hypertriglyceridemia: an excessive amount of triglycerides in the blood.

hypoglycemia: an abnormally low blood glucose level. Hypoglycemia may be caused by hyperfunction of the islets of Langerhans or injection of excessive amounts of insulin.

insulin: the hormone secreted by the beta cells of the islets of Langerhans of the pancreas. Insulin helps transport glucose molecules across cell membranes so that glucose metabolism can occur.

lactose: the sugar found in milk. Lactose breaks down into glucose and galactose.

lipolysis: fat decomposition.

monosaccharide: a simple, six-carbon sugar that is found in many foods. Monosaccharides include glucose, fructose, and galactose.

polydipsia: excessive thirst.

polyphagia: excessive food intake.

polyuria: the excretion of excessive amounts of nearly colorless urine.

pruritus: severe itching.

random blood glucose test: the test of blood glucose on a sample of blood that is collected from a nonfasting patient during a routine visit to the doctor's office.

standard oral glucose-tolerance test (GTT or OGTT): the glucose test in which fasting blood and urine specimens are collected before the test starts to serve as a baseline and then specimens are collected over several hours after consumption of a glucose load. This test is used to screen and diagnose diabetes mellitus.

2-hour postprandial blood sugar (2-hour PPBS) test: the blood glucose test administered 2 hours after the patient has consumed a meal containing 100 grams of carbohydrate or has drunk a 100-gram glucose-load solution.

type 1 diabetes mellitus: Formerly known as insulin-dependent diabetes mellitus (IDDM) or juvenile diabetes. A severe form of diabetes mellitus that usually requires administration of insulin for control. Type 1 is characterized by rapid onset, typically before age 25. Type 1 represents 5 to 10 percent of all DM cases.

type 2 diabetes mellitus: Formerly known as noninsulin-dependent diabetes mellitus (NIDDM) or adult-onset diabetes. A less severe form of diabetes mellitus that may be controlled by diet alone. Type 2 typically has gradual onset after age 40. It is often associated with obesity and represents 90 to 95 percent of all DM cases.

INTRODUCTION

Measuring the blood level of **glucose,** a simple sugar, is probably the most commonly performed blood chemistry test in POLs. This chapter explains how and why blood glucose is measured.

GLUCOSE

To understand why glucose is tested, it is important for you to know what glucose is and how it is normally metabolized and stored in the body.

Defining Glucose

Glucose is one of several **monosaccharides,** or simple, six-carbon sugars, that are found in many foods. Other monosaccharides in food include **fructose,** which is found in fruit and honey and **galactose,** a derivative of milk sugar. These simple sugars are converted to glucose before they are utilized by cells.

Glucose Metabolism and Storage

Glucose is metabolized in the cells, where it is broken down into carbon dioxide and water. When glucose is metabolized, it releases stored energy, which the cells of the body use for virtually all their normal growth and functioning.

> **Where the Energy Stored in Glucose Comes From**
>
> In plants, glucose is formed from water and carbon dioxide with energy from the sun and the help of the plant enzyme chlorophyll. This reaction is known as photosynthesis. The light energy stored in the glucose molecule is released when glucose is metabolized by animals.

When the glucose from food is not needed for energy, it is stored in the form of **glycogen,** a carbohydrate. Most of the glycogen in the body is stored in liver and muscle cells. When these cells become saturated with glycogen, excess glucose is converted to fat and stored as adipose tissue. Fat can be converted back to glucose with the aid of enzymes.

If there is a decrease in the level of blood sugar, the pancreatic hormone **glucagon,** called the fasting hormone, increases. Glucagon is produced by alpha cells in the islets of Langerhans found in the pancreas. It stimulates the liver to increase the breakdown of stored glycogen to glucose in a process called **glycogenolysis.** Although glucagon is important in maintaining blood glucose at normal levels, it cannot do the job alone. The other major pancreatic hormone, **insulin,** also is required.

> **Physiology Note**
>
> In addition to stimulating glycogenolysis, glucagon may enhance the synthesis of glucose from amino acids, found in proteins, and from fatty acids found in lipids. Glucagon also is administered to relieve comas due to excessively low blood sugar.

The Role of Insulin. Insulin controls the rate at which glucose is metabolized because it is needed to transport glucose molecules through cell membranes into the cells, where glucose metabolism occurs. Unless glucose can get from the circulating blood into the cells, it cannot be metabolized. Insulin is produced by the islets of Langerhans in the pancreas, specifically by the beta cells, which make up about 75 percent of the pancreatic structure.

BLOOD GLUCOSE AND DISEASE

The normal glucose level in a random blood sample is 70 to 110 mg/dL. If the patient has fasted before the test, the normal level is 70 to 99 mg/dL. Blood glucose always is lowest in a fasting state. Blood glucose levels outside the normal range may indicate pathology.

An abnormally low blood glucose level is referred to as **hypoglycemia.** It may be caused by hyperfunction of the islets of Langerhans or injection of excessive amounts of insulin. An abnormally high

Table 19-1 Criteria for the Diagnosis of Diabetes Mellitus

1. Symptoms of diabetes plus random plasma glucose concentration ≥200 mg/dl. The classic symptoms of diabetes include polyuria, polydipsia, and unexplained weight loss.
OR
2. Fasting plasma glucose ≥126 mg/dl. Fasting is defined as no caloric intake for at least 8 hours.
OR
3. Two-hour postload glucose ≥200 mg/dL during an oral glucose tolerance test (OGTT). The test should be performed as described by the World Health Organization (WHO) using a glucose load.

Source: American Diabetic Association.

blood glucose level is referred to as **hyperglycemia.** It may be caused by hyperthyroidism or adrenocortical dysfunction but most commonly is due to diabetes mellitus.

Diabetes mellitus is a syndrome caused by inadequate production or utilization of insulin, leading to impaired carbohydrate, protein, and fat metabolism. See Table 19-1 for a list of criteria for the diagnosis of the disease. Diabetes mellitus occurs in two different forms, type 1 and type 2. A third form, **gestational diabetes,** occurs only during pregnancy and generally resolves after delivery.

The more severe form of diabetes, **type 1,** was formerly referred to as insulin-dependent diabetes mellitus (IDDM) or juvenile-onset diabetes. Type 1 comprises only 5 to 10 percent of all cases of diabetes mellitus. It is characterized by rapid onset and typically strikes before age 25. Type 1 diabetes requires administration of insulin to manage the disease. Some characteristics of type 1 include **polyuria** (excessive urination), **polydipsia** (excessive thirst), **polyphagia** (excessive food intake), and rapid weight loss. See Table 19-2 for a complete list of type 1 diabetes characteristics.

In comparison, **type 2** diabetes was formerly referred to as noninsulin-dependent diabetes mellitus (NIDDM) or adult-onset. Type 2 can usually be controlled by diet and oral hypoglycemic medications. It is the less severe form of the disease and the more common, comprising 90 to 95 percent of all cases of diabetes mellitus. It usually has a gradual onset and generally affects adults over age 40. Patients with this form of the disease often are obese.

Table 19-2 Characteristics of Type 1 Diabetes

Clinical characteristics of type 1 diabetes include the following:
• rapid weight loss
• polyuria
• **glycosuria**—presence of glucose in the urine
• polydipsia
• polyphagia
• drowsiness and lethargy
• dehydration
• vomiting
• deep breathing
• a sweet, fruity odor on the breath
• warm but dry skin
• predisposition to infection
• **pruritus**—severe itching
Biochemical characteristics of type 1 diabetes include the following:
• continued secretion of free glucose by the liver, despite hyperglycemia
• inhibited entry of free glucose into muscle and adipose tissue, preventing the storage of glucose as glycogen and fat
• increased **lipolysis**—the breakdown of fat
• entry of uncontrolled amounts of free fatty acids into the blood
• conversion of free fatty acids into ketone bodies, causing a sweet odor on the breath
• severe **acidosis,** an abnormally low blood pH, due to nonmetabolized ketone bodies
• severe **hypertriglyceridemia,** an excessive amount of triglycerides in the blood, due to conversion of some of the free fatty acids to triglycerides, resulting in plasma with the appearance of thick cream
• spillover of glucose into the urine from the blood, which occurs when the plasma glucose level rises above the renal threshold of about 180 mg/dL

BLOOD GLUCOSE TESTS

Blood glucose levels are tested to diagnose diabetes and other abnormalities of carbohydrate metabolism. They also are used to monitor the effects of insulin dosage in type 1 patients. Blood glucose testing can be done in a variety of ways (see Table 19-3).

Table 19-3   Laboratory Tests That Measure Glucose Metabolism

Test	Description
Random blood glucose test	A sample is taken at any time without any preparation.
Fasting blood glucose test	A sample is taken with the patient in a fasting state 8 to 12 hours after the last food and tobacco products have been consumed.
2-hour postprandial blood glucose test	A sample is taken 2 hours after a meal.
Standard oral glucose tolerance test (OGTT) or glucose tolerance test	Fasting blood and urine glucose specimens are taken. Then the patient ingests 100 grams of glucose. Blood and urine specimens are taken at 30 minutes and each hour as decided by the doctor. The test may be shorter but lasts no longer than 6 hours.
Hemoglobin A$_1$C	Tests the glucose residue on hemoglobin to provide a measure of long-term blood glucose levels. Also known as glycosylated hemoglobin test.

Note

The words *blood glucose test* and *blood sugar test* are used interchangeably in the POL.

The Random Blood Glucose Test

In a **random blood glucose test,** a sample of blood is collected from a nonfasting patient during a routine visit to the doctor's office or laboratory. The patient does not require any special preparation, and the length of time since the last meal is not important. The objective is to find out the patient's blood glucose level under normal, ordinary conditions. Diabetes is indicated if the glucose level is greater than 200 mg/dL.

The Fasting Blood Glucose Test

A fasting blood glucose, also known as a **fasting blood sugar (FBS) test,** is performed on a specimen that is collected when the patient is in a fasting state. The patient should not smoke, eat, or drink anything other than water for 8 to 12 hours before the test. It is usually easiest for the patient if the test is scheduled for early morning before the first meal of the day.

A normal FBS test virtually eliminates false positives that are caused by elevated blood glucose in random samples collected after carbohydrates have been consumed. The American Diabetic Association recommends that testing be performed twice in order to confirm diagnosis. Diabetes is indicated if on two or more occasions the venous plasma fasting specimens have glucose levels of greater than or equal to 126 mg/dL.

Glucose Tolerance Tests

When fasting blood glucose levels are not definitive for a diagnosis of diabetes or when there is unexplained glycosuria, a **glucose tolerance test (GTT)** may be ordered. Glucose tolerance tests assess the ability to utilize carbohydrates by measuring the body's response to a challenge load of glucose. The results are interpreted by the physician. Figure 19-1 shows responses to the glucose

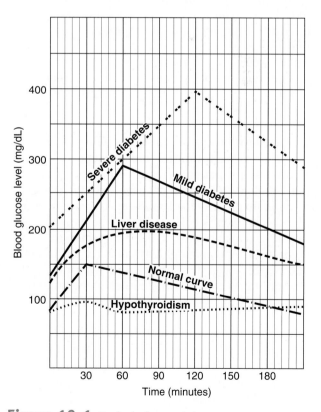

Figure 19-1 Typical glucose tolerance curves, showing the responses of different types of patients.

load in a glucose tolerance test for patients with a variety of conditions.

A glucose tolerance test often is performed when there is some reason to suspect diabetes. Examples include obese patients with family histories of diabetes and patients with unexplained vascular, neurologic, or infectious illnesses. Glucose tolerance tests also may be administered during pregnancy to screen for gestational diabetes, a transient form of diabetes that develops in response to the metabolic and hormonal changes of pregnancy in previously asymptomatic women.

Gestational Diabetes

Gestational diabetes can adversely affect both mother and fetus. Women are considered to be at special risk of developing gestational diabetes if they have one or more of the following:

- a family history of diabetes
- African or Hispanic ancestry
- previous child birth weight over 9 pounds
- a previous fetal loss

Two types of glucose tolerance tests are commonly performed in POLs, the 2-hour postprandial blood sugar test and the standard oral glucose tolerance test. Both glucose tolerance tests require that the patient be in a fasting state for the test. They also require that the patient consume at least 150 grams of carbohydrate per day for 3 days prior to the test. In addition, the patient must have had no alcohol intake.

The 2-Hour Postprandial Blood Glucose Test. In the **2-hour postprandial blood sugar (two-hour PPBS) test,** the patient is required to consume a meal that contains 100 grams of carbohydrate or to drink a 100-gram glucose load solution. Two hours later, a blood specimen is collected from the patient. Some physicians also request a urine specimen to test for glycosuria. A plasma glucose concentration above 200 mg/dL suggests diabetes and warrants further evaluation. Whole blood samples show somewhat lower levels of glucose.

Standard Oral Glucose-Tolerance Test. In the **standard oral glucose tolerance test (GTT or OGTT),** fasting blood and urine specimens are collected before the test starts to serve as a baseline, and then repeated specimens are collected over several hours after consumption of a glucose

load. The glucose load solution usually contains 75 or 100 grams of glucose, but the amount may be tailored to body size. If so, either 1.75 grams of glucose per kilogram of body weight or 50 grams per square meter of body surface are administered.

Urinalysis Note

The collection of urine specimens in the standard oral glucose tolerance test is useful for evaluating how much glucose spills over into the urine at a given level of blood glucose. If glycosuria is observed in the absence of high levels of blood glucose, the patient should be evaluated for abnormal renal tubular function.

Typically in the standard oral glucose tolerance test, blood and urine specimens are collected hourly for up to 6 hours after the glucose is consumed. Most physicians also request a set of half-hourly specimens. Each specimen must be labeled with the exact time of collection. No further specimens are collected once the blood glucose drops back to the baseline level, usually within 3 or 4 hours.

During the test, the patient may drink water but must not consume any food or tobacco. It is common for patients to experience excessive perspiration and some weakness, even fainting, during the test. These are normal reactions to the drop in blood glucose that occurs as insulin is secreted by the pancreas in response to the glucose load.

The standard oral glucose tolerance test is affected by many physiological variables, so careful preparation of patients is necessary for meaningful test results. Patient should be in a normal nutritional state and free of the following drugs: salicylates, diuretics, anticonvulsants, steroids, and oral contraceptives. The doctor will decide whether or not the patient should discontinue these medications when preparing for the test. Patients also should be free of excessive stress for good test results.

A blood glucose level that remains elevated at 2 hours is considered abnormal. A modest 2-hour glucose level that returns to baseline at 3 hours suggests impaired glucose metabolism but does not indicate diabetes. A diagnosis of diabetes mellitus is made when the 2-hour specimen exceeds 200 mg/dL using glucose load.

A very sharp rise in the glucose level after ingestion of the glucose load followed by a decline to subnormal levels may indicate hyperthyroidism or alcoholic liver disease. Patients with gastrointestinal malabsorption may show false-negative results because they cannot absorb the full glucose load.

It is important to take into account the age of patients when interpreting oral glucose tolerance test results because the speed of glucose clearance declines with age. In normal patients, those without diabetes or a family history of the disease, 2-hour blood glucose levels are an average of 6 mg/dL higher for each decade over age 30.

The Hemoglobin A$_1$C Test

The **hemoglobin A$_1$C test,** also known as the **glycosylated hemoglobin test,** detects hyperglycemia that may be missed in type 1 patients who have wide swings in their blood glucose levels.

The hemoglobin A$_1$C test is based on a permanent change in the hemoglobin molecule that occurs when it is exposed to high levels of glucose. A glucose residue attaches to hemoglobin, forming **glycosylated hemoglobin (G-hemoglobin, G-Hgb),** which persists for the remainder of the lifespan of the red cell—an average of 120 days.

> **Physiology Note**
>
> Glycosylation does not impair the oxygen-carrying function of the hemoglobin molecule.

In individuals with repeated periods of hyperglycemia, 18 to 20 percent of the hemoglobin is glycosylated, compared with only 3 to 6 percent in normal individuals. In type 1 patients, a high level of glycosylated hemoglobin indicates inadequate diabetic control in the preceding 3 to 5 weeks. Once blood glucose levels are brought under control, the hemoglobin A$_1$C level returns to normal in about 3 weeks.

USING A GLUCOMETER

Blood glucose frequently is measured in POLs with a **glucose meter** or **glucometer.** The test takes only a few minutes, so glucose meters may be used as initial screening devices, even if a complete panel of blood chemistries including a glucose test is ordered. When used correctly, glucose meters give good, quantitative measures of blood glucose. Many glucose meters can provide results from as low as 10 mg/dL to as high as 600 mg/dL. Some glucose meters are also able to use their memory capabilities to store test results, which can be recalled and averaged.

Glucometer Methods

Each glucose meter utilizes a specific reaction method in order to determine the glucose level. It is important to read the operator's manual included with the glucometer. Information in the manual will explain the specific reaction system, including its weaknesses and sources of errors.

Glucose Meter Controls

CLIA 1988 requires that two glucose control levels be performed each day before a patient's blood glucose is checked on the glucose meter. The controls should include a normal value control and an abnormal value control.

Care of the Instrument and Reagent Strips

Glucose meters are precision instruments that must be handled with care to give accurate results. Dropping may damage the internal electronics and cause a malfunction. Temperature, humidity, and altitude can affect the performance of a glucose meter. The operator's manual can provide more specific information.

Periodic instrument cleaning is required to ensure accurate and reliable operation. The outside should be cleaned with a tissue moistened with clean water, carefully keeping water away from the display window and button. The slot where the reagent strip is placed for reading should be cleaned according to the manufacturer's instructions.

The reagent strips for glucose meters are sensitive to heat, light, and moisture, so they must be properly stored in a cool, dry, dark environment to prevent deterioration. When a test strip is removed from the bottle, the cap should be replaced immediately and kept tight to prevent moisture from entering the bottle. A desiccant in the bottle also helps absorb any excess moisture. Deteriorated test strips appear dark or discolored and should be discarded. Any questionable test strips should be discarded.

PATIENT MONITORING OF BLOOD GLUCOSE

Blood glucose meters are used not only in POLs but also in home monitoring by diabetics. Figures 19-2 and 19-3 show home glucose meters. Home blood glucose monitoring is especially important for type 1 diabetes mellitus patients, for whom regularly scheduled blood testing helps effectively regulate insulin dosage and diet. A fasting blood glucose level performed in the morning before breakfast is probably the best overall indicator of the degree of control in diabetes management. Good management helps type 1 diabetes mellitus patients avoid the extremes of hypoglycemia and hyperglycemia.

The task of instructing patients in diabetes management, including blood glucose testing, frequently is the responsibility of medical assistants. Medical assistants therefore must

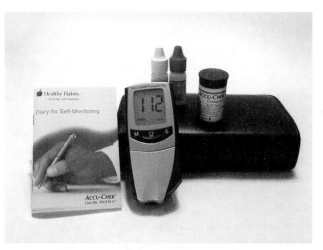

Figure 19-3 An ACCU-CHECK® ADVANTAGE blood glucose meter with a self-monitoring diary, test strips, and level 1 and level 2 controls.

thoroughly understand the proper techniques of collecting and testing samples as well as the importance of quality control checks. In addition to the mechanics of blood glucose testing, diabetic patients must be instructed in the physical and emotional conditions that can affect glucose levels. Then, patients will know when extra testing is needed to ensure that their diabetes is still under control.

Type 1 diabetes patients should keep a permanent log of test results for blood glucose and for urine glucose, if tested. The following information should be recorded in the log for each test:

- the date and time
- the test results
- whether or not a control was run
- whether or not the control was in the accepted range
- the number of hours since last eating
- the time of the last insulin injection or oral hypoglycemic medication
- whether or not the patient was under any physical or emotional stress
- the amount of exercise performed recently by the patient

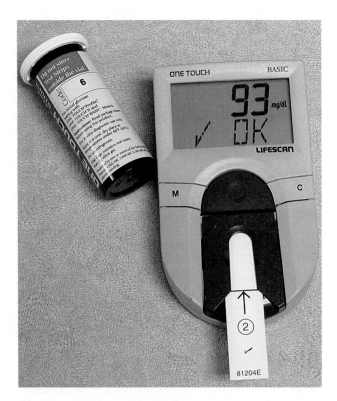

Figure 19-2 A glucometer.

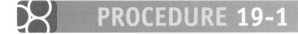

PROCEDURE 19-1

Using a Glucose Meter to Test Blood Glucose

Goal

To correctly determine the blood glucose level of a patient.

Completion Time

15 minutes

Equipment and Supplies

- Disposable gloves
- Impermeable apron, lab jacket, or gown
- Hand disinfectant
- Surface disinfectant
- Alcohol
- Paper towels and tissues
- Biohazard container
- Blood glucose meter
- Blood glucose meter operator guide
- 2 levels of glucose controls
- Glucose test strips
- Lancet for finger puncture
- Pen and notebook

Instructions

Read through the list of equipment and supplies that you will need and the steps of the procedure. Be sure that you understand each step before you begin. Then complete each step correctly and in the proper order. If your completion time is too long, repeat that procedure until you increase your speed.

Steps marked with (*) are critical and must have the maximum points to pass.

Performance Standards	Points Awarded	Maximum Points
1. Put on lab coat.		5
2. Disinfect hands; dry if necessary.		5
3. Put on gloves. Inspect for tears and replace if necessary.		5
4. Collect and prepare the appropriate equipment.		5
5. Read the operator guide for the glucose meter.		10
6. Perform quality control testing per operator's manual instructions.		10
7. Determine if controls are acceptable.		30
8. If any controls are out of range, determine the cause of the problem and correct the problem.		15
9. *Verify specimen identity.		30
10. Explain the fingerstick procedure and encourage the patient to relax.		5
11. Select an appropriate finger site.		10
12. Clean the site with alcohol, using concentric circles.		5
13. Allow the alcohol to completely dry.		5
14. Hold the patient's finger with your nondominant hand and gently apply pressure.		5
15. Quickly puncture the site with the lancet.		10
16. *Engage the lancet's safety mechanism.		30
17. Wipe away the first drop of blood with dry gauze.		10

—table continued

Performance Standards	Points Awarded	Maximum Points
18. Place a drop of blood on the glucose strip testing pad. Apply gentle pressure, but avoid squeezing.		15
19. When glucometer is done analyzing, record the result in the testing log.		20
20. If any error messages are present, refer to the operator's manual and perform any troubleshooting as required.		20
21. Thank and release the patient.		20
22. Discard disposable equipment.		10
23. Return all equipment to storage.		5
24. Wash hands.		5
Total Points		**290**

Overall Procedural Evaluation

Student Name _____

Signature of Instructor _____ Date _____

Comments _____

_____

chapter 19 REVIEW

Using Terminology

Match the terms in the right column with the appropriate definition or description in the left column.

_____ **1.** after meal

_____ **2.** breaking down glycogen

_____ **3.** excessive thirst

_____ **4.** carbohydrate

_____ **5.** hemoglobin A_1C

_____ **6.** hormone from alpha cells

_____ **7.** hormone from beta cells

_____ **8.** increased food intake

_____ **9.** low blood glucose level

_____ **10.** simple sugar

a. glycosylated hemoglobin

b. glucagon

c. glucose

d. glycogen

e. glycogenolysis

f. hypoglycemia

g. insulin

h. polydypsia

i. polyphagia

j. postprandial

Define the following terms in the spaces provided.

11. Acidosis

_____

_____

_____

12. Diabetes mellitus

_____

_____

_____

13. Fructose

_____

_____

_____

14. Gestational diabetes

_____

_____

_____

15. Galactose

_____

_____

_____

16. Hyperglycemia

_____

_____

_____

17. Hypertriglyceridemia

_____

_____

_____

18. Monosaccharide

_____

_____

_____

19. Standard oral glucose tolerance test (GTT or OGTT)

_____

_____

_____

20. Lipolysis

_____

_____

_____

Comparing Type 1 and Type 2 Diabetes

State whether the following are associated with type 1 or type 2 diabetes.

____ **21.** Can be controlled with diet and exercise in some cases

____ **22.** Disease usually develops before the patient turns 25 years old

____ **23.** Primary form of DM that requires insulin for treatment

____ **24.** Gradual onset

____ **25.** Rapid onset

____ **26.** Often associated with obesity

____ **27.** Accounts for 90 to 95 percent of all cases of diabetes

Multiple Choice

Choose the best answer for the following questions.

28. A condition where the fluids of the body are in an acidic condition is known as

a. alkalosis

b. acidosis

c. acidemia

d. hypoglycemia

29. A hormone produced by the alpha cells of the islets of Langerhans of the pancreas, responsible for stimulating the liver cells to break down glycogen, is

a. fructose

b. glucose

c. insulin

d. glucagon

30. A glucose test that assesses the ability of a patient to utilize glucose by measuring a patient's response to a load of glucose is the

a. glucose tolerance test

b. fasting blood glucose

c. hemoglobin A_1C test

d. random blood glucose

31. A test used to detect hyperglycemia in patients with type 1 diabetes that experience wide swings in their blood glucose level is the

a. glucose tolerance test

b. fasting blood glucose

c. hemoglobin A_1C test

d. random blood glucose

32. When glucose from food is not needed for energy, it is stored in the form of _____ in the liver and muscle cells.

a. starch

b. glucose

c. glycogen

d. insulin

33. When glucose from food is not needed for energy, it is stored in the form of _____ throughout the body.

a. fat

b. glucose

c. glycogen

d. insulin

34. Which is NOT a characteristic of type 1 diabetes?

    a. obesity

    b. increased thirst

    c. increased appetite

    d. increased urination

35. Which of the following is NOT a cause of hypoglycemia?

    a. overmedicating with insulin

    b. starvation

    c. overeating

    d. all of the above

36. A glucose test that can be performed at any time without any special patient preparation is the

    a. random blood glucose test

    b. fasting blood glucose test

    c. glucose tolerance test

    d. 2-hour postprandial blood glucose test

37. A glucose test that is performed after a patient has fasted for 8–12 hours but requires no other patient preparation is the

    a. random blood glucose test

    b. fasting blood glucose test

    c. glucose tolerance test

    d. 2-hour postprandial blood-glucose test

38. A glucose test that requires the patient to drink a specified load of glucose and then monitors the body's response is the

    a. random blood glucose test

    b. fasting blood glucose test

    c. glucose tolerance test

    d. 2-hour postprandial blood glucose test

39. A glucose test in which the patient is instructed to eat a meal of 100 grams of carbohydrate and then the patient's glucose level is measured 2 hours later is the

    a. random blood glucose test

    b. fasting blood glucose test

    c. glucose tolerance test

    d. 2-hour postprandial blood glucose test

Acquiring Knowledge

Answer the following questions in the spaces provided below.

40. Where and in what form is glucose stored in the body?

_____

_____

_____

41. What are the normal ranges of blood glucose for nonfasting and fasting samples?

_____

_____

_____

42. What is the criteria for the diagnosis of diabetes mellitus utilizing the standard oral glucose tolerance test?

_____

_____

_____

43. What test is the best overall indicator of control in the management of type 1 diabetes?

_____

_____

_____

44. Explain the role of patient monitoring of blood glucose in the management of type 1 diabetes.

_____

_____

_____

Applying Knowledge—On the Job

Answer the following questions in the spaces provided.

45. The lab where you work does blood glucose tests to monitor pregnant women at risk of developing gestational diabetes. What items of medical history identify those women at special risk?

_____

_____

_____

46. One of your jobs in the physician's office where you work is to give patients instructions in how to prepare for lab tests. What instructions would you give to Ms. Talbot, who is going to have a fasting blood sugar test performed tomorrow morning?

_____

_____

_____

47. What instructions would you give to Mr. Chen, who is going to have a glucose tolerance test in 3 days?

_____

_____

_____

48. Today, in the POL where you work, a patient's glucose concentration remained above 200 mg/dL at the end of the second hour of his glucose tolerance test. How would you interpret this result?

_____

_____

_____

49. The reagent strips that you use with the glucose meter in the POL where you work have turned a dark color. What should you do?

_____

_____

_____

50. A new patient with type 1 diabetes needs instructions in home monitoring of blood glucose levels. The doctor has asked you to explain to the patient how to keep a permanent log of blood glucose testing. What information should you tell the new patient to record in the log?

_____

_____

_____

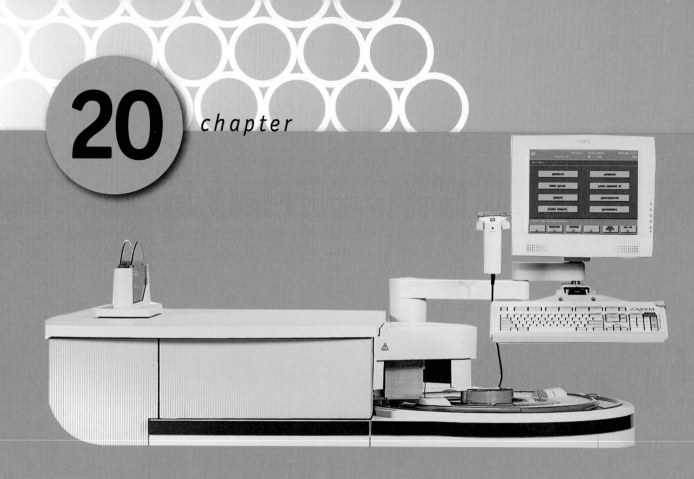

20 chapter

chapter

Chemistry Analyzers and Clinical Application

COGNITIVE OBJECTIVES

After studying this chapter, you should be able to

20.1   use each of the vocabulary terms appropriately.

20.2   state the advantages of using automated chemistry analyzers in the POLs.

20.3   compare discrete and continuous flow analysis systems.

20.4   discuss the role of CLIA with chemistry analyzers.

20.5   describe carbohydrates.

20.6   list the hormones that regulate glucose metabolism and identify how they affect blood glucose levels.

20.7   identify the major causes of hypoglycemia and hyperglycemia.

20.8   distinguish between postprandial hypoglycemia and fasting hypoglycemia.

20.9   describe the three types of biologically important lipids.

20.10   explain the classification of lipoproteins on the basis of density.

20.11   discuss the clinical significance of lipid and lipoprotein levels and proportions.

20.12   describe the composition and role of proteins in the body.

20.13   identify nonprotein nitrogen compounds in the blood that are assessed in POLs.

TERMINOLOGY

acromegaly: a growth abnormality caused by overproduction of growth hormone by the pituitary gland.

adipose tissue: the connective tissue in which fat is stored in cells.

albumin: the most abundant plasma protein. Albumin is responsible for maintaining osmotic pressure at the capillary membrane.

amino acid: one of 20 different compounds in humans that are the building blocks of proteins. Each amino acid contains an amine group and an acidic carboxyl group.

atherosclerosis: the condition in which cholesterol deposits in the blood vessels.

automated chemistry analyzer: an instrument that performs chemistry test procedures automatically.

blood urea nitrogen (BUN): the concentration of nitrogen in the blood, which is used as an indirect measure of urea in the blood.

cholesterol: the sterol of primary biological significance. High levels of cholesterol in the blood are linked with increased risk of cardiovascular disease.

conjugated lipid: a compound made up of fat and another compound such as phosphoric acid (phospholipids) or a carbohydrate (glycolipids).

continuous flow analysis system: a chemistry analyzer in which samples and reagents flow through the instrument one after the other. One test or a variety of tests may be performed on the same sample in a single operation of the instrument.

creatine: a nonprotein nitrogen compound found in muscle tissue. Creatine is synthesized primarily in the liver from three amino acids. It combines readily with phosphate to store energy for muscle contractions.

creatinine: the end product of the metabolism of creatine.

Cushing's syndrome: the condition caused by hypersecretion of the adrenal cortex.

disaccharide: a 12-carbon sugar. Disaccharides include sucrose, lactose, and maltose.

discrete (noncontinuous) analysis system: a chemistry analyzer in which samples and reagents for each test are placed in separate containers, in which the tests are performed. There are two different types: wet chemistry and dry chemistry.

globulin: the second most abundant type of plasma protein. Globulin has a diversity of functions, including transporting other substances and acting as a substrate.

gluconeogenesis: the formation of glycogen from noncarbohydrate sources.

high-density lipoprotein (HDL): a lipoprotein that has high density because it is low in fat content.

hyperthyroidism: hyperactivity of the thyroid gland, leading to increased production of thyroxine.

insulinoma: a tumor of the beta cells of the pancreas.

ion-selective electrode (ISE): a conductor that is sensitive to the activity of a particular ion in solution.

lipid: fat; one of a group of organic compounds made up mainly of carbon, hydrogen, and oxygen. Lipids are used to store energy and as structural materials in the cells.

lipoprotein: a macromolecule of triglycerides, phospholipids, and cholesterol complexed with specialized proteins.

low-density lipoprotein (LDL): a lipoprotein that is low in density because it contains large amounts of fat, primarily in the form of cholesterol.

oral hypoglycemic drug: a drug that decreases the amount of glucose in the blood by stimulating beta cells to secrete more insulin, inhibiting glucose production, or facilitating the transport of glucose to muscle cells.

plaque: a thickened region in an artery wall that prevents blood from flowing freely. Plaques may lead to heart attack or stroke.

polysaccharide: a carbohydrate composed of many molecules of simple sugars. Polysaccharides include starch in plants and glycogen in animals.

potentiometric test: an analytic chemistry test in which the concentration of an analyte is measured by electrical potential.

profile: a group of tests performed to help diagnose pathology of a specific organ or system.

protein: one of a large group of complex, nitrogen-containing organic compounds, consisting of amino acids joined together by peptide bonds.

ribosome: a cellular structure on the surface of rough endoplasmic reticula that synthesizes protein.

saturated fat: a triglyceride in which the fatty acids are saturated with hydrogen atoms. Saturated fats form straight chain molecules that tend to pack together tightly, appearing like the dense white fat in bacon.

thyroxine: the thyroid hormone that raises the level of blood glucose.

triglyceride: a compound made up of fatty acids and glycerol.

unsaturated fat: a triglyceride in which the fatty acids are not saturated with hydrogen atoms. Unsaturated fats tend to be liquids at room temperature.

urea: a small molecule formed from ammonia in the liver that can move freely into both extracellular and intracellular fluid. Urea is concentrated in the urine for excretion.

uremia: a high level of urea in the blood.

uric acid: the end product of the metabolism of purine, an important constituent of nucleic acids.

INTRODUCTION

This chapter describes **automated chemistry analyzers,** instruments that perform a variety of chemistry test procedures automatically. Specific topics include the advantages of automated methods over manual methods, how automated analyzers work, the types of tests they perform, and how quality control is maintained. In addition, this chapter will explore some of the tests performed in the chemistry lab.

THE ADVANTAGES OF AUTOMATION

Automated chemistry analyzers in POLs improve diagnosis and treatment by providing physicians with a great deal of information. Automated analyzers can perform single tests or **profiles,** groups of tests, to help diagnose pathology of a specific organ or system. Automated analyzers increase POL efficiency by reducing turnaround time in test performance. Patients often prefer in-office testing because of its immediate results, allowing the physician to make adjustments in treatment at the patient's side. This is in sharp contrast to the time delay that occurs when specimens are transported to a lab where testing is performed and then the physician is notified of the test results. It is only at that point that a physician can respond to the lab result. This process can take hours to days. As a result of this time delay when sending tests to a reference lab, many physicians have added chemistry testing to their labs. This has been a major influence in the development of chemical analysis instruments for POLs and has led to the production of reliable, simple-to-operate, and relatively inexpensive instruments that are small enough to fit on a lab bench. Many of today's instruments are hand-held and testing can be performed right at the patient's bedside.

> ### Point-of-Care (POC) Testing
>
> Laboratory testing that can be done using a hand-held device at the patient's bedside is referred to as point-of-care testing.

THE TYPES OF CHEMISTRY ANALYZERS

Automated chemistry analyzers are based on one of two types of technology: continuous flow analysis or discrete (noncontinuous) analysis.

Continuous Flow Systems

In **continuous flow analysis systems,** samples and reagents flow through the instrument one after the other. One test or a group of tests may be performed on the same sample in a single operation of the instrument. Samples of whole blood, plasma, serum, or sometimes urine are placed on the analyzer on either straight or circular trays. The analyzer then automatically rotates the specimen into position, introduces the sample, analyzes it, and generates a report. The specific chemical methods used are similar or the same as those used in the manual methods.

These analyzers generally are not used in POLs, but they are common in hospital labs, where larger numbers of samples are tested. Depending on the instrument, continuous flow analyzers can perform over 20 tests on a single specimen.

Discrete Analysis Systems

In **discrete (noncontinuous) analysis systems,** samples and reagents for each test are placed in separate containers, in which the tests are performed. The chemical method used by discrete analysis systems may be either wet chemistry, which involves centrifugal analysis of liquid reagents, or dry chemistry, which involves solid-phase analysis of dry reagents.

Discrete centrifugal analysis uses centrifugation of liquid reagents for wet chemistry procedures. During the centrifugation process, the reagents and the patient sample are mixed together. The instrument analyzes this mixture to generate a result. In comparison, discrete solid-phase analysis utilizes dry reagent layered on slides. Generally, there are at least two layers, each with its own distinct reagent and corresponding reaction. The specimen is added to the slide and reacts with the reagents present. The analyzer interprets this reaction and generates a result.

Additional methods of analysis include **potentiometric tests** in which the concentration of an analyte is measured by electrical potential. Two electrodes are present. The first is the reference electrode that contains a known amount of the ion being tested for. The second electrode is the **ion-selective electrode (ISE)** that is sensitive only to the activity of the ion being tested for. When the patient sample is added, a difference between the amount of the ion in the specimen and the amount of ion in the reference electrode creates an electrical potential. This electrical potential is measured by the instrument and converted into a measurement of the ion concentration of the unknown solution.

> ### Which Chemistry Analyzer to Select
>
> Consider the following questions when selecting a chemistry analyzer for a POL:
>
> - Does the instrument perform tests that are needed frequently for diagnosis?
> - How accurate are the test results?
> - How long does each test take?
> - Will additional staff be required?
> - How difficult is the instrument to maintain?
> - How difficult is the instrument to calibrate?
> - How difficult is the quality control program?
> - What special training is needed to operate the instrument?
> - How much space is needed for the instrument?
> - How long are the reagents stable?
> - Do the reagents require refrigeration or freezer storage?
> - How much does the instrument cost initially?
> - How much do the reagents cost to run each test?
> - How much will Medicaid and Medicare reimburse for each test?
> - Will this addition to the lab be in keeping with the level of complexity at which the lab is certified (i.e., is the test "waived" or "nonwaived")? Check the most recent CLIA regulations.

> ### CLIA Note
>
> CLIA 1988 requires that two levels of control samples for each parameter be performed and recorded each day that a patient sample is tested for that parameter. Control samples should include a normal value and an abnormal value.

Chemistry Testing

The blood transports numerous substances related to metabolic processes. The remainder of this chapter describes the substances most frequently measured in POLs as part of a general assessment of body metabolism. These substances include carbohydrates, lipids, and proteins. Some of the substances analyzed provide information about specific organs or systems, while others reveal the summed effects of numerous metabolic events involving more than one organ or system.

CARBOHYDRATES

Carbohydrates are a large group of sugars, starches, celluloses, and gums that contain only carbon, hydrogen, and oxygen and that are in approximately the proportions 1:2:1, respectively. Carbohydrates are the main source of energy for all body functions and they are needed to process other nutrients. They are formed by all green plants.

Glucose

The body gets most of its energy from the oxidative metabolism of the carbohydrate glucose, a simple, six-carbon sugar or monosaccharide. Glucose is found in the diet most often as part of more complex sugars, including the **disaccharides,** or 12-carbon sugars. Examples of some common disaccharides include sucrose, table sugar, which usually comes from sugar cane; lactose, milk sugar; and maltose, found in malt and sprouting seeds and formed from starch. Glucose also is found in the diet as the major constituent of **polysaccharides,** which are carbohydrates composed of many molecules of simple sugars. Polysaccharides include starch in plants and glycogen in animals.

> ### Fatty Acids as an Energy Source
>
> In addition to glucose, many cells can derive some energy by burning fatty acids, which are acids found in some fats. Fatty acids are a less efficient energy source than glucose, however, and their metabolism generates acid metabolites that are harmful when accumulated.

The body uses enzymes to release glucose from these more complex carbohydrates. Glucose that is not used directly for energy by the cells is stored in the liver and muscles as glycogen or in adipose tissue as **triglycerides.** The latter are compounds made up of fatty acids and glycerol, an alcohol.

Hormones That Regulate Blood Glucose Levels

Because glucose is so important as an energy source, maintaining adequate blood levels of glucose is a high priority for homeostasis, involving many different hormones. The four hormones most significant for glucose regulation are the pancreatic hormones insulin and glucagon, the adrenal hormone epinephrine, and the thyroid hormone **thyroxine.** Insulin acts to lower blood glucose levels, while the other three hormones all work to raise them.

Insulin, which is produced by beta cells in the pancreas, lowers blood glucose levels by

- enhancing the entry of glucose into the cells
- enhancing the storage of glucose as glycogen or fatty acids

- enhancing the synthesis of proteins and fatty acids
- suppressing the breakdown of proteins into amino acids and fat into free fatty acids

Glucagon, which is produced by alpha cells in the pancreas, raises blood glucose levels by

- enhancing the release of glucose from glycogen
- enhancing the synthesis of glucose from amino acids and fatty acids

Epinephrine originates in the medulla of the adrenal gland. It raises blood glucose levels by enhancing the release of glucose from glycogen and fatty acids from adipose tissue. Thyroxine from the thyroid gland raises blood glucose by enhancing the release of glucose from glycogen. It also enhances the absorption of sugars from the intestine.

Abnormal Blood Glucose Levels

Blood glucose levels are measured to assess the adequacy of the hormonal regulation of glucose metabolism and storage. Blood glucose levels that are either too high or too low signal faulty homeostasis and the need to search for causes.

Hyperglycemia. Hyperglycemia refers to a higher-than-normal blood glucose level. Recall that normal, nonfasting blood glucose levels are between 70 and 110 mg/dL. The most common cause of hyperglycemia is diabetes mellitus, which occurs in two forms: type 1 and type 2 diabetes. In type 1 diabetes, the insulin receptors on the cells are normal, but the beta cell mass in the pancreas is markedly reduced. As a result, patients with type 1 diabetes have no measurable circulating insulin. They do not respond to **oral hypoglycemic drugs,** which work in a variety of ways to decrease the amount of glucose in the blood.

> ### Hypoglycemic Drugs
>
> Contrary to popular belief, oral hypoglycemic drugs are not an oral form of insulin, although their purpose is the same—to decrease the amount of glucose in the blood. They work through several mechanisms, including
>
> - stimulating the beta cells of the pancreas to secrete more insulin
> - inhibiting glucose production
> - facilitating the transport of glucose to muscle cells

Instead, patients with type 1 diabetes must take daily insulin injections.

In type 2 diabetes, on the other hand, the beta cell mass is reduced only modestly, and insulin is present in the blood at low, normal, or even high levels. The insulin receptors on the cells are reduced or ineffective. Patients with type 2 diabetes usually respond to oral hypoglycemic drugs and some can control their disease with diet and exercise alone.

In addition to diabetes mellitus, several other conditions can cause hyperglycemia. They include

- **hyperthyroidism,** or hyperactivity of the thyroid gland, which increases the production of thyroxine
- **Cushing's syndrome,** which is caused by hypersecretion of the adrenal cortex
- elevated levels of the hormones estrogen, epinephrine, or norepinephrine
- **acromegaly,** a growth abnormality caused by overproduction of growth hormone by the pituitary gland
- obesity, defined as weight gain of 20 percent greater than ideal weight for height and body build
- treatment with adrenal steroids, thiazide diuretics, or oral contraceptives
- severe liver or kidney damage, which impairs normal carbohydrate metabolism
- alcoholism, which causes liver damage and dysfunction

Hypoglycemia. Hypoglycemia refers to abnormally low levels of glucose in the blood. It is diagnosed only when blood glucose is below 50 mg/dL at the same time that the patient is experiencing symptoms of hypoglycemia. Which specific symptoms are experienced depend on how quickly blood glucose levels fall. When blood glucose falls rapidly, it leads to increased epinephrine secretion, which produces sweating, trembling, weakness, anxiety, and, if prolonged, delirium and loss of consciousness. When blood glucose falls gradually, the symptoms include headache, irritability, and lethargy. In true hypoglycemia, a return to normal blood glucose levels eliminates the symptoms.

The most common cause of hypoglycemia is insulin overdose in patients with unstable type 1 diabetes. Correcting the condition involves ingestion of a source of sugar such as sugar cubes, candy, or orange juice, preferably as soon as symptoms appear. Other conditions that cause high levels of circulating insulin also can produce hypoglycemia. These include large tumors behind the peritoneum and tumors of the beta cells of the pancreas, called **insulinomas.**

There are two types of hypoglycemia: postprandial and fasting hypoglycemia. Postprandial hypoglycemia, also called reactive hypoglycemia, occurs several hours after food is ingested. Symptoms generally last no more than 30 minutes and they resolve without further carbohydrate intake. Postprandial hypoglycemia appears to be due to a delayed or exaggerated response to the insulin that is secreted when sugar is ingested. It may occur early in the development of type 2 diabetes due to a mismatch between pancreatic insulin production and cellular insulin receptors, but most cases have no known physiological cause. The latter cases of postprandial hypoglycemia are considered to be functional disease, that is, disease in which no anatomical changes can be observed to account for the symptoms.

Fasting hypoglycemia is detected by measuring blood glucose levels after a 12- or 24-hour fast. In contrast to postprandial hypoglycemia, fasting hypoglycemia usually is associated with recognizable anatomical changes in an organ or tissue. The major cause is liver disease. Alcoholics, for example, frequently develop fasting hypoglycemia if their carbohydrate intake is low. Their glycogen stores are depleted and alcohol metabolites interfere with **gluconeogenesis**—the formation of glycogen from noncarbohydrate sources. Pancreatic tumors also may cause fasting hypoglycemia.

LIPIDS

Lipids, or fats, are a group of organic compounds made up mainly of carbon, hydrogen, and oxygen. The concentration of energy in lipids is twice that of carbohydrates, so they provide a good source of stored energy for the body. They also are used as structural materials in the cells.

Types of Lipids

Three types of lipids are biologically important: neutral fats, conjugated lipids, and sterols. Neutral fats are triglycerides, fatty acids plus glycerol. **Conjugated lipids** are compounds made up of fat and another compound such as phosphoric acid (phospholipids) or a carbohydrate (glycolipids). Sterols are steroid alcohols. **Cholesterol** is the sterol of primary biological significance.

Triglycerides. Each molecule of triglyceride contains a three-carbon glycerol molecule bonded to three fatty acids. Fatty acids are the major form of fat used by the body to store energy. They are found in **adipose tissue,** which is connective tissue in which fat is stored in cells. Fatty acids enter and leave adipose tissue as needed to provide raw material for gluconeogenesis and direct combustion as an energy source.

Most fatty acids are synthesized by the liver from carbohydrates and proteins. Those that cannot be synthesized are called essential fatty acids because they must be consumed in the diet. They are found in vegetables in the form of linoleic and linolenic acids. One tablespoon per day of corn or olive oil fulfills the daily requirement for essential fatty acids, which are needed for proper functioning of all tissues. Essential fatty acids also are the precursors of prostaglandins, hormonelike fatty acids that perform a number of important functions, including

- stimulating contractility of uterine and other smooth muscles
- lowering blood pressure
- regulating acid secretion of the stomach
- regulating body temperature
- regulating platelet aggregation
- controlling inflammation and vascular permeability

Symptoms of essential fatty acid deficiency include growth retardation, scaliness of the skin, infertility, kidney abnormalities, and increased susceptibility to infections.

There are two basic types of triglycerides: saturated fats and unsaturated or polyunsaturated fats. **Saturated fats** are triglycerides in which the fatty acids are saturated with hydrogen atoms (that is, they are bonded to as many hydrogen atoms as possible). As a result, they form straight chain molecules that tend to pack together tightly, appearing like the dense white fat in bacon. **Unsaturated fats** are triglycerides in which the fatty acids are not saturated with hydrogen atoms. They have kinks—not straight chain structures—so they cannot pack together as tightly. As a result, unsaturated fats tend to be liquids at room temperature. Nutritional research suggests that it is more healthful to consume unsaturated fats like canola, safflower, and olive oils than saturated fats such as butter and lard.

Phospholipids. Phospholipids, which include primarily lecithin, sphingomyelin, and cephalin, comprise the largest fraction of plasma lipids. Circulating phospholipids generally are in the ratio 70 percent lecithin, 20 percent sphingomyelin, and 10 percent cephalin and others. Up to age 30, the plasma concentration of phospholipids is between 150 and 300 mg/dL. While all cells in the body are capable of synthesizing phospholipids, most circulating phospholipids probably are produced in the liver and intestinal mucosa.

Phospholipids play many important roles in body function. They help stabilize other lipids being transported through the blood and are the major constituents of cell membranes. Circulating phospholipids serve as a source of phosphate groups for intracellular metabolism and play an essential role in blood coagulation. Both lecithins and sphingomyelins act as mild detergents. Unlike fatty acids, however, phospholipids seldom are used for energy storage.

Cholesterol. Cholesterol contains a hydroxyl radical (–OH) like all other alcohols. Cholesterol is an important component of cell membrane structure and of the materials that make skin waterproof. The adrenal cortex, ovaries, and testes use cholesterol for the manufacture of steroid hormones, and the liver uses cholesterol to form bile acids, or salts.

It is likely that very little dietary cholesterol enters directly into metabolic reactions. Instead, cholesterol undergoes continuous synthesis, degradation, and recycling in the body. Virtually every type of body tissue can manufacture cholesterol from simple carbon compounds, but those that are particularly active in cholesterol production include the liver, adrenal cortex, ovaries, testes, and intestinal epithelium. The liver is the primary source of cholesterol production.

The rate at which the liver produces cholesterol appears to be related inversely to the amount of circulating chylomicron cholesterol—microscopic cholesterol particles circulating in the blood after fat digestion. When the chylomicron cholesterol level is low, the liver increases its cholesterol production. This occurs with bile duct obstruction, which leads to a reduction in the amount of bile salts reaching the gut to emulsify fats for digestion. As a result, there is less circulating chylomicron cholesterol. The liver responds by doubling or tripling its production of cholesterol.

While the body can synthesize cholesterol with great ease, it has much more difficulty degrading it. Estrogen tends to promote the transport and excretion of cholesterol, while testosterone seems to have the opposite effect or no effect. This hormonal difference in cholesterol excretion may help explain why males have higher rates of **atherosclerosis,** or cholesterol deposits in the blood vessels, than do females, whose estrogen levels are much higher.

Lipoproteins

Lipids are soluble in organic solvents like benzene, chloroform, and ether but insoluble in water. They therefore require transport mechanisms for circulation in the blood. The main lipid components of serum are in the form of **lipoproteins,** which are macromolecules of triglycerides, phospholipids, and cholesterol complexed with specialized proteins. A very small amount of free fatty acids also is present in the blood, complexed with albumin, a simple protein. Lipids are detected and measured in the blood in lipoprotein forms.

Lipoproteins are classified on the basis of density. Because lipids are lower in density and therefore have lower specific gravity than proteins, lipoproteins with many lipid molecules also tend to have low density. Conversely, lipoproteins with only a few lipid molecules have higher density. The three types of biologically significant lipids—triglycerides, phospholipids, and cholesterol—also vary in density, with triglycerides being the least dense. Lipoproteins with very high concentrations of triglycerides have specific gravities below plasma, so they rise to the top of a volume of plasma when centrifuged. See Table 20-1.

Table 20-1   The Composition of Lipoproteins

Lipoprotein	% Triglyceride	% Cholesterol	% Phospholipid	% Protein
Chylomicrons	85 to 95	3 to 5	5 to 10	1 to 2
Very low density (VLDL)	60 to 70	10 to 15	10 to 15	10
Low density (LDL)	5 to 10	45	20 to 30	15 to 25
High density (HDL)	Very little	20	30	50

Lipoproteins with the lowest density are called very-low-density lipoproteins, or VLDL. They consist mainly of fat with very little protein, and virtually all the fat is in the form of triglycerides. **Low-density lipoproteins,** or **LDL,** contain large amounts of fat, primarily in the form of cholesterol. The high cholesterol content is a potential cause of cardiovascular disease. **High-density lipoproteins,** or **HDL,** have the lowest fat content of all the lipoproteins, being composed equally of protein and fat. Research has shown having high levels of LDL is a risk for coronary artery disease (CAD), while a high level of HDL actually has a protective factor against CAD.

Clinical Applications

Many physicians think that an adequate lipid assessment should include the following measurements:

- total cholesterol
- HDL cholesterol
- serum triglyceride level
- LDL cholesterol

The level of LDL cholesterol, the cholesterol content of the LDL fraction, can be determined by measuring the cholesterol remaining after the HDL fraction has been removed by precipitation.

The level of HDL cholesterol is higher, on average, in adult women than in adult men. It also tends to be inversely proportional to total triglyceride level. See Table 20-2.

The clinical significance of lipid measurements still is debated among researchers. While population-based studies reveal clear statistical associations between lipid levels and cardiovascular disease, establishing similar associations in individual patients is not always possible. Nonetheless, populations with high average total cholesterol have high rates of atherosclerosis. High levels of cholesterol in the blood lead to the formation of **plaques,** thickened regions in artery walls that prevent blood from flowing freely. Plaques in arteries of the heart may lead to heart attack and plaques in arteries of the brain may lead to stroke.

Again at the population level, HDL cholesterol concentrations above the normal range are associated with half the average risk for atherosclerosis, while HDL cholesterol concentrations below the normal range are associated with twice or greater the average risk of atherosclerosis. That is why LDL cholesterol sometimes is called "bad cholesterol" and HDL is called "good cholesterol" and why patients with a low proportion of HDL cholesterol are encouraged to adopt healthful lifestyle habits that have been found to raise HDL cholesterol levels.

The American Heart Association has established the following guidelines for each of the cholesterol measurements. Total cholesterol level should be less than 200 mg/dL. Individuals who maintain this cholesterol level are considered to have a "desirable" cholesterol level, indicating that they have a low level of risk for suffering a heart attack, unless they have other risk factors. Individuals whose cholesterol levels are between 200 and 239 mg/dL are considered "borderline high risk," indicating that they need additional evaluation by their physician to determine their specific risk level. Individuals with cholesterol levels greater than 240 mg/dL are "high risk." They are twice as likely to suffer a heart attack or stroke.

LDL cholesterol levels have an even greater predictive value than total cholesterol level when determining an individual's risk for a heart attack or stroke. According to the American Heart Association, the key fact to remember is the lower an individual's LDL, the lower the risk for heart attack or stroke.

HDL is also important in preventing heart attack and/or stroke. Unlike the other cholesterol levels, it is important to have a *high* HDL level. In general, an HDL level less than 40 is considered to be a risk factor for experiencing a stroke or heart attack. See Table 20-3.

Table 20-2   Normal Ranges for HDL Cholesterol

Age/Sex Group	HDL Cholesterol Concentration (mg/dL)
Adult females	50–60
Adult males	40–50

Raising HDL Levels

People who follow these healthful lifestyle habits are likely to increase their level of HDL cholesterol:

- regular exercise
- a diet low in saturated fats and high in foods like vegetables and fish oils
- maintenance of normal weight
- no smoking
- no heavy drinking

Table 20-3   Target Lipid Levels

TOTAL CHOLESTEROL LEVELS	
Desirable	Less than 200 mg/dL
Borderline high risk	200–239 mg/dL
High risk	240 mg/dL and over
LDL CHOLESTEROL LEVELS	
Optimal	Less than 100 mg/dL
Near optimal/above optimal	100 to 129 mg/dL
Borderline high	130 to 159 mg/dL
High	160 to 189 mg/dL
Very high	190 mg/dL and above
HDL CHOLESTEROL LEVELS	
Risk	40 mg/dL
TRIGLYCERIDE LEVEL	
Normal	Less than 150 mg/dL
Borderline high	150–199 mg/dL
High	200–499 mg/dL
Very high	500 mg/dL or higher

Note: American Heart Association recommendations.

PROTEINS

Proteins are a large group of complex, nitrogen-containing organic compounds. The building blocks of proteins are **amino acids,** which are smaller molecules each containing an amine group ($-NH_2$) and an acidic carboxyl group (COOH). Proteins consist of amino acids joined together by peptide bonds between the carbon of one amino acid and the nitrogen of the next. There are 20 different amino acids in humans, and they can be linked together in countless different combinations. As a result, there are numerous different kinds of protein molecules, as compared with just a few kinds of carbohydrate and lipid molecules. We all are different from each other because of our proteins, not because of our carbohydrates or fats.

Protein synthesis and degradation occur continuously in the body. Each day, approximately 20 to 30 grams of protein are irreversibly degraded. As a consequence, this same amount of protein must be ingested to maintain a metabolic steady state, called nitrogen balance. If nitrogen balance is positive, more amino acids are entering the body than are being excreted. If nitrogen balance is negative, on the other hand, excretion of amino acids or their nitrogen-containing metabolites exceeds ingestion. If negative nitrogen balance persists for very long, there will be an eventual loss of essential protein-mediated functions.

Protein synthesis occurs in all body cells on structures called **ribosomes,** located on the surface of rough (granular) endoplasmic reticula (ER). The process is controlled by the genes that are found on the chromosomes within the cell nuclei. Individuals with faulty genes for a particular protein are unable to synthesize that protein correctly. For example, individuals with faulty genes for the blood protein hemoglobin are unable to synthesize normal hemoglobin. Depending on the exact nature of genetic defect, they may synthesize sickle-cell hemoglobin or some other abnormal form of the hemoglobin molecule.

The Role of Proteins in the Body

Because protein molecules are so diverse, they are able to fill a great many different structural and functional roles in the body. Proteins that detect light in the eyes, for example, are very different in composition from proteins that detoxify poisons in the liver.

Structurally, proteins are the main building materials of the body, comprising three-fourths of the solid matter of the body. Proteins are the major components of muscles, blood, skin, hair, nails, and visceral organs.

Functionally, proteins play many important roles. They are needed to

- form hormones, which act as chemical messengers to body organs
- form enzymes, which help biochemical reactions occur faster and control virtually all the life processes that go on in the cells

Diet Essentials

All amino acids enter the body through dietary sources, but 12 of the 20 amino acids also can be synthesized in our cells. The remaining eight amino acids are called essential amino acids because they cannot be synthesized by the human body and must be ingested in foods on a regular basis. Animal sources of protein contain all eight essential amino acids, but most plant sources are lacking in one or more.

- form antibodies, which help protect the body against disease
- transport molecules, which carry substances through the body, such as the hemoglobin protein that transports oxygen in the blood

Blood Proteins

The normal protein content of serum is 6 to 8 g/dL, of which approximately two-thirds is **albumin,** one-third **globulin,** and a few percent fibrinogen. Albumin is responsible for maintaining osmotic pressure at the capillary membrane. Globulin has a diversity of functions, including transporting other substances and acting as a substrate. Fibrinogen is essential for blood clot formation.

Liver cells, called hepatocytes, synthesize fibrinogen and albumin and between 60 and 80 percent of globulin. The remaining globulin consists of immunoglobulins, or antibodies, which are manufactured by the lymphoreticular system.

A general study of blood proteins usually measures total protein and the albumin and nonantibody globulin content of the serum. If either albumin or globulin is measured, the other can be calculated by subtraction from the total protein value. Results are given as the albumin to globulin ratio, A/G.

Most protein determinations actually measure nitrogen, which is found in all amino acids. Nitrogen content then is converted to protein concentration by multiplying by a conversion factor. This provides an accurate estimate of total protein unless hypoalbuminemia and hyperglobulinemia are present. Other lab tests can detect these conditions and provide the diagnostic information needed for patient assessment.

NONPROTEIN NITROGEN COMPOUNDS

Nonprotein compounds in the blood that contain nitrogen include ammonia, urea, uric acid, and creatinine.

Ammonia

Ammonia (NH_3) is a pungent, colorless, alkaline compound that results when proteins are degraded in intracellular protein turnover or in the colon by bacteria that aid in protein digestion. It is formed when amine groups ($-NH_2$) are removed from amino acids in a process called deamination. Ammonia travels to the liver, where it undergoes a series of reactions that convert it to urea.

Urea

Urea is a small molecule that can move freely into both extracellular and intracellular fluid. It is concentrated in the urine for excretion. In stable nitrogen balance, about 25 grams of urea are excreted daily. In the blood, urea levels reflect the balance between urinary excretion of urea and hepatic production of urea from ammonia.

In labs in the United States, urea in the blood is measured indirectly as nitrogen, and the results are expressed as **blood urea nitrogen,** or **BUN.** The normal serum BUN value is 8 to 25 mg/dL. Nitrogen contributes about half of the total weight of urea, and the concentration of urea can be estimated by multiplying the BUN value by 2.14. The BUN may rise slightly following prolonged massive protein intake, but recent dietary intake does not affect random values.

A high level of urea in the blood is called **uremia.** The most common cause is impaired excretion due to renal failure. Postrenal uremia occurs when urea diffuses back into the bloodstream due to urethral obstruction by stones, tumors, or inflammation. Prerenal uremia refers to a high level of urea in the blood that is due to increased protein breakdown. This may be caused by shock, blood loss, dehydration, crush injuries, fever, or burns. A low level of urea in the blood may be caused by liver damage, but damage must be severe to affect BUN values.

Uric Acid

Uric acid is the end product of the metabolism of purine, an important constituent of nucleic acids, which are the building blocks of DNA. Purine is found in the diet, especially in organ meats such as the heart and kidney, legumes, anchovies, and yeast. The turnover of purine occurs continually in the body, producing much of the uric acid, even without purines in the diet. Most uric acid is synthesized in the liver and then carried by the blood to the kidneys, where filtration, absorption, and secretion affect its excretion. Normal daily excretion of uric acid varies from about 0.5 gram on a low-purine diet to about 1.0 gram on a normal-purine diet.

Uric acid dissolves poorly in water, and uric acid salts, or urates, may precipitate as calculi, or stones, in urine that has a high urate concentration. This may occur even if the serum urate concentration is normal. Patients with high serum urate concentrations often have urate deposits in the soft tissues, particularly the joints, producing a painful condition called gout. Conditions that may increase serum uric acid levels include cytolytic treatment of malignancy, especially leukemia and lymphoma; polycythemia; and sickle-cell anemia. Serum levels also are higher when excretion of uric acid is decreased, as it is with alcohol ingestion and renal failure due to any cause.

Creatinine

Creatinine is the end product of the metabolism of **creatine,** a nonprotein nitrogen compound found in muscle tissue. Creatinine is picked up by the blood and transported to the kidneys for excretion. Blood concentration and total urinary excretion of

creatinine fluctuate very little. Blood creatinine rises with kidney failure, but less steeply than the rise in blood urea.

> **Creatine**
>
> Creatine is synthesized in the liver from amino acids. Daily production of creatine remains fairly constant unless a crushing injury or degenerative disease causes massive muscle damage. Creatine combines readily with phosphate to form phosphocreatine, which stores high-energy phosphates necessary for muscle contraction. The reaction is reversible, but small amounts of creatine are irreversibly converted to creatinine during the reaction.

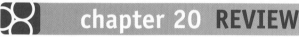

chapter 20 REVIEW

Using Terminology

Match the term on the left with the most appropriate description on the right.

_____ 1. profile
_____ 2. ISE
_____ 3. potentiometric
_____ 4. albumin
_____ 5. amino acid
_____ 6. lipid
_____ 7. disaccharide
_____ 8. creatinine
_____ 9. polysaccharide
_____ 10. triglyceride

a. 12-carbon sugar
b. building block of proteins
c. carbohydrate composed of many molecules of simple sugars
d. group of tests ordered together
e. end product of creatine metabolism
f. compound of fatty acids and glycerol
g. measures the difference in electrical current
h. most abundant plasma protein
i. fat
j. ion-selective electrode

Match the term in the right column with the appropriate definition or description in the left column.

_____ 11. end product of purine metabolism
_____ 12. formation of glycogen
_____ 13. a fraction of plasma lipoproteins
_____ 14. high level of urea in the blood
_____ 15. macromolecule of triglycerides, phospholipids, cholesterol, and specialized proteins
_____ 16. nitrogen concentration in the blood
_____ 17. stores fat
_____ 18. synthesizes protein
_____ 19. thickened regions in artery wall
_____ 20. triglycerides

a. adipose tissue
b. BUN
c. gluconeogenesis
d. HDL cholesterol
e. lipoproteins
f. plaques
g. ribosomes
h. fats
i. uremia
j. uric acid

State the ideal or normal level for the following lipids.

21. Total cholesterol

_____

_____

_____

22. LDL

_____

_____

_____

23. HDL

_____

_____

_____

24. Triglyceride

_____

_____

_____

Multiple Choice

Choose the best answer for the following questions.

25. A chemistry analyzer in which the samples and reagents are packaged in individual containers is referred to as
  a. discrete
  b. continuous
  c. potentiometric
  d. ion-selective electrode

26. An advantage of automated chemistry analysis is
  a. increased speed (turnaround time)
  b. greater consistency of results
  c. ability to perform multiple tests at once
  d. all of the above

27. When evaluating a chemistry analyzer for purchase, you should consider which of the following?
  a. cost of the instrument
  b. whether the testing is "waived" or "nonwaived"
  c. technical difficulty
  d. all of the above

28. A compound that stores energy is
  a. cholesterol
  b. globulin
  c. creatine
  d. glycogen

29. The second most abundant plasma protein is
   a. creatinine
   b. LDL
   c. globulin
   d. urea

30. A group of amino acids joined together by a peptide bond is classified as a
   a. protein
   b. lipid
   c. carbohydrate
   d. saturated fat

31. High levels of total cholesterol act as a _____ a stroke or heart attack.
   a. risk factor for
   b. protective factor against

32. High levels of LDL act as a _____ a stroke or heart attack.
   a. risk factor for
   b. protective factor against

33. High levels of HDL act as a _____ a stroke or heart attack.
   a. risk factor for
   b. protective factor against

Acquiring Knowledge

Answer the following questions in the spaces provided.

34. What hormones regulate glucose metabolism?

_____

_____

_____

35. How do each of the hormones listed in question 34 affect blood glucose levels?

_____

_____

_____

36. What is the major cause of hypoglycemia?

_____

_____

_____

37. What are some of the causes of hyperglycemia?

_____

_____

_____

38. What are the differences between postprandial hypoglycemia and fasting hypoglycemia?

_____

_____

_____

39. How are lipoproteins classified?

_____

_____

_____

40. What are some of the important roles played by proteins in the body?

_____

_____

_____

41. What nonprotein nitrogen compounds are found in the blood?

_____

_____

_____

42. Where does the body get most of its glucose?

_____

_____

_____

43. In what form is most stored energy found in the body?

_____

_____

_____

44. Why is LDL cholesterol called "bad cholesterol" and HDL cholesterol "good cholesterol"?

_____

_____

_____

45. What pathological condition results from high levels of circulating cholesterol over a long period of time?

_____

_____

_____

46. What is the difference between essential and nonessential amino acids?

_____

_____

_____

47. What are the two types of triglycerides? Which group is considered to be more healthful as a dietary component?

_____

_____

_____

48. What three food groups are the basis of most of the body's metabolism?

_____

_____

_____

Applying Knowledge—On the Job

Answer the following questions in the spaces provided.

49. A patient with normal weight came to the laboratory for a repeat cholesterol test. Her previous blood cholesterol level was elevated, and she had been following a special low-fat, low-cholesterol diet recommended by the physician. Why is the physician concerned about the patient's cholesterol level and fat intake?

_____

_____

_____

50. An overweight 50-year-old female has reported for a postprandial blood glucose test. Last week, she had a positive glucose tolerance test. She has been taking oral hypoglycemic medication and following a diet and exercise program prescribed by the doctor. What disease does she most likely have?

_____

_____

_____

51. A male patient with an attack of excruciating joint pain has come to the lab for a blood test. The physician suspects that the patient has gout. What blood test might be performed to help confirm the diagnosis? If the patient has gout, what will the test result likely be?

_____

_____

_____

52. A 6-year-old girl is very low in weight for her age, even though she eats well because she is "always hungry." She also complains of fatigue and excessive thirst. What is the most likely cause of the girl's symptoms? What further testing might be done to confirm the diagnosis?

_____

_____

_____

IMMUNOLOGY AND MICROBIOLOGY

unit

VI

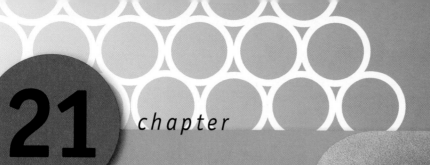

21 chapter

Immunology Tests

21.12 prepare and perform an infectious mononucleosis test using a commercial immunochromatographic test kit.

21.13 prepare and perform individual blood types of the ABO and Rhesus blood groups.

🔳 TERMINOLOGY

ABO blood group: one of two clinically important inherited blood groups; the ABO blood group has two antigens, A and B, and includes four blood types: A, B, AB, and O.

antibody: a protein molecule produced by the lymph system in response to a particular antigen.

antigen: short for antibody generating; a foreign substance that provokes a specific antibody reaction.

autoimmunity: the condition in which the immune system responds inappropriately to the wrong antigens—to self instead of nonself.

B-lymphocyte: B-cell; a lymphocyte that secretes short-lived antibodies involved in humoral immunity.

cell-mediated immunity: the type of specific immunity that is controlled by T-lymphocytes.

chlamydia: a bacterial disease, thought to be the most prevalent sexually transmitted disease in the United States.

complement: a group of proteins in the blood that are important in the immune response; they act by directly lysing organisms and stimulating phagocytosis.

Coombs' test: the antiglobulin test used for monitoring the development of Rh incompatibility in Rh-negative pregnant women.

C-reactive protein (CRP): an abnormal glycoprotein that appears in the acute stage of various inflammatory disorders.

endocytic and phagocytic response: the type of nonspecific immunity in which microorganisms and other foreign matter are engulfed and degraded by body cells.

flocculation: a precipitate in the form of downy tufts.

herpes: the common name for diseases caused by herpesvirus, a family of viruses, including those that cause cold sores and genital ulcers, *Herpes simplex I* and *II*.

human chorionic gonadotropin (hCG): the hormone produced by the villi of the placenta. Detecting it is the basis for early pregnancy tests.

humoral immunity: the type of specific immunity that involves the formation and activity of short-lived antibodies in body fluids.

hypersensitivity: allergy; exaggerated immune response to foreign antigens.

immunity: the body's resistance to foreign invaders, including microorganisms, cancer cells, toxins, and incompatible blood types from other individuals.

immunodeficiency: compromised immune response; the condition in which the immune system is compromised due to a congenital or acquired disorder; characterized by increased susceptibility to disease and poor recovery.

immunology: the branch of medical science that studies the physical and chemical aspects of immunity, or resistance to disease.

immunology test: a lab test that depends on immune reactions for results. Immunology tests include tests for pregnancy, many diseases, and blood types.

inflammatory response: a complex series of events triggered by a wound or invasion by microorganisms, leading to redness, swelling, heat, and pain. Inflammatory response reduces the spread of infection and promotes healing.

Lyme disease: a bacterial disease transmitted by deer ticks.

nonspecific immunity: innate immunity; the general resistance to disease that characterizes a particular species. In humans, nonspecific immunity includes physical and anatomical barriers, physiological barriers, endocytic and phagocytic responses, and the inflammatory response.

physical and anatomical barriers: a type of nonspecific immunity; the body's first line of defense against foreign invaders. Physical and anatomical barriers include the skin, mucous membranes, body secretions, and benevolent bacteria.

physiological barrier: a type of nonspecific immunity; a chemical factor that kills pathogens gaining access to the body.

Rhesus (Rh) blood group: one of two clinically important inherited blood groups. Rh-positive blood has the D antigen; Rh-negative blood does not.

rheumatoid arthritis (RA): a chronic systemic autoimmune disease characterized by inflammation in the joints and crippling.

rubella: German measles; a mild systemic disease caused by the Rubella virus.

sensitivity: the ability of a lab test for a particular disease to identify correctly those who have the disease.

specific immunity: acquired immunity; immunity to a specific foreign antigen that is acquired after exposure to it.

specificity: the ability of a lab test for a particular disease to identify correctly those who do not have the disease.

syphilis: a devastating, sexually transmitted disease caused by the spirochete *Treponema pallidum.*

systemic lupus erythematosus (SLE): a systemic autoimmune disease that affects connective tissues and injures the skin, joints, kidneys, nervous system, and mucous membranes.

titer: the highest dilution, or lowest concentration, capable of producing an observable reaction.

T-lymphocytes: T-cells; the basis of cell-mediated immunity.

toxin: poison.

INTRODUCTION

This chapter describes how the immune system protects individuals from disease and how immune reactions are used in POLs to diagnose disease and to type blood.

IMMUNOLOGY AND IMMUNITY

Immunology is the branch of medical science that studies the physical and chemical aspects of **immunity**—the body's resistance to foreign invaders. Foreign invaders include, most commonly, disease-causing microorganisms like bacteria and viruses. They also include cancer cells and **toxins.** While transfused blood and transplanted tissue cells from other individuals serve beneficial purposes, because of the foreign antigens present, they are viewed as "foreign invaders" by the immune system.

Interest in immunity dates back to the earliest written accounts. A large volume of sacred scriptures outlined health laws and practices to avoid contamination such as segregating individuals with certain diseases. Over the past 300 years, the research

of scientists like Leeuwenhoek, Jenner, Pasteur, and Koch has provided knowledge that led to modern laws of sanitation and aseptic medical practices.

The typing of blood began in the first part of the twentieth century and laid the foundation for safe and effective blood transfusions. Today's understanding of the immune system has been increased greatly by research on organ transplants and HIV, the virus that causes AIDS, a disease of the immune system.

HOW THE IMMUNE SYSTEM WORKS

The human immune system is a complex system of cells and molecules that act in concert to distinguish foreign invaders from the body's own cells and to eliminate foreign invaders from the body. Immune system responses fall into two broad categories: nonspecific immunity and specific immunity.

Nonspecific Immunity

Nonspecific immunity, or innate immunity, is the general resistance to disease that characterizes a particular species. In humans, it consists of four types of defense against foreign invaders: physical and anatomical barriers, physiological barriers, endocytic and phagocytic responses, and the inflammatory response.

Physical and Anatomical Barriers. Physical and anatomical barriers are the body's first line of defense against attack from foreign invaders, preventing most microorganisms from entering the body. They include

- the skin
- mucous membranes
- body secretions like tears, saliva, and mucus
- benevolent bacteria

More specifically, the skin is somewhat acidic, thus preventing the growth of most microorganisms on its surface. Ciliated epithelial cells of the mucous membranes sweep microorganisms away from the respiratory and gastrointestinal tracts. Tears, saliva, and mucus all contain proteins that kill the microorganisms swept away. The gut and vagina have protective colonies of benevolent

---

The Case of Smallpox

Smallpox is a good example of how knowledge of immunity has advanced through time. The practice of immunizing against smallpox and thereby provoking the body into an immune response to the disease was begun many centuries ago. By the end of the 1700s, Edward Jenner began using the milder and safer cowpox vaccine to immunize against smallpox.

It was not until the twentieth century, with advances in microbiology and biochemistry, that the physiological mechanisms underlying vaccination were understood. By 1969, thanks to efforts in public health, the World Health Organization declared the world to be free of the smallpox virus, the first pathogen to have been eradicated by human efforts. Cultures of the smallpox virus now are kept in only a limited number of research laboratories. It is currently debated whether these last remaining smallpox organisms should be destroyed or kept for potential future research.

bacteria that prevent pathogenic strains from gaining a foothold in these areas.

Physiological Barriers. If microorganisms do gain entry to the body, they are met with a variety of **physiological barriers**—chemical factors that kill pathogens. For example, the very acidic environment of the stomach kills most microorganisms that reach it. Soluble chemical factors, which consist of a variety of proteins in the body, attack viruses and bacteria. Interferon, which is a protein formed when cells are exposed to viruses or tumor cells, helps protect noninfected cells against viral infection. **Complement,** a series of enzymatic proteins in serum, causes lysis of microorganisms and enhances the inflammatory response.

Endocytic and Phagocytic Responses. Microorganisms that evade the first two sets of barriers and penetrate blood or tissue are subject to **endocytic and phagocytic responses,** in which they are engulfed and degraded by body cells. Most body cells are able to ingest and degrade foreign molecules. Phagocytes can engulf and consume whole bacteria. Phagocytes include

- *macrophages:* large cells of the reticuloendothelial system that are found in loose connective tissues and various organs of the body
- *monocytes and neutrophils:* two types of white blood cells

The Inflammatory Response. The **inflammatory response** is a complex series of events triggered by a wound or invasion by microorganisms. It leads to redness, swelling, heat, and pain. This response isolates foreign matter and keeps it from spreading to other parts of the body. It also promotes healing.

Specific Immunity

Specific immunity, or acquired immunity, refers to immunity from a specific foreign invader that is acquired after exposure to it. Specific immunity primarily involves lymphocytes.

The Basis of Specific Immunity. Specific immunity depends on the ability of the immune system not only to distinguish self from nonself but to "remember" encounters with foreign invaders. Because of this "memory," having once encountered a foreign molecule or microorganism, the immune system is capable of inducing a heightened state of immune reactivity when it encounters the foreign invader again.

The Antigen-Antibody Reaction. Foreign substances that provoke a specific immune reaction are called **antigens.** Most often, antigens are large protein molecules found on the surfaces of microorganisms,

but they also include toxins and molecules on foreign blood cells and other tissues. The word *antigen* is short for "antibody generating." **Antibodies,** in turn, are protein molecules produced by the lymph system in response to a particular antigen.

> **Note**
>
> Antibodies are the globulin portion of serum proteins. Antibodies also are called immunoglobulins. They are classified into the subgroups IgA, IgD, IgE, IgG, and IgM on the basis of molecular size and other characteristics.

Antibodies usually are specific for a particular antigen; that is, a given antigen stimulates the production of antibodies that react against just that antigen. Each type of antigen-antibody bonding is unique, like a lock and key, as Figure 21-1 shows.

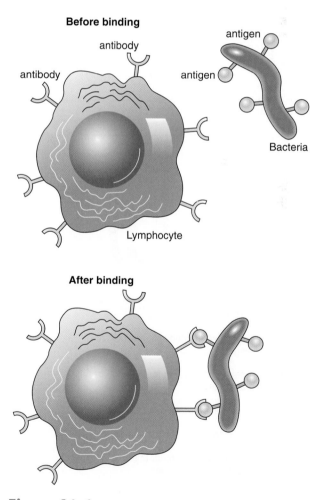

Figure 21-1 The antigen-antibody complex. This schematic representation shows the immune antibodies of the lymphocyte reaching out to the antigens on the bacterium.

Even closely related microorganisms elicit somewhat different antibodies in a human host.

Once bonded, the antigen-antibody complex can be neutralized by precipitation or agglutination. Alternatively, antibodies may "tag" antigens for destruction by phagocytes or lysis by complement.

Types of Specific Immunity. Specific immune responses are divided into two types: humoral immunity and cell-mediated immunity. **Humoral immunity** is the formation and activity of short-lived antibodies in the body's "humors," that is, in body fluids. Humoral antibodies are found in blood, lymphatic fluid, lymph nodes, the spleen, spinal fluid, and saliva. The lymphocytes involved in humoral immunity are **B-lymphocytes,** or B-cells. They originate in the bone marrow and then migrate to various lymphoid tissue where they proliferate and differentiate into antibody-secreting cells.

Cell-mediated immunity is controlled by **T-lymphocytes,** or T-cells, which also arise in the bone marrow. While still immature, T-cells migrate to the thymus, where they mature and become immunocompetent, that is, capable of responding to foreign invaders. Immunocompetence is indicated by the appearance of antigen-specific receptors on the surfaces of mature T-cells. Immunocompetent T-cells leave the thymus and migrate to the lymph nodes and spleen, where antigens bind to their surface receptors. This binding event sensitizes the T-cells to grow and multiply rapidly. They soon form an army of identical cells, called clones.

Some members of the T-cell clone become killer T-cells. These kill virus-infected, cancer, or foreign tissue cells by binding to them and releasing toxic chemicals (see Figure 21-2). Other members of the clone become helper T-cells, also called effector

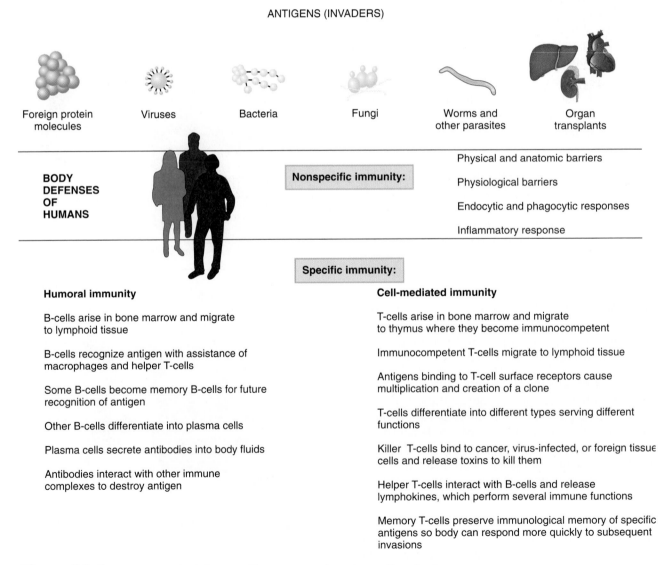

Figure 21-2 How the body defenses of humans attack antigens (invaders).

T-cells. These interact with B-cells and release chemicals, called lymphokines, that perform a number of immune functions, including

- stimulating killer T-cells and B-cells to grow and divide
- attracting other types of white blood cells, such a neutrophils, into the area
- enhancing the ability of macrophages to ingest and destroy microorganisms

Finally, a few members of each T-cell clone become memory cells. These are long-lived cells that provide immunological memory of the antigen so that the body can respond more quickly to its subsequent invasions. There are also memory B lymphocytes. This is how the immune system "remembers" encounters with foreign invaders.

DISEASES OF THE IMMUNE SYSTEM

Because the immune system is crucial to good health, when it becomes dysfunctional, serious illness usually results. Dysfunctions of the immune system include immunodeficiency, autoimmunity, and hypersensitivity.

Immunodeficiency

Immunodeficiency, or compromised immune response, is characterized by

- persistent or recurrent infections by organisms that do not ordinarily cause disease
- incomplete recovery from infections
- undue susceptibility to certain forms of cancer

Some immunodeficiency diseases result from congenital defects that interfere with normal development of the immune system. Others result from acquired conditions that damage the function of the immune system. An example of congenital immunodeficiency is hypogammaglobulinemia, an inherited deficiency of one or more types of immunoglobulin. Examples of acquired immunodeficiency include the weakening of body defenses by severe malnutrition, many types of cancer, and HIV. Immunodeficiency also can result from the administration of immunosuppressant drugs, which are prescribed to prevent rejection of transplanted organs.

Autoimmunity

Autoimmunity refers to an inappropriate immune response to the wrong antigens—to self instead of nonself. The cause of autoimmune diseases is poorly understood, but several theories have been proposed, including

- Mutations, viruses, drugs, or injuries alter body tissues so that they are no longer recognized as self.
- Normally inaccessible tissue antigens leak into areas where they come into contact with the immune system and stimulate the production of antibodies.

The inappropriate immune response in an autoimmune disease may be either localized or systemic. Systemic lupus erythematosus (SLE) is a systemic autoimmune disease. Hashimoto's thyroiditis, on the other hand, is localized. It affects just the thyroid gland. These and other human autoimmune diseases and the organs or systems that they affect are listed in Table 21-1.

Hypersensitivity

Hypersensitivity is an exaggerated immune response to foreign antigens. Hypersensitive reactions also are called allergic reactions. They may be systemic or localized.

There are two types of hypersensitivity: immediate hypersensitivity and delayed hypersensitivity. Immediate hypersensitivity, which involves B-cells, occurs within minutes after a sensitive individual is exposed to an antigen. Reactions range from mild to life threatening. Exposure to an antigen may cause temporary, localized hives, for example, or it may cause anaphylaxis, a potentially

Table 21-1   Human Autoimmune Diseases

Disease	Organ or System Affected
Addison's disease	Adrenal cells
Autoimmune hemolytic anemia	Red blood cell membrane
Grave's disease	Thyroid gland
Hashimoto's thyroiditis	Thyroid gland
Type 1 diabetes	Pancreatic beta cells
Multiple sclerosis (MS)	Central nervous system
Pernicious anemia	Gastric parietal cells
Rheumatoid arthritis	Connective tissue
Spontaneous infertility	Sperm
Systemic lupus erythematosus	Connective tissue, any organ of the body

fatal, systemic hypersensitivity with symptoms of edema and choking. Delayed hypersensitivity, which involves T-cells, develops over a period of 12 to 24 hours. It is usually induced by infections of fungi, viruses, bacteria, and other microorganisms.

LABORATORY TESTS UTILIZING IMMUNE REACTIONS

Lab tests that depend on immune reactions for results are called **immunology tests.** Pregnancy, autoimmune diseases, diseases caused by microorganisms, and blood types are among the conditions that can be detected by immunology tests. CLIA waived test kits are used in POLs to test for some of these conditions. Others usually are referred to reference laboratories.

Historical Note

The first tests involving immune reactions were called serological tests because serum was the body fluid tested when these tests were pioneered at the beginning of the twentieth century. Now, other body fluids, cells, tissues, and urine are tested for immune reactions, but the term *serology* is still used interchangeably with immunology.

Sensitivity and Specificity

The advances in monoclonal antibody–based technology have increased the accuracy of immunology tests. Manufacturers of immunology tests often include information in their product inserts about the accuracy of their test products, frequently using the terms *sensitivity* and *specificity*. To judge the accuracy of these tests used in many POLs, it is important to be familiar with the meaning of these two terms.

The **sensitivity** of a lab test for a particular disease refers to the ability of the test to identify correctly those who have the disease. If a test has a high degree of sensitivity, virtually all patients who have the disease will test positive. There will be few, if any, false negatives—people who have the disease but test negative—although the test may produce false positives—people who do not have the disease but test positive.

The **specificity** of a lab test for a particular disease refers to the ability of the test to identify correctly those who do not have the disease. If a test has a high degree of specificity, virtually all those who do not have the disease will test negative. There will be few, if any, false positives, although the test may produce false negatives.

The most accurate lab tests are both highly sensitive and highly specific, producing very few false positive or false negative results. Such tests identify virtually everyone who has the disease and seldom if ever misidentify those who do not. Although most tests in POLs are not both highly sensitive and highly specific, they still give useful results when combined with other clinical findings. For example, a quick, inexpensive test with a high degree of sensitivity, but not specificity, may be used to screen individuals who are at risk of a disease. Being highly sensitive, the test is unlikely to produce false negatives, that is, to miss anyone who actually has the disease. False positives can be eliminated with a follow-up test that is more specific—and often more expensive and difficult.

Immunology Tests

Basically, all immunology tests consist of an antigen-antibody reaction and some form of measurable, often visible, indicator of the reaction. Based on the type of reaction and how it is detected, immunology tests can be placed in the following categories, which are described in detail below:

- *radioimmunoassay:* an antigen binds to a radioactive isotope and the level of radioactivity is measured
- *enzyme-linked immunosorbent assay (ELISA):* an antigen or antibody binds to an enzyme, producing a colored reaction; also known as enzyme immunoassay (EIA)
- *precipitin reaction:* antigen-antibody complexes precipitate out of solution, producing a visible residue
- *agglutinin reaction:* antigen-antibody complexes agglutinate, or clump together, in solution
- *lysing reaction:* antigen-antibody reaction causes lysis of cells

Radioimmunoassay. A radioimmunoassay tags an antigen with a radioactive isotope and then tests its presence or quantity in antigen-antibody reactions. This type of test is extremely sensitive, but it is available for use only in large laboratories.

Enzyme-Linked Immunosorbent Assay. In an enzyme-linked immunosorbent assay (ELISA), an antigen or antibody binds to an enzyme. The enzyme then generates a colored reaction product. The colored reaction may occur in a tube, coated on a dipstick or latex beads, or printed on a membrane. Unlike radioimmunoassays, ELISA tests are simple to use and are available in several different test kits for use in POLs. Most CLIA waived immunology testing devices use the enzyme immunoassay method known as immunochromatography in which antigen or antibodies are detected when the specimen migrates across a membrane leaving a colored reaction. Pregnancy and HIV are examples of these types of test procedures.

Precipitin Reactions. Precipitin reactions depend on the formation of a precipitate when the antigen and antibody are in solution together. If a soluble antigen and antibody are placed in solution in optimal amounts, minute flakes or granules precipitate, which are visible to the naked eye. Precipitation may occur in the form of a ring at the bottom of the tube. The size of the ring indicates the quantity of antigen or antibody present, but it is not very precise. Some types of precipitin reactions produce **flocculation,** a precipitate in the form of downy tufts.

Agglutinin Reactions. Agglutinin reactions depend on the formation of clumps of antigen-antibody complexes in solution. Agglutinin reactions are common in tests of bacteria, yeast, and molds. They also occur in blood typing. Agglutinin reactions often are preferred to precipitin reactions because agglutination is easier to see than is precipitation. Agglutinin reactions also are far more sensitive. Precipitin reactions can be converted to agglutinin reactions by adsorbing antigens onto latex beads, red blood cells, or other particles.

Passive agglutinin reactions include an additional step. Two consecutive antigen-antibody reactions are used, the second to test if the first has occurred. Some drug tests use passive agglutinin reactions.

Lysin Reactions. In lysin reactions, cells are lysed by an antigen-antibody reaction coupled with complement (serum enzymes). Red blood cells are lysed in transfusions of incompatible blood and in hemolytic disease of the newborn. Lysis also occurs when a bacterial membrane is destroyed by an attacking antibody.

> **Note**
>
> Different types of tests may be used for the same antigen-antibody reaction. For example, an antigen-antibody reaction that normally causes precipitation may be caused to agglutinate instead by adsorbing antigen into a medium such as latex beads or red blood cells. The same reaction may have an enzyme complex attached to it that changes color when the reaction occurs. The choice of test for a particular antigen-antibody reaction depends on factors like accuracy, simplicity, cost, and time.

Quantitative Measurement of Immune Reactions

Most POL immunology tests are qualitative—the results are only positive or negative, indicating presence or absence of an antigen or antibody. To understand the course or severity of disease, sometimes it is important to know the quantity of an antigen or antibody. For example, a positive rheumatoid arthritis agglutination should be retested and reported quantitatively.

> **Note**
>
> CLIA waived immunology tests are qualitative—the results are only positive or negative. For those test results in which the severity of the disease or condition must be monitored, quantitative results are needed. These quantitative tests are CLIA nonwaived and are usually performed in hospital or reference labs.

Quantitative reports of antigen-antibody reactions are expressed as **titers.** The titer is the highest dilution, or lowest concentration, still capable of producing an observable reaction. For an agglutinin reaction, for example, the titer is the highest dilution capable of producing agglutination.

In determining the titer, dilutions generally are graduated, with each dilution twice as great as the one before. Tubes for the desired number of dilutions are set up and labeled with their dilutions, and the same amount of diluent is added to each. Then, an equal amount of specimen is added to the first tube, producing a 1:2 dilution. After the first tube is mixed, a new pipette is used to move half the solution from the first tube to the second tube, then half the solution from the second tube is moved to the third tube, and so on, until the last tube is reached. Diluting in this manner ensures that each tube is twice as dilute, or half as concentrated, as the tube preceding it. The tubes then have the dilutions 1:2, 1:4, 1:8, 1:16, and so on. An alternative method sometimes used produces dilutions of 1:10, 1:20, 1:40, and so on.

> **Note**
>
> Manufacturer's inserts in test kits have the instructions needed for making dilutions for determining titers when using their products.

After the dilutions of a positive testing specimen are prepared, each dilution is tested and read for a positive reaction, such as agglutination or color change, depending on the test. The highest dilution that still gives a positive reaction is the titer that is reported.

Quality Control

As with all tests performed in POLs, controls must be run on immunology tests to check reagents and test procedures. Quality control results of immunology controls should be written in the quality control records for documentation purposes.

The Use of Controls. Controls may be supplied with the test kits. Some test procedures have internal controls, built-in controls, but also recommend external controls to be run with each newly opened kit, new lot number, and new laboratory employee, and whenever problems are identified. Each laboratory should establish criteria for performing controls and document in the control logs. Positive controls indicate if the test is working. Negative controls show if reactions are caused by some substance other than test sera. Both positive and negative controls also are used as standards for reading and interpretation of patient test results.

Caution!

Treat controls with the same caution as you do patient specimens. Some are derived from human blood, so it is possible that they are biologically hazardous, even though they have been tested for HBV and HIV.

Batch Size. Batches of tests must not be so large that there is too great a time lag between the reading of the first and last specimens. If there is a difference in the readings of controls run at the beginning and end of the batch, the batch size should be reduced.

The Manufacturer's Instructions. Clinical laboratory tests are researched thoroughly by large research laboratories, and manufacturer's instructions must be followed precisely to ensure accurate patient test results. Variables such as temperature, humidity, and lighting must be as close as possible to those recommended by the manufacturer.

Most antigen-antibody tests must be performed at room temperature, so reagents and patient specimens must be allowed to come to room temperature before testing. If the climate is extremely dry, the humidity level may have to be increased.

Lighting is important for reading test results accurately. A black background is best for reading the agglutination of white latex beads, for example, while a white background is best for reading agglutination of dark colors. Reflected light usually is specified, but lighted translucent panels are used in reading blood-type agglutinations.

Other Considerations. Cross-contamination between patient specimens and controls must be avoided by using separate stirrers and pipettes for each specimen and control. Wooden applicator sticks may be used as disposable stirrers. Care must be taken to replace the correct caps on reagent bottles because switching caps also can produce cross-contamination.

Reagents should be mixed well but not overmixed or shaken too vigorously, especially if the reagent is fragile. Latex beads and blood cells have protein coatings that may be damaged if mixing is too vigorous.

Patient specimens should not be lipemic or hemolyzed. If test results are questionable for particular specimens, they should be retested using the same method or a different method, or they should be sent to a referral laboratory for testing. If questions still remain, the manufacturer of the test kit or reagent should be contacted for assistance.

Conditions Tested with Antigen–Antibody Test Kits

Producing the reagents needed for tests of antigen-antibody reactions is beyond the scope of POLs, so test kits from medical supply houses are used. Table 21-2 lists some of the immunology tests for which kits are available.

Storing Test Kits

Many immunology test kits should be stored in the refrigerator between uses, but some may be stored at room temperature. Refrigerated kits generally have a longer period of use before the expiration date. Always check the expiration date and discard out-of-date test kits.

Pregnancy. Pregnancy can be ascertained as early as 10 days after conception by testing for **human chorionic gonadotropin (hCG)**, a hormone produced by the chorionic villi of the placenta. Most commercial test kits for this hormone use the immunochromatographic (see Figures 21-3 and 21-4) method on either serum or urine specimens. Several pregnancy tests may be run at once, but

Table 21-2 Antigen-Antibody Test Kits Available for Use in POLs

Test	Disease or Condition
hCG	Pregnancy (hormone)
RPR (rapid plasma reagin)	Syphilis (bacteria)
Epstein-Barr (Heterophile antibodies)	Infectious mononucleosis (virus)
GAS (Group A strep)	Strep throat (bacteria)
GBS (Group B strep)	Neonate infection (bacteria)
Rheumatoid arthritis factor	Rheumatoid arthritis (autoimmunity)
Respiratory syncytial virus	Respiratory infection (virus)
Herpes simplex I and *II*	Cold sores and genital ulcers (virus)
Chlamydia	Sexually transmitted disease (bacteria)
Lyme disease	Disease transmitted by ticks (bacteria)
Allergens (miscellaneous)	Hypersensitivity (immunity)
Autoimmune antibodies	Systemic lupus erythematosus (autoimmunity)
Candida	Yeast infections (fungus)
C-reactive protein (CRP)	Acute inflammatory condition
Rubella	Rubella (German measles) (virus)
Febrile agglutinations	Typhoid, paratyphoid, brucellosis, *Proteus* infections, tularemia (bacteria)
Trichomonas	Sexually transmitted disease (protozoan)
Legionella	Legionaires (bacteria)
HIV	Human immunodeficiency virus
H. pylori	*Helicobacter pylori* (bacteria)
Bladder Tumor Antigen	Bladder cancer

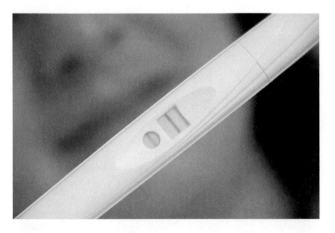

Figure 21-3 Test results from ready-purchased kits are easy to read. This particular pregnancy test shows up as a color development of a plus (positive or +) or minus (negative or −) sign. This test is negative.

separate pipettes must be used. Otherwise, hCG may be transferred from one test pad to another.

If urine is used, a first morning specimen is preferred because it contains higher levels of hCG, but any random specimen may be used. Urine should be collected in a clean, dry glass or plastic container. If serum is used, the specimen must not be hemolyzed. For both serum and urine, the specimen should be tested immediately, refrigerated for up to 48 hours, or frozen for later testing.

Chlamydia. The bacterial disease **chlamydia** is thought to be the most prevalent sexually transmitted disease in the United States. It also may be transmitted to infants from infected mothers through direct contact during or after birth. Chlamydia causes both urogenital disease and eye disease. Worldwide, it is the single leading cause of

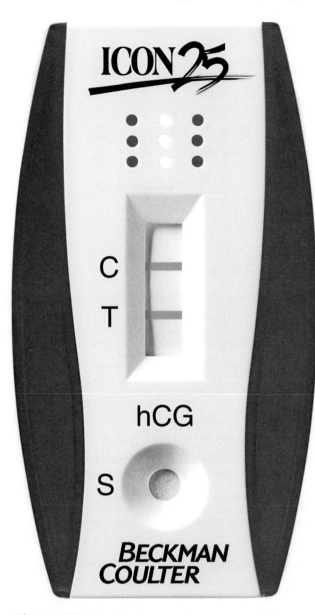

Figure 21-4 This CLIA waived testing device is an example of a positive urine hCG test showing both the control and test color development. (ICON™, Beckman Coulter, Fullerton, CA)

blindness. Because chlamydia is a bacterial disease, infections can be cured with broad-spectrum antibiotics and sulfonamides. However, chlamydia is hard to diagnose. The bacteria are very small and live only within the host's cells. An ELISA test is available for chlamydia testing in POLs.

Strep Throat. Strep throat is caused by Group A strep (GAS), a hemolytic strain of *Streptococcus* bacteria that causes strep throat and, less commonly, rheumatic fever, an autoimmune disease. The latter may lead to endocarditis, or inflammation of the inner lining of the heart, and permanent damage to the heart valves. Other organs, including the kidneys and nerves, also may be affected. Without prompt treatment of the original strep infection with antibiotics, autoimmune disease may result.

The Group A strep (GAS) test is a lateral-flow immunoassay test that is easy to perform, but the steps must be followed precisely. Care should be taken not to mix up the reagents or use them out of order. First, the throat is swabbed with a sterile, nonabsorbent rayon-fiber swab, supplied with the test kit. The swab is inserted into a testing device and treated with reagents to extract the Strep A antigen. If the Strep A antigen is present, it will bind with the specific antibody in the testing medium and create a color change that is easy to interpret. (See Figure 21-5.)

> **Note**
>
> Group B strep (GBS) is the nonhemolytic strain of *Streptococcus* that causes severe infections in newborns and infants. There is a separate test for this pathogen.

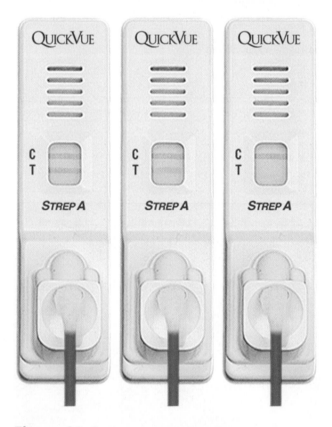

Figure 21-5 Testing devices that are used for rapid detection of Group A *Streptococcus* infections. Throat swab specimens are obtained and antigen is extracted; results can be reported in less than 10 minutes. (Quick-Vue In-Line Strep A Quidel, San Diego, CA)

Infectious Mononucleosis. Also called "mono" and abbreviated IM, this serious disease most often affects teenagers and young adults. Because it is thought to be transmitted orally, infectious mononucleosis is sometimes also called the "kissing disease." It is caused by the Epstein-Barr virus, and it has flulike symptoms, including fever, fatigue, weakness, swollen lymph nodes, sore throat, and headache. Symptoms may be prolonged and lead to involvement of the liver, spleen, or other organs.

Test procedures for the detection of the Epstein-Barr virus include agglutination, EIA, and lysin reaction. The CLIA waived screening test is EIA and uses immunochromatographic lateral flow as in the pregnancy test procedures (see Figure 21-6). The more complex test is likely to be performed in a larger reference or hospital laboratory. It uses lysis of red blood cells through several dilutions of serum to give the titer of the heterophile antibody, which reacts with the Epstein-Barr virus.

> **Note**
>
> The infectious mononucleosis antibody may be present even in the absence of symptoms. This may occur for several months after the acute, febrile phase of the illness has passed or if the case is subclinical.

Syphilis. The devastating STD **syphilis** is caused by the spirochete, or spiral bacterium, *Treponema pallidum.* Without antibiotic treatment, syphilis persists for many years, leading to involvement of many organs and systems and, ultimately, death.

The immune system produces complex antibodies to the bacteria, and these provide the basis for the diagnostic tests. A screening test used in POLs is the RPR, rapid plasma reagin. This is a flocculation test.

False positives are frequent with syphilis screening tests, so positive results generally are verified with more accurate tests performed in larger labo-

ratories. False positives may be caused by malaria, advanced pulmonary tuberculosis, pregnancy, or old age. False negatives also occur. They may be caused by a nonfunctioning immune system, alcohol consumption, or syphilis infection that is too recent to have triggered antibody production.

Rheumatoid Arthritis. The chronic systemic disease **rheumatoid arthritis (RA)** is characterized by inflammatory changes in joints and related structures that result in crippling deformities. The specific cause of rheumatoid arthritis is unknown, but generally it is thought that the pathological changes in the joints are related to an autoimmune antigen-antibody reaction.

> **Note**
>
> Rheumatoid arthritis shows great variation in the symptoms and the course of the disease. In some patients, there is lung involvement.

The diagnostic test for rheumatoid arthritis detects the presence of rheumatoid factor, an immunoglobulin (IgM) found in the sera of many rheumatoid arthritis patients. The test uses agglutination on a latex-fixation slide to detect the presence of the immunoglobulin. False positives may be caused by acute viral infections and old age. When the rheumatoid arthritis test is positive, the serum is diluted and retested, and the result is reported as a titer.

Systemic Lupus Erythematosus. Systemic lupus erythematosus (SLE) is an inflammatory disorder primarily affecting women ages 20 to 40 years. Depending on the severity of the disease, almost any organ of the body may be affected. SLE is considered to be an autoimmune disease that arises spontaneously, but viral infections and certain drugs also may be causal factors.

Laboratory tests for patients with SLE show a decrease in WBC and RBC counts and in the platelet count, along with an increased sedimentation rate. Diagnosis is confirmed by positive test results for the presence of antinuclear antibodies (ANA).

> **Tests for Autoimmune Disorders**
>
> Panels of screening tests for autoimmune antibodies may be used for rheumatoid arthritis, systemic lupus erythematosus, and other autoimmune disorders. The screening panels have several chemical reagent pads on one plastic test strip.

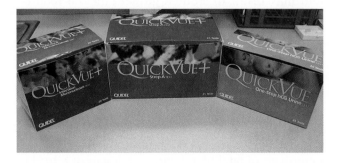

Figure 21-6 The QuickVue+ Infectious Mononucleosis test aids in the diagnosis of infectious mononucleosis and uses chromatographic immunoassay to detect IgM heterophile antibodies.

Lyme Disease. Lyme disease is caused by the spirochete *Borrelia burgdorferi,* which is transmitted from host to host by small deer ticks. Symptoms, which are not definitive of Lyme disease, include fever, severe headache, fatigue, and muscle aches. Without antibiotic treatment, the disease may progress to arthritis and involvement of the heart and nervous system. Diagnosis is made with an ELISA test.

Herpes. Herpes is the common name for diseases caused by herpesvirus, a family of viruses including those that cause cold sores (*Herpes simplex I*), genital ulcers (*Herpes simplex II*), shingles (*Herpes zoster*), and chicken pox (*Varicella*). After the primary infection, herpesvirus may remain dormant for years and then establish a latent infection. The virus lives within the nerve cells, where it is protected from the immune system. It may become activated by any of a variety of factors, including stress, trauma, allergic reactions, and illness. Once activated, the virus multiplies and emerges as a sore on the skin. Cold sores commonly occur around the mouth. Genital ulcers occur on the penis in the male and on the perineum, vagina, and cervix in the female. Genital herpes is a sexually transmitted disease. An ELISA test is available for diagnosing active herpes. The procedure is similar to that for the GAS test described earlier.

Rubella. Rubella, or German measles, is a mild systemic disease caused by the *Rubella* virus. Symptoms include slight fever, drowsiness, swollen lymph nodes, sore throat, and a characteristic rash. The disease is similar to but generally milder than rubeola (measles). If a woman contracts rubella during the first trimester of pregnancy, the virus may damage the fetus, producing mental retardation, microcephaly, deafness, cardiac abnormalities, or generalized growth retardation. An agglutination card test is available to POLs to test for rubella.

Inflammatory Conditions. The acute stage of various inflammatory disorders is characterized by an abnormal glycoprotein, called **C-reactive protein (CRP)**. CRP is a general test for inflammation and is useful when correlated with other diagnostic information. A latex agglutination test is available for CRP testing in POLs.

Human Immunodeficiency Virus (HIV). This is a virus that infects and destroys the human immune system. Eventually, in most cases it leads to acquired immunodeficiency syndrome (AIDS), which is fatal. The virus attacks and destroys helper T-cells, which are lymphocytes that are vital in protecting the body from infection. As these cells are destroyed, it increases the risk of infection from opportunistic microorganisms—those that a normal immune system could fight. The greatest risk factor for contracting HIV infection is unprotected sexual activity. The virus can be found in body fluids including semen, vaginal secretions, and blood.

Diagnosis depends upon demonstrating the presence of antibodies in the blood due to the response to infection with HIV. Rapid HIV tests have been developed and approved by the FDA and are available as CLIA waived kits used as screening. These tests are interpreted visually and require no instrumentation. HIV antigens are affixed to the test strip or membrane. If HIV antibodies are present in the specimen, they bind to the antigen and a color reaction appears. There may be false positives due to cross reaction with other viruses; therefore confirmatory tests such as the Western blot test or the immunofluorescent antibody test should be performed.

Helicobacter pylori. *H. pylori,* formerly known as *Campylobacter pyloridis,* is a spiral-shaped bacillus that has been associated with a variety of gastrointestinal diseases including chronic gastritis, gastric (peptic) ulcers, and duodenal ulcers. Symptoms of these ulcers include abdominal pain with some relief after eating. The bacteria were originally identified through cultures taken from gastric biopsy specimens. The invasive endoscopic procedure used to diagnose this infection is expensive and creates a risk to the patient. The immunochromatographic tests use serum to rapidly detect antibodies to *H. pylori*. Patients with positive test results accompanied by gastric symptoms are treated with antibiotics.

Hemolytic Disease of the Newborn. Also known as *erythroblastosis fetalis,* hemolytic disease of the newborn (HDN) causes severe jaundice in newborns and may result in stunted growth, mental retardation, or death. The cause of HDN was unknown until the discovery of the **Rhesus (Rh) blood group.** It generally occurred only in second and succeeding pregnancies, not firstborn infants. It is now known that HDN is due to a blood-type incompatibility between mother and fetus. Rhesus antigen in the Rh-positive fetus stimulates production of maternal antibodies in the Rh-negative woman, who lacks the antigen. The maternal antibodies may cause severe hemolysis of fetal blood and high levels of bilirubin by the time of birth. Severely affected infants must be given a blood exchange to replace the hemolyzed blood with normal blood.

HDN has a chance of occurring whenever an Rh-negative woman has an Rh-postive child because there may be an accidental exchange of blood between fetus and mother. Pregnant women routinely have Rhesus blood-type determinations to see if they are Rhesus negative and thus at risk for HDN. If the father tests negative for Rhesus antigen, there is no risk. If the father tests Rh positive, then the woman should be given HDN vaccine to prevent HDN in future pregnancies.

HDN vaccine contains antibodies from Rh-negative individuals who have been sensitized to the Rh antigen. The vaccine is given to the Rh-negative mother immediately after the birth of her first Rh-positive child, before her immune system has had time to develop antibodies to the Rhesus antigen. As a result of the vaccine, the Rh-negative mother's immune system does not produce the antibodies itself and develops no "memory" for the antigen. The vaccine antibodies are short lived so that, by the time of the next pregnancy, the woman no longer has circulating Rhesus antibodies.

Coombs' Test. Coombs' test, also known as the antiglobulin test, is used for monitoring the development of Rh incompatibility in at-risk pregnant women. It detects the presence of antierythrocyte antibodies on their red blood cells. If antibodies are present, red blood cells have been sensitized in vivo to the D antigen, and their fetuses are at risk of HDN.

To perform a Coombs' test, red blood cells of the patient are washed in a saline solution to remove the plasma, which has interfering substances. Then the red blood cells are mixed with antiglobulin serum that has been obtained from a medical supply house, centrifuged, and checked for agglutination. Agglutination indicates that antibodies are present and sensitization has occurred. When the test result is negative, the sample is left for a few minutes at room temperature and then recentrifuged. If there is still no agglutination, a negative test result is reported. A control of red blood cells known to be sensitized is tested along with the patient's cells.

CLINICALLY IMPORTANT INHERITED BLOOD TYPES

The Rhesus blood group is one of two clinically important inherited blood groups. The other is the **ABO blood group.** Although there are many other inherited blood groups, these two cause most of the problems with incompatibility.

When a transfusion of Rh-positive blood is given to an Rh-negative-sensitized patient, the same hemolytic reaction may occur as the one just described for hemolytic disease of the newborn. In this case, the Rh-negative individual most likely was sensitized by a previous transfusion of Rh-positive blood. An Rh-negative patient can receive only one exposure to Rh-positive blood without a notable transfusion reaction. Therefore, only Rh-negative blood can be given safely.

Exposure to incompatible ABO blood-group antigens occurs in ways in addition to transfusions of incompatible blood. By adulthood, most of us are sensitized to antigens of incompatible ABO blood types through exposure to bacteria that contain the same antigenic molecules.

In POLs, slide tests are sufficient for typing the ABO and Rhesus blood groups for screening and diagnostic purposes. In blood banks, where blood is prepared for transfusions, a more complete analysis of blood compatibility is necessary. This includes tube typing and tube cross-matches, which analyze both antigens and antibodies. Blood transfusions are prepared only by qualified technicians with specialized training in blood banking.

Understanding Blood Types

To understand why some blood types are compatible and others are not, you need to know more about the ABO and Rhesus blood groups. Keep in mind that Rh incompatibility must be considered separately from ABO incompatibility. A patient's own blood type is always preferred for a transfusion. Other blood types, if compatible, may be substituted during emergencies or shortages.

ABO. The ABO blood group has four different blood types: A, B, AB, and O. The letters signify the type of antigen that each type of blood has on the surface membranes of its red blood cells. Type A blood has A antigen, type B blood has B antigen, and type AB blood has A and B antigens equally. Type O blood has neither type A antigen nor type B antigen.

People with blood types A, B, and O produce antibodies against the antigens they do not carry—type A against antigen B, type B against antigen A, and type O against antigens A and B. Therefore, patients with type A blood never should receive transfusions of type B or AB blood. Similarly, patients with type B blood cannot receive type A blood or type AB blood, and type O patients cannot receive type A, B, or AB blood. As Table 21-3 shows, Type O blood can be accepted by anyone.

Table 21-3 Compatible ABO Blood Types

Recipient ABO Blood Type	Recipient Antigens	Recipient Antibodies	Compatible Donor Blood Types
AB	A, B	None	AB, A, B, O
A	A	B	A, O
B	B	A	B, O
O	None	A, B	O

Table 21-4 Compatible and Incompatible Rhesus Blood Types

Recipient Rhesus Blood Type	Recipient Antigen	Recipient Antibodies	Compatible Donor Rh Blood Types
Rh positive	D	None	Rh positive & Rh negative
Rh negative	None	Anti-D	Rh negative only

This is because it lacks both A antigens and B antigens. It is also why type O people are called universal donors. By contrast, people of type AB blood can accept blood of any type because they produce no antibodies. This is why they are called universal recipients.

Rhesus. Over 50 Rhesus antigens have been identified; however, most complications arise from the Rh antigens D, C, c, E, and e. Antigen D is the most common and causes the strongest antibody reaction, so it is the most clinically significant. People with antigen D are called Rh positive; people without it are called Rh negative. About 15 percent of Euro-Americans are Rh negative. People with Rh-negative blood cannot receive blood transfusions of Rh-positive blood. People with Rh-positive blood, on the other hand, can receive transfusions of either Rh-positive or Rh-negative blood see Table 21-4.

Testing for Blood Type

POL tests for blood type are based on agglutinin reactions because blood group antigen-antibody complexes normally agglutinate. These tests are CLIA nonwaived.

ABO and Rhesus Blood Types. ABO and Rhesus blood types usually are tested in POLs by the slide method. A drop of blood cells, either fresh or suspended in their plasma, is mixed with commercial antiserum and inspected for agglutination. Table 21-5 and Figure 21-7 show agglutination of different blood types.

Table 21-5 Slide Reactions to Commercial Typing Antisera

Patient Blood Type	Anti-A-Sera	Anti-B-Sera	Rh D Positive Sera
A positive	Agglutinated	—	Agglutinated
B positive	—	Agglutinated	Agglutinated
AB positive	Agglutinated	Agglutinated	Agglutinated
O positive	—	—	Agglutinated
A negative	Agglutinated	—	—
B negative	—	Agglutinated	—
AB negative	Agglutinated	Agglutinated	—
O negative	—	—	—

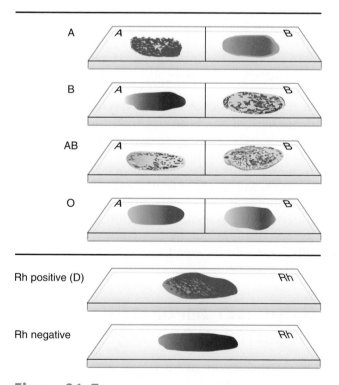

Figure 21-7 The agglutination of different ABO and Rhesus blood types with antisera.

PROCEDURE 21-1

Pregnancy Test Using EIA Method

Goal

After successfully completing this procedure, you will be able to prepare and perform a human chorionic gonadotropin (hCG) determination with urine for detection of pregnancy by the EIA or immunochromatographic method.

Completion Time

15 minutes

Equipment and Supplies

- Disposable gloves
- Goggles or face shield
- Impermeable jacket, gown, or apron
- Hand disinfectant
- Surface disinfectant
- Paper towels and tissue
- Biohazard container
- Chromatographic immunoassay pregnancy test kit (Beckman Coulter ICON hCG)
- Patient urine or serum sample
- Paper and pen

Instructions

Read through the list of equipment and supplies that you will need and the steps of the procedure. Be sure that you understand each step before you begin. Then complete each step correctly and in the proper order.

*Steps marked with (*) are critical and must have the maximum points to pass.

Performance Standards	Points Awarded	Maximum Points
1. Put on a protective jacket, gown, or apron; put on face shield or goggles; wash your hands with disinfectant, dry them, and put on gloves.		10
2. Follow standard precautions.		10
3. Collect and prepare the appropriate equipment. The test includes internal controls and confirms sufficient sample volume and correct procedural technique. Follow guidelines recommended for running external controls for test kit.		5
4. *Verify the identification of the patient specimen and label the container.		15
5. Bring the pouch to room temperature and then open the pouch and remove the test device.		5
6. Place the test device on a clean and level surface. Hold the dropper vertically and transfer 3 full drops of urine or serum to the sample well (S) of the test device.		10
7. Start the timer.		5
8. Wait for the red line(s) to appear. Read the result at 3 minutes for urine or 5 minutes for serum.		10
9. *Record the test as positive if two distinct red lines appear, one at the (C) and one at the (T). Record the test as negative if one red line appears in the (C) region. No apparent line appears in the (T) region.		10
10. Record the results on the laboratory report form. Document in the patient chart, control log, and master log according to laboratory guidelines.		10
11. Dispose of the patient sample and disposable equipment following waste disposal guidelines for biohazardous waste.		5
12. Disinfect other equipment and return to storage.		5
13. Clean the work surfaces following standard precautions.		5
14. Remove your gloves, dispose, and wash your hands.		5
Total Points		110

Overall Procedural Evaluation

Student Name _____

Signature of Instructor _____ Date _____

Comments _____

_____

 PROCEDURE 21-2

Infectious Mononucleosis Test

Goal

After successfully completing this procedure, you will be able to prepare and perform an infectious mononucleosis test for the qualitative detection of human heterophile antibodies in serum, plasma, or whole blood using a commercial immunochromatographic test kit (Quidel QuickVue + ®).

Completion Time

15 minutes

Equipment and Supplies

- Disposable gloves
- Face shield or goggles
- Impermeable jacket, gown, or apron
- Hand disinfectant
- Surface disinfectant
- Paper towels and tissue
- Biohazard container
- Chromatographic immunoassay test kit (QuickVue+®)
- Patient blood sample (serum, plasma, or whole blood)
- Paper, pen, and laboratory requisition form

Instructions

Read through the list of equipment and supplies that you will need and the steps of the procedure. Be sure that you understand each step before you begin. Then complete each step correctly and in the proper order. Document properly.

*Steps marked with (*) are critical and must have the maximum points to pass.

Performance Standards	Points Awarded	Maximum Points
1. Put on a protective jacket, gown, or apron; put on face shield or goggles; wash your hands with disinfectant, dry them, and put on gloves.		10
2. Follow standard precautions.		10
3. Collect and prepare the appropriate equipment. Internal controls are included with the testing device. Positive and negative external controls are included and should be tested with each new lot or shipment and by recommended guidelines.		5
4. *Verify the identification of the patient specimen and match with laboratory requisition form.		15
5. Remove the testing device from the pouch and place on a well-lit and level surface. Locate the "Test Complete" and the "Read Result" windows and the "Add" well.		5
6. Using patient serum or plasma, add one drop of specimen to the "Add" well using the pipette provided.		5
7. Holding the Developer bottle vertically, add 5 drops of Developer to the "Add" well and start the timer.		5

8.	Read the results in 5 minutes. "Test Complete" line must be visible by 10 minutes (the internal control).	10
9.	*Record the test as positive if there is any shade of a blue vertical line forming a "+" sign in the "Read Result" window along with the blue "Test Complete" line. Record as negative if there is no blue vertical line in the "Read Result" window along with the blue "Test Complete" line.	15
10.	Record the results on the laboratory report form. Document in patient chart, control log, and master log according to laboratory guidelines.	10
11.	Dispose of the patient sample and disposable equipment following waste disposal guideline for biohazardous waste.	5
12.	Disinfect other equipment and return to storage.	5
13.	Clean the work surfaces following standard precautions.	5
14.	Remove your gloves, dispose, and wash your hands.	5
	Total Points	**110**

Overall Procedural Evaluation

Student Name _____

Signature of Instructor _____ Date _____

Comments _____

_____

PROCEDURE 21-3

ABO and Rhesus Blood Type Determination

Goal

After successfully completing this procedure, you will be able to prepare and perform individual blood types for ABO (Part 1) and Rhesus (Part 2) blood groups.

Completion Time

20 minutes

Equipment and Supplies

- Disposable gloves
- Face shield or goggles
- Impermeable jacket, gown, or apron
- Hand disinfectant
- Surface disinfectant
- Paper towels and tissue
- Biohazard container
- Glass microscope slides
- Commercial antisera for blood typing (anti-A, anti-B, and anti-D)
- Wooden applicator sticks
- View box with built-in light
- Watch with second hand
- Wax pencil
- Disposable transfer pipette
- EDTA blood specimen
- Paper, pen, and laboratory requisition form

Instructions

Read through the list of equipment and supplies that you will need and the steps of the procedure. Be sure that you understand each step before you begin. Then complete each step correctly and in the proper order. Document properly.

*Steps marked with (*) are critical and must have the maximum points to pass.

Performance Standards	Points Awarded	Maximum Points
1. Put on a protective jacket, gown, or apron; put on face shield or goggles; wash your hands with disinfectant, dry them, and put on gloves.		10
2. Follow standard precautions.		10
3. Collect and prepare the appropriate equipment.		5
4. *Verify the identification of the specimen and match with laboratory requisition form.		15
Part 1: ABO Blood Type		
5. Divide a clean glass slide into two equal parts with a wax pencil and label the left side "A" and the right side "B."		5
6. Holding the dropper about one-half inch from the slide, place a drop of A antiserum on the left (A) side of the slide. Do not contaminate the dropper by letting it touch the slide.		5
7. In the same manner, place a drop of B antiserum on the right (B) side of the slide.		5
8. Using a transfer pipette, place a drop of whole blood beside the antiserum on the left side of the slide; the drop should be about the same size as the drop of antiserum. Do not allow the pipette to touch the slide or antiserum.		10
9. Repeat step 8 on the right side of the slide.		10
10. Using circular motion and a wooden applicator stick, thoroughly mix the blood and A antiserum together on the left side of the slide. Dispose of the applicator stick in biohazard container.		5
11. Repeat step 10 for the right side of the slide using a new wooden applicator stick. Dispose in biohazard container.		5
12. Turn on the view box and note the time. Rock the slide on the view box gently back and forth for two minutes while observing the red blood cells for agglutination. (Note: If a view box is unavailable, improvise with a strong light.)		5
13. *If agglutination occurs on the left side only, record the blood type as type A. If agglutination occurs on the right side only, record the blood type as type B. If agglutination occurs on both sides, record the blood type as type AB. If no agglutination occurs on either side, record the blood type as type O.		15
14. Discard the glass slide in the appropriate biohazard container.		5
Part 2: Rhesus Blood Type		
15. With a wax pencil, label a clean, dry glass slide with "Rh."		5
16. Holding the dropper about one-half inch from the slide, place a drop of Rh (D) antiserum on the slide. Do not contaminate the dropper by touching the slide.		5
17. Using a transfer pipette, place a drop of whole blood beside the Rh D antiserum. Make the drop about the same size as the blood drop. Do not let the pipette touch the slide or the antiserum.		5
18. Using a circular motion and a disposable wooden applicator stick, thoroughly mix the blood and the antiserum together on the slide. Then dispose of the wooden applicator in the biohazard container.		5
19. Place the slide on the view box that has warmed to between 40 and 50 degrees Celsius. The slide should warm to about 37 degrees Celsius.		5
20. For 2 minutes, rock the slide gently back and forth while observing for agglutination.		5

21.	*If agglutination occurs, record the Rh as positive on the laboratory report. If no agglutination occurs, record the blood type as Rh negative.	15
22.	Dispose of the slide and other disposable equipment following waste disposal guidelines for biohazardous waste.	5
23.	Refrigerate the antisera.	5
24.	Disinfect other equipment and work area following standard precautions.	5
25.	Remove your jacket, gown, or apron, and gloves; wash your hands with disinfectant and dry.	5
	Total Points	175

Overall Procedural Evaluation

Student Name _____

Signature of Instructor _____ Date _____

Comments _____
_____

chapter 21 REVIEW

Using Terminology

Match the term in the right column with the appropriate definition or description in the left column.

_____ **1.** allergy
_____ **2.** antiglobulin test
_____ **3.** an autoimmune disease
_____ **4.** cell-mediated immunity
_____ **5.** C-reactive protein
_____ **6.** precipitation
_____ **7.** humoral immunity
_____ **8.** increased susceptibility to disease
_____ **9.** rapid plasma reagin
_____ **10.** pregnancy hormone

a. B-lymphocytes
b. Coombs' test
c. CRP
d. flocculation
e. hCG
f. hypersensitivity
g. immunodeficiency
h. RA
i. RPR
j. T-lymphocytes

Multiple Choice

Choose the best answer for the following questions.

11. Which of the following would be considered the body's first line of defense against antigens?
 a. gastric HCl
 b. interferon
 c. complement
 d. benevolent bacteria

12. The immune response triggered by a wound that keeps the pathogen from spreading and promotes healing is the
 a. specific immunity
 b. inflammatory response
 c. antibody response
 d. endocytic response

13. Protein molecules produced by the lymph system in response to a particular antigen are called
   a. enzymes
   b. foreign
   c. antibodies
   d. macrophages

14. Which of the following is an autoimmune disorder?
   a. HIV
   b. AIDS
   c. RA
   d. Pregnancy

15. A lab test procedure that has a high degree of sensitivity will
   a. identify those patients that have the disease
   b. have a high number of false positives
   c. identify those patients with interfering antigens
   d. never need confirmatory testing

Acquiring Knowledge

Mark the following statements as true or false and rewrite the false statements to make them true.

16. Specific immunity is the general resistance to disease that characterizes a particular species.

_____

_____

_____

17. Interferon is a protein that helps protect uninfected cells from viral infection.

_____

_____

_____

18. Innate immunity refers to immunity acquired after exposure to a foreign invader.

_____

_____

_____

19. Foreign substances that provoke a specific immune reaction are called antibodies.

_____

_____

_____

20. A few members of each T-cell clone become memory cells.

_____

_____

_____

21. False positives are people who have the disease but do not test positive.

_____

_____

_____

22. In a radioimmunoassay, an antigen binds to a radioactive isotope and the level of radioactivity is measured.

_____

_____

_____

Answer the following questions in the spaces provided.

23. What are four types of nonspecific immune defenses in humans?

_____

_____

_____

24. What role do physical and anatomical barriers play in defending bodies from microorganisms? What are some examples?

_____

_____

_____

25. What are the physiological barriers of nonspecific immunity?

_____

_____

_____

26. Describe the inflammatory response.

_____

_____

_____

27. What is the role of antigen-antibody reactions in specific immunity?

_____

_____

_____

28. Distinguish between humoral immunity and cell-mediated immunity.

_____

_____

_____

29. What is autoimmunity and what are some possible causes?

_____

_____

_____

30. What conditions may bring about immunodeficiency?

_____

_____

_____

31. What characterizes patients with immunodeficiency?

_____

_____

_____

32. What distinguishes immediate hypersensitivity and delayed hypersensitivity?

_____

_____

_____

33. How do sensitivity and specificity relate to accuracy?

_____

_____

_____

34. For each of the following types of immunology tests, describe the reaction that occurs and give an example of a disease or condition that is diagnosed with that type of test: a. ELISA, b. precipitin reaction, c. agglutinin reaction, d. lysin reaction.

_____

_____

_____

35. How are immune reactions measured quantitatively?

_____

_____

_____

36. Discuss quality control in immunology testing in POLs.

_____

_____

_____

37. Describe the ABO blood group, including all of the antigens and blood types.

_____

_____

_____

38. Which ABO blood types may donate to which types?

_____

_____

_____

39. Describe the Rhesus blood group and blood types.

_____

_____

_____

40. What Rhesus blood types can be received by an Rh-positive patient? by an Rh-negative patient?

_____

_____

_____

41. When and why does hemolytic disease of the newborn (HDN) occur?

_____

_____

_____

42. List four diseases or conditions that are tested by immunological methods.

_____

_____

_____

43. Why is blood typed for Rh in POLs?

_____

_____

_____

44. What causes the color reaction in an ELISA test?

_____

_____

_____

45. What is the most common sexually transmitted disease?

_____

_____

_____

Applying Knowledge—On the Job

Answer the following questions in the spaces provided.

46. You have just received a request for a rheumatoid arthritis test. What controls should you run with the patient test to be certain that the reagents are reacting as they should?

_____

_____

_____

47. A teenage patient came to the laboratory for a CBC, blood chemistries, and an immunology test. He has been very sick with flulike symptoms and is not recovering well. When you examine the stained blood differential slide, you find many large, abnormal lymphocytes. What antigen-antibody test might the physician order to help diagnose this patient's condition?

_____

_____

_____

48. A small child has been brought to the laboratory for a throat smear. The mother told you that the physician prescribed antibiotics to prevent a possible occurrence of rheumatic fever. What bacterial infection does the physician suspect? What immunology test might the physician order to diagnose it?

_____

_____

_____

49. One of the patients in the clinic received an allergy shot, and in just a few minutes she began to choke from severe edema of the larynx. What type of reaction did the patient have?

_____

_____

_____

50. You have just typed a pregnant woman's blood for both ABO and Rhesus blood groups. There were no agglutinations. What is her blood type?

_____

_____

_____

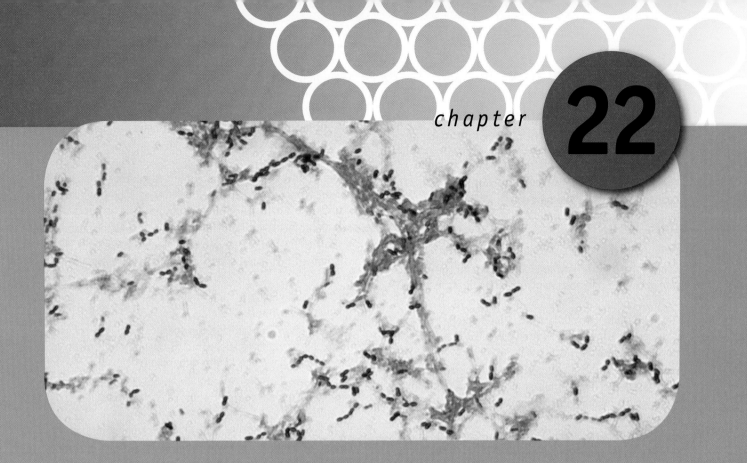

chapter **22**

Microbiology

COGNITIVE OBJECTIVES

After studying this chapter, you should be able to

22.1 use each of the vocabulary terms appropriately.

22.2 explain the relevance of microbiology to POLs.

22.3 describe how infectious diseases are diagnosed.

22.4 list the reasons that viral diseases often are difficult to diagnose and treat.

22.5 discuss differences that aid in the identification of bacteria species.

22.6 describe the requirements of bacterial growth.

22.7 discuss the role of sensitivity testing in selecting antibiotics for bacterial infections.

22.8 identify several human diseases caused by fungal, protozoan, and helminth microorganisms.

22.9 list aseptic techniques for working with microorganisms in POLs and explain why these techniques are important.

PERFORMANCE OBJECTIVES

After studying this chapter, you should be able to

22.10 prepare a heat-fixed bacterial smear.

22.11 prepare a Gram stain from an unstained bacterial smear.

22.12 examine a prepared Gram stained smear and classify the microorganisms by their morphology and Gram stain reaction.

TERMINOLOGY

antibiotic: a drug administered to kill or inhibit the growth of bacteria.

aseptic technique: a lab technique that ensures the isolation of pathogenic microorganisms, including personal protective equipment and sterilization.

bacillus: a rod-shaped bacterium. Bacilli include the bacteria that cause tuberculosis and diphtheria.

bacitracin: an antibiotic used in cultures to give an early indication of the presence of Group A strep.

bacteria: single-celled microorganisms in the kingdom *Monera*. Bacteria cause many different infections in humans.

catalase test: the lab test in which hydrogen peroxide is added to urine cultures to distinguish *Streptococcus* from *Staphylococcus* infections.

coagulase test: the lab test that demonstrates the presence of an enzyme produced by pathogenic *Staphylococcus* organisms, thereby distinguishing them from nonpathogenic strains of *Staphylococcus*.

coccus: a spherical or oval bacterium. Cocci include *Streptococcus* and *Staphylococcus*.

culture media: substances containing nutrients used to grow bacteria; may be liquid or solid.

direct culture: a primary culture; a culture grown by inoculating patient specimens directly onto the culture medium.

fastidious bacterium: a bacterium that has very precise nutritional and environmental requirements for growth, including *Niesseria gonorrhoeae*.

fungus: a plant of the phylum Fungi, which lacks chlorophyll. Fungi are microorganisms that include yeasts and molds, some of which cause disease.

gram negative: bacteria that stain pink or red with Gram stain, including *Escherichia coli* and *Neisseria gonorrhoeae*.

gram positive: bacteria that stain deep purple with Gram stain, such as *Staphylococcus* and *Streptococcus* organisms.

Gram stain: the most commonly used stain for bacterial smears. Gram stain separates organisms into two clinically meaningful groups: gram negative organisms and gram positive organisms.

helminth: a true worm. Several species parasitize the human intestinal tract, including tapeworms and hookworms.

microbiology: the branch of science that studies microscopic organisms.

oxidase test: the lab test in which oxidase reagent is added to a colony of suspected *Niesseria gonorrhoeae* to confirm the presence of this organism.

protozoan: a single-celled animal. Several species of protozoa are pathogenic to humans, including *Giardia lamblia*.

pure culture: a culture that is grown from a single colony of bacteria that was taken from a direct culture. A pure culture serves to further isolate the pathogen.

spiral bacteria: bacteria that include the bacteria that cause syphilis and Lyme disease.

urinary tract infection (UTI): an infection of the organs of the urinary tract system caused by any of several different bacteria. A UTI is diagnosed when the urine bacteria concentration exceeds 100,000 organisms per milliliter.

virus: a simple organism that causes many diseases in humans, including colds and herpes. Viruses live and reproduce within the cells of a host.

INTRODUCTION

Microbiology is the branch of science that studies microscopic organisms. This chapter shows how microbiology is relevant to POLs, describes disease-causing microorganisms, and outlines microbiology procedures.

MICROBIOLOGY

The relevance of **microbiology** to POLs lies primarily in isolating and identifying disease-causing microorganisms. This is necessary for diagnosis and treatment of many infectious diseases.

How Infectious Diseases Are Diagnosed

As is true with any disease, when a patient presents with an infectious disease, signs and symptoms often provide physicians with a tentative diagnosis. For example, measles, a viral disease, often is diagnosed by its characteristic rash.

A tentative diagnosis may be followed up with a lab test to confirm the diagnosis. A simple blood test may confirm the presence of a virus through detection of an antigen-antibody reaction. If a bacteria pathogen is suspected, as in a wound, a specimen from the infected area may be examined directly in a stained smear. Alternatively, culturing may be necessary to produce sufficient bacteria for identification.

Advances in microbiology identification with immunoassay techniques and nucleic acid hybridization methods have made it possible to assist the physician in the diagnosis of infections faster and easier than traditional cultures. Tuberculosis, caused by the species *Mycobacterium tuberculosis,* can now be detected using DNA probe technique in hours instead of several weeks.

Clinical Applications

Few of today's POLs use all of the procedures for identifying microorganisms that are outlined in this chapter. Some POLs depend entirely on reference laboratories for microbiology testing. Nonetheless, the contents of this chapter are important for all POL workers for the following reasons:

* understanding the diagnosis and treatment of patients with infectious diseases
* practicing correct collection and handling of patient microbiology specimens
* following safety practices for microbiological hazards

To understand the diagnosis and treatment of patients with diseases caused by microorganisms, you should know the types of organisms involved and their characteristics and requirements. Knowledge of correct specimen-collection and specimen-handling procedures is important because virtually all POL workers collect and handle microbiology specimens, even when the testing is done in reference labs. The reports from reference labs can be only as good as the specimens they receive.

For their own safety and the safety of their patients, POL workers must follow appropriate aseptic practices when handling infectious disease organisms. In addition to the rise of HIV and hepatitis, several other infectious diseases have made a resurgence over the past decade—tuberculosis, measles, and antibiotic-resistant strains of *Streptococcus* and *Staphylococcus,* among others.

DISEASE-CAUSING MICROORGANISMS

Most disease-causing microorganisms, like other living things, are part of the Linnaean system of classification, in which organisms are grouped according to their similarities. Organisms also may be classified clinically into pathogenic, disease-causing,

and nonpathogenic, nondisease-causing, groups. Human pathogenic microbes include viruses, bacteria, fungi, and protozoa. In addition, large internal parasites such as tapeworms, hookworms, and pinworms produce microscopic eggs.

Classification of Living Things

In the Linnaean system of classification, the largest subdivision of living things is the kingdom, followed by the phylum, class, order, family, genus, and species. The kingdom includes organisms that are only generally similar, whereas, at the other end of the hierarchy, the species includes only organisms of the same type. The scientific name of an organism consists of its genus and species names. *Candida albicans,* for example, is the genus and species of a yeast that causes vaginal infections.

Viruses

Although hundreds of **viruses** have been identified to date, there still is debate over their classification. Many scientists do not place them in any of the kingdoms of living organisms because they do not consider them to be true organisms. Why? Viruses are simpler than bacteria, which are the simplest true organisms known today. Viruses also are the smallest living things, measuring about one-twenty-billionth of a meter in diameter. In addition, viruses do not have cells or metabolic machinery. An individual virus particle, or virion, consists of nothing more than a thin protein coat wrapped around either RNA or DNA. All other living things have both RNA and DNA.

How do viruses grow and reproduce? They invade the cells of other organisms for shelter, nutrients, and the missing nucleic acids. Within a host cell, they take over the metabolic machinery, thrive, and multiply. When the host cell dies, they spread through the fluids surrounding the cell and infect new host cells. Some viruses can survive in the outside environment before infecting a new host.

The fact that viruses live within their hosts' cells makes viral illnesses difficult to treat. There are few effective virucides, drugs that kill viruses, because most chemicals that destroy viruses are toxic to the cells of the host. Antibiotics are useless against viruses, although they may be prescribed for opportunistic bacterial infections that sometimes occur when the body is weakened by viral infection. Viruses also get a head start on treatment because most viral infections do not produce symptoms until multiplication of the virus is under way. In addition, viruses that can survive extremes of humidity and temperature may be difficult to eliminate from the environment.

Some viruses produce a passing acute infection in the host. Rhinovirus, for example, which causes colds, generally produces an acute, self-limiting infection. Other viruses infect the host for life. Herpesvirus, for example, may produce cold sores throughout the life of the host, whenever the host's immunity is weakened. Similarly, the varicella virus that causes chicken pox may remain dormant in the host for years and resurface later in life as the disease shingles.

Because of their small size, viruses are not visible under light microscopes. Viruses are highly antigenic, however, so many can be identified immunologically. As you saw in Chapter 21, the viruses that may be detected in POLs with immunological tests include those that cause German measles, herpes, infectious mononucleosis, and AIDS. Other viral diseases seen in physicians' offices include colds (rhinovirus), mumps, influenza, hepatitis, chicken pox, shingles, encephalitis, and warts.

More About Warts

Warts are caused by the papilloma virus and are spread from person to person by direct contact. Plantar's warts grow underneath the epidermis of the soles of the feet and often are very painful. Venereal warts are found on the genitals and are sexually transmitted.

Bacteria

Bacteria are single-celled microorganisms that previously were classified as plants but now are placed in a kingdom of their own, the *Monera*. The smallest bacteria are only two-ten-millionths of a meter (0.2 micrometer) in diameter. The size of bacteria puts them just within the range of light microscopes, so they may be observed directly in smears.

Bacteria reproduce by cell division at a very high rate—about once every 20 minutes for some species. It has been estimated that trillions of bacteria are in and on the average human body. Clearly, the total number of bacteria in the world must be astonishingly high. Fortunately, most bacteria are either beneficial or nonpathogenic to humans as long as they stay in their usual environments. However, most bacteria also are capable of causing disease if they breach the body's defenses. Any bacteria grown from a normally sterile site should be regarded as pathogenic until proven otherwise.

Bacterial species differ from one another in several ways. These ways include size, shape, appendages, motility, staining characteristics, chemical characteristics, and population growth patterns. Many of these differences are useful in determining which species are causing disease in patients. Identification is important for the administration of the appropriate antibiotic treatment. Bacteria also vary greatly in the type of environment and nutrients that they require for growth. Lab personnel must take these differences into account when culturing bacteria.

Morphology. As Figure 22-1 illustrates, bacteria have three principal shapes: spherical or oval (cocci), rod-shaped (bacilli), and spiral (spirilla and spirochetes).

The **cocci** (spherical or oval bacteria) may appear singly (micrococci) or in pairs (diplococci), chains (streptococci), or irregular grapelike clusters (staphylococci). They also may occur in square or cubical groupings (sarcinae). Cocci are incapable of independent motion. They include the bacteria that cause common strep and staph infections.

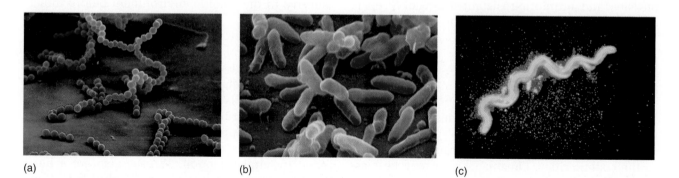

(a)   (b)   (c)

Figure 22-1 The three principal shapes of bacteria: (a) cocci (round); (b) bacilli (rods); and (c) spiral (spirochetes and spirilla).

The **bacilli** (rod-shaped bacteria) may appear single or attached end to end in chains (streptobacilli). Bacilli also may occur in palisades, that is, attached side to side like boards in a fence. Most bacilli have appendages allowing independent motion. The appendages may be single or multiple, occurring either as whips or as tufts. They may be located at just one end of the organism, at both ends, or protruding from all surfaces. Bacilli include the bacteria that cause tuberculosis, typhoid fever, diphtheria, and leprosy.

The **spiral bacteria** may be comma-shaped (vibrio), rigid and spiral (spirilla), or very coiled and flexible (spirochetes). The flexible spiral bacteria move by flexing, snapping, or bending. Spiral bacteria include the bacteria that cause syphilis, yaws, and Lyme disease.

Staining Characteristics. Another way of identifying bacteria is by their staining characteristics. Staining also is necessary to enhance the visibility of features of an individual bacterium. The most commonly used stain is the **Gram stain,** named for its originator. Using Gram stain is a four-step procedure (see Figure 22-2):

- staining with crystal violet, a deep purple dye
- intensifying the purple stain with iodine
- decolorizing with alcohol
- counterstaining with safranin, a pink dye

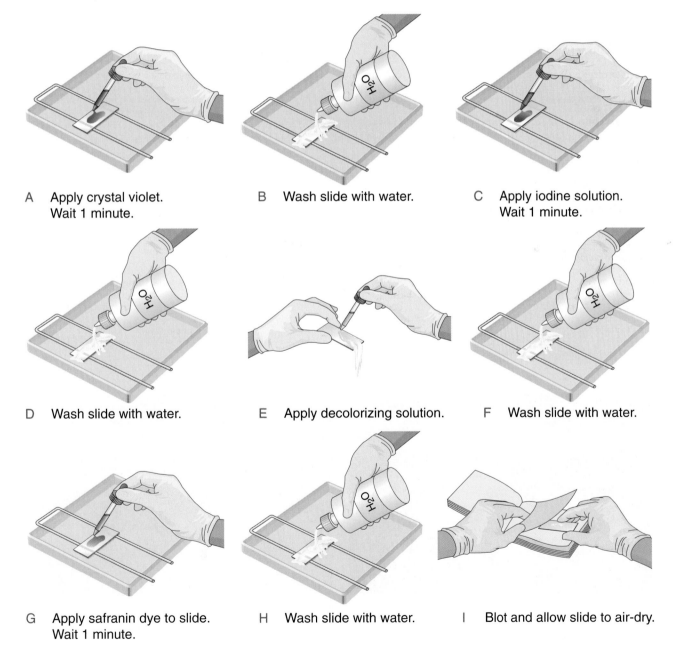

A Apply crystal violet. Wait 1 minute.

B Wash slide with water.

C Apply iodine solution. Wait 1 minute.

D Wash slide with water.

E Apply decolorizing solution.

F Wash slide with water.

G Apply safranin dye to slide. Wait 1 minute.

H Wash slide with water.

I Blot and allow slide to air-dry.

Figure 22-2 Gram stain procedure.

Technique Tip

Beware: Gram positive bacteria can be decolorized if the timing of the decolorization step of the procedure is too long.

On the basis of their staining affinities with Gram stain, bacteria can be divided into two groups: gram positive and gram negative (see Table 22-1). **Gram positive** bacteria stain deep purple with crystal violet because their thick cell walls retain the dye even when alcohol is added to the slide. **Gram negative** bacteria are decolorized by the addition of alcohol because their cell walls are thinner. Instead, they stain pink or red with the safranin. (See Figure 22-3.)

The classification of bacteria into gram positive and gram negative groups is very useful clinically. Gram positive and gram negative bacteria not only react differently to chemical tests but also have different antibiotic sensitivities as well.

Table 22-1   Examples of Gram Positive and Gram Negative Bacteria

Bacteria	Shape	Disease
Gram Positive (stain deep purple)		
Streptococcus pneumoniae	Cocci in pairs	Pneumonia
Staphylococcus aureus	Cocci in clusters	Abscesses, wound infections, boils, toxic shock syndrome
Streptococcus pyogenes	Cocci in chains	Strep throat
Clostridium tetani	Bacilli	Tetanus
Clostridium perfringens	Bacilli	Gas gangrene
Gram Negative (stain pink or red)		
Escherichia coli	Bacilli	Urinary tract infections
Neisseria gonorrhoeae	Cocci in pairs	Gonorrhea
Proteus mirabilis	Bacilli	Urinary tract infections
Pseudomonas aeruginosa	Bacilli	Infections in debilitated patients
Salmonella typhi	Bacilli	Typhoid fever
Helicobacter pylori	Spiral	Gastric ulcers

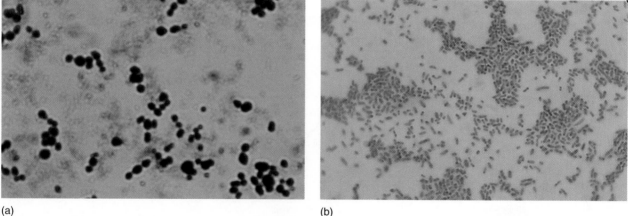

(a)   (b)

Figure 22-3 (a) Gram positive organisms appear blue or deep purple after staining. (b) Gram negative organisms appear pink or red.

Capsule Formation

Many bacteria form a layer of slimy, mucous-like material around each cell, called a capsule. The presence of a capsule is associated with the virulence of some pathogenic bacteria. Capsules can be seen in stained smears of bacteria.

Bacterial Metabolism. Bacteria produce enzymes that break down complex organic matter into simpler compounds. Some bacteria, called fermenters, break down sugars and other carbohydrates into alcohol and carbon dioxide. Other bacteria break down complex proteins into simpler nitrogenous compounds in a process called putrefaction. In the absence of air, these bacteria create foul odors in wound abscesses.

Enzymatic reactions such as these may be used to distinguish bacteria that have the same shape and staining characteristics. The nitrite test on the urine dipstick, for example, tests for the breakdown of nitrates into nitrites by bacteria present in the urine. Other such tests are conducted in culture tubes. A bacterial species may be identified by the type of sugar that it ferments, for example, or the color it produces when a particular chemical is added to the culture medium.

Toxin Production. Many bacteria produce toxins that are detrimental to the human host. Exotoxins are given off by the living bacterial cell to the surrounding tissues. Endotoxins are released as the bacteria die and disintegrate. Diseases caused by bacterial toxins include diphtheria, tetanus, and botulism (see Table 22-2).

Table 22-2 Some Exotoxin-Producing Bacteria and Related Diseases

Bacterial Species	Diseases
Bacillus cereus	Food poisoning
Clostridium botulinum	Botulism (food poisoning)
Clostridium tetani	Tetanus
Corynebacterium diphtheriae	Diphtheria
Escherichia coli	Urinary tract infections
Staphylococcus aureus	Pyogenic (pus-forming) infection
Streptococcus pyogenes	Strep throat, scarlet fever
Salmonella typhi	Typhoid fever

Bacterial Growth. Like all living things, bacteria have the property of growth in a favorable environment. Aspects of the environment important for bacterial growth include nutrition, temperature, humidity, and pH. Knowledge of bacterial growth is essential in POLs, where colonies of bacteria may be grown from just one organism to supply enough bacteria to identify the species. Some bacteria have very precise nutritional and environmental requirements for growth. These are called **fastidious bacteria.** An example is *Neisseria gonorrhoeae,* which causes gonorrhea. It requires an atmosphere of 3 to 10 percent carbon dioxide and special nutrients, including hemolyzed blood. In addition, inhibitors must be added to the culture medium to prevent rampant growth of nonpathogenic bacteria that also grow in the genitourinary tract.

When bacteria are grown under ideal conditions, the pattern of population growth of the colony may help in its identification. Many bacteria, such as *Escherichia coli,* multiply every 20 minutes, producing an exponential rate of growth. Growth will continue at this rate until nutrition is exhausted or the environment is altered unfavorably.

Figure 22-4 shows an idealized population growth curve for a colony of bacteria. Following are the phases of population growth:

I. *Lag phase:* population growth is not yet apparent

II. *Exponential phase:* the population is experiencing very rapid growth, doubling each time it reproduces

III. *Stationary period:* the population growth ceases as a balance is reached between cell division and cell death

IV. *Death acceleration:* the death rate accelerates as nutrients are depleted and/or waste materials collect

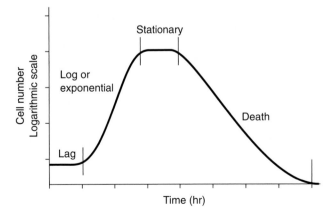

Figure 22-4 Population growth curve for colony of bacteria.

Most bacteria derive their food from organic sources; however, some live on nonliving organic matter and are referred to as saprophytes. Saprophytic bacteria are nonpathogenic and are considered to be benevolent because necessary processes of decay depend on them. Bacteria that survive on living organic matter are called parasites. They often cause disease in their hosts.

Most bacteria require free oxygen to live. Bacteria of this type are called aerobes. Some aerobes prefer free oxygen but can survive on oxygen obtained from chemical compounds. Other bacteria are called anaerobes. They are able to grow in the absence of oxygen (O_2). Obligate anaerobes can grow only in the absence of oxygen. Facultative anaerobes, on the other hand, prefer an atmosphere without oxygen but can grow in oxygen as well. These distinctions are important for culturing bacteria because an oxygen-free environment must be provided for anaerobes.

The fastidious bacterial species *Neisseria gonorrhoeae* that causes gonorrhea is capnophilic, meaning it requires carbon dioxide for optimal growth. Atmospheric carbon dioxide for the organism can be produced in several ways:

- a carbon dioxide–producing tablet inserted into an airtight plastic bag containing the culture
- a lighted candle placed in the upper part of an airtight jar containing the culture
- a vacuum pump that removes the oxygen, which is replaced with carbon dioxide (only in larger POLs)

If the bag or jar is opened to inspect the culture, a new tablet or lighted candle must be used to reestablish the carbon dioxide atmosphere.

Most pathogenic bacteria prefer a temperature near human body temperature (35–37 degrees Celsius), but many saprophytic bacteria have optimum growth over a wider range of temperatures. Some species of bacteria can survive in temperatures that range from subfreezing to 70 degrees Celsius. The typhoid bacterium, *Salmonella typhi,* for example, can remain frozen for months and, after thawing, it still can cause disease.

Moisture is essential for the growth of all bacteria, although different species vary in their ability to tolerate dryness. Moisture is needed in order for nutrients to enter the cells and wastes to leave them because these processes depend on diffusion. Diffusion is the passing of molecules in aqueous solution through a membrane from a region of high concentration to a region of lower concentration.

The majority of human pathogenic bacteria living on the skin and in the body cavities prefer a pH near neutral—7.2 to 7.5. Although an occasional pathogenic bacterial species can withstand extremely acidic or alkaline conditions, generally strong acids and bases are quickly lethal to microorganisms.

Antibiotics. Antibiotics are drugs that are administered to either kill bacteria (bactericides) or inhibit their growth by preventing reproduction (bacteriostatic antibiotics). Sensitivity tests determine which particular antibiotic to use against a given bacterial pathogen.

In sensitivity tests, the antibiotics being considered for treatment are placed in a culture medium. If the culture does not grow, the drug is considered to be effective. If the culture grows in abundance, the drug is considered to be ineffective. This mode of testing is based on the assumption that bacteria will respond to antibiotics in vivo (in the body) in the same way they have been demonstrated to respond in vitro (in an artificial environment). Antibiotic sensitivity testing is not recommended for POLs unless quantitative dilutions of the drug and pathogen are used. The amounts of both pathogen and drug affect the outcome. (See Figure 22-5.)

Antibiotic sensitivity testing is important in preventing the development of antibiotic-resistant strains of bacteria, which is a major treatment problem. Because bacteria reproduce so quickly and exchange DNA molecules, they can evolve multiple drug-resistant strains. This is most likely to occur when patients are treated with ineffective antibiotics or when they prematurely discontinue treatment with antibiotics that are effective.

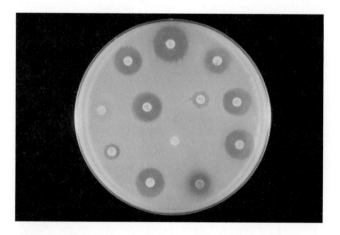

Figure 22-5 Antibiotic sensitivity test. The clear zones surrounding the disks indicate sensitivity to the antibiotic.

Culturing Bacteria. When bacteria are not easily seen on a direct smear, a culture may be performed. Common bacteriology specimens such as throat swabs, urine specimens, cervical or urethral exudates, or simple wound cultures can be performed in POLs. Because of limitations in staff, space, and equipment, many cultures are sent to reference or hospital microbiology labs. Other specimens such as sputum, eye and ear exudates, skin lesions, stools, or body fluids should be collected properly and sent to a referral laboratory. Culturing these specimens requires more complex methods of identification and current CLIA regulations have explicit guidelines addressing these specifically.

The type of **culture medium** selected to culture a specimen depends on the type of specimen collected. It may be a liquid broth or solid agar. Agar provides a good base for isolating bacterial colonies. One such medium is blood agar, which uses 5 percent sheep blood as the nutrient. Specialized media may be made by adding ingredients that inhibit or promote the growth of individual bacterial species or have other special functions. Examples of culture media include the following (see Figure 22-6):

- *Selective media* contain deterrents that discourage growth of microbes other than those being studied. One example is mannitol salt agar (MSA) for isolation and identification of most *Staphylococcus aureus* strains.

- *Enriched media* have additives to encourage the growth of fastidious organisms. An example is chocolate agar containing 1 percent hemoglobin and supplements for such bacteria as *Neisseria* and *Haemophilus.*

- *Differential media* contain additives that permit visual differentiation of bacteria; an example is MacConkey agar containing lactose to distinguish lactose-fermenting *Escherichia coli* (red or pink) and non–lactose fermenting gram negative enteric bacilli.

- *Transport media* protect pathogens during transport; they may contain charcoal to absorb bactericidal waste substances. An example is JEMBEC (Becton Dickinson) transport system for growing *Neisseria gonorrhoeae.*

- *Carbohydrate-metabolism media* have a specific carbohydrate and indicator added; examples of carbohydrates include lactose, sucrose, and glucose.

- *Proteolysis media* are a variety of media that test for the splitting of various proteins into their components; they often have colored indicators that depend on a secondary chemical reaction.

A colony is a group of bacteria grown from a single parent cell. Sometimes colonies are divided and grown on several types of media to study their growth patterns. Bacterial colonies can be described in terms of their shapes in cross sections, their patterns of growth, and the types of margins that they have. In cross section, the shape of a bacterial colony may be flat, convex, pulvinate (very convex), or umbilicate (dimpled). The growth pattern of a colony may be crenated (notched), circular, filamentous, spindle-shaped, or irregular. The margin of the colony may be swarming (covers the entire plate), lobed, undulating (wavy), filamentous, curled, or eroded.

Automated Systems for Bacterial Identification. Automated panels are available for use in larger POLs for testing bacteria for both identification and antibiotic sensitivities. One such system is the Vitek® 2 Compact (bioMerieux, Inc., Durham, North Carolina [800-682-2666]). Another is the MicroScan® (Siemens Medical Solutions USA, Malvern, Pennsylvania [800-743-6367]) (see Figure 22-7), in which a suspected pathogen is isolated and identified as gram positive or gram negative. Then a colony is transferred to a broth medium, allowed to grow to a standardized turbidity, and then inoculated into the appropriate panel—gram positive or gram negative.

The microcuvettes used in the panels contain dehydrated nutrients and chemicals to support various growth patterns and chemical reactions of bacteria. On the gram negative panel, for example, the chemical reactions include the fermenting of

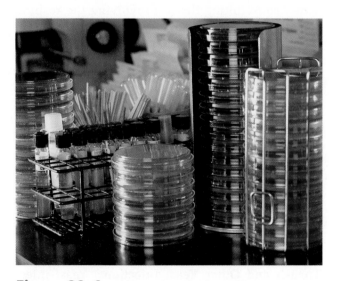

Figure 22-6 Examples of culture media.

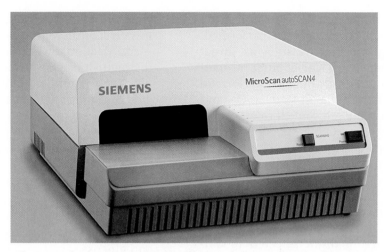

Figure 22-7 Automated system for bacterial identification: AutoScan4 System (Siemens Medical Solutions USA, Malvern, PA).

different sugars. The panels are incubated for 18 to 24 hours and then read manually, with results recorded on a worksheet or by the MicroScan® Microdilution Viewer that interprets the color or reaction as positive or negative. The particular combination of positive cuvettes that result identify the microbe being investigated. Antibiotic susceptibility panels also can be inoculated and incubated. Again, panels are available for both gram positive and gram negative bacteria.

Fungi

Fungi are a group of microorganisms that includes yeasts and molds. Figure 22-8 shows some examples. Only a few species cause disease in humans. Fungi that cause disease often are divided into dermatophytes, which infect only the skin, and systemic fungi, which can cause disease within deeper tissues and organs of the body. Diseases caused by parasitic fungi include histoplasmosis, coccidioidomycosis, and dermatomycosis. Yeast is part of the normal flora of the intestines and skin, but overgrowths commonly cause infections. Thrush is a common infection caused by overgrowth of yeast.

Histoplasmosis. Histoplasmosis is a systemic respiratory disease acquired by inhaling dust contaminated with *Histoplasma,* a genus of parasitic fungi. *Histoplasma* is especially common in the rural Midwest. The disease ranges from a mild, self-limiting infection to a fatal disease. Antibiotic treatment is prescribed.

Coccidioidomycosis. Also known as San Joaquin Valley fever, coccidioidomycosis is caused by a fungus that grows in hot, dry areas, especially in the southwestern United States. It ranges from an

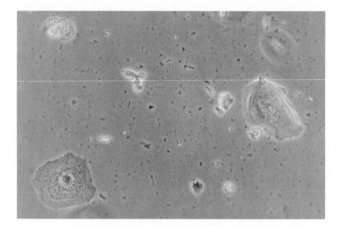

Figure 22-8 *Candida albicans* is an example of fungi.

acute, self-limiting disease involving the respiratory organs to a progressive, chronic disease that may involve almost any part of the body. Antibiotic treatment is needed for the progressive form of the disease.

Dermatomycosis. Dermatomycosis is any fungus infection of the skin. It may occur on various parts of the body. There are several common names for skin infections caused by fungi, depending on the part of the body infected. Athlete's foot refers to a fungal skin infection of the foot; jock itch refers to a fungal infection of the groin and perineum. The fungi thrive on moisture, so the affected areas should be kept clean and dry. Treatment generally is with topical fungicides.

Thrush and Other Yeast Infections. Yeast infections frequently are seen in POLs. Generally yeast infections are caused by *Candida albicans,* a gram positive pathogenic strain. Thrush is a yeast infection of the mouth that often occurs in infants. Vaginal yeast infections also are common, especially in pregnancy, with antibiotic use, and in patients with diabetes mellitus. In addition to a well-balanced diet and good hygiene, treatment of these infections includes fungicidal drugs and antibiotics.

Tests for Fungal Infections. To test for fungal infections of the nails, skin, and vagina, a specimen is collected from the infected area. Vaginal specimens are described here, but the same general procedure applies to specimens from other parts of the body.

The physician collects the vaginal specimen by holding two swabs together and swabbing the cervix, fornix, and vaginal walls. The specimen is placed in a small amount (about 0.5 mL) of saline solution in a tube. The swabs are mixed and squeezed against the wall of the tube to make certain that the solution contains the entire collected specimen. Then, a drop of the saline solution is transferred with one of the swabs to a microscope slide. One drop of 10 percent potassium hydroxide (KOH) solution is added to the drop on the slide. The liquid on the slide is covered immediately with a coverslip, and the underside of the slide is heated over a light bulb or flame. Boiling is avoided.

After the slide cools, it is examined under both low power and dry high power objectives for fungal cells, hyphae (mold filaments), and yeast cells. Under the microscope, fungi may appear as a tangled mat. Fungal cells generally are larger than are bacterial cells, and they have definite, thick walls. Fungal cells vary in both size and shape (round, ovoid, or elongated). Hyphae look like filamentous, branching chains. Although yeast has a characteristic appearance (rounded single cells with buds), it may be mistaken for red blood cells in urine specimens. Closer inspection reveals different cell sizes and budding.

Protozoa

Protozoa are single-celled organisms in the animal kingdom. There are several species pathogenic to humans, including *Entamoeba histolytica, Giardia lamblia,* and *Trichomonas vaginalis.*

Entamoeba histolytica. This **protozoan** parasite causes amoebic dysentery, which is characterized by diarrhea, intestinal bleeding, and fatigue. It is spread by contaminated water and food and by flies. Amoebic dysentery is common in third-world countries, and occasional cases are seen in the United States.

Similar nonpathogenic organisms may be confused with this pathogen. Diagnosis is made from stool specimens in reference laboratories.

Giardia lamblia. This protozoan may cause malabsorption syndrome and weight loss as well as diarrhea and gastrointestinal discomfort. Stool specimens processed by POLs may be analyzed in a reference laboratory for the presence of cyst and trophozoite stages of the giardia's life cycle. (See Figure 22-9(a).)

Trichomonas vaginalis. This protozoan is transmitted sexually. It infects the vagina of females and the prostate gland of males. While it may be asymptomatic in males, in females it causes profuse vaginal discharge, with intense burning, chafing, and itching. Once diagnosed, both sexual partners are treated for infection. Although asymptomatic, a male may reinfect his female partner if he is not treated.

Trichomonas pathogens are easy to observe microscopically in a wet mount preparation of saline solution under a coverslip. The specimen should be examined immediately because the parasites quickly lose their mobility and then resemble white blood cells. Occasionally, *Trichomonas* are seen alive in urinary sedimentation examinations. It is a relatively large microorganism, with four anterior antennae and an undulating membrane (see Figure 22-9(b)).

Helminths

Helminths are true worms as opposed to the larval forms of insects. A number of helminth species parasitize the human intestinal tract, including tapeworms, hookworms, pinworms, whipworms, and roundworms. The majority of worm infestations occur in tropical areas, but they may be found worldwide.

Diagnosis of helminth infestation involves identifying either the microscopic eggs or the adult worms, most commonly in fecal specimens. Without specialized training, it is difficult to distinguish the eggs from other fecal matter. Except for detection of pinworms, which is an easy test, fecal specimens should be analyzed in reference laboratories. State, regional, and local health departments often provide diagnostic services for helminth infestations as well. Mailing tubes usually are supplied by the diagnostic laboratory, but they also can be purchased from supply houses.

Tapeworms. Tapeworm infestations are caused by several different species of worms in the subclass *Cestoda.* Tapeworms vary in length from a few

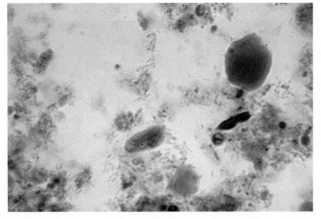

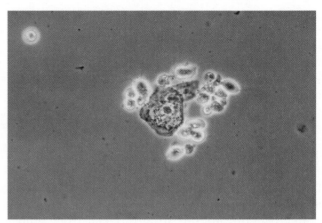

(a) (b)

Figure 22-9 (a) *Giardia lamblia* cyst; (b) *Trichomonas vaginalis.*

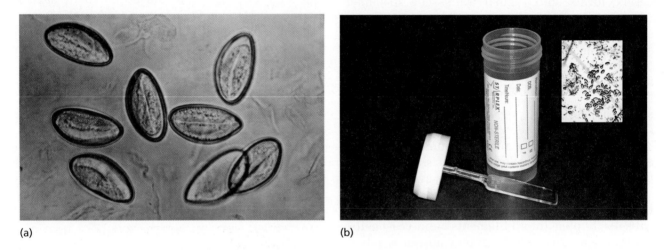

(a) (b)

Figure 22-10 (a) *Enterobius vermicularis* (pinworm) eggs. (b) Pinworm paddle collection device.

millimeters to several meters. Adult tapeworms live in the small intestine, anchored to the intestinal wall by a scolex—the so-called head, which has hooks and suckers for attachment. Tapeworms absorb food from the intestinal tract of the host through their skin. Their eggs are excreted in the host's feces and may be ingested by intermediate vertebrate hosts such as cows, pigs, or fish. The eggs develop into larvae in the muscle tissues of the intermediate hosts. Human infection occurs when inadequately cooked meat from an infected animal is eaten.

Hookworms. Hookworm infestations are caused by species belonging to the class *Nematoda.* Larval forms enter the body through bare feet and then migrate through the blood stream to the lungs. Eventually, the larvae are coughed up and then swallowed, thereby entering the intestinal tract. In the intestines, they attach to the intestinal wall

and suck blood for nourishment. Hookworm infestations can cause lethargy, abdominal pain, and microcytic hypochromic anemia.

Pinworms. Pinworm infestations are caused by the species *Enterobius vermicularis* (see Figure 22-10(a)), also in the class *Nematoda.* They live in the colon unattached to the host. The eggs are deposited in the perianal region, where they may cause itching and come into contact with the hands and fingernails of the host. From there, they may be carried to the mouth, where they are swallowed and reinfect the host's intestinal tract. Other family members may be infected through contaminated clothing and bedding. Infections are more common in children than in adults. Good hygiene is the best prevention for pinworm infestations.

Diagnosis of pinworm infestation is based on the microscopic detection of the eggs or worms trapped on pinworm paddles. (See Figure 22-10(b).)

Collection of pinworm specimens should be made by the patient or parents of the patient. To collect a pinworm specimen, press the sticky side of the paddle device to the perianal area. The paddle is then inserted into the cuvette for transport to the lab. Some pinworm tape strips can be placed directly on the stage of the microscope and scanned for eggs or larvae.

Roundworms. Roundworm infestations are caused by the species *Ascaris lumbricoides,* a large nematode. Eggs are passed in the feces of infected hosts, incubate in the soil, and are ingested by new hosts. The adult form lives in the small intestine and may cause abdominal pain and vomiting.

MICROBIAL TECHNIQUES

This section describes procedures and materials needed to identify microorganisms in POLs. Because safety is of primary importance when dealing with potentially infectious microorganisms, this subject is addressed first.

Safety

Safety must always be a top priority in microbiology work. Even when the strains of microorganisms being handled are not considered highly pathogenic, there is risk of serious infection. The best safeguards against accidental microbial infection in POLs are knowledge of the dangers involved and careful attention to aseptic techniques.

Aseptic Technique. The practice of **aseptic techniques** ensures that pathogens remain isolated. Isolation prevents accidental exposure of lab workers and patients as well as contamination of specimens by unwanted organisms from the outside. When dealing with potentially infective microorganisms, lab workers always should wear appropriate personal protective equipment, including

- disposable gloves
- plexiglass face shields to protect the face from spatters
- laboratory jackets, aprons, or gowns to absorb spatters

When performing microbiology collections and procedures, all spills should be wiped up immediately with disinfectant. Counters, work surfaces, and refrigerators should be disinfected daily with surface disinfectant. All contaminated equipment and instruments should be sterilized as they are used. Specimens and cultures should be sterilized by autoclave or incineration. The wire loop that is used to manipulate specimens and cultures should be sterilized with an electric incinerator. (See Figure 22-11(c).) Alternatively disposable plastic loops may be used. These save time and labor. Sterile containers always should be used, as should sterile media and swabs, which are available from supply houses.

Tools Needed for Microbiology Procedures

Several specialized instruments and supplies are needed for microbiology procedures in POLs. Some are reusable, but many supplies are disposable.

Loops and Needles. Loops are used to manipulate very small amounts of specimen. They come in different sizes, most commonly 10 μL (0.01 mL) and 1.0 μL (0.001 mL). There are reusable wire loops and disposable plastic loops. Wire loops may be made of platinum iridium, a very expensive metal, or nickel chromium, which is cheaper. Loops always must be sterile. (See Figure 22-11(a).)

By touching a colony with a loop, lab personnel can lift small amounts of microorganisms from one solid medium onto another and can streak the microbes in thin ribbons on the second medium to start a new culture. The loop can be used to move colonies to and from broth for incubation and study. It also can be used to transfer drops of water or saline solution to slides to mix with bacteria for smears.

Alternatively, needles are used for inoculating media with microorganisms for culturing. The same precautions should be taken in using inoculating needles as other needles used in POLs. Needles also should be sterilized after every use.

Swabs and Media. The swabs and media used in microbiology work in POLs usually are purchased sterile and prepackaged from commercial supply houses. Both must remain sterile and free of all contaminants until use. Only then can lab workers be certain that the growth of bacteria on culture media is of pathogens and not contaminants. In addition, media should be kept in a dark refrigerator until just before use, when they should be allowed to come to room temperature. (See Figure 22-11(b).)

Testing Microbiology Specimens

After a microbiology specimen is collected, care must be taken not to contaminate the specimen or allow it to dry out. It must be transported in a sterile container.

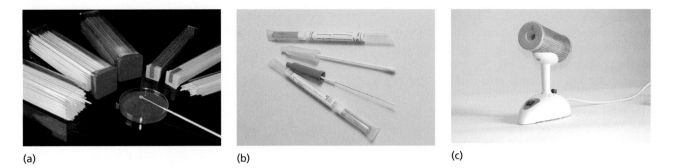

(a)   (b)   (c)

Figure 22-11 (a) Disposable plastic loops. (b) Disposable sterile swabs come in various sizes. (c) Electric incinerator.

Smears. In order to study microbes under the microscope, a smear must be made. This may be a direct smear, made from a swab of the affected area to provide a quick view of the specimen, or the specimen may be cultured first and then a smear made from the cultured organisms.

A direct smear is made by rolling a specimen swab across the surface of a sterilized glass slide. The smear should be air dried and then fixed, either by heat or by methanol fixation. Fixing the smear coagulates the protein in the bacteria, adhering them to the slide so that they will not wash away when the smear is stained.

After the slide has cooled, the smear is stained with Gram stain. Then, the slide is examined under the oil-immersion objective of the microscope. The morphology, stain affinity, density, and other notable characteristics of the specimen are reported.

A smear from a culture is made by first preparing the slide to accept the pathogen. A small drop of distilled water is added with a sterile loop to the top of the slide. Then, the loop is resterilized and touched to an isolated culture, and a very small amount is withdrawn and mixed with the water on the slide to make an emulsion. The emulsion is spread thinly on the slide so that it is about as wide as a dime or nickel. Then it is fixed, stained, and viewed in the same way as a direct smear.

Cultures. A **direct culture,** or primary culture, is grown by inoculating patient specimens directly onto the culture medium. The specimen swab is rolled on the medium to get as much as possible of the specimen from the swab. A **pure culture** is one that is grown from a single colony of bacteria that was taken from the direct culture. Pure cultures generally are preferred to direct cultures because they further isolate the pathogen.

> **Technique Tip**
>
> When removing covers from sterile containers such as the caps of tubes, hold them in your other hand. Do not lay them down. If you must lay a cover down, make sure to face the inner surface upward, away from the counter. Dispose of waste immediately without touching the counter.

Throat Cultures for Group A *Streptococcus*

While viruses cause some sore throats, Group A strep is considered to be the major cause of sore throats due to bacterial infection. If possible, the diagnosis of strep throat is made during the patient's office visit with an antigen-antibody test. However, if only a few strep organisms are present, a false negative may result. In this case, a confirmatory test is made by culturing for the Group A strep organism. Diagnosis is based on hemolysis of blood in the culture medium by streptolysin, an enzyme produced by the strep organism that lyses red blood cells.

Collecting and Handling Specimens. A sufficient sample of microorganisms must be collected to grow a representative throat culture. This is done by taking a throat swab with a sterile Dacron or calcium alginate swab. A cotton swab should not be used because it may inhibit the growth of the strep organism.

With the tongue held down with a tongue depressor, the specimen should be taken directly from the back of the throat and tonsils. The swab should be rubbed on these areas, not just patted. This can be accomplished quickly and relatively easily by using a horizontal, or lazy eight, motion or a large O with the swab. Two swabs should be

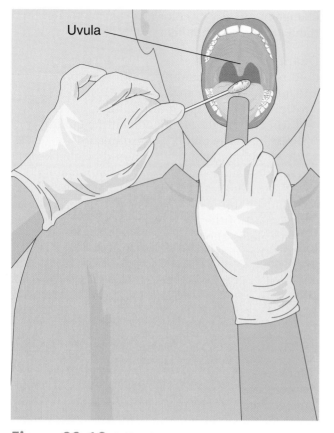

Uvula

Figure 22-12 Collecting and processing a throat culture: swab the throat area; swab any white patches on the tonsils.

To inoculate the throat swab onto the blood-agar plate, follow these steps:

* Label the bottom of the agar plate with the patient's name and chart number. (The container will be stored upside down.)
* Using the throat swab, inoculate a small area of the plate by rolling the swab over it. Then discard the swab in disinfectant or a biohazard container.
* Use a sterile loop to streak one-fifth of the outside area of the plate, overlapping some of the area where the swab was rolled.
* Without sterilizing or withdrawing the loop, proceed to the next area.
* Continue around the plate in a clockwise direction until you cover most of the outside surface. Make the final quadrant into a "fish-tail" streak. (See Figure 22-13.)
* Immediately sterilize the loop if it is wire or discard it into disinfectant or a biohazard container if it is plastic. Do not lay the contaminated loop down on the counter.

done at the same time so that if one swab is used for the enzyme test and is negative, the second swab is available for a culture to be planted. This is especially important with children and patients with a sensitive gag reflex. (See Figure 22-12.)

The teeth and inside of the mouth must be avoided when the swab is inserted and withdrawn. If the swab touches them, the culture may be representative of the flora of the mouth, not the throat.

If the specimen is to be forwarded to a reference laboratory, the swab should be placed immediately in the sterile container with transport media. The tube should be labeled with the patient's name and chart number, and the specimen should be processed according to the instructions provided by the reference laboratory.

Culturing Specimens. Throat cultures are grown on 5 percent sheep-blood agar. This medium provides good growth potential and is best for showing the hemolytic activity of Group A strep. The culture medium may have inhibitors added to suppress the growth of normal throat flora for better growth of the strep organism.

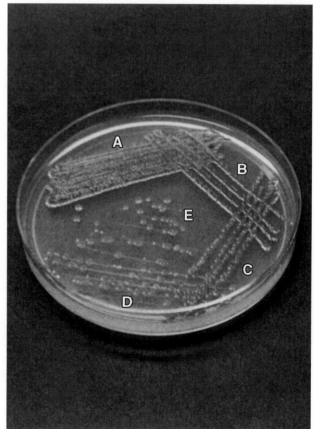

Figure 22-13 Inoculate the throat culture by rolling the swab over a small area of the plate. Using a sterile loop, streak the plate as in the figure. Proper streaking yields colonies of bacteria isolated as in areas D and E.

Place a disk of the antibiotic **bacitracin** in the center of the first quadrant of the agar plate to give an early indication of the presence of Group A strep. A zone of growth inhibition around the disk is indicative of Group A strep because bacitracin inhibits the growth of this organism.

For a pure culture, a single colony of the pathogen is taken from the first culture with a sterile loop. The colony then is streaked onto a new blood-agar plate. A bacitracin disk is placed in the center of the streaked area. If need be, pure cultures for more than one patient can be grown on the same agar plate. (See Figure 22-14.)

Interpreting the Results. Cultures are read for evidence of Group A strep after they incubate for 18 to 24 hours. Diagnosis is based on beta hemolysis of the blood agar by the streptolysin enzyme. Blood agar normally is semiopaque, and beta hemolysis makes it translucent. After beta hemolysis, there are large, colorless, translucent zones surrounding the colonies, both on the surface of the agar and within the stabs. The colonies themselves appear translucent to slightly opaque and are about the size of pinpoints.

Other bacteria, including *Staphylococcus,* produce beta hemolysis, but their colony morphology is different from that of strep. Normal throat bacteria produce a different type of hemolysis, called alpha hemolysis, which leads to distinctive greenish zones around the colonies. Colonies with no change in opacity or color in the agar surrounding them are those of nonhemolytic organisms.

Quality Control. Quality control for strep throat cultures requires careful attention to procedures and manufacturer's instructions. It also involves proficiency testing, maintenance of quality-culturing materials, and documenting quality control results in the quality control records.

New shipments of media should be checked on arrival for visible signs of contamination and deterioration such as cracking, drying, hemolysis, leaking, and bubbling. Media lot numbers should be kept as part of the quality control record. Sleeves of agar plates should be stored agar-side up and kept in the plastic sleeves until needed. Opening too soon can allow drying or contamination. Each new vial of bacitracin disks should be checked for effectiveness by testing a disk on a known beta Group A strep culture.

Genitourinary Cultures for Gonorrhea

Gonorrhea is a prevalent, sexually transmitted disease caused by the bacterium *Neisseria gonorrhoeae.* Symptoms include inflammation and pus. Early diagnosis is important for successful treatment because, without treatment, gonorrhea can lead to sterility and other complications.

> **Note**
>
> This section only applies to genitourinary tract specimens, not those collected from the eye, rectum, or throat. Specimens from the latter areas should be sent to a reference laboratory.

By law, a positive test for gonorrhea in POLs must be reported to the state health department. A positive POL test for gonorrhea also should be confirmed by a reference laboratory if

- it appears to be an antibiotic-resistant strain
- the clinical picture is at odds with the test result
- legal issues are involved (for example, the patient is a child)

Culturing *Neisseria gonorrhoeae.* Gonorrhea often can be diagnosed from a direct smear of penile exudate, but when a direct smear fails to reveal the organism, a culture may be made. For a specimen culture of suspected gonorrhea, Thayer-Martin or NYC agar medium should be used. Both are enrichment media that enhance the growth of *Neisseria*

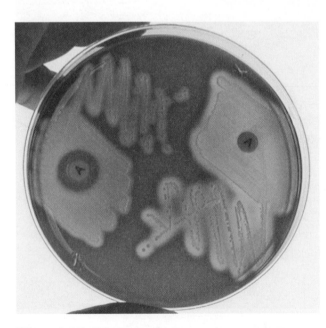

Figure 22-14 Group A strep on blood agar. The bacitracin disk on the left indicates presumptive positive for *Streptococcus pyogenes.* The bacitracin-resistant test on the right is not Group A.

gonorrhoeae while inhibiting competitive organisms from the genitourinary area. The media may be purchased separately or as part of self-contained kits that also contain carbon dioxide–generating capsules. Recall that this pathogen requires a carbon dioxide atmosphere.

The specimen swab should be plated as soon as possible after the sample is collected because the pathogen can survive just 30 minutes away from the moisture and warmth of the human body or a substitute medium. This also is why *Neisseria gonorrhoeae* specimens and cultures never should be refrigerated. If there is a delay in transporting the specimen to the laboratory, a transport medium such as the JEMBEC® should be used. (See Figure 22-15.) This rectangular plate contains a modified Thayer-Martin transport medium. After the specimen has been inoculated onto the plate, the plate and a CO_2 tablet are placed in a zipper storage bag. Moisture in the medium activates the CO_2 tablet, creating a carbon dioxide atmosphere in the bag. The culture can then be placed in the 35-degrees-Celsius incubator and observed for any growth.

In inoculating the plate, all areas of the swab are rolled over the medium, which has been brought to room temperature. Then, the swab is discarded into a biohazard container. A sterile loop is used to streak the specimen back and forth across the medium. The inoculated plate should be placed immediately in the incubator at 35 degrees Celsius in an atmosphere of 3 to 10 percent carbon dioxide.

After the culture has incubated for 24 to 48 hours, it is examined for the presence of *Neisseria gonorrhoeae*. If the culture is negative, it should be incubated for another 24 hours (or a total of 72 hours) and examined again before being discarded.

Identifying *Neisseria gonorrhoeae*. Colonies of *Neisseria gonorrhoeae* are small, smooth, translucent, and grayish. However, colony morphology is insufficient for positive identification of the pathogen. Several other microorganisms, including both bacteria and yeast, may grow on the inhibitory media and present a similar appearance. Positive identification of *Neisseria gonorrhoeae* must be based on additional factors, including

- test gram negative and look like coffee beans facing each other
- test positive on the oxidase test

In the **oxidase test,** oxidase reagent is added to a colony of suspected *Neisseria gonorrhoeae*. One or two drops of reagent may be added directly to the colony on the culture. Alternatively, one or two drops of reagent may be used to moisten filter paper and a loop may be used to smear microbes on the moistened paper. Instructions from the manufacturer of the oxidase reagent should be followed. If a black or dark blue color occurs within 30 seconds of adding the reagent, the result is positive and the organism is *Neisseria gonorrhoeae*. (See Figure 22-16.)

> **Caution!**
>
> Certain wire loops may give positive results on the oxidase test because iron in the wire reacts with the reagent.

Quality Control. Quality control in *Neisseria gonorrhoeae* testing requires adherence to proper techniques, occasional proficiency testing of unknown samples, and maintenance of the quality of the culture media and oxidase reagent. Remember to document the quality control results in the quality control journal.

Each new batch of culture media must be tested by inoculation with both *Escherichia coli* and *Neisseria gonorrhoeae*. The media should grow *Neisseria gonorrhoeae* and inhibit *Escherichia coli* after 24 hours of incubation. Alternatively, pretested media can be obtained from reference laboratories, which also supply documentation of the quality control testing. This documentation must be kept in the quality control records of POLs.

The oxidase reagent must be checked each day it is used. This is done by testing a known sample of *Neisseria gonorrhoeae*.

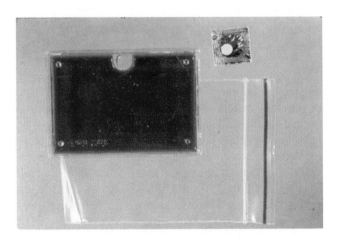

Figure 22-15 JEMBEC® transport culture medium for inoculation of *Neisseria*.

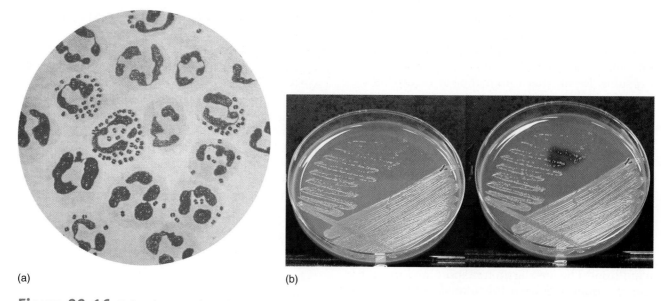

(a)

(b)

Figure 22-16 *Neisseria gonorrhea.* (a) Gram negative intracellular diplococci; (b) oxidase-positive test on the right.

Urine Cultures

Urine cultures usually are made to diagnose **urinary tract infection (UTI).** The urinary tract is predisposed to infection because urine has nutrients capable of supporting bacterial growth. If urine is not completely voided from the bladder at each urination (as occurs in some medical conditions), bacteria may grow in the bladder. The ureter is only about 1.5 inches long in adult females, so their bladders are relatively accessible to bacteria. That is why UTIs are more common in women than in men.

Urine cultures differ from strep throat and gonorrhea cultures in that the number of bacteria present are more important in diagnosis than are the type of bacteria present. A bacterial concentration of over 100,000 organisms per milliliter indicates UTI, while a concentration below 10,000 per milliliter is often insignificant. A concentration between 10,000 and 100,000 organisms per milliliter is inconclusive and must be confirmed by another culture or by clinical evidence.

Microorganisms That Cause Urinary Tract Infections. Most UTIs result from migration of the patient's own intestinal tract flora to the urinary tract. Intestinal tract flora are predominantly gram negative. *Escherichia coli,* a gram negative organism, accounts for 80 percent of UTI. Most of the remaining 20 percent of UTIs are due to the gram negative species *Kiebsiella pneumoniae, Enterobacter aerogenes,* and species of *Proteus* and *Pseudomonas.* Gram positive organisms like strep and staph account for very few UTIs.

> ### Reducing the Risk of UTI
>
> Female patients should be encouraged to follow hygienic practices that reduce the risk of UTIs. After using the toilet, they always should wipe from front to back. This helps prevent contamination of the ureter by bacteria from the intestinal tract.

Collecting and Handling Specimens. Patients must be instructed in how to obtain a clean-catch, midstream urine specimen. The urine specimen should not be centrifuged before culturing. Other urinalysis tests of the same specimen should be postponed until after the culture is made in order to prevent contamination of the culture.

Gram Staining. A Gram stain can provide a valuable guide to the type of antibiotic that should be prescribed for a UTI. Antibiotics are classified according to the type of bacteria against which they are most effective. Some antibiotics are most effective against gram negative organisms, while others are most effective against gram positive organisms.

Several methods are available for culturing urine for a Gram stain test. In the traditional method, a known amount of uncentrifuged urine is measured with either a 0.01 mL or 0.001 mL loop and placed on two different media:

- general-purpose sheep-blood agar
- gram positive-inhibiting media (either MacConkey or EMB medium)

The media are streaked in a crisscross pattern and incubated for 24 hours. Then, the colonies are counted and the concentration of bacteria is calculated with the following formula:

$$\text{Bacteria/mL} = \text{Number of colonies} \times \text{Conversion factor}$$

where the conversion factor is 100 for the 0.01 mL loop and 1,000 for the 0.001 mL loop.

Two types of commercial culture kits are available for urine testing: the dipstick paddle and the coated tube. The dipstick paddle has a selective medium for gram negative organisms on one side and a nonselective medium on the other side that grows both gram negative and gram positive organisms. The media are inoculated by pouring urine over the paddle or by dipping the paddle in urine. After inoculation, the paddle is replaced in its sterile bottle and incubated at 37 degrees Celsius for 18 to 24 hours.

The coated-tube culture has a special enriched medium and color indicators on its inner surface. Urine is poured into the tube and then poured out. The cap is placed on the tube, and the urine residue is incubated in the same way as in other urine cultures.

For both commercial culture kits, the manufacturer's inserts include color charts and instructions for counting colonies and calculating bacteria concentration. When identification and colony counts are made from the comparison chart, the growth should be reported as "presumptive." This is particularly important when Gram stains and isolation of the bacteria are not performed as additional tests. (Precise identification requires more complex testing to differentiate between strains of bacteria.) The term "presumptive" is a precaution in keeping with CLIA and the registration status of moderate-level POLs. It indicates to the medical staff the extent of testing. If needed, bacteria grown with the kits may be used for additional testing, transferred to other cultures, or sent to reference laboratories for further study.

Contaminated Cultures

Individual UTIs usually are caused by one type of bacteria. If a culture shows a mix of three or more different organisms, then you should suspect contamination.

Chemical Tests. Chemical tests are available to identify the organisms found in urine cultures. The **catalase test** uses hydrogen peroxide to distinguish *Streptococcus* from *Staphylococcus,* both gram positive organisms. Staph produces bubbles when exposed to 30 percent hydrogen peroxide. Strep does not.

The **coagulase test** demonstrates the presence of an enzyme produced by pathogenic staph organisms. Nonpathogenic strains, such as those found on the skin, lack the enzyme and test negative. In the test, staph organisms are mixed with a drop of rabbit plasma. Clotting indicates a positive result—the presence of the enzyme.

Latex slide kits are also available for rapid presumptive tests for *Staphylococcus aureus.* These are latex agglutination tests that use red blood cells and anti–*S. aureus* to react with suspected colonies from a culture. Results are fast and convenient for use in POLs.

Note

Forward unusual organisms growing in a urine culture to a reference laboratory for further identification.

Another bacterial identification system is Enterotube® (Roche, Inc., Nutley, New Jersey). The Enterotube identification kit is a multitest system designed to confirm the identification of various pure culture isolates. Each tube contains eight types of differential agar that allows for biochemical testing at one time. Changes in color can confirm the identity of pathogenic bacteria. This testing procedure takes from 24 to 48 hours to complete. (See Figure 22-17.)

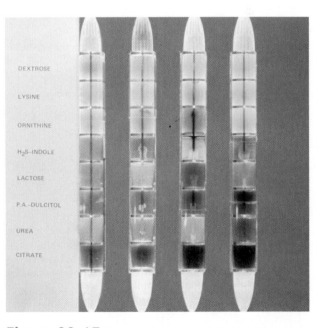

Figure 22-17 Enterotube® is used to identify bacteria from pure cultures.

Quality Control. Quality control in urine cultures is maintained by the same general methods used in other types of cultures. Media quality is maintained by visual inspection, proper storage, and usage before the expiration date. Reagent quality is maintained by testing. Vials of catalase and coagulase should be checked upon receipt. Catalase can be checked with a known staph species or a drop of blood. Coagulase is checked with *Staphylococcus aureus.* Remember to document your quality-control results in the quality control journal.

> **Caution!**
>
> Treat all urine cultures as biohazardous at all times and discard them in a biohazard container.

PROCEDURE 22-1

Fixing a Bacterial Smear for Staining

Goal

After successfully completing this procedure, you will be able to prepare a heat-fixed bacterial smear with microorganisms supplied by the instructor or from a swab of normal microflora in your mouth.

Completion Time

15 minutes

Equipment and Supplies

- Disposable gloves
- Impermeable apron or laboratory jacket
- Face shield
- Hand disinfectant
- Surface disinfectant
- Paper towels and tissues
- Biohazard container
- Source of microorganisms
- Bunsen burner or hot plate
- Glass slides
- Sterile cotton swab or sterilized loop
- Distilled water or saline solution
- Forceps

Instructions

Read through the list of equipment and supplies that you will need and the steps of the procedure. Be sure that you understand each step before you begin. Then complete each step correctly and in the proper order.

*Steps marked with (*) are critical and must have the maximum points to pass.

Performance Standards	Points Awarded	Maximum Points
1. Put on a protective jacket, gown, or apron; wash your hands with disinfectant, dry them, and put on gloves and face protection.		10
2. Follow standard precautions.		10
3. Collect and prepare the appropriate equipment.		5
4. Using a sterile loop or swab, place one loop or a small drop of water or saline solution on a clean glass slide.		5
5. With a sterile swab, rub your teeth and gums gently, turning the swab to cover all sides with mouth microflora. Alternatively, use a sterile loop or swab to obtain a small sample of microorganisms from your instructor. If you use a nondisposable loop, sterilize it before and after in an incinerator until red hot and sterile.		10
6. Place the mouth swab, or the microorganism specimen, in the drop of water or saline on the slide; turn the swab gently to mix the microorganism into the liquid.		10

7.	Stir the liquid and mouth microflora, or microorganism specimen, until they form a thin emulsion about the size of a dime or nickel.		5
8.	Set aside the slide and allow it to air dry to avoid scattering microorganisms; do not wave or blow on the slide.		5
9.	After the slide has air dried, heat fix it by passing it two or three times over the laboratory burner or allow to heat fix with a slide warmer. Do not let the slide get too hot.		5
10.	Lay the slide aside to cool before staining.		5
11.	Discard disposable supplies in the biohazard container.		5
12.	Disinfect other equipment and return it to storage.		5
13.	Remove your gloves, dispose, and wash your hands.		5
	Total Points		**85**

Overall Procedural Evaluation

Student Name _____

Signature of Instructor _____ Date _____

Comments _____

_____

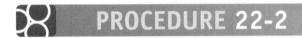

PROCEDURE 22-2

Gram Staining a Bacterial Smear

Goal

After successfully completing this procedure, you will be able to prepare a Gram stained smear from an unstained heat-fixed bacterial smear.

Completion Time

15 minutes

Equipment and Supplies

- Disposable gloves
- Impermeable apron or laboratory jacket
- Face shield
- Hand disinfectant
- Surface disinfectant
- Paper towels and tissues
- Biohazard container
- Unstained, heat-fixed smear of microorganisms
- Staining rack
- Squeeze bottle or beaker of tap water
- Gram stain kit containing reagents (crystal violet, iodine, ethyl alcohol or acetone, and safranin)
- Eyedropper or Pasteur pipette
- Forceps

Instructions

Read through the list of equipment and supplies that you will need and the steps of the procedure. Be sure that you understand each step before you begin. Then complete each step correctly and in the proper order.

*Steps marked with (*) are critical and must have the maximum points to pass.

Performance Standards	Points Awarded	Maximum Points
1. Put on a protective jacket, gown, or apron; wash your hands with disinfectant, dry them, and put on gloves and face shield		10
2. Follow standard precautions.		10

—table continued

Performance Standards	Points Awarded	Maximum Points
3. Collect and prepare the appropriate equipment.		5
4. Place the unstained, fixed smear on the staining rack, with the smear side up.		5
5. Flood the slide with crystal violet solution and let it stand one minute.		5
6. At the end of one minute, rinse the stain off with tap water from a plastic squeeze bottle; drain off the excess water.		5
7. Flood the smear with iodine solution and let it stand for one minute.		5
8. At the end of 1 minute, wash the smear with tap water. Drain off the excess water.		5
9. Pick up the slide and decolorize (ethyl alcohol or acetone) for about 5 seconds until the dye no longer runs off the smear except in the thickest portion.		5
10. Wash the slide briefly with tap water.		5
11. Apply safranin for 1 minute to counterstain.		5
12. Wash it gently and briefly with tap water. Clean the back of the slide and blot the front dry with paper towel. Let air dry.		5
13. Clean the work surfaces following standard precautions.		5
14. Remove your gloves, dispose, and wash your hands.		5
Total Points		**80**

Overall Procedural Evaluation

Student Name _____

Signature of Instructor _____ Date _____

Comments _____

_____

PROCEDURE 22-3

Microscopic Examination of a Gram Stained Smear

Goal

After successfully completing this procedure, you will be able to examine a prepared Gram stained smear and report the morphology and Gram stain reaction of the microorganisms.

Completion Time

15 minutes

Equipment and Supplies

- Disposable gloves
- Impermeable apron or laboratory coat
- Hand disinfectant
- Surface disinfectant
- Paper towels and tissues
- Biohazard container
- Microscope
- Immersion oil
- Lens paper
- Gram stained bacterial slide

Instructions

Read through the list of equipment and supplies that you will need and the steps of the procedure. Be sure that you understand each step before you begin. Then complete each step correctly and in the proper order.

*Steps marked with (*) are critical and must have the maximum points to pass.

Performance Standards	Points Awarded	Maximum Points
1. Put on a protective jacket, gown, or apron; wash your hands with disinfectant, dry them, and put on gloves.		10
2. Follow standard precautions.		10
3. Collect and prepare the appropriate equipment.		5
4. Secure the slide, stained side up, on the microscope stage.		5
5. Focus the slide under the 10X objective.		5
6. Focus the slide under the 45X objective.		5
7. Move the 45X objective out of the way and place a drop of immersion oil on the slide.		5
8. Move the 100X objective into place and focus with the fine-focus adjustment knob until the bacteria come into view. Adjust the light as necessary.		10
9. If you cannot adjust the focus, check to see that the slide is right-side up, then return to the 10X objective and repeat steps 5 through 8.		5
10. Scan the slide to find a thin area. Thick areas do not show cell morphology well.		5
11. Identify the type of bacteria by shape such as coccus, bacillus, and spirochete and describe any other morphology, such as chains, clusters, and palisades. Record the results.		10
12. Classify the bacteria by stain reaction (purple are gram positive and pink or red are gram negative). Record the results.		10
13. To save the slide, wipe the immersion oil off the slide with a soft tissue.		5
14. Discard disposable supplies and equipment in a biohazard container.		5
15. Clean and store the microscope in its proper storage area.		5
16. Clean work area using standard precautions.		5
17. Remove your jacket, gown, or apron, and gloves; wash your hands with disinfectant and dry them.		5
Total Points		**110**

Overall Procedural Evaluation

Student Name _____

Signature of Instructor _____ Date _____

Comments _____

_____

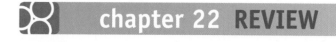

chapter 22 REVIEW

Using Terminology

Define the following terms in the spaces provided.

1. Virus

_____

_____

_____

2. Coccus

_____

_____

_____

3. Spiral bacteria

_____

_____

_____

4. Gram positive

_____

_____

_____

5. Gram negative

_____

_____

_____

6. Fastidious bacteria

_____

_____

_____

7. Catalase test

_____

_____

_____

8. Coagulase test

_____

_____

_____

9. Helminth

_____

_____

_____

10. Fungus

_____

_____

_____

11. Protozoan

_____

_____

_____

12. Aseptic technique

_____

_____

_____

13. Pure culture

_____

_____

_____

14. Oxidase test

_____

_____

_____

15. Bacitracin

_____

_____

_____

16. Antibiotic

_____

_____

_____

17. Bacteria

_____

_____

_____

Multiple Choice

Choose the best answer for the following questions.

18. All of the following are examples of microorganisms that are visible under light microscopes except
    a. bacteria
    b. viruses
    c. protozoa
    d. yeast

19. The chemical test that distinguishes *Streptococcus* from *Staphylococcus* infections is the
    a. coagulase
    b. culture
    c. bacitracin
    d. catalase

20. Which of the following microbes are rod-shaped bacteria?
    a. *Staphyloccus*
    b. *Lactobacillus*
    c. *Streptococcus*
    d. *Giardia lamblia*

21. In microscope examination of a Gram stain smear, dark blue spherical-shaped bacteria arranged in chains were observed. They are most likely
    a. *Streptococcus*
    b. *Staphylococcus*
    c. *E. coli*
    d. rhinovirus

22. All of the following diseases are caused by viruses except
    a. common cold
    b. herpes
    c. infectious mononucleosis
    d. syphilis

Acquiring Knowledge

Answer the following questions in the spaces provided.

23. Identify several types of microorganisms that cause disease in humans and name some of the diseases that they cause.

    _____

    _____

    _____

24. Explain the relevance of microbiology to POLs.

    _____

    _____

    _____

25. Describe how infectious diseases are diagnosed.

    _____

    _____

    _____

26. Why are viral diseases sometimes difficult to diagnose and difficult to treat?

_____

_____

_____

27. Discuss the use of Gram stain in identifying bacteria.

_____

_____

_____

28. Besides staining and morphology, what differences among bacterial species aid in their identification?

_____

_____

_____

29. What factors must be appropriate for optimal growth of a given bacterial species?

_____

_____

_____

30. What temperature do most pathogenic bacteria prefer? Why?

_____

_____

_____

31. Discuss the role of sensitivity testing in selecting antibiotics for bacterial infections.

_____

_____

_____

32. Identify several human diseases caused by fungi.

_____

_____

_____

33. What treatment usually is prescribed for fungal infections?

_____

_____

_____

34. What diseases in humans are caused by protozoan microorganisms?

_____

_____

_____

35. What are some helminth infestations in humans?

_____

_____

_____

36. List the aseptic techniques for working with microorganisms in POLs.

_____

_____

_____

37. Why are aseptic techniques important when working with microbial pathogens?

_____

_____

_____

Applying Knowledge—On the Job

Answer the following questions in the spaces provided.

38. A suspected gonorrhea specimen has been collected in the clinic where you work. How should you process it?

_____

_____

_____

39. You have been asked to examine a blood-agar culture for the growth of Group A strep. What should you look for?

_____

_____

_____

40. Your laboratory just received a new supply of media for bacterial cultures. Where and how should you store them until they are used?

_____

_____

_____

41. The physician has requested that a Gram stain be made of the discharge from an infected sore to determine if the infecting organism is _Staphylococcus_. How should you make and stain the smear? What do you expect to see if it is a staph infection?

_____

_____

_____

APPENDICES

Standard Precautions and Other Laboratory Safety Information

STANDARD PRECAUTIONS

1. Treat all biological material as biohazardous and capable of transmitting HIV, HBV, HCV, and other diseases. Isolate and contain biological material from collection, through testing, to disposal.

2. Utilize the best personal protective equipment and engineering controls available. Wear gloves and laboratory coats. Wear a face shield if spatters are likely. Keep specimens enclosed when possible in covered containers. Use a biological safety cabinet for procedures that produce aerosols or droplets.

3. Sanitize equipment and work surfaces before and after procedures, after spills, and at the end of the day. Apply the principles of sanitation to all general laboratory work. Avoid careless techniques that scatter pathogenic contaminants through the laboratory.

4. Decontaminate blood and body fluid spills immediately. Use 10 percent household bleach or another approved disinfectant.

5. Do no pipetting by mouth. Avoid sharp instruments. Do not handle used needles with your hands. Do not recap used needles and do not remove used needles from syringes.

6. Wash your hands often—between each activity and whenever you touch biohazardous material. Contaminated hands provide a bridge for pathogens to escape from one area to another.

7. Keep your hands, pencils, and so forth away from your face and hair. Touching one's face is often a habit—a dangerous one. The eyes, nose, and mouth are lined with mucous membranes, which may be penetrated by pathogens.

8. Do not eat, drink, groom, or mix nonlaboratory activities within the laboratory even when relaxing or saving time. Do not store food, drink, or other nonlaboratory items in the laboratory area used for collecting, testing, or reagent storage. Leave pencils, laboratory jackets, and work gear in the laboratory. These provide bridges for pathogens to escape from the work area.

9. Keep informed about current developments concerning serious communicable diseases, including HIV (human immunodeficiency virus), HBV (hepatitis B), HCV (hepatitis C), and tuberculosis. Know the infection probability, the means of prevention, and the effectiveness of treatment. Consider the benefits of hepatitis B vaccination.

10. Keep safety in mind. Incorporate into your laboratory routine a safety review schedule that provides automatic reminders.

CHEMICAL SAFETY

1. Respect chemicals. Treat them as toxic unless they are known to be harmless.

2. Store chemicals in appropriate containers and cabinets. Flammable chemicals should be stored in fireproof cabinets. Reactive and caustic chemicals should be stored separately, in shatterproof containers.

3. Wear appropriate personal protective equipment. This includes suitable shoes to protect your feet, long sleeves, and gloves, where needed.

4. Avoid fumes and physical contact with chemicals. Never smell or taste a chemical. Wash your hands after handling chemicals.

5. Discard unidentified, contaminated, questionable, or out-of-date chemicals.

6. Use good inventory and storage techniques. Keep on hand only what is needed in an up-to-date inventory.

PHYSICAL SAFETY

1. Avoid electrical and physical accidents by anticipating and removing hazards before accidents happen.

2. Maintain an emergency plan. Display a drawing of the fire-escape routes in the building.

3. Do not block exits with furniture or storage. In case of fire, these items present a hazard.

4. Maintain a safety manual and review it periodically.

OSHA Bloodborne Pathogens Standard

(29 C.F.R. § 1910.1030)

Some of the most basic requirements of the OSHA Bloodborne Pathogens standard include

- A written exposure control plan, to be updated annually
- Use of standard precautions
- Consideration, implementations, and use of safer, engineered needles and sharps
- Use of engineering and work practice controls and appropriate personal protective equipment (gloves, face and eye protection, gowns)
- Hepatitis B vaccine provided to exposed employees at no cost

- Medical follow-up in the event of an exposure incident
- Use of labels or color coding for items such as sharps disposal boxes and containers for regulated waste, contaminated laundry, and certain specimens
- Employee training
- Proper containment of all regulated waste

www.osha.gov

Sample Blood and Body Fluid Exposure Report Form

Exposure Event Number _____

Sample Blood and Body Fluid Exposure Report Form

Facility name: _____

Name of exposed worker: Last _____ First: _____ ID #: _____

Date of exposure: _____ / _____ / _____   Time of exposure: _____ : _____ AM   PM (Circle)

Job title/occupation: _____   Department/work unit: _____

Location where exposure occurred: _____

Name of person completing form: _____

Section I. Type of Exposure *(Check all that apply.)*

❏ **Percutaneous (Needle or sharp object that was in contact with blood or body fluids)**
   (Complete Sections II, III, IV, and V.)

❏ **Mucocutaneous** *(Check below and complete Sections III, IV, and VI.)*
   ___ **Mucous Membrane**   ___ **Skin**

❏ **Bite** *(Complete Sections III, IV, and VI.)*

Section II. Needle/Sharp Device Information

(If exposure was <u>percutaneous</u>, provide the following information about the device involved.)

Name of device: _____   ❏ Unknown/Unable to determine

Brand/manufacturer: _____   ❏ Unknown/Unable to determine

Did the device have a sharps injury prevention feature, i.e., a "safety device"?

❏ Yes   ❏ No   ❏ Unknown/Unable to determine

If yes, when did the injury occur?

❏ Before activation of safety feature was appropriate   ❏ Safety feature failed after activation

❏ During activation of the safety feature   ❏ Safety feature not activated

❏ Safety feature improperly activated   ❏ Other: _____

Describe what happened with the safety feature, e.g., why it failed or why it was not activated: _____

_____

Section III. Employee Narrative *(Optional)*

Describe how the exposure occurred and how it might have been prevented:

_____

_____

_____

Section IV. Exposure and Source Information

A. Exposure Details: *(Check all that apply.)*

   1. Type of fluid or material (For body fluid exposures _only_, check which fluid in adjacent box.)

   ❏ Blood/blood products

   ❏ Visibly bloody body fluid*

   ❏ Non-visibly bloody body fluid*

   ❏ Visibly bloody solution (e.g., water used to clean a blood spill)

*Identify which body fluid		
— Cerebrospinal	— Urine	—Synovial
— Amniotic	—Sputum	—Peritoneal
— Pericardial	—Saliva	—Semen/vaginal
— Pleural	—Feces/stool	—Other/Unknown

   2. Body site of exposure. *(Check all that apply.)*

   ❏ Hand/finger   ❏ Eye   ❏ Mouth/nose   ❏ Face

   ❏ Arm   ❏ Leg   ❏ Other (Describe: _____)

   3. If percutaneous exposure:

   Depth of injury *(Check only one.)*

   ❏ Superficial (e.g., scratch, no or little blood)

   ❏ Moderate (e.g., penetrated through skin, wound bled)

   ❏ Deep (e.g., intramuscular penetration)

   ❏ Unsure/Unknown

   Was blood visible on device before exposure?   ❏ Yes   ❏ No   ❏ Unsure/Unknown

   4. If mucous membrane or skin exposure: *(Check only one.)*

   Approximate volume of material

   ❏ Small (e.g., few drops)

   ❏ Large (e.g., major blood splash)

   If skin exposure, was skin intact?   ❏ Yes   ❏ No   ❏ Unsure/Unknown

B. Source Information

1. **Was the source individual identified?**   ❏ Yes   ❏ No   ❏ Unsure/Unknown

2. **Provide the serostatus of the source patient for the following pathogens.**

	Positive	Negative	Refused	Unknown
HIV Antibody	❏	❏	❏	❏
HCV Antibody	❏	❏	❏	❏
HbsAg	❏	❏	❏	❏

3. **If known, when was the serostatus of the source determined?**

❏ Known at the time of exposure

❏ Determined through testing at the time of or soon after the exposure

Section V. Percutaneous Injury Circumstances

A. What device or item caused the injury?

Hollow-bore needle

❏ Hypodermic needle

— Attached to syringe — Attached to IV tubing
— Unattached

❏ Prefilled cartridge syringe needle

❏ Winged steel needle (i.e., butterfly type devices)
— Attached to syringe, tube holder, or IV tubing
— Unattached

❏ IV stylet

❏ Phlebotomy needle

❏ Spinal or epidural needle

❏ Bone marrow needle

❏ Biopsy needle

❏ Huber needle

❏ Other type of hollow-bore needle (type: _____)

❏ Hollow-bore needle, type unknown

Suture needle

❏ Suture needle

Glass

❏ Capillary tube

❏ Pipette (glass)

❏ Slide

❏ Specimen/test/vacuum

❏ Other: _____

Other sharp objects

❏ Bone chip/chipped tooth

❏ Bone cutter

❏ Bovie electrocautery device

❏ Bur

❏ Explorer

❏ Extraction forceps

❏ Elevator

❏ Histology cutting blade

❏ Lancet

❏ Pin

❏ Razor

❏ Retractor

❏ Rod (orthopaedic applications)

❏ Root canal file

❏ Scaler/curette

❏ Scalpel blade

❏ Scissors

❏ Tenaculum

❏ Trocar

❏ Wire

❏ Other type of sharp object

❏ Sharp object, type unknown

Other device or item

❏ Other: _____

B. Purpose or procedure for which sharp item was used or intended.

(Check <u>one procedure</u> type and complete information in corresponding box as applicable.)

❏ Establish intravenous or arterial access (Indicate type of line.) ⟶

❏ Access established intravenous or arterial line
(Indicate type of line <u>and</u> reason for line access.) ⟶

❏ Injection through skin or mucous membrane
(Indicate type of injection.)

❏ Obtain blood specimen (through skin)
(Indicate method of specimen collection.)

❏ Other specimen collection

❏ Suturing

❏ Cutting

❏ Other procedure

❏ Unknown

Type of Line
___ Peripheral   ___ Arterial
___ Central   ___ Other

Reason for Access
___ Connect IV infusion/piggyback
___ Flush with heparin/saline
___ Obtain blood specimen
___ Inject medication
___ Other: _____

Type of Injection
___ IM injection   ___ Epidural/spinal anesthesia
___ Skin test placement   ___ Other injection
___ Other ID/SQ injection

Type of Blood Sampling
___ Venipuncture   ___ Umbilical vessel
___ Arterial puncture   ___ Finger/heelstick
___ Dialysis/AV fistula site ___ Other blood sampling

C. When and how did the injury occur? (From the left-hand side of page, select the point during or after use that most closely represents when the injury occurred. In the corresponding right-hand box, select *one or two* circumstances that reflect how the injury happened.)

❏ During use of the item ⟶

Select one or two choices:
___ Patient moved and jarred device
___ While inserting needle/sharp
___ While manipulating needle/sharp
___ While withdrawing needle/sharp
___ Passing or receiving equipment
___ Suturing
___ Tying sutures
___ Manipulating suture needle in holder
___ Incising
___ Palpating/Exploring
___ Collided with co-worker or other during procedure
___ Collided with sharp during procedure
___ Sharp object dropped during procedure

❏ After use, before disposal of item ⟶

Select one or two choices:
___ Handling equipment on a tray or stand
___ Transferring specimen into specimen container
___ Processing specimens
___ Passing or transferring equipment
___ Recapping (missed or pierced cap)
___ Cap fell off after recapping
___ Disassembling device or equipment
___ Decontamination/processing of used equipment
___ During clean-up
___ In transit to disposal
___ Opening/breaking glass containers
___ Collided with co-worker/other person
___ Collided with sharp after procedure
___ Sharp object dropped after procedure
___ Struck by detached IV line needle

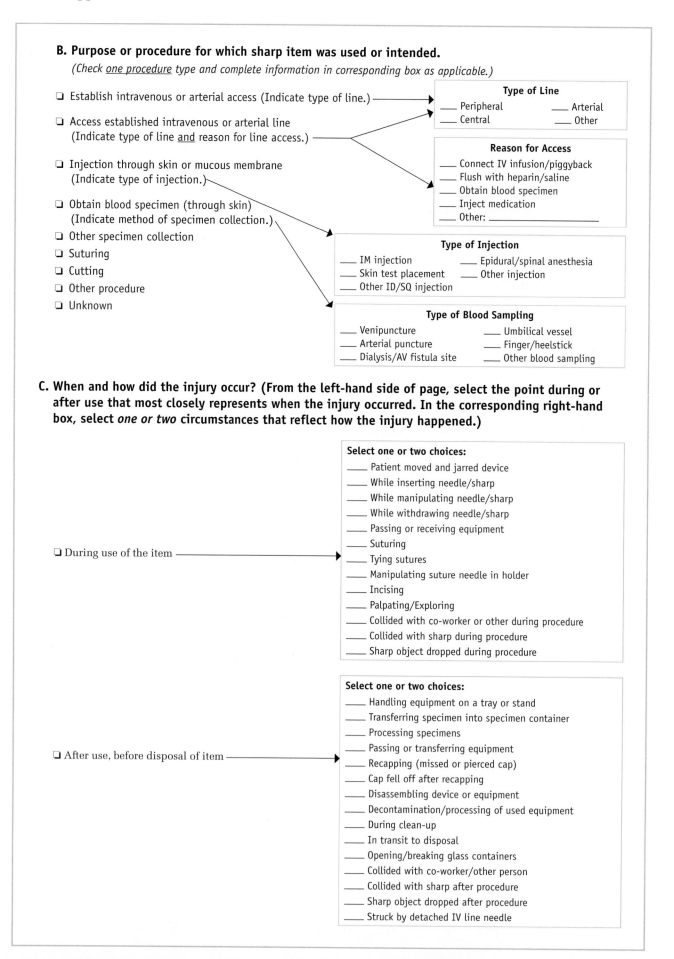

❏ During or after disposal of item ——————————➤

❏ Other (Describe): _____
_____
_____

❏ Unknown

Select one or two choices:
____ Placing sharp in container:
   ____ Injured by sharp being disposed
   ____ Injured by sharp already in container
____ While manipulating container
____ Overfilled sharps container
____ Punctured sharps container
____ Sharp protruding from open container
____ Sharp in unusual location:
   ____ In trash
   ____ In linen/laundry
   ____ Left on table/tray
   ____ Left in bed/mattress
   ____ On floor
   ____ In pocket/clothing
   ____ Other unusual location
____ Collided with co-worker or other person
____ Collided with sharp
____ Sharp object dropped
____ Struck by detached IV line needle

Section VI. Mucous Membrane Exposure Circumstances

A. What barriers were used by worker at the time of the exposure? *(Check all that apply.)*

❏ Gloves   ❏ Goggles   ❏ Eyeglasses   ❏ Face Shield   ❏ Mask   ❏ Gown

B. Activity/Event when exposure occurred (Check one.)

❏ Patient spit/coughed/vomited
❏ Airway manipulation (e.g., suctioning airway, inducing sputum)
❏ Endoscopic procedure
❏ Dental procedure
❏ Tube placement/removal/manipulation (e.g., chest, endotracheal, NG, rectal, urine catheter)
❏ Phlebotomy
❏ IV or arterial line insertion/removal/manipulation
❏ Irrigation procedure
❏ Vaginal delivery
❏ Surgical procedure (e.g., all surgical procedures including C-section)
❏ Bleeding vessel
❏ Changing dressing/wound care
❏ Manipulating blood tube/bottle/specimen container
❏ Cleaning/transporting contaminated equipment
❏ Other:
❏ Unknown

Comments: _____
_____
_____
_____

NOTE: This is not a CDC or OSHA form. This form was developed by CDC to help healthcare facilities collect detailed exposure information that is specifically useful for the facilities' prevention planning. Information on this page (#1) may meet OSHA sharps injury documentation requirements and can be copied and filed for purposes of maintaining a separate sharps injury log. Procedures for maintaining employee confidentiality must be followed.

CLIA'S Levels of Certification

CLIA established three categories of tests: *waived, moderate complexity* (which includes the subcategory of provider-performed microscopy (PPM) procedures), and *high complexity*. Each laboratory must be either CLIA-exempt or possess one the types of CLIA certificates listed below. The Centers for Medicare and Medicaid Services (CMS) has primary responsibility under CLIA for regulating laboratories.

Laboratories certified for waived testing can perform only those procedures determined to be waived by CMS. Laboratories that certify as moderate complexity may do moderate level tests and waived tests. Laboratories certified as high complexity may do high complexity, moderate complexity, and waived testing. The nonwaived laboratories are subject to CLIA regulations, surveys, and inspections.

TYPES OF CLIA CERTIFICATES

Certificate of Waiver

This certificate is issued to a laboratory to perform only waived tests.

Certificate for Provider-Performed Microscopy Procedures (PPMP)

This certificate is issued to a laboratory in which a physician, midlevel practitioner, or dentist performs no tests other than the microscopy procedures. This certificate permits the laboratory to also perform waived tests.

Certificate of Registration

This certificate is issued to a laboratory that enables the entity to conduct moderate or high complexity laboratory testing or both until the entity is determined by survey to be in compliance with the CLIA regulations.

Certificate of Compliance

This certificate is issued to a laboratory after an inspection that finds the laboratory to be in compliance with all applicable CLIA requirements.

Certificate of Accreditation

This is a certificate that is issued to a laboratory on the basis of the laboratory's accreditation by an accreditation organization approved by Health and Human Services.

www.cms.gov

Preparing the Physician's Office Laboratory for Inspection

Preparation for a CLIA or state inspection should begin 6 to 18 months ahead of the inspection date. OSHA inspections are unannounced.

The following documentation should be reviewed to ensure that it is adequate and up-to-date.

PERSONNEL FILES

Each employee file should include the following:

❏ Job application
❏ Training/orientation checklist

❏ Copies of diplomas and/or certifications

❏ Annual performance evaluations

❏ Continuing education

In a separate employee safety file, the following documents should be stored:

❏ Job classification and biohazardous task list for each employee

❏ Hepatitis B immunization documentation or signed waiver of vaccination

❏ Proof of biological safety training

❏ Documentation of any employee's accidental occupational exposure to biohazards or toxic chemicals. Records of medical follow-up should be included.

PROCEDURE MANUAL

❏ Includes a SOP for every test performed at that laboratory, including specimen requirements, specimen handling, and test result interpretation

INSTRUMENT MAINTENANCE MANUALS

❏ Logs of all maintenance (daily, weekly, monthly, yearly, etc.)

❏ Maintenance performed should meet or exceed the manufacturer's recommendations

QUALITY CONTROL MANUAL

❏ Includes documentation of all quality control performed

❏ Should include QC testing for each day that patient testing is performed

❏ Should include any QC problems and documentation of how that problem was resolved

❏ Calibration also should be included

SAFETY MANUAL

The safety manual includes an adequate safety program that includes

❏ A written plan to reduce occupational exposure to bloodborne pathogens and to hazardous chemicals

❏ OSHA personnel categorization files that show the level of exposure to bloodborne pathogens for each job level

❏ Sanitation, waste-disposal, and housekeeping plans

TEMPERATURE LOG

❏ Must include daily temperature logs of the room, refrigerators, freezers, incubators as required

PATIENT TESTING LOG

❏ Includes all patient test results

PATIENT RECORDS

Each patient record includes

❏ All ordering information

❏ Signed requisitions

❏ Copies of final test results that include the physical address of the laboratory

PROFICIENCY TESTING

❏ Documentation that the laboratory is enrolled in proficiency testing

❏ Documentation that all laboratory personnel have participated in proficiency testing

OTHER REQUIRED DOCUMENTATION

❏ Name of qualified laboratory director

❏ List of job titles of personnel who perform tests, as well as their certification and education

❏ List of specialty areas of testing (hematology, chemistry, microbiology, etc.)

❏ List of the number of patient tests performed annually in each specialty area

appendix **F**

Example of Laboratory Requisition Form

Family Practice Medical Group, Inc.
101 Anywhere, Anycity, ST 00000
Tel (000)123-4567
Fax (000)321-7654

Laboratory Requisition Form

Patient's Name (Last)	(First)	(Middle)
(Date of Birth)		
Address	Phone number ( )	
City	State	Zip
Social security number	Physician	Specimen collection Date & Time

Insurance Co Name	Policy Holder
Address	
Policy Number	Relationship:
Group #	
	Patient or Guardian Signature:	Date:

Check Test Ordered **Provide ICD-9 Code**

Panels	ICD-9		ICD-9		ICD-9		ICD-9
Basic Metabolic		Cholesterol Total		PSA		Chlamydia screen	
Thyroid		Chol HDL		TSH		GC Screen	
Electrolytes		Chol LDL		T3		Gram Stain	
Liver Function		CK		T4		Grp A Beta Strep	
Lipid Profile		CMV		Uric Acid		Strep A Culture	
Renal Function		ESR		WBC		Throat Culture	
		EBV		WBC with diff		Urine Culture	
Test		Glucose		Bleeding Time		Viral Culture	
ACE		Hemoglobin		Blood Gases		Wound Culture	
ADH		Hematocrit				OC&P	
ALT		Hgb Alc		**Urine Tests**			
AFP		HIV		Glucose			
Amylase		Iron		HCG			
AST		LDH		Ketone			
Bilirubin		PKU		U/A Routine			
BUN		Protein, Total					
CEA		Protein, Albumin		**Microbiology**			
Calcium		Protime		AFB Culture			
		PTT		C & S			

Normal Values of Common Laboratory Tests

This section provides a list of normal ranges for a variety of laboratory tests. Normal ranges also may be referred to as reference values or ranges. Each laboratory is responsible for establishing its own normal value range. Variations are based on the specific equipment and procedure utilized. In addition, different populations and localities also can create variations in the normal ranges. Therefore, when evaluating patient results, it is important to compare the patients' results with the normal ranges established by the laboratory performing the testing.

Please note that the same test value may be expressed in different metric units or SI units.

Routine Urinalysis	Normal Values	Clinical Significance
Albumin	Negative	Kidney function
Bilirubin	Negative	Liver function
Blood, occult	Negative	Kidney function
Glucose	Negative	Carbohydrate metabolism
Hemoglobin	Negative	Kidney function
Ketones	Negative	Fat metabolism disorder
pH	4.6–8.0	Acid/base balance
Protein	Negative	Kidney function
Urobilinogen	0.1–1.0 E.U.*/dL	Liver function

* Ehrlich units

Test	Normal Values	Clinical Significance
CBC		
Hemoglobin	Varies with age: Ten years = 12–14.5 g/dL Adult female = 12.5–15 g/dL Adult male = 14–17 g/dL	Increases with polycythemia, high altitude, chronic pulmonary disease Decreases with anemia, hemorrhage
Hematocrit	Varies with age: Newborn = 50–62% One year old = 31–39% Adult female = 36–46% Adult male = 42–52%	Increases with dehydration and polycythemia Decreases with anemia and hemorrhage
White blood cell count	Varies with age: Adults = 4,500–12,000/mm^3	Increases with acute infection, polythycemia, and other diseases Extremely high counts in leukemia Decreases in some viral infections and other conditions

—*table continued*

Test	Normal Values	Clinical Significance
Red blood cell count	Varies with age: Adult female = 4.0–5.5 million/mm^3 Adult male = 4.5–6.0 million/mm^3	Increases with polythycemia and dehydration Decreases with anemia, hemorrhage, and leukemia
Erythrocyte sedimentation rates		
Sediplast (Westergren autozero system)	F < age 50 = 0–20 mm/1 hour F > age 50 = 0–30 mm/1 hour M < age 50 = 0–15 mm/1 hour M > age 50 = 0–20 mm/1 hour	Increased in infections, inflammatory disease, and tissue destruction Decreased in polythycemia and sickle-cell anemia
Wintrobe sedimentation rate	F 0–15 mm/1 hour M 0–7 mm/1 hour	Increased in infections, inflammatory disease, and tissue destruction Decreased in polythycemia and sickle-cell anemia

Test	Normal Values	Clinical Significance
Platelets	140,000–400,000/mm^3	Increases with hemorrhage Decreases with leukemias
Blood Chemistries		
Albumin	3.2–5.5 g/dL	Decreases in kidney disease and severe burns
Alkaline phosphatase	30–115 mU*/mL	Assists in diagnosis of liver and bone disease
ALT (SGPT)	0–45 mU*/mL	Used to detect liver disease
Amylase	25–125 U*/L	Elevated in acute pancreatitis, mumps, intestinal obstructions
AST (SGOT)	0–41 mU*/mL	Used to detect tissue damage Increases with myocardial infarction and other conditions Decreases in some diseases
Total bilirubin (serum)	0.3–1.1 mg/dL	Increases in conditions causing red blood cell destruction or biliary obstruction
BUN (blood urea nitrogen)	8–25 mg/dL	Used in diagnosis of kidney disease, liver failure, other diseases
Calcium	8.5–10.5 mg/dL	Used to assess parathyroid functioning and calcium metabolism and to evaluate malignancies
Total cholesterol	Average = 120–200 mg/dL[†] (varies with age and sex of individual)	Cardiovascular disease Increases in diabetes mellitus and hypothyroidism Decreases in hyperthyroidism, acute infections, and pernicious anemia

[†] A cholesterol level of less than 200 mg/dL is recommended by the American Heart Association for both males and females of all ages.

HDL cholesterol	30–85 mg/dL[†]	

[†] Varies with age and sex of individual

LDL cholesterol	50–210 mg/dL[†]	

[†] Varies with age and sex of individual

Creatinine	0.4–1.5 mg/dL	Used as a screening test of renal functioning
Fasting blood sugar	70–110 mg/100mL	Used as a screening test for carbohydrate metabolism

GTT (glucose-tolerance test)	FBS 70–110 mg/dL 30 min 120–170 mg/dL 1 hr 120–170 mg/dL 2 hr 100–140 mg/dL 3 hr less than 125 mg/dL	Used to detect disorders of glucose metabolism
LDH (Lactase dehydrogenase)	100–225 mU*/mL	Assists in the diagnosis of myocardial infarction and differential diagnosis of muscular dystrophy and pernicious anemia
Triglycerides	40–170 mg/dL	Used to evaluate suspected atherosclerosis
Uric acid	2.2–9.0 mg/dL	Used to evaluate renal failure, gout, leukemia
Electrolytes		
Carbon dioxide (CO_2)	22–26 mEq/L	Diagnosis of acid/base imbalance
Chloride	96–110 mEq/L	Helps in diagnosing disorders of acid/base balance
Potassium	3.5–5.5 mEq/L	Used to diagnose disorders of water balance and acid/base imbalance
Sodium	135–145 mEq/L	Diagnosis of acid/base imbalance occurring in many conditions

* U = Unit (international enzyme unit)

appendix **H**

Vocabulary of the Clinical Laboratory

Clinical laboratories, like other medical specialties, have their own standard vocabulary to be mastered for efficient work. Accuracy and efficiency that promote quality assurance are emphasized. Variation is not permitted if it hinders work or might result in misunderstanding. However, standard abbreviations are used routinely for both tests and reagents. The rules of standard medical terminology, with root words, prefixes, and suffixes, apply to many terms. These may describe laboratory equipment, tests, and the diseases being treated. Reagents are named by the rules of chemistry.

Laboratory vocabulary can be divided into the general areas of metric measurement, laboratory equipment, reagents, tests, and clinical diseases. The general types of vocabulary within each division follow:

- Metric measurement (SI) uses the prefixes and units of the metric system. The prefixes designate the multiple or fraction of the metric unit. These prefixes, units, or abbreviations must always use the correct letter and capitalization.
- Laboratory equipment is often named by prefixes and word roots based on the rules of medical terminology. (An example is the photometer, which consists of two root words: *photo,* meaning light, and *meter,* meaning measure.) However, automated instruments and test kits are often known by the trade names assigned by the manufacturer.
- Laboratory reagents are denoted by their chemical names, symbols (which are chemical abbreviations), or initials. Trade names also may be used. Inorganic compounds are generally identified by their chemical symbols or name. Complex organic compounds are often designated by the initials or names of their chief components. The concentration level of a reagent, if needed, is included along with the name.
- Tests are generally signified by the analyte or parameter being measured. However, the name may be derived from the procedure itself.
- Names of the clinical diseases associated with particular tests often follow the rules of standard medical terminology. (These rules may be found in medical terminology textbooks. Abbreviated lists of word roots, prefixes, and suffixes are found in various medical textbooks and medical dictionaries.)

427

Common abbreviations in the physicians' office laboratory:

A1c: hemoglobin A1c, glycosylated hemoglobin

ACE: angiotensin-converting enzyme

AFB: acid fast bacillus

A/G ratio: albumin/globulin ratio

AIDS: acquired immunodeficiency syndrome

ALL: acute lymphocytic leukemia

ALP: alkaline phosphate

ALT: alanine aminotransferase (SGPT)

AML: acute myelogenous leukemia

aPTT: activated partial thromboplastin time

AST: aspartate aminotransferase (SGOT)

B-cell: a type of lymphocyte

BMP: basic metabolic panel

BNP: brain natriuretic peptide

BUN: blood urea nitrogen

Ca: chemical symbol for calcium

CBC: complete blood cell count

CDC: Centers for Disease Control and Prevention

CEA: carcinoembryonic antigen

CK: creatine kinase

Cl: chemical symbol for chloride

CLIA '88: Clinical Laboratory Improvement Amendment of 1988

CLL: chronic lymphocytic leukemia

CMA: certified medical assistant

CML: chronic myelogenous leukemia

CMV: cytomegalovirus

CNS: central nervous system

CO_2: carbon dioxide

CPK: creatine phosphokinase

CRP: C-reactive protein

C&S: culture and sensitivity

CSF: cerebral spinal fluid

DNA: deoxyribonucleic acid

EBV: Epstein-Barr virus

EDTA: a blood anticoagulant (ethylenediaminetetraaceticacid)

epith: epithelial

ESR: erythrocyte sedimentation rate

GTT: glucose-tolerance test

Hb, Hgb: hemoglobin

HBV: hepatitis B virus

HCG: human chorionic gonadotropin hormone

Hct: hematocrit

HCV: hepatitis C virus

HDL: high-density lipoproteins

HDN: hemolytic disease of the newborn

HIV: human immunodeficiency virus

H_2O: water

HPF: high-power field of the microscope

IDDM: insulin-dependent diabetes mellitus

IM: infectious mononucleosis

INR: international normalized ratio, prothrombin time

ITP: idiopathic thrombocytopenia purpura

IU: international unit

K: chemical symbol for potassium

LDH lactate dehydrogenase

LDL: low-density lipoproteins

LPF: low-power field of the microscope

mEq: milliequivalent (a chemical measurement)

MI: myocardial infarction

MLT: medical laboratory technician

MRSA: methicillin-resistant *Staphylococcus aureus*

MT (ASCP): medical technologist certified by the American Society of Clinical Pathologists

Na: chemical symbol for sodium

NIDDM: noninsulin-dependent diabetes mellitus

O&P: ova and parasites

OSHA: Occupational Safety and Health Administration

pH: a measure of acidity or alkalinity (hydrogen ion concentration)

PKU: phenylketonuria

POCT: point-of-care test

POL: physician's office laboratory

PPBS: postprandial blood sugar

PPE: personal protective equipment

PSA: prostate specific antigen

PT: prothrombin time

QNS: quantity not sufficient

RA: rheumatoid arthritis

RBC: red blood cell, also called erythrocyte

RF: rheumatoid factors

RIA: radioimmunoassay

RMA: registered medical assistant

RMT: registered medical technologist

RNA: ribonucleic acid

sp gr: specific gravity

staph: *Staphylococcus*

stat: immediately (emergency)

STD: sexually transmitted disease

strep: *Streptococcus*

T-cell: a type of lymphocyte, a white blood cell

TIA: transient ischemic attack

TIBC: total iron-binding capacity

UA: urinalysis

UTI: urinary tract infection

VDRL: Venereal Disease Research Laboratory

VLDL: very-low-density lipoprotein

WBC: white blood cell, also called leukocyte

Common Laboratory Equipment and Glassware

1. Petri dishes—used for holding agar for bacterial cultures

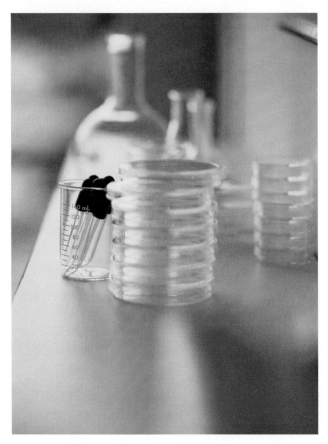

3. Serological pipettes—used for measuring smaller amounts of liquids

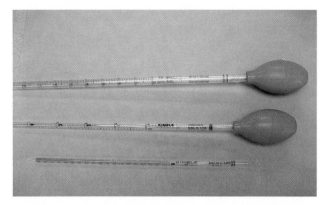

4. Transfer pipettes—plastic, disposable dropper pipettes for transferring liquids

2. Beakers, graduated cylinders, flasks—used for measuring and holding liquids

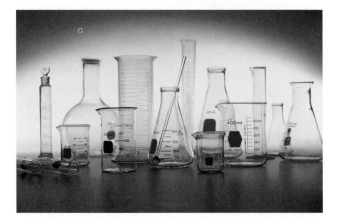

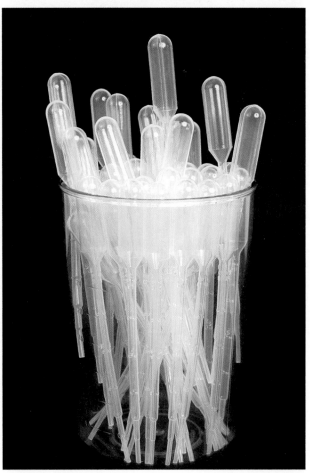

5. Auto pipettes—used to withdraw and dispense small amounts of liquids automatically

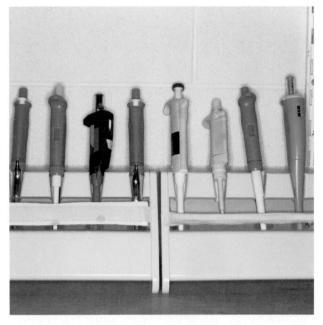

6. Centrifuges—used to separate materials into different layers by spinning at high speeds

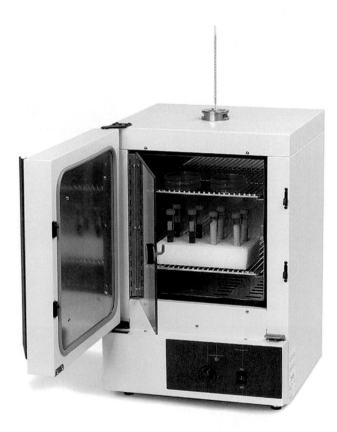

7. Autoclave—used to sterilize materials and equipment by using steam under pressure

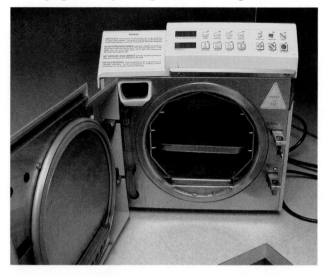

8. Incubators—cabinets used to keep bacterial cultures at specific temperatures for optimal growth

Glossary

A

ABO blood group   one of two clinically important inherited blood groups; the ABO blood group has two antigens, A and B, and includes four blood types: A, B, AB, and 0.

absolute polycythemia   erythrocytosis; an increase in the number of red blood cells because of increased red blood cell production.

accuracy   how close a test result comes to the true value of the substance being measured. Asks the question—are the results correct?

acid   a chemical that donates hydrogen ions (H+), lowers the pH of solutions, and reacts with bases to form water and chemical salts.

acidosis   acidity of body fluids; abnormally low blood pH. The blood is more acidic than normal.

acromegaly   a growth abnormality caused by overproduction of growth hormone by the pituitary gland.

action value   also called panic value or critical value; a patient lab test result requiring immediate medical attention. Action values fall outside the normal test value range, although not all abnormal values require immediate action.

activated partial thromboplastin time (aPTT)   a coagulation procedure that tests for coagulation factors II, V, VIII, IX, X, XI, and XII, all of which are involved in the intrinsic pathway of coagulation. It is used to evaluate the effect of the administration of anticoagulant drugs.

acute lymphocytic leukemia   predominantly a children's disease, in which the blood-forming tissues produce an excessive number of lymphocytes.

adipose tissue   the connective tissue in which fat is stored in cells.

adjustable ocular   usually, the eyepiece on the left. It can be adjusted to correct the focus for the individual's visual acuity.

adult hemoglobin   hemoglobin A.

aerobic   microorganisms that prefer or require an oxygen-rich environment for growth.

aerosolization   the conversion of a liquid, such as blood or blood products, or a solid, such as a powdered chemical, into a fine mist that travels through the air.

agglutination   a clumping together, as of red blood cells.

agranulocytes   the third of white blood cells, including both monocytes and lymphocytes, that have few, if any, visible granules.

agranulocytosis   an acute disorder characterized by severe sore throat, fever, complete exhaustion, and an extreme reduction in the number of neutrophils.

albumin   the most abundant plasma protein. Albumin is responsible for maintaining osmotic pressure at the capillary membrane.

alkalosis   abnormally high blood pH. The blood is more alkaline than normal.

amino acid   one of 20 different compounds in humans that are the building blocks of proteins. Each amino acid contains an amine group and an acidic carboxyl group.

anaerobic   microorganisms that prefer or require a carbon-dioxide-rich environment for growth.

analyte   a substance that is tested for in a laboratory procedure for its presence or quantity in a patient or quality control specimen.

anemia   the condition in which there is a deficiency in the amount of hemoglobin in the blood, thus reducing the oxygen-carrying capacity of the blood.

anisocytosis   the excessive variation in the size of cells, especially red blood cells.

anoxia   a deficiency of oxygen.

antecubital   in the inner arm at the bend of the elbow; the most common site for venipuncture.

antibiotic   a drug administered to kill or inhibit the growth of bacteria.

antibody   a protein molecule produced by the lymph system in response to a particular antigen.

anticoagulant   an agent that prevents the clotting of blood, such as oxalate, citrate, EDTA, or heparin.

antigen   short for antibody generating; a foreign substance that provokes a specific antibody reaction.

431

anuria   the complete absence of urine excretion.

aperture (microscope)   in a microscope, the opening through which the light passes such as in the stage or iris diaphragm.

aperture   an opening, as in the probe of an electrical impedance or electron-optical cell counter, through which blood cells and other formed elements in diluting solution pass in single file.

aplastic anemia   anemia caused by deficient red blood cell production, due to disorders of the bone marrow.

artifact   an extraneous, nontissue feature that contaminates specimen slides.

ascorbic acid   vitamin C.

aseptic technique   a lab technique that ensures the isolation of pathogenic microorganisms, including personal protective equipment and sterilization.

atherosclerosis   the condition in which cholesterol deposits in the blood vessels.

autoclave   a device utilizing steam under pressure to sterilize medical instruments and laboratory specimens.

autoimmunity   the condition in which the immune system responds inappropriately to the wrong antigens—to self instead of nonself.

automated chemistry analyzer   an instrument that performs chemistry test procedures automatically.

B

bacillus   a rod-shaped bacterium. Bacilli include the bacteria that cause tuberculosis and diphtheria.

bacitracin   an antibiotic used in cultures to give an early indication of the presence of Group A strep.

bacteria   single-celled microorganisms in the kingdom *Monera*. Bacteria cause many different infections in humans.

bacteriuria   the presence of bacteria in the urine.

balanitis   inflammation of the glans penis, most often due to *Trichomonas vaginalis, Herpes,* or *Chlamydia trachomatis.*

base   a chemical that yields hydroxide ions (OH⁻) when dissolved in water (e.g., sodium hydroxide). Bases raise the pH of a solution and react with acids to form chemical salts and water.

basophil   the least common type of granular white blood cell, containing large cytoplasmic granules that stain blue-black with alkaline dyes.

Bence Jones protein   an abnormal protein found in patients with multiple myeloma and other conditions. The reagent strip test for urinary protein is not sensitive to it.

bevel   sheared opening at the anterior end of the needle. Needles should enter the vein with the bevel side of the needle "up" or visible to the lab personnel.

bias   the skewing of test results away from the true value.

bilirubin   a product of the breakdown of red blood cells. A high serum level of bilirubin may result in excretion through the kidneys, in addition to the usual route of excretion through the intestines.

bilirubinemia   a high level of bilirubin in the blood.

bilirubinuria   the presence of bilirubin in the urine.

binocular   literally, pertaining to two eyes; a microscope with two eyepieces, one for each eye.

biohazard   a biological specimen containing blood or other body fluid that has the potential for transmitting disease.

biological specimen   a specimen that originates from a living organism. Examples are blood, blood products, other body fluids such as cerebrospinal fluid or urine, biopsy samples, bacterial smears, and bacterial cultures.

bladder   stores the urine produced by the kidneys.

bleeding time   the time it takes a small, standardized incision to stop bleeding.

blood urea nitrogen (BUN)   the concentration of nitrogen in the blood, which is used as an indirect measure of urea in the blood.

bloodborne pathogens   microorganisms that cause disease and can be transmitted through blood or other body fluids. HIV is an example.

B-lymphocyte   B-cell; a lymphocyte that secretes short-lived antibodies involved in humoral immunity.

brucellosis   a bacterial disease primarily of cattle, which leads to an increase in lymphocytes and a decrease in neutrophils.

buffy coat   the 0.5 to 1.0 mm thick, whitish-tan layer of white blood cells and platelets that forms between the packed red blood cells and plasma when whole blood is centrifuged.

butterfly needle   also known as a "winged infusion set." A modified venipuncture needle that is shorter in length, is held by its "butterfly wings," and has a tubing attached to the posterior portion of the needle that can be attached to a needle holder or syringe.

C

calculus urinary stone. Also known as renal calculi.

calibration verification testing calibrators (known substances) in the same manner as patient specimens to ensure the accuracy of the results throughout the reportable range.

calibration the testing and adjustment of an instrument to establish that the results reported by the test reflect the actual concentration of the sample.

calibrator a known solution of an analyte obtained from a manufacturer or professional organization and used as a measuring stick to set instruments to read test results correctly. Calibrators are used during calibration procedures.

capillary a small blood vessel that connects arterioles and venules. Contains a mixture of arterial and venous blood.

capillary puncture the puncture of a capillary for the purpose of collecting a blood specimen.

carotenemia the presence of carotene in the blood.

casts, urinary microscopic solid forms created from protein precipitates in the renal tubules and voided in the urine.

catalase test the lab test in which hydrogen peroxide is added to urine cultures to distinguish *Streptococcus* from *Staphylococcus* infections.

catheterization, urinary the process of inserting a tube through the urethra into the urinary bladder to obtain a urine specimen.

caustic burning or corrosive; usually destructive to living tissue.

CDC Centers for Disease Control and Prevention.

cell counter a manual counter for differential white blood cell counts with keys for each type of white cell.

cell-mediated immunity the type of specific immunity that is controlled by T-lymphocytes.

cerebrovascular accident stroke. A cerebrovascular accident is characterized by the sudden loss of consciousness followed by possible paralysis. Cerebrovascular accidents may be caused by an embolus or thrombus that occludes a cerebral artery, among other causes.

Certificate for Provider-Performed Microscopy Procedures (PPMP) a certificate issued to a laboratory in which a physician, midlevel practitioner, or dentist performs only microscopy procedures. This certificate permits the laboratory to also perform waived tests.

Certificate of Accreditation a certificate issued to a laboratory on the basis of the laboratory's accreditation by an accreditation organization approved by the Health Care Financing Administration (HCFA).

Certificate of Compliance a certificate issued to a laboratory after an inspection that finds the laboratory to be in compliance with all applicable CLIA requirements.

Certificate of Registration a certificate issued to a laboratory that enables the entity to conduct moderate or high-complexity laboratory testing or both until the entity is determined by survey to be in compliance with the CLIA regulations.

Certificate of Waiver certificate that allows a laboratory to only perform waived tests.

chain of transmission the unbroken line of transmission of a disease from one host with the disease to a new host.

chemical hazard a source of danger from exposure to chemicals.

chlamydia a bacterial disease, thought to be the most prevalent sexually transmitted disease in the United States.

cholesterol the sterol of primary biological significance. High levels of cholesterol in the blood are linked with increased risk of cardiovascular disease.

chronic granulocytic leukemia a type of chronic leukemia caused by a chromosomal abnormality, leading to an overproduction of basophils in the bone marrow.

clean-catch, midstream urine specimen a urine specimen collected midstream after thoroughly cleaning the surrounding area to prevent contamination of the specimen; used when urine is to be cultured.

clotting disorder a coagulation disease in which clots form in the blood spontaneously.

coagulase test the lab test that demonstrates the presence of an enzyme produced by pathogenic *Staphylococcus* organisms, thereby distinguishing them from nonpathogenic strains of *Staphylococcus*.

coagulation the process of clotting, which depends on the presence of several coagulation factors, including prothrombin, thrombin, thromboplastin, fibrinogen, and calcium.

coagulation factor one of 12 compounds required for the coagulation process. Coagulation factors must be present in appropriate amounts for clotting to occur effectively.

coagulation studies   tests performed to see how fast and how well a patient is capable of forming a clot.

coarse adjustment   the first step in focusing, in which the distance between the specimen and the lens (working distance) is covered very quickly, either by lowering the objective or raising the stage.

coccus   a spherical or oval bacterium. Cocci include *Streptococcus* and *Staphylococcus.*

coefficient of variation (CV)   also called the relative standard deviation; the standard deviation expressed as a percent of the mean.

colorimeter   an instrument for measuring intensity of color. It identifies the wavelengths of colored light in nanometers.

common denominator   a common multiple of the denominators of two or more fractions.

complement   a group of proteins in the blood that are important in the immune response; they act by directly lysing organisms and stimulating phagocytosis.

complete blood count (CBC)   a battery of hematological tests often requisitioned in POLs. It includes hemoglobin concentration, hematocrit, red and white blood cell counts, differential white blood cell count, and sometimes erythrocyte indices.

concentrate   a substance, either liquid or solid, that is strong because it has had fluid removed from it.

concentration   the strength of a chemical in a solution.

condenser   also called the substage. Located just below the opening in the mechanical stage and above the light source, the condenser controls the amount of light.

confirmation test   also known as a confirmatory test; a more precise and specific test used to confirm the results of a screening test. In urinalysis, the screening test is usually the urinalysis strips.

conjugated lipid   a compound made up of fat and another compound, such as phosphoric acid (phospholipids) or a carbohydrate (glycolipids).

contamination   the pollution of an area or substance with unwanted extraneous material such as pathogens or hazardous chemicals.

continuous flow analysis system   a chemistry analyzer in which samples and reagents flow through the instrument, one after the other. One test or a variety of tests may be performed on the same sample in a single operation of the instrument.

control   a sample used to maintain accuracy and quality in a procedure. Its concentration is known within very accurate limits and its variability is ascertained by the manufacturer. It is used as part of daily quality control procedures.

conversion factor   a ratio that relates the same measure in the systems of units; used to convert from one unit to another.

Coombs' test   the antiglobulin test used for monitoring the development of Rh incompatibility in Rh-negative pregnant women.

coumarin   a group of drugs, including warfarin, used to prevent and treat clotting disorders. Coumarin drugs act in the liver, where they interfere with the synthesis of vitamin K–dependent coagulation factors (II, VII, IX, and X).

coverslip   small, thin glass used to cover liquid specimens on slides to protect the microscope and stabilize the specimen. A special coverslip is manufactured for use by the hemacytometer.

C-reactive protein (CRP)   an abnormal glycoprotein that appears in the acute stage of various inflammatory disorders.

creatine   a nonprotein nitrogen compound found in muscle tissue. Creatine is synthesized primarily in the liver from three amino acids. It combines readily with phosphate to store energy for muscle contractions.

creatinine   the end product of the metabolism of creatine.

crenated   usually used to refer to shrunken red blood cells that appear small and scalloped around the edges.

culture and sensitivity (C & S)   microbiology testing used to determine the bacteria causing infection and make a determination regarding which antibiotics are effective.

culture media   substances containing nutrients used to grow bacteria; may be liquid or solid.

Cushing's syndrome   the condition caused by hypersecretion of the adrenal cortex.

cyanmethemoglobin   a very stable cyanide and hemoglobin compound that results when a solution of potassium ferrocyanide and potassium cyanide is added to blood, lysing the red blood cells and releasing their hemoglobin content.

cylindruria   the condition characterized by large numbers of casts in the urine.

cystitis   inflammation of the urinary bladder.

D

decantation   the process of pouring off fluid. In urinalysis, it usually refers to the pouring off of the liquid portion of urine after it has been centrifuged.

decimal   any number expressed in base 10, or a fraction in which the denominator is a power of 10.

dehydration   the loss of body water in excess of intake, resulting in a net deficiency of water in the tissues. Dehydration is caused by either decreased intake or increased loss of water and may be due to excessive vomiting, diarrhea, sweating, or uncontrolled diabetes.

denominator   the part of a fraction that is at the bottom of a fraction. It functions as a divisor.

desquamation   the shedding of layers of cells or skin.

diabetes mellitus (DM)   a syndrome caused by inadequate production or utilization of insulin, leading to impaired carbohydrate, protein, and fat metabolism. Diabetes mellitus occurs in two major forms. Type 1 is formerly known as insulin-dependent or juvenile-onset. Type 2 is formerly known as noninsulin-dependent or adult-onset. A third form, gestational diabetes, only occurs in pregnant women.

differential white blood cell count   differential or "diff"; a determination of the percent of each type of white blood cell out of a total of 100 white blood cells observed under magnification by the oil immersion objective (100X) on a stained blood smear. Also can be calculated by automated CBC analyzer.

diluent   an agent that reduces the strength of a substance to which it is added.

dilution   a solution that has been weakened by addition of a diluent.

dimensional analysis   a method of problem solving in which units of measure are carried through all calculations. This method ensures the answer has the desired units.

direct culture   a primary culture; a culture grown by inoculating patient specimens directly onto the culture medium.

disaccharide   a 12-carbon sugar. Disaccharides include sucrose, lactose, and maltose.

discrete (noncontinuous) analysis system   a chemistry analyzer in which samples and reagents for each test are placed in separate containers, in which the tests are performed.

There are two different types: wet chemistry and dry chemistry.

disinfection   any practical procedure for reducing the pathogen contamination in the inanimate environment, as in the air, on work counters, or on equipment.

distal convoluted tubule   the part of the coiled renal tubule that begins after the loop of Henle.

diuretic   agent that increases urine production.

dividend   a number to be divided.

divisor   the number by which a dividend is divided.

E

electrical impedance cell counter   an automated hematology instrument, such as the Beckman Coulter and Abbot Cell Dyn instruments, that analyzes formed elements in the blood on the basis of their impedance of an electrical current.

electrical impedance method   the method of studying the formed elements in the blood that depends on their resistance to the flow of an electrical current.

electrolyte   ion that is positively or negatively charged.

embolism   the sudden obstruction of a blood vessel by an embolus.

embolus   an undissolved mass in a blood or lymphatic vessel. It is usually a blood clot but may consist of fat globules, bacteria, or other debris. About 75 percent of emboli arise in the deep veins of the legs.

endocarditis   the inflammation of the lining of the heart. Endocarditis may be associated with an increase in the number of monocytes.

endocytic and phagocytic response   the type of nonspecific immunity in which microorganisms and other foreign matter are engulfed and degraded by body cells.

engineering control   a device that keeps biohazards away from laboratory personnel.

English system   the foot–pound–ounce system of units of measurement that most of us use every day.

eosin   a red-orange acidic dye used to stain blood smears for microscopic examination.

eosinophil   a granular white blood cell with a bilobed nucleus and cytoplasmic granules that stain brilliant red-orange with eosin dye. Increased numbers of eosinophils are associated with allergies and internal parasitic infections.

epinephrine   adrenaline; an adrenal gland hormone that stimulates the sympathetic nervous system.

equation   a mathematical statement that expresses equality between two expressions on either side of an equals sign.

equivalent fractions   fractions that look different but have the same quantity.

erythremia   polycythemia vera.

erythrocyte   a red blood cell.

erythrocyte count   red blood cell count.

erythrocyte indices   three indicators of the size or hemoglobin content of the red blood cells that are used in the diagnosis of anemia. They include the mean cell volume (MCV), the mean cell hemoglobin (MCH), and the mean cell hemoglobin concentration (MCHC).

erythrocyte sedimentation rate (ESR or sed rate)   the rate at which red blood cells settle out of plasma when placed in a vertical tube.

erythrocytosis   absolute polycythemia.

erythropoiesis   the formation of red blood cells.

erythropoietin   the kidney hormone that triggers red blood cell formation. It is produced whenever hemoglobin concentration or oxygen saturation declines.

evacuated tube system   a vacuum tube system for drawing blood by venipuncture. It allows multiple samples to be drawn with a single puncture.

exponent   a symbol written above and to the right of a number. An exponent indicates how many times the number is multiplied by itself.

exposure incident   a situation in which laboratory personnel are exposed to a potentially hazardous substance, such as blood or a toxic chemical.

eyepiece   *see* ocular.

F

false negative   when the test result is negative and the patient has the disease or condition.

false positive   when the test result is positive, but the patient does not have the disease or condition.

fastidious bacterium   a bacterium that has very precise nutritional and environmental requirements for growth, including *Niesseria gonorrhoeae*.

fasting blood-sugar (FBS) test   the blood glucose test performed on a specimen collected after the patient has fasted for 8 to 12 hours. The FBS test is usually scheduled for early morning, before the first meal of the day.

fatty cast   renal cast that contains fat droplets because of chronic renal disease.

fetal hemoglobin   hemoglobin F.

fibrin   the whitish, filamentous protein formed by the action of thrombin on fibrinogen. Other formed elements in the blood become entangled in the interlacing filaments of fibrin, thus forming a blood clot.

fibrinogen   coagulation factor I; a compound in plasma that is converted to fibrin by thrombin in the presence of calcium.

fine adjustment   the step in focusing in which only small changes are made in the working distance between the lens and the specimen.

fingerstick   puncturing the soft pad of the ring or middle finger in order to collect a blood specimen.

first morning urine specimen   also called 8-hour, overnight, early morning, or first morning specimen; a urine specimen collected as soon as the patient arises in the morning, consisting of urine that has collected in the bladder during the night.

flocculation   a precipitate in the form of downy tufts.

flow cytometry   a technique that analyzes cells as they are forced through a detector system; this system could be an electric current, a light or laser beam, or fluorescent dyes.

foam test   a test to detect the presence of bilirubin in urine that appears yellow-orange.

formula   a rule written in mathematical symbols and numbers. A formula expresses the relationship between two or more quantities.

fraction   a numerical representation of the quotient of two numbers.

fructose   a simple, six-carbon sugar in fruit and honey.

fungus   a plant of the phylum Fungi, which lacks chlorophyll. Fungi are microorganisms that include yeasts and molds, some of which cause disease.

G

galactose   a simple (six-carbon) sugar formed from the breakdown of lactose (milk sugar).

galactosemia   the presence of galactose in the blood. Galactosemia is the condition in which galactose is not converted to glucose due to a lack of the enzyme galactase. If left undetected in children, it can lead to failure to thrive and ultimately can lead to death.

gauge the diameter of the needle. The smaller the gauge, the larger the diameter.

general policy manual a laboratory manual that contains the overall policies for every aspect of laboratory operation, particularly as they relate to employees, their qualifications, job duties, and job benefits.

gestational diabetes a transient form of diabetes that develops in response to the metabolic and hormonal changes of pregnancy in previously asymptomatic women. Gestational diabetes generally resolves after delivery.

globulin the second most abundant type of plasma protein. Globulin has a diversity of functions, including transporting other substances and acting as a substrate.

glomerular filtrate fluid formed in the kidneys when the entering, or afferent, arteriole is larger than the exiting, or efferent, arteriole, thus creating a higher blood pressure than is found in most capillaries. The hydrostatic pressure forces water and other substances out of the blood, forming the glomerular filtrate. The glomerular filtrate has about the same composition as tissue fluid elsewhere in the body.

glomerulonephritis a condition in which the glomerular capillaries are inflamed and become permeable to protein.

glucagon the hormone produced by the alpha cells in the islets of Langerhans of the pancreas; called the fasting hormone because it increases when blood glucose levels are low and stimulates the liver to break down stored glycogen.

gluconeogenesis the formation of glycogen from noncarbohydrate sources.

glucose a simple, six-carbon sugar found in many foods. Glucose metabolism provides most of the energy needed for normal growth and functioning.

glucose meter (glucometer) an instrument to measure blood glucose "at the patient's bedside," allowing patients to monitor their glucose levels at home.

glucose tolerance test (GTT) a test of the ability to metabolize glucose, in which the patient is tested for blood and urine glucose at short intervals after consuming a known quantity of glucose in solution. See also standard oral glucose tolerance test.

glucosuria (glycosuria) the condition in which there is glucose in the urine.

glycogen a carbohydrate formed from excess glucose that is stored in liver and muscle cells. Glycogen serves as a source of stored energy for the body.

glycogenolysis the process for breaking down stored glycogen into glucose. Glycogenolysis occurs in the liver when stimulated by the hormone glucagon.

glycosuria the presence of glucose in the urine.

glycosylated hemoglobin (G-hemoglobin hemoglobin A1C, G-Hgb) hemoglobin with an attached glucose residue.

gram (g) the basic metric unit for weight or mass. A gram equals 0.03527 ounce in the English system.

gram negative bacteria that stain pink or red with Gram stain, including *Escherichia coli* and *Neisseria gonorrhoeae.*

gram positive bacteria that stain deep purple with Gram stain, such as *Staphylococcus* and *Streptococcus* organisms.

Gram stain the most commonly used stain for bacterial smears. Gram stain separates organisms into two clinically meaningful groups: gram negative organisms and gram positive organisms.

granular cast fine-or coarse-grained dark renal cast that has degenerated from a hyaline or waxy cast. An increase in the number of granular casts may indicate pyelonephritis.

granulocyte a polymorphonuclear white blood cell that contains granules in its cytoplasm. This class includes neutrophils, eosinophils, and basophils.

H

hazardous chemical list a list maintained by OSHA that identifies toxic chemicals used in laboratories. It may be consulted to determine the toxicity of a chemical.

HBV (hepatitis B virus) the virus that causes hepatitis B, a type of severe hepatitis transmitted by sexual contact, by needle sharing, or through contaminated blood, blood products, or other body fluids.

HCV (hepatitis C virus) previously known as Non-A Non-B hepatitis virus; the virus that causes hepatitis C, a serious type of hepatitis transmitted by contaminated blood and blood products, needles, and sexual contact. There is presently no vaccine for HCV.

Health Insurance Portability and Accountability Act (HIPAA) federal regulation that established a national baseline for protecting patient's health information.

heelstick   puncturing the lateral portion of the heel in infants in order to collect a blood specimen. This may only be done on infants who have not yet begun to walk.

helminth   a true worm. Several species parasitize the human intestinal tract, including tapeworms and hookworms.

hemacytometer   a counting device or counting chamber to count cells such as red or white blood cells.

hematocrit (Hct or "crit")   the volume of red blood cells packed by centrifugation in a given volume of blood. It is given as a percent.

hematology   the study of blood and blood-forming tissues.

hematology calibrator   a hematology control that is certified to be highly stable over its entire life; used to set the electronics of automated hematology instruments.

hematology control   an artificial blood, containing both human and animal cells, that is used to check the stability of electronic settings of automated hematology instruments.

hematology test   a blood test, including hematocrit, hemoglobin concentration, and red and white blood cell counts, among others.

hematoma   a subcutaneous mass of blood at a venipuncture site. Also known as a bruise.

hematuria   the presence of erythrocytes (red blood cells) in urine. Hematuria can be caused by several different conditions and may be a sign of a serious clinical condition.

hemoconcentration   the increased concentration of red blood cells due to decreased plasma volume.

hemoglobin (Hgb)   the oxygen-carrying protein of red blood cells.

hemoglobin A   the normal adult hemoglobin. It develops by 6 months of age to replace hemoglobin F, or fetal hemoglobin.

hemoglobin A_1C test (glycosylated hemoglobin test)   a recently developed blood glucose test based on the amount of glycosylated hemoglobin in the blood. The glycosylated hemoglobin test detects hyperglycemia that may be missed in type 1 patients who have wide swings in their blood glucose levels. There is a direct correlation between the amount of hemoglobin A_1C and the average glucose level in the patient's blood over the last 3 months.

hemoglobin C   an abnormal hemoglobin that is more prevalent in African Americans. It causes chronic hemolytic anemia, splenomegaly, arthralgia, and abdominal pain.

hemoglobin E   an abnormal hemoglobin that is prevalent in India, Southeast Asia, and Southeast Asian immigrants in the United States. It causes a mild form of hemolytic anemia.

hemoglobin F   fetal hemoglobin. This hemoglobin is found in fetuses and infants until 6 months of age. It is replaced by hemoglobin A, or adult hemoglobin.

hemoglobin S   sickle-cell hemoglobin.

hemoglobin S-C disease   the disease in individuals heterozygous for hemoglobins S and C. The symptoms, which usually appear after age 40, include hematuria and pain in the bones, joints, abdomen, and chest.

hemoglobinopathy   any disease caused by abnormal hemoglobin.

hemoglobinuria   the presence of hemoglobin in the urine.

hemolysis   the breakdown of red blood cells, with the release of hemoglobin into the plasma or serum. In general, hemolyzed specimens are not acceptable for testing.

hemolytic anemia   the anemia that is due to the breakdown of red blood cells.

hemolyze   the destruction of red blood cells, which releases the hemoglobin.

hemophilia   one of a group of diseases in which excessive bleeding occurs because of inherited deficiencies in blood coagulation factors; characterized by uncontrolled hemorrhaging, possibly even from the slightest injury.

hemophilia A   classic hemophilia; the most common type of hemophilia, caused by a recessive sex-linked gene that leads to the inability to synthesize coagulation factor VIII, antihemophilic factor (AHF).

hemophilia B   Christmas disease; the second most common type of hemophilia, caused by a recessive sex-linked gene that leads to the inability to synthesize coagulation factor IX, plasma thromboplastin component (PTC).

hemophilia C   a relatively uncommon type of hemophilia, caused by a dominant autosomal gene, leading to the inability to synthesize factor XI, plasma thromboplastin antecedent (PTA).

hemorrhagic disease   any of several diseases in which excessive bleeding occurs because blood fails to clot.

hemorrhagic disease of the newborn   a bleeding disease due to lack of vitamin K–producing intestinal flora in less than 1 percent of newborns, occurring between the second and seventh day after birth. Hemorrhagic disease of the newborn is treated by administration of vitamin K. Vitamin K is necessary to the formation of several clotting factors, including prothrombin.

hemostasis   the arrest of bleeding.

heparin sodium   a widely used anticoagulant drug for the management of clotting disorders. It works by inhibiting the conversion of prothrombin to thrombin.

herpes   the common name for diseases caused by herpesvirus, a family of viruses, including those that cause cold sores and genital ulcers, *Herpes simplex I* and *II.*

heterozygous   pertaining to the inheritance of different forms of a gene from each parent.

high density lipoprotein (HDL)   a lipoprotein that has high density because it is low in fat content.

histogram   a graph derived from sampling showing frequency distributions.

HIV (human immunodeficiency virus)   the virus that causes AIDS (acquired immunodeficiency syndrome).

homeostasis   an equilibrium state of the body maintained by feedback and internal regulation of body processes. Homeostasis helps keep individuals healthy by returning their physical state to normal following stress or trauma.

homozygous   pertaining to the inheritance of the same form of a gene from each parent.

human chorionic gonadotropin (hCG)   the hormone produced by the villi of the placenta. Detecting it is the basis for early pregnancy tests.

humoral immunity   the type of specific immunity that involves the formation and activity of short-lived antibodies in body fluids.

hyaline cast   the most common type of renal cast. Hyaline casts are colorless, homogeneous, and semitransparent. An increase in the number of hyaline casts indicates damage to the glomerular capillary membrane, permitting leakage of protein.

hyperbilirubinemia   the presence of a high level of bilirubin in the blood.

hyperchromic   having excess hemoglobin; refers to red blood cells with excess hemoglobin that appear darker in color when stained with dye.

hyperglycemia   an abnormally high blood glucose level, most commonly caused by diabetes mellitus.

hypersegmented   having a nucleus with more than five segments, or lobes; used to describe certain neutrophils.

hypersensitivity   allergy; exaggerated immune response to foreign antigens.

hypersthenuria   the production of urine with high specific gravity. Hypersthenuria may be caused by several different diseases.

hyperthyroidism   hyperactivity of the thyroid gland, leading to increased production of thyroxine.

hypertonic urine   a concentrated urine with a specific gravity of 1.030 or greater.

hypertriglyceridemia   an excessive amount of triglycerides in the blood.

hypochromic   having too little hemoglobin; refers to red blood cells that appear lighter in color when stained with dye.

hypoglycemia   an abnormally low blood glucose level. Hypoglycemia may be caused by hyperfunction of the islets of Langerhans or injection of excessive amounts of insulin.

hyposthenuria   the production of urine with low specific gravity. Hyposthenuria may be caused by several different diseases.

hypotonic urine   a diluted urine with a specific gravity of 1.003 or less.

I

ICP (infection control program)   a program that provides the maximum protection for health care workers against occupational sources of disease.

icteric   jaundiced; characterized by a high level of bilirubin. Icteric serum and plasma look dark yellow or greenish.

immunity   the body's resistance to foreign invaders, including microorganisms, cancer cells, toxins, and incompatible blood types from other individuals.

immunodeficiency   compromised immune response; the condition in which the immune system is compromised due to a congenital or acquired disorder; characterized by increased susceptibility to disease and poor recovery.

immunology   the branch of medical science that studies the physical and chemical aspects of immunity, or resistance to disease.

immunology test   a lab test that depends on immune reactions for results. Immunology tests include tests for pregnancy, many diseases, and blood types.

in control   a phrase used to indicate that the quality system that measures the accuracy of a procedure is within acceptable limits.

index   the small *i* under the summation sign. The index indicates the range over which the summation is to be performed.

infectious lymphocytosis   a rare disorder, probably of viral origin, that leads to an increase in the number of small lymphocytes.

infectious mononucleosis   an acute infectious disease in which lymphocytes are both more numerous and larger than normal and often contain vacuoles, causing them to resemble monocytes—hence the name of the disease.

inflammatory response   a complex series of events, triggered by a wound or invasion by microorganisms, leading to redness, swelling, heat, and pain. Inflammatory response reduces the spread of infection and promotes healing.

instrument calibration and maintenance manual   a laboratory manual that contains instructions and dated records of laboratory instrument calibration and maintenance.

insulin   the hormone secreted by the beta cells of the islets of Langerhans of the pancreas. Insulin helps transport glucose molecules across cell membranes so that glucose metabolism can occur.

insulinoma   a tumor of the beta cells of the pancreas.

international normalized ratio (INR)   a method of reporting PT results for patients on oral anticoagulant therapy.

International System of Units (SI)   the world's most widely used modern form of the metric system of units.

inventory control manual   a laboratory manual that contains a file of supply house contact information and orders and a calendar for keeping a tally of supplies on hand.

inverse   opposite or reverse. The inverse of a fraction is created by turning it upside down.

ion-selective electrode (ISE)   a conductor that is sensitive to the activity of a particular ion in solution.

iris diaphragm   located in the condenser, the iris diaphragm is the aperture that controls the amount of light entering through the opening in the stage by contracting or enlarging like the iris of the eye.

iron-deficiency anemia   the anemia resulting from lack of or the inability to utilize available iron in the body.

isosthenuria   the production of urine with consistently low specific gravity regardless of fluid intake. Isosthenuria is a sign of marked impairment of renal function.

isotonic   having the same osmotic pressure. An isotonic solution with the same osmotic pressure as red blood cells is used to prepare blood for red blood cell counts.

J

jaundice   yellowing of the eyes and skin caused by excess bilirubin in the blood. Urine may appear burnt-brown to orange.

K

ketoacidosis   an acid condition of the body marked by the presence of ketones.

ketone   an intermediary product of fat metabolism. Ketones can appear in the urine during periods of starvation, fever, and dieting.

ketonuria   the presence of ketones in the urine.

kidney   structure responsible for forming the urine. Most individuals are born with two.

kidney stone (calculus)   a hard stone that forms in the hollow passages of the urinary system in some individuals.

kilogram (kg)   the metric unit of weight or mass that is equal to 1,000 grams and to 2.2 pounds in the English system.

kilometer (km)   the metric unit of length that equals 1,000 meters. A kilometer equals 0.62137 mile in the English system.

L

lactose   the sugar found in milk. Lactose breaks down into glucose and galactose.

lancet   a sharp, piercing device used to puncture a finger or heel in order to obtain a capillary specimen.

leukemia   a disease characterized by unrestrained production of white blood cells.

leukocyte   a white blood cell.

leukocyte count   white blood cell count.

leukocytosis   an abnormally high white blood cell count.

leukopenia   an abnormally low white blood cell count, usually below 4,500/mm^3.

Levey-Jennings chart   a chart on which control values are plotted daily. It is divided into areas of acceptable, low, and high values, enabling lab workers to easily assess the normalcy of test results.

light scattering (optical counting) method   the method of studying formed elements in the blood that depends on their interruption of a beam of light from a laser lamp.

linearity a measure of an instrument's ability to measure test results in an accurate manner. Test results plotted in a straight line on a graph indicate accuracy.

lipemia the presence of an abnormal amount of fat in the blood.

lipemic having an abnormally high level of fat. Specimens are cloudy or milky in appearance.

lipid fat; one of a group of organic compounds made up mainly of carbon, hydrogen, and oxygen. Lipids are used to store energy and as structural materials in the cells.

lipiduria the presence of fat in the urine.

lipolysis fat decomposition.

lipoprotein a macromolecule of triglycerides, phospholipids, and cholesterol complexed with specialized proteins.

liter (L) the basic unit of volume in the metric system. A liter equals 1.0567 quarts in the English system.

low density lipoprotein (LDL) a lipoprotein that is low in density because it contains large amounts of fat, primarily in the form of cholesterol.

Lyme disease a bacterial disease transmitted by deer ticks.

lymphocyte a nongranular white blood cell with a single nucleus. It is the most common of all white blood cells in children; typically small and round with a nonsegmented nucleus and no cytoplasmic granules.

lyse to break down a formed substance, such as red blood cells.

M

macrocyte a red blood cell that is unusually large (greater than 12 microns in diameter).

manual a laboratory handbook that contains instructions and recording forms for a particular aspect of laboratory work. Examples include safety and quality control manuals.

maple-syrup urine disease a very rare inborn error of metabolism that is fatal if not treated. The urine of patients with this disorder has a maple-syrup odor.

mean the arithmetic average of a sample of values.

mean cell hemoglobin (MCH) the average weight of hemoglobin in red blood cells in a sample (also called mean corpuscular hemoglobin).

mean cell hemoglobin concentration (MCHC) average concentration of hemoglobin in a given volume of packed red blood cells in a sample (also called mean corpuscular hemoglobin concentration).

mean cell volume (MCV) the average volume of red blood cells in a sample (also called mean corpuscular volume).

mechanical stage a platform that holds the slide. The mechanical stage can be moved in four directions so that any part of the slide may be viewed.

median the middle value in an ordered sample of values, with the same number of values below and above it.

median cephalic vein one of the major veins of the inner arm. It is used frequently in venipuncture.

median cubital vein a short vein of the inner arm just below the elbow. It is used frequently in venipuncture.

megakaryocyte a large bone marrow cell with large or multiple nuclei. Megakaryocytes give rise to platelets, which are cytoplasmic fragments of megakaryocytes.

meter (m) the basic unit of length in the metric system. A meter equals 1.0936 yards in the English system.

methylene blue a blue alkaline dye used to stain blood smears for microscopic examination.

metric system the system of measurement based on the meter, in which each unit is related to a basic unit of volume, length, or mass by a power of 10.

microbiology the branch of science that studies microscopic organisms.

microcontainer a blood collection system used with capillary puncture.

microcyte a red blood cell that is unusually small (less than 6 microns in diameter).

microhematocrit a method of determining the hematocrit. It uses just two or three drops of blood collected in a capillary tube.

microscope an instrument that uses a lens or combination of lenses to enlarge very small objects for viewing.

microscopy the use of a microscope.

micturition also called urination; the voiding, or passing, of urine from the bladder through the urethra.

milligram (mg)   the metric unit of weight or mass obtained by dividing the gram by 1,000.

millimeter (mm)   the metric unit of length obtained by dividing the meter by 1,000.

mode   the value that occurs most often in a sample.

monocular   literally, pertaining to one eye; a microscope in which there is only one eyepiece.

monocyte   the largest type of cell in the blood; an agranulocyte that has gray-blue cytoplasm when stained with the appearance of ground glass.

monocytic leukemia   a form of acute leukemia in which abnormal monocytes proliferate and invade the blood, bone marrow, and other tissues.

mononuclear   having an undivided nucleus, such as lymphocytes and monocytes.

monosaccharide   a simple, six-carbon sugar that is found in many foods. Monosaccharides include glucose, fructose, and galactose.

MSDS (Material Safety Data Sheet)   included with all chemical shipments describing precautions and disposal information.

myocardial infarction   an infarct, or area of necrosis (tissue death), in the myocardium. Myocardial infarction is usually due to occlusion of a coronary artery. Myocardial infarction is associated with pain, shock, cardiac failure, and frequently death.

myocardium   the middle, muscular layer of the walls of the heart.

myoglobinuria   the presence of myoglobin in the urine. Myoglobulin can appear in the urine during periods of muscle damage.

N

needle holder   Also known as hub or adapter; the plastic holder into which the posterior end of the needle is secured.

needlestick   the act of puncturing yourself with a used needle.

neoplasm   an abnormal growth of tissue, such as a tumor.

nephrology   the study of the structure and function of kidneys.

nephron   the basic functional unit of the kidneys, composed of a renal corpuscle and proximal and distal convoluted renal tubules. Each kidney has over a million nephrons.

neutropenia   a decrease below normal in the number of neutrophils in the blood, due to certain drugs, some acute infections, radiation, or certain diseases of the spleen or bone marrow.

neutrophil   the most common type of white blood cell; a granulocyte with a multilobed nucleus and cytoplasm filled with fine pink granules when stained with dye. Also the most commonly found type of white blood cell in urine sediment.

NFPA Diamond   a symbol, issued by the National Fire Protection Association, in the shape of a diamond with four colored quadrants that can be used in laboratories to label hazardous materials to show the type and level of hazard.

nonspecific immunity   innate immunity; the general resistance to disease that characterizes a particular species. In humans, nonspecific immunity includes physical and anatomical barriers, physiological barriers, endocytic and phagocytic responses, and the inflammatory response.

nonwaived tests   tests with more complicated steps and procedures in which the risk of erroneous results is higher. Previously defined as "moderate" or "high-complexity" tests.

normochromic   normal in color; used to describe red blood cells that have the normal amount of hemoglobin.

normocyte   an average-sized red blood cell, about 7.5 micrometers (µm) in diameter.

nosepiece   a rotating, circular apparatus on the microscope that holds the objectives and moves them into position as needed.

nucleated red blood cell (RBC)   a red blood cell that contains a nucleus. It resembles a white blood cell under low power magnification and may inflate the white blood cell count.

numerator   in any fraction or ratio, the number at the top of a fraction.

O

objective   the lens of the microscope that collects the image from the slide, magnifies it, and transmits it to the eyepiece lens, or ocular.

occult blood   blood that cannot be detected with the naked eye. It must be detected by chemical or microscopic analysis.

ocular   also called eyepiece. The ocular lens collects the image from the objective lens and magnifies it 10X in most oculars.

oil-immersion objective   the lens with the highest power of magnification (about 100X). The oil-immersion objective clarifies the image by using a layer of oil between the specimen and the objective to refract the light into the lens.

oliguria   the excretion of less than 400 mL of urine in 24 hours in adults. Oliguria is a life-threatening condition requiring immediate correction.

opalescence   the milky appearance in urine due to bacteria or lipids.

optical counting method   light scattering method.

oral hypoglycemic drug   a drug that decreases the amount of glucose in the blood by stimulating beta cells to secrete more insulin, inhibiting glucose production, or facilitating the transport of glucose to muscle cells.

orthostatic proteinuria   increased levels of protein in the urine when the patient is in a standing position.

OSHA (Occupational Safety and Health Administration)   a federal agency within the U.S. Department of Labor. OSHA works to assure the safety and health of workers.

out of control   the description given to a quality system when test results are beyond the upper or lower limits of the accepted range or when they are on only one side of the mean, showing a shift or trend pattern.

oxidase test   the lab test in which oxidase reagent is added to a colony of suspected *Niesseria gonorrhoeae* to confirm the presence of this organism.

P

palpating   touching or feeling.

pathogen   disease-causing microorganism.

patient testing log   daily, chronological journal of all of the work that is performed in the lab. Logs can be either manual or computerized.

percent   "out of a hundred"; a fraction with 100 as the denominator.

perineum   the outside area of the body immediately surrounding the rectum and urethra.

peritoneum   a membrane lining the abdominal cavity.

pernicious anemia   a potentially fatal form of anemia that may be due to deficiency or malabsorption of vitamin B_{12}. Pernicious anemia is associated with an abnormally low white blood cell count.

pH   the degree of acidity or alkalinity (basic) expressed in hydrogen ion concentration. It can range from 0 to 14. Acids have a pH less than 7.0. Bases have a pH greater than 7.0.

phase microscopy   the type of microscopy in which differences in the refractive index are translated into differences in brightness; used to view unstained specimens.

phenylketonuria (PKU)   an inborn error of protein metabolism that results in mental retardation if not treated. The urine of patients with PKU often has a distinctive mousy odor.

phlebotomy   blood collection by venipuncture.

physical and anatomical barriers   a type of nonspecific immunity; the body's first line of defense against foreign invaders. Physical and anatomical barriers include the skin, mucous membranes, body secretions, and benevolent bacteria.

physical hazard   a source of danger in the environment, such as shock, housekeeping accidents, and falls.

physiological barrier   a type of nonspecific immunity; a chemical factor that kills pathogens gaining access to the body.

plaque   a thickened region in an artery wall that prevents blood from flowing freely. Plaques may lead to heart attack or stroke.

plasma   the pale yellowish liquid part of whole blood.

platelet   a small round or oval disk-shaped blood cell that assists in blood clotting.

platelet plug   a clump of platelets that adhere to an injured vessel to help stop bleeding; often sufficient to stop the flow of blood in capillary wounds.

poikilocytosis   a condition in which many red blood cells have abnormal or multiple types of shapes.

point-of-care (POC) testing   laboratory tests that can be performed at the patient's bedside, rather than sending the specimen to the lab for testing. Requires a very small amount of specimen.

POL   physician's office laboratory.

policy   a management plan based on the goals of the lab or of particular aspects of lab work. Policies guide decision making and plans of action.

polychromatic stain   a stain containing dyes of two or more colors, such as Wright's stain, which contains methylene blue and eosin.

polycythemia   an increase above normal in the number of red blood cells in circulation.

polycythemia vera   erythremia; a chronic, usually fatal disease of the bone marrow that results in greatly elevated red blood cell counts.

polydipsia   excessive thirst.

polymorphonuclear   having a multilobed nucleus; used to describe cells such as granulocytes.

polyphagia   excessive food intake.

polysaccharide   a carbohydrate composed of many molecules of simple sugars. Polysaccharides include starch in plants and glycogen in animals.

polyuria   the excretion of excessive amounts of nearly colorless urine. Polyuria is confirmed by a 24-hour urine volume greater than 2,000 mL.

post-exposure evaluation   a set of procedures required by OSHA as a follow-up to exposure incidents.

post-exposure prophylaxis   preventive treatment for exposure to possible pathogenic microorganisms, HIV, HBV, and HCV, for example.

postprandial urine specimen   an after-meal specimen; used most often to test for the presence of glucose in urine.

potentiometric test   an analytic chemistry test in which the concentration of an analyte is measured by electrical potential.

PPE (personal protective equipment)   clothing and other equipment that shield workers from outside contaminants. PPE includes gloves, uniforms, fluid-proof aprons, masks, and eye-shields.

precision   the ability to repeatedly get the same result.

primary standard   a quality control sample that is of the highest possible quality and accuracy.

procedure   the steps of a particular test or assay. They should be written so someone doing the test the first time can accurately perform the test.

proficiency testing   a component of the quality system that tests the accuracy of laboratory procedures and staff.

proficiency testing manual   a permanent record of proficiency test results that augment the quality control record.

profile   a group of tests performed to help diagnose pathology of a specific organ or system.

prostatitis   inflammation of the prostate.

protein   one of a large group of complex, nitrogen-containing organic compounds, consisting of amino acids joined together by peptide bonds.

proteinuria   a condition in which protein appears in the urine.

prothrombin   coagulation factor II; a compound in circulating blood that is converted to thrombin by the action of thromboplastin.

prothrombin time (PT)   a coagulation procedure that tests for coagulation factors I, II, VII, and X, all of which are involved in the extrinsic pathway of coagulation. Prothrombin time is used to evaluate the effect of the administration of anticoagulant drugs.

protozoan   a single-celled animal. Several species of protozoa are pathogenic to humans, including *Giardia lamblia*.

pruritus   severe itching.

pseudoagglutination   the clumping together of red blood cells as in the formation of rouleaux but differing from true agglutination in that the clumped cells can be dispersed by shaking.

pure culture   a culture that is grown from a single colony of bacteria, which was taken from a direct culture. A pure culture serves to further isolate the pathogen.

pyogenic   pus producing; includes organisms such as staphylococcus and streptococcus.

pyuria   the presence of white blood cells in the urine.

Q

QBC (quantitative buffy coat) calibration check tube   the tube used with a QBC instrument to perform a daily quality control check. It gives a set of expected values and acceptable deviation values for each parameter.

QBC (quantitative buffy coat) instrument   an automated hematology instrument that centrifuges nondiluted blood samples and estimates blood parameters such as hemoglobin, hematocrit, platelet counts, and WBC counts on the basis of differences in density and fluorescence.

qualitative tests   tests that produce a yes or no, positive or negative type result.

quality assessment   a set of policies implemented to give patients the very best medical care possible. Quality assessment covers every aspect of medical care.

quality control (QC)   any measure that ensures consistent laboratory procedures and accurate test results.

quality control manual   a laboratory manual that contains written descriptions of quality control procedures and records of quality control test results, the latter usually recorded on Levey-Jennings charts.

quality system   all of the laboratory's policies, processes, procedures, and resources needed to achieve quality testing.

quantitative tests   tests that provide a numerical number to indicate an amount.

quantity not sufficient (QNS)   when the amount of specimen is not adequate and therefore testing cannot be performed.

quick-stain method   a method of staining blood smears in which the smear is dipped sequentially in fixative, acidic stain, and alkaline stain; also called the three-step method.

quotient   the number resulting from the division of one number by another.

R

random blood glucose test   the test of blood glucose on a sample of blood that is collected from a nonfasting patient during a routine visit to the doctor's office.

random error   unpredictable error with no obvious pattern.

random urine specimen   a urine specimen that is taken at any time of day or night, usually during a visit to the physician's office.

range   the difference between the largest and smallest values in a sample.

ratio   the relationship in size or quantity between two things.

reagent   a substance used to produce a chemical reaction.

reconstitute   to add liquid to a dried powder to return it to its original liquid form.

record   a written account of a procedure or past event.

red blood cell (RBC) count   erythrocyte count; the number of red blood cells per cubic millimeter of blood; performed manually by counting red blood cells under high power magnification on a hemacytometer. Whole blood is diluted with an isotonic solution that prevents lysing of red blood cells.

reduction test   also called Benedict's test. It tests for simple sugars such as lactose, galactose, fructose, and pentose, not just for glucose, in the urine.

reference range   also called normal, or expected, values. The range of values that are expected in a healthy person. About 95 percent of normal, healthy individuals will test in this range.

refractometer   an instrument for measuring the refractive index, which is the ratio of the velocity of light in air to the velocity of light in a solution such as urine. It is used to determine the specific gravity of a liquid.

relative polycythemia   an increase in red blood cells relative to plasma volume. It occurs due to dehydration.

reliability   the accuracy and precision of a testing procedure or instrument.

renal   pertaining to the kidney.

renal cast   the tube-shaped element in urine sediment, formed in the tubules of the kidney by the deposition of protein.

renal threshold   spillover point; the concentration of a substance in the blood above which the substance is not reabsorbed and remains in the urine for excretion; often used with reference to glucose.

renal tubular acidosis   a condition in which the renal tubules are unable to excrete hydrogen ions that increase body acidity.

reproducibility   the ability to repeat test results.

requisition   a printed form used by a physician to request a laboratory test for a patient.

resolution   the ability of a set of lenses to distinguish fine detail; the most important gauge of a microscope's quality.

reticulocyte   an immature red blood cell, which retains traces of endoplasmic reticula.

reticulocytopenia   the lowering of the number of circulating reticulocytes; usually found in patients with pernicious anemia, aplastic anemia, or bone marrow failure.

reticuloendothelial cell   cell of the spleen or bone marrow in which hemoglobin from lysed red blood cells is degraded to bilirubin.

rheostat   a device that controls the amount of current entering an electrical circuit. A rheostat controls the light on a microscope.

Rhesus (Rh) blood group   one of two clinically important inherited blood groups. Rh-positive blood has the D antigen; Rh-negative blood does not.

rheumatoid arthritis (RA)   a chronic systemic autoimmune disease characterized by inflammation in the joints and crippling.

ribosome   a cellular structure on the surface of rough endoplasmic reticula that synthesizes protein.

rouleaux   a clump of red blood cells that appear to be stacked like a roll of coins.

rubella   German measles; a mild systemic disease caused by the Rubella virus.

S

safety manual   a laboratory manual containing safety regulations, safety procedures, and policies, particularly as they relate to biological and chemical hazards, exposure incidents, and waste disposal.

saturated fat   a triglyceride in which the fatty acids are saturated with hydrogen atoms. Saturated fats form straight chain molecules that tend to pack together tightly, appearing like the dense white fat in bacon.

scientific notation   a system of writing decimals. In scientific notation, 10 raised to some power is used to specify where the decimal should be placed.

screening tests   initial, noninvasive, inexpensive tests that can test large numbers of patients for health problems such as diabetes and kidney disease.

secondary standard   a quality control sample that is developed in comparison with a primary standard.

semiquantitative tests   tests that provide results that represent a range.

sensitivity   the ability of a lab test for a particular disease to identify correctly those who have the disease.

serotonin   a potent vasoconstrictor that is released by platelets adhering to a wounded blood vessel.

serum   the yellow liquid portion of blood after the blood has been allowed to clot; it does not contain fibrinogen; the fibrinogen is in the clot.

sickle-cell anemia   a life-threatening disease that occurs in individuals homozygous for the sickle-cell hemoglobin gene.

sickle-cell hemoglobin   the most common type of abnormal hemoglobin in the United States. It is found primarily in African Americans. Sickle-cell hemoglobin is so named because it causes red blood cells to become sickle shaped under conditions of low oxygen tension, thus producing sickle-cell anemia.

sigma (Σ,σ)   the eighteenth letter in the Greek alphabet; used in statistics to represent the standard deviation (lowercase, σ) or summation (uppercase, Σ).

simplify   to express a fraction as a ratio between smaller numbers.

solute   the substance dissolved in a liquid to form a solution.

solution   the liquid containing a dissolved substance or substances.

solvent   the liquid in which substances are dissolved to form a solution.

specific gravity (SG) of urine   the density of urine relative to the density of distilled water. The concentration of dissolved substances gives urine greater specific gravity because these substances give urine greater weight.

specific immunity   acquired immunity; immunity to a specific foreign antigen that is acquired after exposure to it.

specificity   the ability of a lab test for a particular disease to identify correctly those who do not have the disease.

specimen   a small amount of body tissue (e.g., urine, blood, or tumor biopsy) taken for purposes of examination. The sample is assumed to represent the whole and to provide meaningful results for the total individual.

specimen collection manual   a laboratory manual containing all of the information needed to collect specimens for the various tests performed in the POL or its referral laboratory, including the types of collection apparatus required for each test and special handling requirements for specimens. The same information is often found in a chart posted near the specimen collection site.

specimen log   a daily, chronological log of all of the specimens collected and received by the laboratory.

sperm   male reproductive cells.

spherocytosis   a condition in which red blood cells assume a spherical shape.

spiral bacteria   bacteria that include the bacteria that causes syphilis and Lyme disease.

splenomegaly   the enlargement of the spleen. Splenomegaly is due to abnormal hemoglobin, among other possible causes.

stage   the platform on a microscope that supports the glass slide and specimen for viewing. The stage may move up and down for focusing.

standard deviation (*s* or σ)   a measurement of the variation from the mean in a sample of values.

standard operating procedure (SOP) manual   a lab manual containing instructions for each procedure performed in the POL. Includes detailed instructions that standardize the way a test is performed.

standard oral glucose-tolerance test (GTT or OGTT)   the glucose test in which fasting blood and urine specimens are collected before the test starts to serve as a baseline and then specimens are collected over several hours after consumption of a glucose load. This test is used to screen and diagnose diabetes mellitus.

Standard Precautions guidelines that use the CDC Universal Precautions and OSHA Blood-borne Pathogen Standards to direct health care workers in protection against pathogens transmitted by infectious patients.

standard a rule by which test results are measured; a quality control sample manufactured and analyzed to very exact measurements.

stationary ocular usually, the eyepiece for the right eye. It is adjusted for focus first using the coarse and fine adjustment knobs.

statistics the branch of mathematics that deals with the collection, analysis, and interpretation of numerical data.

STD sexually transmitted disease.

summation represented by uppercase sigma, Σ; indicates addition of the numbers or variables that follow.

supernatant fluid remaining at the top of a specimen after centrifugation.

supravital stain dye added to cells while they are living to make them easier to see. It is a stain that stains only living cells, not dried blood smears.

syphilis a devastating, sexually transmitted disease caused by the spirochete *Treponema pallidum.*

syringe an instrument with a needle used for drawing blood from a vein.

systematic error a noticeable pattern of errors.

systemic lupus erythematosus (SLE) a systemic autoimmune disease that affects connective tissues and injures the skin, joints, kidneys, nervous system, and mucous membranes.

T

target value the value given by the manufacturer of a quality control sample as the expected quality control result.

template method (Ivy bleeding time) a method of testing bleeding time. The template method standardizes the size and depth of the incision.

thrombin an enzyme formed from the conversion of prothrombin by thromboplastin and other coagulation factors. Thrombin joins soluble fibrinogen molecules into long, hairlike molecules of insoluble fibrin.

thrombocytopenia a hemorrhagic disease due to a deficiency of platelets, which results in many small hemorrhages.

thrombophlebitis the inflammation of a vein due to a blood clot. Thrombophlebitis is a common problem in elderly, immobile patients.

thromboplastin coagulation factor III; the immediate initiator of the blood-clotting mechanism. Thromboplastin interacts with other coagulation factors to convert prothrombin to thrombin.

thrombosis the formation of a blood clot, or thrombus, within the vascular system. Thrombosis is treated with anticoagulants.

thrombus a blood clot within the vascular system.

thyroxine the thyroid hormone that raises the level of blood glucose.

timed urine specimens urine specimens collected at timed intervals. Often used to diagnose diabetes or to assess the rate of renal clearance.

titer the highest dilution, or lowest concentration, capable of producing an observable reaction.

T-lymphocytes T-cells; the basis of cell-mediated immunity.

total volume the amount of a solution, including both solute and solvent.

tourniquet a constrictor band used to distend veins to facilitate venipuncture.

toxic poisonous.

toxin poison.

transfer device mechanical device used to assist in the transfer of blood from a syringe into the specimen tubes.

triglyceride a compound made up of fatty acids and glycerol.

true value or gold standard the value for a test result that is based on the results obtained from the best qualified laboratories using the purest reagents, the most refined methods, and the best technology.

turbidity cloudiness in a solution due to suspended particles, which scatter light and produce the cloudy appearance.

24-hour urine specimen a collective specimen that includes the total urine output of a patient for a 24-hour period; usually collected by the patient at home and often used for quantitative analysis.

2-hour postprandial blood sugar (2-hour PPBS) test the blood glucose test administered 2 hours after the patient has consumed a meal containing 100 grams of carbohydrate or has drunk a 100 gram glucose-load solution.

2-hour urine specimen   the total urine output of a patient for a 2-hour period.

type 1 diabetes mellitus   Formerly known as insulin-dependent diabetes mellitus (IDDM) or juvenile diabetes. A severe form of diabetes mellitus that usually requires administration of insulin for control. Type 1 is characterized by rapid onset, typically before age 25. Type 1 represents 5 to 10 percent of all DM cases.

type 2 diabetes mellitus   Formerly known as noninsulin-dependent diabetes mellitus (NIDDM) or adult onset diabetes. A mild form of diabetes mellitus that may be controlled by diet alone. Type 2 typically has gradual onset after age 40. It is often associated with obesity and represents 90 to 95 percent of all DM cases.

U

Universal Precautions   a set of recommendations formulated by the CDC to protect workers against HIV and other pathogens. The precautions impose isolation of all specimens of blood, blood products, and other body fluids capable of transmitting pathogens.

unsaturated fat   a triglyceride in which the fatty acids are not saturated with hydrogen atoms. Unsaturated fats tend to be liquids at room temperature.

urea   a small molecule, formed from ammonia in the liver, that can move freely into both extracellular and intracellular fluid. Urea is concentrated in the urine for excretion.

uremia   a high level of urea in the blood.

ureteritis   inflammation of the ureters.

ureters   carry the urine from the kidneys to the bladder.

urethra   carries the urine out of the body.

-uria   a suffix that denotes urine or urination.

uric acid   the end product of the metabolism of purine, an important constituent of nucleic acids.

urinalysis (UA)   the clinical analysis of urine to determine its physical, chemical, and microscopic properties.

urinalysis strips   also known as urine reagent strips and/or urine dipsticks; test strip impregnated with reagents that provide a quick and easy way to assess a variety of chemical characteristics of the urine. Strips can provide information about glucose, protein, ketones, and other analytes.

urinary sediments   solid substances found in standing urine specimen. Can include bacteria, red blood cells, white blood cells, urinary casts, etc.

urinary tract infection (UTI)   an infection of the organs of the urinary tract system caused by any of several different bacteria. A UTI is diagnosed when the urine bacteria concentration exceeds 100,000 organisms per milliliter.

urine control   a pretested specimen, the result and value of which are known and can be used to test the variability of the POL's procedures, reagents, and equipment in performing urinalysis.

urine sediment   the solid material that settles to the bottom of urine when it stands or is centrifuged.

urobilinogen   a colorless derivative of bilirubin; formed by the action of intestinal bacteria.

urobilinogenuria   excess urobilinogen in the urine.

urochrome   the yellow pigment that causes the characteristic yellow color of urine.

V

vacuole   a clear space in cell cytoplasm that is filled with fluid or air.

validity   ability of a test to correctly determine those who have a disease or condition and those patients who do not have the disease or condition.

variability   the tendency for objects and procedures to change, or deviate, from their original state or from some standard.

vascular phenomenon   one of three major components of hemostasis. The term *vascular phenomenon* refers to the vascular response to bleeding, which is vasoconstriction.

vasoconstriction   the constricting, or narrowing, of a blood vessel.

vector   a carrier, such as an insect, of a pathogen.

venipuncture   the puncture of a vein for therapeutic purposes or for drawing blood.

virus   a simple organism that causes many diseases in humans, including colds and herpes. Viruses live and reproduce within the cells of a host.

visual acuity   clarity of vision.

W

waived test   defined by CLIA as "simple laboratory examination and procedures that have an insignificant risk of erroneous results."

warfarin   one of the coumarin group of anticoagulants used to prevent and treat clotting disorders. Warfarin also is used as rodent poison.

waxy cast   the renal cast that is yellowish, with irregular broken ends.

white blood cell (WBC) count   leukocyte count; the number of white blood cells per cubic millimeter of blood; counted manually under low-power magnification on a hemacytometer. Whole blood is diluted with a solution that lyses red blood cells.

working distance   the distance between the specimen and the objective. It is important to check this distance frequently to avoid bringing the lens into contact with the slide.

work-practice control   a method that incorporates safety into laboratory procedures.

Wright's stain   a polychromatic stain for fixing and staining blood smears. It contains eosin and methylene blue dyes in a methyl alcohol solution.

PHOTO CREDITS

Chapter 1
Opener: © Getty RF; 1-1: © Ken Lax; 1-2: Courtesy and © Becton, Dickinson and Company; 1-3a (left & right): © Global Scientific, Inc.; 1-3b: © Matt Meadows; 1-3c: © The McGraw-Hill Companies, Inc., photographer Suzie Ross; 1-4: © Getty RF; 1-5a, b: © The McGraw-Hill Companies, Inc., photographer Suzie Ross; 1-6, 1-7: © Getty RF; 1-8: Courtesy Tyco/Healthcare/Kendal; 1-11: © Phyllis Cox.

Chapter 2
Opener: © Corbis RF; 2-1: © Olympus Corporation; 2-3: © Getty RF; 2-5: © Matt Meadows.

Chapter 3
Opener: © Vol. 170/Corbis RF.

Chapter 4
Opener: © Matjaz Boncina/istockphoto.com.

Chapter 5
Opener: © The McGraw-Hill Companies, Inc.,/Suzie Ross, photographer; 5-1: © Comstock/Jupiter RF; 5-12: © Will & Deni McIntyre/Photo Researchers.

Chapter 6
Opener: © The McGraw-Hill Companies, Inc., photographer John Thoeming

Chapter 8
Opener: © Leesa Whicker; 8-1: Courtesy and © Becton, Dickinson and Company; 8-3: © O Damika/Mediscan; 8-4, 8-6: © Cliff Moore; 8-7: © Mediscan.

Chapter 9
Opener: © Getty RF; 9-2, 9-3: Courtesy of University of Iowa Hospitals and Clinics, Department of Pathology; 9-5: © Leesa Whicker; 9-6a-c: Courtesy of University of Iowa Hospitals and Clinics, Department of Pathology; 9-11: © Leesa Whicker.

Chapter 10
Opener: © Jim Arbogast/Getty RF; 10-1: © Total Care Programming, Inc.; 10-3a, b: Courtesy of University of Iowa Hospitals and Clinics, Department of Pathology; 10-4d: © Photo Alto RF; 10-13: © Total Care Programming, Inc.; 10-14: Courtesy of Centers for Disease Control; 10-15: © Alfred Pasieka/SPL/Photo Researchers.

Chapter 11
Opener and 11-1: © Total Care Programming, Inc.; 11-2: Courtesy of University of Iowa Hospitals and Clinics, Department of Pathology; 11-3a, b: © Total Care Programming, Inc.; 11-4a-c, 11-5: Courtesy and © Becton, Dickinson and Company; 11-7: © Total Care Programming; 11-9: © Photodisc/Getty RF; 11-10, 11-11: © Total Care Programming, Inc.

Chapter 12
Opener: © Mediscan/Corbis; 12-1a: Courtesy and © Becton, Dickinson and Company; 12-1b: © Scott Camazine/Phototake; 12-2: © Dumas/Mediscan; 12-6a,b: Courtesy and © Becton, Dickinson and Company; 12-7a,b: © Leesa Whicker; 12-8: © Total Care Programming, Inc.

Chapter 13
Opener, 13-3, 13-6a: © Total Care Programming, Inc.; 13-6b-e: © Terry Wild Studio; 13-7: © Phyllis Cox; 13-8: © Total Care Programming, Inc.

Chapter 14
Opener: © Phyllis Cox.

Chapter 15
Opener: © The McGraw-Hill Companies Inc., Al Telser, photographer; 15-1: Reproduction of *Morphology of Human Blood Cells*/ has been granted with approval of Abbott Laboratories, all rights reserved by Abbott Laboratories.; 15-5b: © Phyllis Cox; 15-6, 15-7: Reproduction of *Morphology of Human Blood Cells* has been granted with approval of Abbott Laboratories, all rights reserved by Abbott Laboratories.; 15-8 Courtesy Control Concepts Inc.; 15-9a, 15-11, 15-13: © Ed Reschke.

Chapter 16
Opener: © Liquidlibrary/PictureQuest RF; 16-1a: © Abbott Diagnostics; 16-1b: © Beckman Coulter; 16-8: © QBC Diagnostics.

Chapter 17
Opener: © Corbis RF; 17-3a: © Polymedco, Inc.; 17-3b: © Diesse, Inc.; 17-4: © Leesa Whicker; 17-7: Reproduction of *Morphology of Human Blood Cells* has been granted with approval of Abbott Laboratories, all rights reserved by Abbott Laboratories.

Chapter 18
Opener: © Corbis RF; 18-2 © SPL/Photo Researchers; 18-4a, b, 18-5a: © ITC Products; 18-5b: © Roche Diagnostics Corporation; 18-6: © Beckman Coulter.

Chapter 19
Opener: © Sergey Laventev/iStockphoto.com; 19-2: © Total Care Programming, Inc.; 19-3: © The McGraw-Hill Companies, Inc.

Chapter 20
Opener: © Abbott Diagnostics.

Chapter 21
Opener: © Phyllis Cox; 21-3: © Getty RF; 21-4: © Beckman Coulter; 21-5: © Quidel Corporation; 21-6: © Total Care Programming, Inc.

Chapter 22
Opener: Image courtesy of the Centers for Disease Control and Prevention, Dr. Mike Miller; 22-1a, b: © Oliver Meckes/Photo Researchers; 22-1c: © Volker Stegner/Peter Arnold; 22-3a, b: © Martin M. Rotker; 22-5: Courtesy Centers for Disease Control; 22-6: © Corbis RF; 22-7: Courtesy of Siemens; 22-8: Courtesy Centers for Disease Control and Prevention/Dr. Stuart Brown; 22-9a: CDC/ Dr. Theo Hawkins; 22-9b: © Morendum Animal Health, Ltd./Photo Researchers; 22-10a: Courtesy Centers for Disease Control and Prevention; 22-10b: © 2009 David M. Raymondo; 22-11a: © Hardy Diagnostics. www.HardyDiagnostics.com; 22-11b: © Cliff Moore; 22-11c: © McCormick Scientific; 22-13: © Courtesy Josephine A. Morello; 22-14: Courtesy Neal R. Chamberlain, Ph.D. and Betty J. Cox, M.A.; 22-15: © Courtesy Josephine A. Morello; 22-16a: Courtesy Centers for Disease Control and Prevention; 22-16b: Courtesy Neal R. Chamberlain, Ph.D. and Betty J. Cox, M.A.; 22-17: Courtesy Centers for Disease Control and Prevention/Dr. Theo Hawkins.

Appendix I:
Photo 1, 2: © Getty RF; Photo 3: © Phyllis Cox; Photo 4: © Big Stock Photo; Photo 5: Getty RF; Photo 6,7: © Total Care Programming, Inc.; Photo 8: © Thermo Fisher Scientific Inc.

Index

Note: Page numbers followed by f indicate figures and t, tables.

A

Abbott Laboratories, 268, 286
Abbreviations, 428
  in metric system, 49t
  for standard deviation, 63, 73
ABO blood group, 363, 375–376
  compatible types in, 376t
  testing for, 376, 376f, 376t, 379–381
Absolute number of reticulocytes, 307
Absolute polycythemia, 245, 250–251
ACCU-CHECK ADVANTAGE blood
    glucose meter, 338f
Accuracy, 70, 72, 73f
ACETEST for ketones, 150
Acetic acid test for urine protein,
    148–149
Acid-base balance, 141–142
Acid urine, 142, 175f, 176t
Acidosis, 134, 142, 332
  diabetes and, 334t
  ketones and, 143
Acids, 3, 14, 111
ACL 100 Coagulation Analyzer, 323, 323f
Acromegaly, 346, 350
AcT Diff Hematology Analyzer, 286
Action value, 92, 95, 101
Activated partial thromboplastin time
    (aPTT), 315–316, 322–323, 323f
Acute lymphocytic leukemia, 263, 271
Addis, Thomas, 119
Addition
  of decimals, 46
  of exponents, 47
  of fractions, 45
ADH; see Antidiuretic hormone (ADH)
Adipose tissue, 347, 351
Adjustable ocular, 25, 29
Adult hemoglobin, 228, 232
AD-VIA, 286
Aerobic blood culture, 191, 191f
Aerobic microorganisms, 185, 394
Aerosolization, 3, 7
Agar, 395
Agglutination, 246
  of blood types, 376, 376f, 376t
  red blood cell count and, 251
Agglutinin reaction, 368, 369
Agranulocytes, 263, 264–265

Agranulocytosis, 263, 272
AIDS; see Human immunodeficiency
    virus (HIV)
Albumin, 144, 347, 355
Alcohol
  for capillary puncture, 215
  hand rubs with, 195
  methyl, 267
  for venipuncture, 187, 189, 196
Alkaline urine, 142, 175f, 176t
Alkalosis, 134, 142
Allergic reactions, 10, 186–187, 367–368
American Heart Association, 353
Amino acids, 347, 354
Ammonia, 355
Amoebic dysentery, 397
Anaerobic blood culture, 191, 191f
Anaerobic microorganisms, 185, 394
Analytes, 70, 78
Anaphylaxis, 367–368
Anemia, 228, 231
  aplastic, 246, 251
  drugs and, 251
  erythrocyte indices in, 298, 299
  hemolytic, 229, 232
  iron-deficiency, 229, 231, 236
  pernicious, 246, 247
  red blood cell count in, 250, 250f, 251
  reticulocytopenia in, 307
  sickle-cell, 229, 232
Anisocytosis, 263, 272
Anoxia, 246, 247
Antecubital fossa, 185, 186, 195–196, 196f
Antibiotics, 388
  Gram staining for, 404
  sensitivity testing for, 125, 394, 394f
  viruses and, 389
Antibodies, 363, 365–366, 365f, 366f
Anticoagulant drugs, 320
Anticoagulants, 185
  blood collection tubes with, 190, 191,
    192
  for blood smears, 265
Antidiuretic hormone (ADH), 113
Antidote for warfarin poisoning, 320
Antigen-antibody reaction, 365–366, 365f
  in immunology tests, 368–369
  quantitative measurement of, 369–370
Antigen-antibody test kits, 370–375

Antigens, 363, 365, 366f
Antiseptics, 187–188
Antisera, blood typing, 376, 376f, 376t
Anuria, 118, 121
Aperture
  of electrical impedance cell counter,
    285, 286, 286f
  of microscope, 25, 28, 28f
Aplastic anemia, 246, 251
aPTT; see Activated partial
    thromboplastin time (aPTT)
Arm of microscope, 26, 26f
Arterial blood specimens, 185
Arteries vs. veins, 196, 197
Artifacts, 25, 26, 170
Ascaris lumbricoides, 399
Ascorbic acid, 134, 143
Aseptic technique, 388, 399
Aspirin, 320, 321
Atherosclerosis, 347, 352, 353
Attitudes, personnel, 15–16
Autoclave, 3, 11
Autoimmune diseases, 367t, 373
Autoimmunity, 363, 367
Automated chemistry analyzers, 346,
    347, 348
  advantages of, 348
  substances measured by, 349
    carbohydrate, 349–351
    lipid, 351–353, 353t, 354t
    nonprotein nitrogen compound,
      355–356
    protein, 354–355
  terminology for, 346–347
  types of, 348–349
Automated coagulation analyzers, 323,
    323f
Automated ESR analyzers, 301, 302f
Automated hematology instruments, 284,
    285
  for hemoglobin measurement, 232
  quality control for, 290–291
  requiring diluted samples, 286–289,
    286f, 289f
  requiring undiluted samples, 289–290,
    289f, 290f
  terminology for, 285
  tests performed with, 286
Automated systems for bacterial
    identification, 395–396, 396f
Automated urinalysis, 141

453